I0057366

Gynecological Surgery: New Frontiers

Gynecological Surgery: New Frontiers

Editor: Vivian Stone

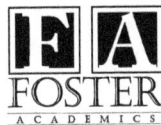

FA
FOSTER
ACADEMICS

www.fosteracademics.com

www.fosteracademics.com

FA
FOSTER
ACADEMICS

Cataloging-in-Publication Data

Gynecological surgery : new frontiers / edited by Vivian Stone.
    p. cm.
Includes bibliographical references and index.
ISBN 978-1-63242-815-8
1. Generative organs, Female--Surgery. 2. Gynecology. 3. Generative organs, Female--Diseases. I. Stone, Vivian.
RG104 .G85 2019
618.105 9--dc23

© Foster Academics, 2019

Foster Academics,
118-35 Queens Blvd., Suite 400,
Forest Hills, NY 11375, USA

ISBN 978-1-63242-815-8 (Hardback)

This book contains information obtained from authentic and highly regarded sources. Copyright for all individual chapters remain with the respective authors as indicated. All chapters are published with permission under the Creative Commons Attribution License or equivalent. A wide variety of references are listed. Permission and sources are indicated; for detailed attributions, please refer to the permissions page and list of contributors. Reasonable efforts have been made to publish reliable data and information, but the authors, editors and publisher cannot assume any responsibility for the validity of all materials or the consequences of their use.

Trademark Notice: Registered trademark of products or corporate names are used only for explanation and identification without intent to infringe.

Contents

Preface

Surgery of the female reproductive system is known as gynecological surgery. Gynecology involves the study of the health of the breasts and the female reproductive system, which includes the uterus, vagina and ovaries. A speculum is often used for the purpose of gynecological examination. Hysterectomy, oophorectomy and tubectomy are some of the common gynecological surgical procedures. The surgical removal of the uterus is known as hysterectomy. Oophorectomy is a type of gynecological surgery related to the surgical removal of the ovaries. Tubectomy refers to the surgical procedure for sterilization in which a woman's fallopian tubes are blocked and sealed in order to prevent the eggs from reaching the uterus for implantation. It is a permanent and effective method of birth control. The objective of the book is to give a general view of the different areas of gynecological surgery. It elucidates the concepts and innovative models around prospective developments with respect to gynecological surgery. The extensive content of this book provides the readers with a thorough understanding of the subject.

This book is the end result of constructive efforts and intensive research done by experts in this field. The aim of this book is to enlighten the readers with recent information in this area of research. The information provided in this profound book would serve as a valuable reference to students and researchers in this field.

At the end, I would like to thank all the authors for devoting their precious time and providing their valuable contribution to this book. I would also like to express my gratitude to my fellow colleagues who encouraged me throughout the process.

Editor

Total laparoscopic hysterectomy for benign disease: outcomes and literature analysis

Liliana Mereu[1*], Roberta Carlin[1], Alice Pellegrini[1,2], Francesca Guasina[1], Valeria Berlanda[1,2] and Saverio Tateo[1]

Abstract

Objective: To analyze surgical outcomes of total laparoscopic hysterectomy (TLH) for benign disease.

Methods: Retrospective analysis of 361 consecutive cases, prospectively collected from January 2012 to June 2016, of women who underwent TLH in St. Chiara Hospital in Trento, Italy. Clinical, demographic, surgical, and intra and perioperative data were recorded. Complications were graded on the Clavien-Dindo morbidity scale. Data were compared with literature. Statistical analysis was performed with SPSS (SPSS Chicago, IL).

Findings: Main indication for TLH was uterine fibromatosis (78.6%). Mean uterine size was 327 ± 249 g (range 30–1800 g). Mean operating time was 115 ± 36 min. No laparotomy conversion occurred. Mean length of hospital stay was 2.6 ± 1.1 days (range 1–12 days).
Complications requiring surgical intervention in general anesthesia occurred in 3 patients (0.8%): 1 (0.3%) hydroureteronephrosis, 1 (0.3%) bowel adhesions, and 1 (0.3%) port side hernia; complication requiring surgical intervention without general anesthesia occurred in 6 patients (1.6%): 2 (0.6%) hydroureteronephrosis, 1 (0.3%) vaginal cuff dehiscence, and 3 (0.8%) vaginal cuff bleeding.

Conclusions: Total laparoscopic hysterectomy is a procedure with a low incidence of complications. Our data compare favorably with the data of the other listed studies.

Keywords: Total laparoscopic hysterectomy, Complications, Outcomes, Benign disease, Total hysterectomy

Introduction

Hysterectomy is the most frequent gynecological procedure performed, and in most cases, the laparoscopic approach may avoid the need for laparotomy.

The benefits of laparoscopic hysterectomy (LH) versus abdominal hysterectomy (AH) are a quicker return to normal activities, a lower intraoperative blood loss, a smaller drop in hemoglobin, a shorter hospitalization, and less infections. The drawbacks are more injuries to the urinary tract and longer operation time [1]. However, the wider use of the laparoscopic approach and the improvement of surgeons' skills can decrease the incidence of complications [2]. The purpose of this study is to evaluate our total laparoscopic hysterectomy (TLH) surgical technique, analyzing the intra and postoperative surgical results and complications with a simple and reproducible classification and to compare the results with data in the literature.

Materials and methods

This is a retrospective analysis of a prospectively collected database (Oxford CEBM level 3), conducted by the Department of Gynecology and Obstetrics of St. Chiara Hospital in Trento (Italy). The data concern a number of consecutive cases of women who underwent TLH between January 2012 and June 2016.

The data on the patient's age, body mass index (BMI), parity, comorbidities, menopause status, previous surgery, surgical indication, surgical procedures, uterine weight, and intra and postoperative outcomes (duration of procedure, blood loss, hospital stay, and complications) were collected in a database. The duration of procedure was calculated from the beginning to the end of surgery, and the concomitant surgical procedures were included.

* Correspondence: liliana_mereu@yahoo.com
[1]Department of Gynecology and Obstetrics, St. Chiara Hospital of Trento, Trento, Italy
Full list of author information is available at the end of the article

Inclusion criteria are as follows: age > 18 years, signed written informed consent, uterine benignant disease, and indication for laparoscopic hysterectomy.

Exclusion criteria were malignant disease, adnexal pathology with suspicion of malignancy, genital prolapse, and contraindications to laparoscopy. Patients were subsequently examined 4 to 6 weeks after surgery and if needed even before or after. Patient's clinical data were collected from the hospital clinical database: SIO (Sistema Informatico Ospedaliero); exams, hospitalization, and visits performed in the district are available for a follow-up period of 6 months. Patient's consensus was asked during the hospitalization.

Ethical approval for the study was obtained from the Institutional Review Board.

Surgeries were performed by two expert surgeons (ST and LM).

TLH surgical technique

Before surgery, patients underwent routine examinations, including blood tests, gynecological examination, gynecological ultrasound scanning, and endometrial biopsy. Patients received antibiotic prophylaxis (with cephalosporin given following anesthetic induction) and thromboprophylaxis with low molecular weight heparin. All patients were routinely catheterized at the beginning of operation, with the catheter being removed the day after, as soon as the patient could independently reach the toilet. Bladder was filled with 20 ml of Sodium Indigotin Disulfonate 40 mg/10 ml diluted in 250 ml of saline. The patient was placed in supine position under endotracheal general anesthesia. The abdomen and vagina were disinfected. The patient was draped and placed in the Trendelenburg position. The peritoneum entry was performed with a modified open technique or with a Veress needle. The surgical technique follows the one described by Clermont-Ferrand [3] using cold scissors, bipolar forceps, and the Hohl uterine manipulator (Karl Storz GmbH, Tuttlingen, Germany). In case of large uterus, until 2015, the organ was vaginally removed after cold blade laparoscopic morcellation, since 2015 vaginal morcellation of the uterus inside an endobag was undertaken. In case of big uterus that did not fit into the endobag, a minilaparotomy for extraction was performed. In most cases, suture was performed using barbed suture or polyglactin 2/0 interrupted suture. TLH with bilateral salpingo-ovariectomy was suggested to menopausal patients, and prophylactic bilateral salpingectomy was offered to the other patients.

Classification of complications

Complications were recorded and divided into intraoperative and postoperative and further distinguished according to the structure involved.

Each postoperative complication was graded on the Clavien-Dindo 5-grade morbidity scale [4]. Grade I: any deviation from the normal postoperative course not requiring therapy (allowed therapeutic regimens are drugs as antiemetics, antipyretics, analgesics, diuretics, electrolytes, and physiotherapy, wound infections opened at the bedside). Grade II: issues requiring pharmacological treatment with drugs other than those allowed for grade I complications. Blood transfusions and total parenteral nutrition are also included. Grade III: issues requiring surgical, endoscopic, or radiological intervention. Grade IIIA: issues requiring intervention not under general anesthesia. Grade IIIB: issues requiring intervention under general anesthesia. Grade IV: life-threatening complication (including CNS complications) requiring IC/ICU management. Grade IVA: single organ dysfunction (including dialysis). Grade IVB: multiorgan dysfunction. Grade V: death of the patient. The time of occurrence of complication was indicated with "D" if it occurred after discharge, "E" if it had an early onset (< 30 days), and "L" if it had a late onset (≥ 30 days).

Statistical analysis

Statistical analysis was performed with SPSS (SPSS Chicago, IL).

Normally distributed data are presented as mean ± SD, and skewed data as median (range). Categorical variables are reported as absolute values and percentages. Categorical variables were compared using the X^2 test. P values < .05 were considered to be statistically significant.

Literature analysis

Studies were selected from a literature analysis, exploring the PubMed database with a combination of the keywords "hysterectomy," "laparoscopic," "total laparoscopic," "complication," and "outcome"; cases dealing with total laparoscopic hysterectomy were selected. We took into consideration studies published after 2007 on total laparoscopic hysterectomy for benign disease, with a number of patients ≥ 200 and considering overall complications, including all uterus weights and patients' characteristics.

Results

The baseline characteristics of 361 women who underwent TLH are summarized in Table 1. Indication for TLH was uterine symptomatic fibromatosis in 284 (78.7%) patients, metrorrhagia in 19 (5.2%) patients, endometrial hyperplasia with atypia 31 (8.5%) patients, endometrial hyperplasia without atypia in 6 (1.7%) patients, CIN 3 in 2 (0.3%) patients, adenomyosis in 9 (2.5%), and other indications in 14 (3.9%) patients. Seventy-six out of 361 patients (21.1%) were menopausal, and the surgical indications for TLH in this subgroup were 37 symptomatic myomas, 28 endometrial hyperplasia, 2 CIN3, and 9 other conditions.

Table 1 Characteristics of patients (n = 361)

Characteristics	Data
Age, years	49.6 ± 6.5 (37–83)
Comorbidity	
Diabetes	14 (3.9)
Hypertension	61 (16.9)
Smoke	34 (9.4)
Cardiopathy	11 (3.0)
Body mass index	25.8 ± 5.6 (17–51)
Menopause	76 (21.1)
Previous abdominal surgery	
Laparoscopy	
1	61 (16.9)
≥ 2	9 (2.5)
Laparotomy	
1	127 (35.2)
≥ 2	22 (6.1)

Values are given as mean ± SD (range) or number (percentage) unless stated otherwise
Abbreviation: BMI body mass index (calculated as weight in kilograms by the square of height in meters)

Table 2 describes intraoperative outcomes. No conversion to laparotomy for complication occurred. There were 2 (0.6%) intraoperative complications: 1 (0.3%) blood transfusion and 1 (0.3%) bladder injury. Postoperative complications are described in Table 3. Mean hospital stay was 2.6 ± 1.1 days. Postoperatively, complication grade V (death) or

Table 2 Intraoperative outcomes (n = 361)

Outcomes	Data[a]
Mean operating times, min	113 ± 36 (45–240)
Mean blood loss, ml	44 ± 79 (10–500[c])
Mean uterine size, g	327 ± 249 (30–1800)
Morcellement	198 (54.8)
Minilaparotomy	3 (0.8)[d]
Complications	
Bladder injury	1 (0.3)
Blood transfusion	1 (0.3)[c]
Concomitant procedure	
Bilateral salpingectomy	211 (58.4)
Bilateral annessectomy	118 (32.7)
Lysis of adhesions	70 (19.4)
Ovarian cyst enucleation	19 (5.3)
Other surgical procedure[b]	23 (6.4)

[a]Values are given as mean ± SD (range) or number (percentage) unless stated otherwise
[b]Included: mammary nodule removal, colecystectomy, endometriosis heradication, and hernioplasty
[c]Uterus weight 1800 mg and preoperative anemia
[d]To remove surgical pieces

grade IV (life-threatening complication) did not occur. There were 3 (0.8%) grade IIIB complications that arose after discharge: 1 hydroureteronephrosis, 1 port side hernia, and 1 bowel adhesions. 6 (1.7%) grade IIIA complications occurred after discharge: 1 vaginal cuff dehiscence, 3 vaginal cuff bleeding, and 2 hydrouretheronephosis (Table 3).

Results of literature analysis
Six studies with TLH population have been selected from the literature analysis: Kim et al. [5], Wallwiener et al. [6], Twijnstra et al. [7], Boosz et al. [8], Morelli et al. [9], and Ng et al. [10]. Table 4 shows the comparison of intraoperative outcomes while Table 5 shows intra and postoperative findings.

Discussion
Laparoscopy has been performed in gynecological surgery for more than 20 years, and its use is increasing. In most countries, the proportion of LHs has gradually increased over the years [1].

Many classifications of laparoscopic hysterectomy have been proposed, the most used being the 2003 one by Reich [11], which divides the laparoscopic hysterectomy procedure into LAVH (laparoscopically assisted vaginal hysterectomy), LH (laparoscopic hysterectomy), and TLH (total laparoscopic hysterectomy), the latter being when the entire operation is performed laparoscopically, with no vaginal component except the removal of the uterus. However, some authors have described the total laparoscopic hysterectomy technique with suture of the cuff by vaginal route [12]. This variety of techniques and definitions, added to the different stratification classifications of complications in various studies, makes it difficult to compare data in literature.

For these reasons, we decided to (1) include in this study only TLH with suture of the vaginal vault by laparoscopic approach, (2) use the Clavien-Dindo morbidity scale, which is a reproducible simple system to grade complications, based on the therapy required to treat them, (3) select from the TLH literature only recent studies published after 2007, and with a sizable number of patients (> 200). The present study includes 361 consecutive patients who underwent laparoscopic hysterectomy for benign disease and is one of the largest monocentric series present in the literature. Analyzing patients' characteristic, the mean BMI of the patients of the present study (25.8) was in line with that of the majority of the other studies [5–9], as only the series of Ng et al. had a quite low BMI: 19.2 [10].

A large number of women included in the study had undergone previous laparotomy (41.3%) and 24.1% one or more previous cesarean section. Previous abdominal surgery is no longer a contraindication to the laparoscopic

Table 3 Postoperative complications (graded by Dindo-Clavien score)

Dindo-Clavien score	Description	N, onset time
IIIB	Hydroureteronephrosis	1
	Pre-discharge	0
	Post-discharge	1, E
	Port side hernia	1
	Pre-discharge	0
	Post-discharge	1, L
	Bowel adhesions	1
	Pre-discharge	0
	Post-discharge	1, L
Total		3 (0.8)
IIIA	Vaginal cuff bleeding	3
	Pre-discharge	0
	Post-discharge	3, E
	Vaginal cuff dehiscence	1
	Pre-discharge	0
	Post-discharge	1, E
	Hydroureteronephrosis	2
	Pre-discharge	0
	Post-discharge	2, (1E, 1L)
Total		6 (1.6)
II	Urinary infection	14
	Pre-discharge	5, E
	Post-discharge	9, E
	Vaginal cuff hematoma	1
	Pre-discharge	0
	Post-discharge	1, E
	Cardiac arrhythmia	2
	Pre-discharge	2, E
	Post-discharge	0
	Pelvic abscess	1
	Pre-discharge	0
	Post-discharge	1, E
	Wound infection	4
	Pre-discharge	0
	Post-discharge	4, E
	Vaginal cuff infection	4
	Pre-discharge	0
	Post-discharge	4 (2E-2 L)
	Postoperative blood transfusion	2
	Pre-discharge	1, E
	Post-discharge	1, E
Total		28 (7.8)
I	Wound hematoma	2
	Pre-discharge	2, E
	Post-discharge	0
	Paresthesia	3
	Pre-discharge	1, E
	Post-discharge	2, E
	Vaginal cuff bleeding	4
	Pre-discharge	0
	Post-discharge	4 (3E-1L)

Table 3 Postoperative complications (graded by Dindo-Clavien score) *(Continued)*

Dindo-Clavien score	Description	N, onset time
	Vaginal cuff dehiscence	2
	Pre-discharge	0
	Post-discharge	2, E
	Wound dehiscence	4
	Pre-discharge	0
	Post-discharge	4, E
	Wound infection	1
	Pre-discharge	0
	Post-discharge	1, L
Total		16 (4.4)

Values are given as number (percentage) unless stated otherwise
E early onset (< 30 days), *L* late onset (≥ 30 days)

approach, even if number of previous caesarian sections could be a risk factor for bladder lesions [13].

The surgical approach to hysterectomy as well as the average weight of uteri removed by laparoscopic approach still depends on the surgeon. The proportion of AH compared to LH for benign disease in our department was 8.6%. The value is not reported in the studies selected, but it can vary considerably, from 2–5% [14] to 64% [15]. The average weight of the uteri removed was 327 g; this value is higher (more than 60 g) than the mean uterus weight reported by other authors (217–259 g) [5–8]. For this reason, morcellation with laparoscopic cold knife was necessary in 54.8% of cases, to remove the uterus.

The literature shows a prevalence of uterine sarcoma in presumed uterine fibroids from 0.00 to 0.49% [16]. In the present, the incidence of incidentally diagnosed sarcoma was 0.8%: 2 leiomyosarcomas and 1 endometrial stromal sarcoma. Even if the comparisons of the different study populations in the literature is difficult, one hypothesis to explain this finding could be that,as myoma size is considered a risk factor for sarcoma, in the present study, the mean weight and related size of the removed uteri is higher than those reported by other studies on hysterectomy and prevalence of uterine sarcoma.

Mean operative time was 113 min, which is comparable to other series [6–8] despite a higher mean uterine weight. It is quite longer if we consider two reference centers for laparoscopic surgery, with a mean operative time of 90 and 80 min [17, 18].

All the procedures in the present series were performed by two senior surgeons adopting the TLH technique described by Wattiez et al. [19] that requires a uterine manipulator to reduce ureteral injury and to facilitate a correct exposition of the pelvis area: pouch of Douglas, posterior fornix, and uterine vessels.

Concerning the hospitalization time, our data favorably compare with literature [5, 6, 9, 10]; however, hospital stay does not always reflect the postoperative course, since it is often influenced by rules related to

Table 4 Comparison with literature: baseline characteristics

Authors	N. Pt		Mean age (year)[a]	Mean BMI[a]	Mean uterus weight (g)[a]	Mean operative time (min)[a]	Mean hospital stay (days)[a]
Kim 2015 [5]	366	Retrospective study	47.7 ± 7.4	24.9 ± 2.6	259 ± 149	149.3 ± 59	5.5 ± 2.0
Wallwiener 2013 [6]	294	Prospective study	48.4 ± 8.5	25.6 ± 5.1	220 ± 205	103 ± 36	4.9 ± 2.8
Twijnstra 2012 [7]	960	Cohort analysis	48.8 ± 11.3	27.5 ± 5.7	217 ± 196	118 ± 40	–
Boosz 2011 [8]	567	Retrospective study	47.9 ± 9.1	26.2 ± 5.3	243 ± 198	104 ± 44	–
Morelli 2007 [9]	200	Randomized trial	41.2 ± 4.4	26.3 ± 3.7	–	86 ± 3	2.9 ± 1.4
Ng 2007 [10]	435	Retrospective study	47.5 (34–72)[b]	19.2 (12–34)[b]	–	136(40-257)[b]	2.7(1-20)[bc]
Present study	361	Prospective study[d]	49.6 ± 6.5	25.8 ± 5.6	327 ± 249	113 ± 36	2.6 ± 1.1 (1–12)[b]

[a]Mean ± SD
[b]Mean (range)
[c]Data considered for 427 patients with a successful TLH (no laparotomy conversion)
[d]Retrospective analysis of a prospective collected database

economic aspects, department procedures, territory, and patient's expectations. In many countries, early discharge policies are implemented and there are several studies of total laparoscopic hysterectomies performed in Day Surgery with analgesic therapy after discharge [20].

Only 2 (0.6%) intraoperative complications occurred: 1 bladder injury (0.3%) recognized and sutured during the intervention with a good outcome and 1 (0.3%) blood transfusion (uterus weight of 1800 g) due to intraoperative blood loss of 500 ml and preoperative anemia (Hb 9.2 g/dl).

In the majority of the studies in the literature, the intraoperative complications are not taken into account as a specific group and these in the overall record of complications. An unrecognized intraoperative minor complication could become a postoperative major complication requiring reintervention. For this reason, even if the risk of intraoperative complications is very low (0.6%), routinely filling the bladder with Sodium Indigotin Disulfonate is a cost-effective procedure in case of total hysterectomy.

There were 3 (0.8%) grade IIIB complications, these arose after discharge. A ureteral occlusion appeared early with fever and hydroureteronephrosis in a patient who had undergone TLH for acute urine retention caused by a very large fibroma. This was treated with ureteral replanting. A late onset port side hernia required a hernioplasty procedure and late onset bowel adhesions required a laparoscopic lysis.

Grade IIIA complications occurred in 6 (1.7%) patients after discharge: an early vaginal cuff dehiscence was solved with outpatient positioning of stitches, 3 early vaginal cuff bleeding, 2 of which required readmissions and 1 that required blood transfusion and 2 ureteral occlusions that were treated uneventfully with the endoscopic positioning of a double J catheter. No ureteral fistula occurred.

The majority of complications (35/53: 66.3%) arose after discharge, within 1 month after surgery; during the recovery in the postoperative period 11 (20.8%), complication occurred: 5 urinary infections, 2 cardiac arrhythmias, and 1 anemia, resolved with medical treatment.

The Clavien-Dindo score is also useful to categorize the "minor" complications in a more detailed way, as is important in a controlled clinical activity.

In our series, 28 (7.8%) patients required additional medical treatment for postoperative complications and 16 (4.4%) patients had mild postoperative conditions

Table 5 Comparison with literature: intraoperative and postoperative complications

	Bladder injury[a]	Ureteral Injury[a]	Bowel injury[a]	Vascular injury[a]	Vaginal cuff dehiscence[a]	Mini laparotomy[a]	Laparotomy[a]	Total laparotomies[a]	Blood transfusion[a]	Reoperation[a]
Kim 2015 [5]	4 (1.1)	5 (1.4)	3 (0.8)	0 (0)	9 (2.5)	0 (0)	17 (4.6)*	17 (4.6)*	–	–
Wallwiener 2013 [6]	0 (0)	0 (0)	0 (0)	1 (0.3)	2 (0.7)	–	–	19 (6.5)*	–	19 (6.4)[c]*
Twijnstra 2012 [7]	13 (1.4)	4 (0.4)	5 (0.5)	1 (0.1)	–	–	–	46 (4.8)*	–	15(1.6)
Boosz 2011 [8]	4 (0.7)	1 (0.2)	1 (0.2)	–	4 (0.7)	1 (0.2)	0 (0)	1 (0.2)	–	10 (1.8)
Morelli 2007 [9]	7 (3.5)*	5 (2.5)	1 (0.5)	–	–	–	–	10 (5)*	14 (7.0)*	2 (1)
Ng 2007 [10]	1 (0.2)[b]	1 (0.2)[b]	4(0.9)[b]	0 (0)[b]	0 (0)	3 (0.7)	5 (1.1)	8 (1.8)	17 (4.0)[b,*]	–
Present study	1 (0.3)	1 (0.3)	0 (0)	0 (0)	0 (0)	3 (0.8)	0 (0)	3 (0.8)	3 (0.8)	4 (1.1)[d]

[a]Values are given as number (percentage) unless stated otherwise
[b]Data considered for 427 patients with a successful TLH (no laparotomy conversion)
[c]Operations for pelvic abscess, pelvic peritonitis, or hematoma are included
[d]Reoperation for bowel adhesions and port side hernia are included
*The difference with the data of the present study is statistically significant (p < 0.05)

that required treatment, mostly conservative, visits, or unplanned medications.

In the literature, complications are frequently classified as "major" or "minor," although this can lead to subjective interpretations, with a tendency to underestimate the event.

To compare our data with the literature, we had to consider major complications grouped by the organ involved. Our data compare favorably with those reported in the literature.

In the present study, we had only 1 bladder lesion (0.3%), in line with the data reported by other authors [5–8, 10, 17, 21] except for Morelli et al. [9], that reported a significantly higher percentage (3.5%) of bladder injury, probably related to the high numbers of patients with previous cesarean section (> 50%).

Ureteral injuries occurred in 3 cases (0.8%), just 1 of them needing surgical intervention (0.3%); these data are in line with those reported in the other series [5–10] and with the gynecological laparoscopic literature [17, 21].

Vaginal vault complications in laparoscopic surgery may occur, even though they are rare [22]. It is believed that the risk of vaginal cuff dehiscence is correlated to the chosen approach to hysterectomy and to suture. The suture of the cuff by vaginal route is associated with a lower risk of complications and a shorter operative time [23]. However, different sutures laparoscopically performed can differ in operative time and complications [14]. In our series, in 83.3% of cases, a laparoscopic vaginal cuff closure has been performed with a continuous barbed suture; we identified 7 (1.9%) cases of bleeding and 3 (0.8) cases of dehiscence, 4 (1.1%) requiring reintervention without general anesthesia, while 6 (1.6%) had complications that were considered minor and did not require any medical or surgical intervention. These findings are in line with the 0–3.3 percentage of dehiscence reported in recent suture dehiscence literature [24, 25]. Regarding vaginal bleeding: 3 major (0.8%) and 4 minor (1.1%) instances were recorded, with a prevalence in the present study comparable with those reported in the literature: 1.4–32.5 [15] and even lower considering that the majority of the studies do not consider Clavien-Dindo grade 1 vaginal bleeding.

Conversion to laparotomy due to complications or surgical difficulties did not become necessary. A minilaparotomy to remove the calcific specimen was necessary in 3 cases (0.8%). Data from similar series [5–7, 9, 10] revealed a mean rate of conversion of 4.5% (range 1.8–6.5%) while Boosz et al. reported a percentage of conversion of 0.2% [8]. Blood transfusion was necessary in only 3 (0.8%) cases evidencing a statistical significant difference in comparison with the 7% rates reported by Morelli et al. [9] and the 3% by Ng et al. [10].

Conclusion

This study confirmed that total laparoscopic hysterectomy is a procedure with a low incidence of complications. Moreover, the technological evolution of the last few years, in terms of type of endoscope, multifunctional instruments, ultra MinInvasive accesses, and the possibility of completing courses in surgical technique and anatomy, have allowed its large-scale diffusion, extending its indications to difficult cases in a frail older population, with improvements also in term of indirect health costs.

Abbreviations
AH: Abdominal hysterectomy; BMI: Body mass index; LAVH: Laparoscopically assisted vaginal hysterectomy; LH: Laparoscopic hysterectomy; TLH: Total laparoscopic hysterectomy

Acknowledgements
None

Funding
None

Authors' contributions
LM is a surgeon who supervised the study. RC analyzed the data and wrote the article. AP collected the data. FG analyzed the data and revised the final version of the article. VB collected the data and wrote the article. ST is a surgeon who analyzed the data and provided the original idea. All authors read and approved the final manuscript.

Competing interests
The authors declare that they have no competing interests.

Author details
[1]Department of Gynecology and Obstetrics, St. Chiara Hospital of Trento, Trento, Italy. [2]Department of Gynecology and Obstetrics, University of Verona, Verona, Italy.

References
1. Aarts JW, Nieboer TE, Johnson N, Tavender E, Garry R, Mol BW et al (2015) Surgical approach to hysterectomy for benign gynaecological disease. Cochrane Database Syst Rev:CD003677 0.1002/14651858.CD003677
2. Mäkinen J, Brummer T, Jalkanen J, Heikkinen AM, Fraser J, Tomás E et al (2013) Ten years of progress improved hysterectomyoutcomes in Finland1996–2006: a longitudinal observation study. BMJ Open 3(10):28
3. Velemir L, Azuar AS, Botchorishvili R, Canis M, Jardon K, Rabischong B et al (2009) Optimizing the role of surgeons assistants during a laparoscopic hysterectomy. Gynecol Obstet Fertil 37:74–80
4. Clavien PA, Sanabria JR, Strasberg SM (1992) Proposed classification of complications of surgery with examples of utility in cholecystectomy. Surgery 111:518–526
5. Kim SM, Park EK, Jeung IC, Kim CJ, Lee YS (2015) Abdominal, multi-port and single-port total laparoscopic hysterectomy: eleven-year trends comparison

of surgical outcomes complications of 936 cases. Arch Gynecol Obstet 291: 1313–1319

6. Wallwiener M, Taran FA, Rothmund R, Kasperkowiak A, Auwärter G, Ganz A (2013) Laparoscopic supracervical hysterectomy (LSH) versus total laparoscopic hysterectomy (TLH): an implementation study in 1,952 patients with an analysis of risk factors for conversion to laparotomy and complications, and of procedure-specific re-operations. Arch Gynecol Obstet 288:1329–1339

7. Twijnstra AR, Blikkendaal MD, van Zwet EW, van Kesteren PJ, de Kroon CD, Jansen FW (2012) Predictors of successful surgical outcome in laparoscopic hysterectomy. Obstet Gynecol 119:700–708

8. Boosz A, Lermann J, Mehlhorn G, Loehberg C, Renner SP, Thiel FC (2011) Comparison of re-operation rates and complication rates after total laparoscopic hysterectomy (TLH) and laparoscopy-assisted supracervical hysterectomy (LASH). Eur J Obstet Gynecol Reprod Biol 158:269–273

9. Morelli M, Caruso M, Noia R, Chiodo D, Cosco C, Lucia E (2007) Total laparoscopic hysterectomy versus vaginal hysterectomy: a prospective randomized trial. Minerva Ginecol 59(2):99–105

10. Ng CC, Chern BS, Siow AY (2007) Retrospective study of the success rates and complications associated with total laparoscopic hysterectomy. J. Obstet. Gynaecol Res 3(4):512–518

11. Reich H, Roberts L (2003) Laparoscopic hysterectomy in current gynaecological practice. Rev Gynaecol Pract 3:32–40

12. Ghezzi F, Uccella S, Cromi A, Siesto G, Serati M, Bogani G (2010) Postoperative pain after laparoscopic and vaginal hysterectomy for benign gynecologic disease: a randomized trial. Am J Obstet Gynecol 203(118):e1–e8

13. Pillet MCL, Leonard F, Chopin N, Malaret JM, Borghese B, Foulot H et al (2009) Incidence and risk factors of bladder injuries during laparoscopic hysterectomy indicated for benign uterine pathologies: a 14.5 years experience in a continuous series of 1501 procedures. Hum Reprod 24(4):842–849

14. Karacan T, Ozyurek E, Usta T, Odacilar E, Hanli U, Kovalak E, Dayan H (2018) Comparison of barbed unidirectional suture with figure-of-eight standard sutures in vaginal cuff closure in total laparoscopic hysterectomy. J Obstet Gynaecol 24:1–6. https://doi.org/10.1080/01443615.2017.1416597

15. Jacoby VL, Autry A, Jacobson G, Domush R, Nakagawa S, Jacoby A (2009) Nationwide use of laparoscopic hysterectomy compared with abdominal and vaginal approaches. Obstet Gynecol 114:1041–1048

16. Cui RR, Wright JD (2016) Risk of occult uterine sarcoma in presumed uterine fibroids. Clin Obstet and Gynecol 59:103–118

17. Wattiez A, Soriano D, Cohen SB, Nervo P, Canis M, Botchorishvili R (2002) The learning curve of total laparoscopic hysterectomy: comparative analysis of 1647 cases. J Am Assoc Gynecol Laparosc 9:339–345

18. Malzoni M, Perniola G, Perniola F, Imperato F (2004) Optimizing the total laparoscopic hysterectomy procedure for benign uterine pathology. J Am Assoc Gynecol Laparosc. 11:211–218

19. Thoma V, Salvatores M, Mereu L, Chua I, Wattiez A (2007) Laparoscopic hysterectomy: technique, indications. Ann Urol (Paris) 41:80–90

20. Maheux-Lacroix S, Lemyre M, Couture V, Bernier G, Laberge PY (2015) Feasibility and safety of outpatient total laparoscopic hysterectomy. JSLS 19:1–6

21. Donnez O, Jadoul P, Squifflet J, Donnez J (2009) A series of 3190 laparoscopic hysterectomies for benign disease from 1990 to 2006: evaluation of complications compared with vaginal and abdominal procedures. BJOG 116:492–500

22. Uccella S, Ghezzi F, Mariani A, Cromi A, Bogani G, Serati M, Bolis P (2011) Vaginal cuff closure after minimally invasive hysterectomy: our experience and systematic review of the literature. Am J Obstet Gynecol 205(119e):1–12

23. Uccella S, Cromi A, Bogani G, Casarin J, Formenti G, Ghezzi F (2013) Systematic implementation of laparoscopic hysterectomy independent of uterus size: clinical effect. J Minim Invasive Gynecol 20:505–516

24. Uccella S, Malzoni M, Cromi A, Seracchioli R, Ciravolo G, Fanfani F, Shakir F, Gueli Alletti S, Legge F, Berretta R, Corrado G, Casarella L, Donarini P, Zanello M, Perrone E, Gisone B, Vizza E, Scambia G, Ghezzi F (2018) Laparoscopic vs transvaginal cuff closure after total laparoscopic hysterectomy: a randomized trial by the Italian Society of Gynecologic Endoscopy. Am J Obstet Gynecol 218(5):500.e1–500.e13. https://doi.org/10.1016/j.ajog.2018.01.029

25. Bogliolo S, Musacchi V, Dominoni M, Cassani C, Gaggero CR, De Silvestri A, Gardella B, Spinillo A (2015) Barbed suture in minimally invasive hysterectomy: a systematic review and meta-analysis. Arch Gynecol Obstet 292(3):489–497

Effects of salpingectomy during abdominal hysterectomy on ovarian reserve: a randomized controlled trial

Afsaneh Tehranian[1*], Roghayeh Hassani Zangbar[1], Faezeh Aghajani[1], Mahdi Sepidarkish[2], Saeedeh Rafiei[1] and Tayebe Esfidani[1]

Abstract

Background: The aim of this study was to investigate the effect of salpingectomy on ovarian function by measuring AMH.

Methods: This study was a balanced, single-center, double-blind, randomized, controlled trial in Ruin Tan Arash Hospital, Tehran, between May 2013 and November 2014. A total of 30 patients undergoing elective abdominal hysterectomy were randomized into two groups, 15 with salpingectomy and 15 without salpingectomy. The primary objective of this study was to compare mean difference of anti-Mullerian hormone (AMH) between two groups. The secondary outcomes measured were follicle-stimulating hormone (FSH), operative time, and blood loss.

Results: Serum AMH levels decreased at 3 months after hysterectomy in all patients (pre AMH 1.32 ± (0.91); post AMH 1.05 ± (0.88), $P < 0.001$), the salpingectomy group (pre AMH 1.44 ± (0.94); post AMH 1.13 ± (0.86), $P < 0.001$), and no salpingectomy group (pre AMH 1.2 ± (0.9); post AMH 0.97 ± (0.92), $P < 0.001$). The rate of decline of AMH levels after surgery did not differ between the two groups (25% (17–33%) vs. 26% (15–36%), $P = 0.23$) among the women with salpingectomy versus without salpingectomy, respectively. There was no difference in the mean operative time (mean difference 0.33, 95% CI − 22.21 to 22.86, $P < 0.92$), mean blood loss (mean difference − 0.66, 95% CI − 15.8 to 14.46, $P < 0.97$), and post FSH (mean difference 0.34, 95% CI − 1.2 to 1.88, $P < 0.65$) between both groups.

Conclusions: Salpingectomy with abdominal hysterectomy is a safe treatment that does not have a deleterious effect on ovarian reserve.

Keywords: Salpingectomy, Hysterectomy, Ovarian reserve, Anti-Mullerian hormone

Background

Hysterectomy is one of the most common surgeries in women worldwide [1]. It is applied for the treatment of various problems, such as pelvic pain, menstrual problems, tumors, and other related diseases. However, based on the patient's problem, in addition to the uterus, removal of the fallopian tubes, ovaries, or cervix may be necessary [2]. Every year, 600,000 women are undergoing hysterectomy surgery in the USA [3]. The surgery is done as abdominally and vaginally, but from 1980 onwards, it is also done by laparoscopy, which plays a major role in the treatment of gynecologic malignancies, uterine leiomyoma, endometrial hyperplasia, and uterine prolapse [3, 4].

Hysterectomy may have complications. One of the most important complications is reduced ovarian function, which is not dependent on the type of surgery and is very important for women of reproductive age [1, 5]. Previous studies have shown that women undergoing hysterectomy experience menopausal symptoms faster

* Correspondence: afsanehtehranian@yahoo.com
[1]Department of Obstetrics and Gynecology, Roointan-Arash Women's Hospital, Tehran University of Medical Sciences, Tehran, Iran
Full list of author information is available at the end of the article

and compared with other women have lower number of follicles, lower serum progesterone levels, and higher levels of follicle-stimulating hormone (FSH) [6]. The measures for preserving ovarian function after hysterectomy are always important.

Salpingectomy is a procedure for sterilization and with hysterectomy leads to good results, especially in recent decades [7, 8]. Salpingectomy can be due to different reasons, including treatment of ectopic pregnancy, infections in the fallopian tubes, and fallopian tube prolapse treatment after hysterectomy [9]. It seems that preserving ovarian function after hysterectomy is very important. Hysterectomy preserves the both ovaries and tubes through salpingectomy close to the uterus to preserve blood supply to the mesosalpinx of ovaries [10]. Many gynecologists refuse to perform salpingectomy at the time of hysterectomy due to blocking uterine blood flow to the ovaries and disrupting its function [11]. There is no agreement on the effect of salpingectomy, and some studies revealed the devastating impact of salpingectomy [12]. Interestingly, findings of studies have shown that the primary source of ovarian cancer is fallopian tubes and if hysterectomy is along with salpingectomy, cancer progression may be prevented. The preferred surgery is removing tubes associated with hysterectomy in women who have high levels of uterine cancer [13]. It can be proved in practice that hysterectomy with salpingectomy has no harmful effects on ovarian function and is used as a suitable technique for hysterectomy. The aim of this study was to investigate the effect of salpingectomy on ovarian function by measuring anti-Mullerian hormone (AMH) (as a substitute for ovarian reserve). Therefore, the mean AMH was compared between the two groups of hysterectomy and hysterectomy with salpingectomy within 3 months after surgery.

Methods

This study was a balanced, single-center, double-blind, randomized, controlled trial in Ruin Tan Arash Hospital, Tehran, between May 2013 and November 2014.

The participants were premenopausal women aged 18 to 45 years who were undergoing abdominal hysterectomy for non-malignant gynecologic disease with preservation of the ovaries. All patients gave written informed consent before any study-related tests were done. Ethics approval was obtained from the Tehran University of Medical Sciences Clinical Research Ethics Board. Date of approval was January 31, 2015. The study was registered in Iranian Registry of Clinical Trials (www.IRCT.ir) by the number of IRCT2014123118866N4.

The inclusion criteria were age < 45 years, elective hysterectomy (without oophorectomy), absence of menopausal symptoms, and baseline FSH value of <10 IU/mL. Women with the following characteristics were excluded

prior to enrollment: a history of pelvic surgery, cystic (> 10 mm) or any solid ovarian mass in transvaginal ultrasound, hormone replacement treatment and/or hormonal contraception for the last 6 months, a history of pelvic surgery, and a present or past smoking history.

After their consent was obtained, patients were randomly assigned in two groups, using a random number sequence, generated with a proprietary computer application, according to a randomized block design. The randomization list was created by the clinical trial's epidemiologist, who kept the codes until completion of the study. Allocation concealment was maintained by having procedure indicator cards inside a set of numbered opaque sealed envelopes. Patients were allocated to treatment by the author opening the next numbered envelope, after screening, in the presence of the patient. None of the staff or patients had access to the randomization codes during the study. A patient's treatment assignment would only be unblended when knowledge of the treatment was essential for the further management of the patient. The surgeon performing the procedures was blinded to the treatment allocation until the time of surgery.

Group 1 patients (salpingectomy) underwent total hysterectomy with removal of the fallopian tubes bilaterally. Caution was given to avoid injury to the ovarian vessels and to divide the mesosalpinx as close to the fallopian tube as possible. In group 2 (without salpingectomy), the fallopian tubes were divided in the proximal tubal isthmus.

The primary objective of this study was to compare mean difference of anti-Mullerian hormone (AMH) between two groups. The secondary outcomes measured were follicle-stimulating hormone (FSH), operative time, and blood loss.

The serum samples were collected preoperatively and at 3 months after the surgery from each patient. All hormonal measurements were performed in the same reference laboratory. Blood samples were obtained by venipuncture, and the sera extracted by centrifuge. Serum FSH and LH levels were measured by enzyme-linked fluorescent assay (VIDAS, BioMerieux SA) according to the manufacturer's instructions. Serum AMH level was measured by enzyme-linked immunosorbent assay (ELISA) kit according to the manufacturer's instructions (AMH Gen II ELISA; Immunotech) and reported as nanograms per milliliter with the detection limit of 0.006 ng/mL. The intraassay and interassay coefficients of variation (CV) were 4.38 and 5.64% for FSH, 4.14 and 4.86% for AMH, and 4.23 and 5.48% for LH, respectively.

The study required the enrollment of 30 patients in each group to have at least 80% power to detect mean difference of 0.5 between two groups with regard to main outcome (with two-sided test and type 1 error of 5%).

All analyses were performed on an intent-to-treat basis. Summaries of continuous and categorical measures were presented as the mean± (SD) and N (%) respectively. We compared a difference between baseline characteristics of patients and after randomization into the two groups with a chi-square test for categorized data and with Student's t test for continuous variables. GLM (general linear model) (family = Gaussian, link = identity) was used to compare the two study arms for the primary and secondary end point at 3 months after the surgery. The model included treatment as main effects and age, body mass index (BMI), pre AMH, parity, pre FSH, and pre LH as covariates. Testing was performed at a 95% significance level. Results were presented as the mean difference with 95% confidence intervals. Statistical tests were two tailed. Data were analyzed using Stata software version 13 (Stata Corp, College Station, TX, USA). The conduct and analysis of the trial adhered to the 2010 CONSORT guidelines.

Results

In this study, 114 patients were recruited between January 2, 2014 and November 3, 2014. Eighty-four patients did not meet the criteria for participation. Ultimately, 30 patients were randomized into two groups: 15 women with salpingectomy and 15 women without salpingectomy. There were no complications directly attributable to performing salpingectomy. The study profile is shown in Fig. 1.

The mean age of patients was 40.13 (95% CI 38.88–41.38). The mean BMI of participants was 28.22 (95% CI 26.86–29.58) kg/m2 and mean uterine weight of 289.66 (95% CI 233.71–345.61) grams. Mean age in the salpingectomy group

was 39.08 years (SD 3.72) and 40.46 years (SD 3.02) in the without salpingectomy group. Baseline and surgical characteristics in two groups are described in Table 1. The study groups were well matched with respect to demographics and disease characteristics.

Serum AMH levels were decreased at 3 months after hysterectomy in all patients (pre AMH 1.32 ± (0.91); post AMH 1.05 ± (0.88), $P < 0.001$), the salpingectomy group (pre AMH 1.44 ± (0.94); post AMH 1.13 ± (0.86), $P < 0.001$), and without salpingectomy group (pre AMH 1.2 ± (0.9); post AMH 0.97 ± (0.92), $P < 0.001$). The rate of decline of AMH levels after surgery did not differ between the two groups (25%(17–33%) vs. 26%(15–36%), $P = 0.23$) among the women with salpingectomy versus without salpingectomy respectively (Fig. 2). Also in multivariate analysis, there was no significant difference between two groups at 3 months after operation (mean difference 4.46, 95% CI – 0.19 to 0.04, $P < 0.21$).

There was no difference in the mean operative time (mean difference 0.33, 95% CI -22.21 to 22.86, $P < 0.92$), mean blood loss (mean difference – 0.66, 95% CI – 15.8 to 14.46, $P < 0.97$), and post FSH (mean difference 0.34, 95% CI – 1.2 to 1.88, $P < 0.65$) between both groups.

Discussion

The findings of this study confirmed the results of previous studies that showed that salpingectomy with hysterectomy cannot cause to a devastating effect on the ovarian reserve and 3 months after treatment, no significant difference was seen in the levels of AMH between the two treatments. Also, no significant differences were observed between the two groups in terms of surgical time and blood loss, and compared with hysterectomy, salpingectomy was not associated with any complications [14–16].

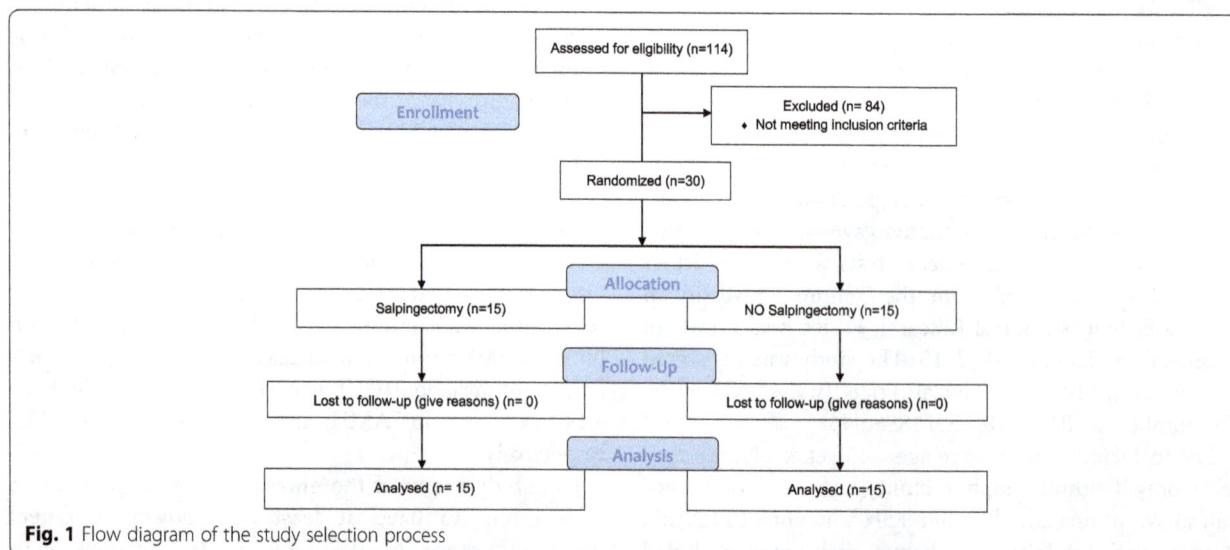

Fig. 1 Flow diagram of the study selection process

Table 1 Baseline demographics and clinical characteristics

	Salpingectomy (n = 15)	No salpingectomy (n = 15)	P value
Age (years)	39.8 ± (3.72)	40.46 ± (3.02)	0.59
BMI	27.51 ± (4.14)	28.94 ± (3.02)	0.29
Parity	3.13 ± (0.51)	2.86 ± (0.99)	0.36
Pre AMH	1.2 ± (0.9)	1.44 ± (0.94)	0.47
Pre FSH	7.48 ± (1.84)	7.21 ± (2.48)	0.74
Pre Hb	12.26 ± (0.91)	11.82 ± (1.06)	0.24
Diameter ovarian	12.26 ± (1.09)	12.06 ± (1.16)	0.63
Uterine weight (g)	263.33 ± (118.12)	316 ± (176.26)	0.34

In a study by Sezik et al. in 2007, 24 patients were randomly divided into two groups (12 subjects in each group). In one of the groups, hysterectomy was performed with removal of both tubes, but in another group, the tubes were partially removed. One and 6 months after the intervention, patients were compared according to hormonal profile. The mean levels of hormones FSH, LH, estradiol, and ovarian volume were similar in both groups [14]. Morelli et al. in 2013 compared 158 patients retrospectively. A group of patients underwent hysterectomy without salpingectomy, and another group was women who had hysterectomy with salpingectomy. In the present study, no significant difference was observed between the two groups based on the levels of hormones AMH, FSH, antral follicle count, and the mean ovarian volume and peak systolic velocity was same in both groups [15]. A pilot study was conducted in North Carolina on 30 women aged 18 to 45 years were under laparoscopic hysterectomy along with bilateral salpingectomy or without salpingectomy. The AMH

level was measured 3, 4 and 6 months after the intervention and then compared between the two groups. A significant decrease was not seen within groups at the baseline in AMH levels compared with after the intervention. Also, there was no significant difference between the two groups after intervention in both measurement times [17].

In keeping with the findings of the study, mean operative time and blood loss between the two groups were not significantly different. Although consistent results were obtained in line with other studies, contrary to the findings several studies reported an adverse effect of salpingectomy on the ovarian reserve [18–20]. In a retrospective study by Xu-ping Ye et al. on 198 women who were eligible for IVF-ET (in vitro fertilization—embryo transfer), AMH levels were compared among three groups of unilateral salpingectomy (83 subjects), bilateral salpingectomy (41 subjects), and no tubal surgery (54 subjects). The mean AMH in the group without tubal surgery was higher than the bilateral salpingectomy group. (183.48 vs. 127.11 fmol/ml, P = 0.037). The mean FSH was significantly higher in the bilateral salpingectomy group than the group without tubal surgery (7.85 vs 9.13 mLU/ml, P = 0.048) [21]. Findings from consequences of 288 IVF-ET cycles in 251 women with tubal factor infertility from January 2001 to December 2011 revealed that there was no significant difference between none ovarian response parameters in the two groups with and without salpingectomy [10].

The disagreement among studies can be attributed to the following reasons. One of the reasons may be due to different designs in these studies. Given that the best evidence comes from randomized clinical trial (RCT), more information can be cited from this type of studies

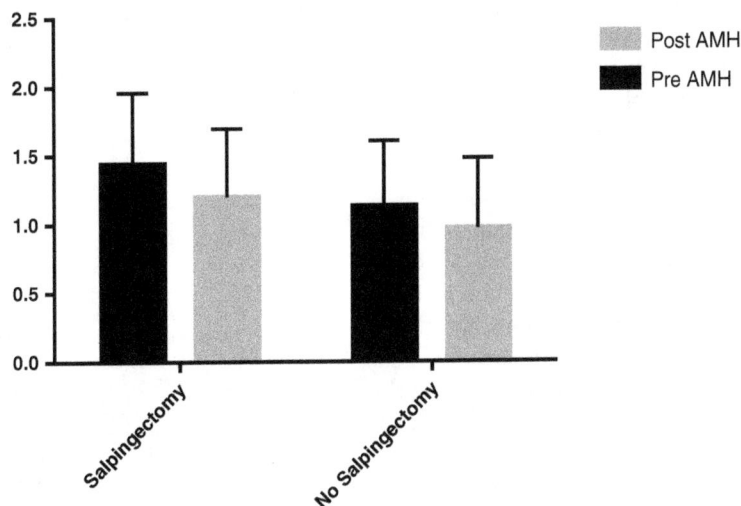

Fig. 2 The rate of decline of AMH levels after surgery among the women with salpingectomy vs no salpingectomy

[22]. Of abovementioned studies, one of them was RCT and others were retrospective cohort and case-control. The present study was conducted as RCT with relatively satisfactory sample size that confirmed the results of others studies and did not report a harmful effect of salpingectomy. Another reason was the use of different markers of ovarian reserve in the studies [22]. In the retrieved studies, reported measures included duration of gonadotropin stimulation, the amount of used gonadotropin, follicle count, the number of retrieved oocytes, fertility rate, and hormone levels (FSH, LH, estradiol, and AMH).

AMH is a glycoprotein dimer mainly secretes from granulocytes of preantral and small antral follicles. AMH levels are relatively constant throughout the menstrual cycle and have a very strong correlation with the number of follicles and ovarian reserve and are an important indicator of fertility [23, 24]. Previous studies have shown that AMH compared with other hormone markers is better predictive factor and is less affected by manipulating the endogenous gonadotropin. In the present study, AMH measured best predict ovarian reserve [25].

Some studies have shown that an effect of salpingectomy is harmful in infertile patients undergoing IVF-ET. In these studies, confounding factors affecting ovarian reserve and the process of infertility treatment (eligibility for IVF) were not adjusted. Infertile individuals undergoing ART is specific and cannot be a representative of all women of reproductive age [10]. Therefore, the results of these studies can be influenced by selection bias. Another factor that could contradict the results of these studies is due to measurement bias the skill of the surgeon.

It seems that if salpingectomy is done with minimum damage to the ovarian microvascularization, blood flow to the ovaries will be complete and the ovary function remains undisturbed. Adequate amounts of blood flow have a vital role in the follicular maturation, either spontaneously or stimulated, by influencing the synthesis of steroid hormones [18]. Ovarian blood flow is provided from two basic sources: ovarian artery originated from the aorta and ramus ovaricus that comes from the uterine artery. The blood flow of the tubes arises from ovarian artery and ramus ovaricus. Studies that found harmful effect of salpingectomy concluded based on decreased blood flow to the ovaries and reduction in its efficiency [12]. One of the important reasons for the phenomenon is expertise and skill of the surgeons.

The strengths of this study included study design (RCT), measuring objective outcomes and high prediction, and relatively desirable sample size. The most important limitation of the study was lack of long-term follow-up that causes to no tracking medium-term and long-term effects of hysterectomy and salpingectomy in

menopause patients and their ovarian function. The lack of uterine blood flow measurement is the limitations of this study.

Conclusions
Salpingectomy with abdominal hysterectomy is a safe and convenient treatment that does not have a deleterious effect on ovarian reserve. It is suggested that multicenter RCT studies with higher sample size and longer duration of follow-up are done to extract more accurate and reliable results about the effects of salpingectomy on fertilization.

Key message
The findings of this study confirmed the results of previous studies that showed that salpingectomy with hysterectomy cannot cause to a devastating effect on the ovarian reserve and 3 months after treatment, no significant difference was seen in the levels of AMH between the two treatments.

Authors' contributions
AT contribute to the conception and design of the work, interpretation of data. RH participated in the design of the study and performed the statistical analysis. FA participated in the sequence alignment and drafted the manuscript. MS participated in the design of the study and performed the statistical analysis. SR participated in data gathering, drafting the work and revising it critically for content. TE conceived of the study and participated in its design and coordination. All authors read and approved the final manuscript.

Competing interests
The authors declare that they have no competing interests.

Author details
[1]Department of Obstetrics and Gynecology, Roointan-Arash Women's Hospital, Tehran University of Medical Sciences, Tehran, Iran. [2]Department of Epidemiology and Reproductive Health, Reproductive Epidemiology Research Center, Royan Institute for Reproductive Biomedicine, ACECR, Tehran, Iran.

References
1. Hammer A, Rositch AF, Kahlert J, Gravitt PE, Blaakaer J, Sogaard M (2015) Global epidemiology of hysterectomy: possible impact on gynecological cancer rates. Am J Obstet Gynecol 213(1):23–29
2. Asante A, Whiteman MK, Kulkarni A, Cox S, Marchbanks PA, Jamieson DJ (2010) Elective oophorectomy in the United States: trends and in-hospital complications, 1998–2006. Obstet Gynecol 116(5):1088–1095
3. Wu JM, Wechter ME, Geller EJ, Nguyen TV, Visco AG (2007) Hysterectomy rates in the United States, 2003. Obstet Gynecol 110(5):1091–1095
4. Chhabra S, Kutchi I, Bhavani M, Mehta S (2015) Trends in morbidity mortality associated with hysterectomy for benign gynaecological disorders in low resource settings. Current Women's Health Reviews 11(2):152–156
5. Escobar DA, Botero AM, Cash MG, Reyes-Ortiz CA (2016) Factors associated with hysterectomy among older women from Latin America and the Caribbean. Women Health 56(5):522–39

6. Hodges KR, Davis BR, Swaim LS (2014) Prevention and management of hysterectomy complications. Clin Obstet Gynecol 57(1):43–57

7. Kwon JS (2015) Ovarian cancer risk reduction through opportunistic salpingectomy. J Gynecol Oncol 26(2):83–86

8. Kwon JS, McAlpine JN, Hanley GE, Finlayson SJ, Cohen T, Miller DM et al (2015) Costs and benefits of opportunistic salpingectomy as an ovarian cancer prevention strategy. Obstet Gynecol 125(2):338–345

9. Minig L, Chuang L, Patrono MG, Cardenas-Rebollo JM, Garcia-Donas J (2015) Surgical outcomes and complications of prophylactic salpingectomy at the time of benign hysterectomy in premenopausal women. J Minim Invasive Gynecol 22(4):653–657

10. Almog B, Wagman I, Bibi G, Raz Y, Azem F, Groutz A et al (2011) Effects of salpingectomy on ovarian response in controlled ovarian hyperstimulation for in vitro fertilization: a reappraisal. Fertil Steril 95(8):2474–2476

11. Bradley MS, Visco AG (2015) Role of salpingectomy at the time of urogynecologic surgery. Curr Opin Obstet Gynecol 27(5):385–389

12. Dar P, Sachs GS, Strassburger D, Bukovsky I, Arieli S (2000) Ovarian function before and after salpingectomy in artificial reproductive technology patients. Hum Reprod 15(1):142–144

13. Daly MB, Dresher CW, Yates MS, Jeter JM, Karlan BY, Alberts DS et al (2015) Salpingectomy as a means to reduce ovarian cancer risk. Cancer Prev Res 8(5):342–348

14. Sezik M, Ozkaya O, Demir F, Sezik HT, Kaya H (2007) Total salpingectomy during abdominal hysterectomy: effects on ovarian reserve and ovarian stromal blood flow. J Obstet Gynaecol Res 33(6):863–869

15. Morelli M, Venturella R, Mocciaro R, Di Cello A, Rania E, Lico D et al (2013) Prophylactic salpingectomy in premenopausal low-risk women for ovarian cancer: primum non nocere. Gynecol Oncol 129(3):448–451

16. Verhulst G, Vandersteen N, Van Steirteghem AC, Devroey P (1994) Bilateral salpingectomy does not compromise ovarian stimulation in an in vitro fertilization/embryo transfer programme. Hum Reprod 9(4):624–628

17. Findley AD, Siedhoff MT, Hobbs KA, Steege JF, Carey ET, McCall CA et al (2013) Short-term effects of salpingectomy during laparoscopic hysterectomy on ovarian reserve: a pilot randomized controlled trial. Fertil Steril 100(6):1704–1708

18. Chan CCW, Ng EHY, Li CF, Ho PC (2003) Impaired ovarian blood flow and reduced antral follicle count following laparoscopic salpingectomy for ectopic pregnancy. Hum Reprod 18(10):2175–2180

19. Gelbaya TA, Nardo LG, Fitzgerald CT, Horne G, Brison DR, Lieberman BA (2006) Ovarian response to gonadotropins after laparoscopic salpingectomy or the division of fallopian tubes for hydrosalpinges. Fertil Steril 85(5):1464–1468

20. Orvieto R, Saar-Ryss B, Morgante G, Gemer O, Anteby EY, Meltcer S (2011) Does salpingectomy affect the ipsilateral ovarian response to gonadotropin during in vitro fertilization-embryo transfer cycles? Fertil Steril 95(5):1842–1844

21. Ye X-P, Yang Y-Z, Sun X-X (2015) A retrospective analysis of the effect of salpingectomy on serum anti Mullerian hormone level and ovarian reserve. Am J Obstet Gynecol 212(1):53 e1-. e10

22. Chow SC, Liu JP (2008) Design and analysis of clinical trials: concepts and methodologies. Wiley

23. Broer SL, Mol BWJ, Hendriks D, Broekmans FJM (2009) The role of antimullerian hormone in prediction of outcome after IVF: comparison with the antral follicle count. Fertil Steril 91(3):705–714

24. Depmann M, Eijkemans MJC, Broer SL, Scheffer GJ, van Rooij IAJ, Laven JSE, et al. (2016) Does anti-Mullerian hormone predict menopause in the general population? Results of a prospective ongoing cohort study. Human Reproduction 31(7):1579–1587

25. Shaw CM, Stanczyk FZ, Egleston BL, Kahle LL, Spittle CS, Godwin AK et al (2011) Serum antimullerian hormone in healthy premenopausal women. Fertil Steril 95(8):2718–2721

Endometrial cancer in a woman undergoing hysteroscopy for recurrent IVF failure

Pietro Gambadauro[1,2,3]* and Johannes Gudmundsson[1,3]

Abstract

Background: Hysteroscopy, despite being the undisputed gold standard for the examination of the uterine cavity, is controversial as a routine procedure in infertile women. However, benign intrauterine conditions are common in women suffering repeated in vitro fertilization (IVF) failure, and growing evidence suggests a unique diagnostic and therapeutic role for hysteroscopy. Endometrial malignancy, on the contrary, is unreported by large published series of women with repeated IVF failures undergoing hysteroscopy, and its impact on fertility, for obvious reasons, has not been studied.

Results: An unsuspected endometrial cancer was diagnosed in an asymptomatic 38-year-old woman undergoing hysteroscopy because of several repeated failures of in vitro fertilization and embryo transfer.

Conclusions: Endometrial cancer can be found at hysteroscopy in young women with repeated IVF failures. The possibility of repeatedly unsuccessful fertility treatments should be taken into account when counseling infertile women about conservative treatment of endometrial cancer.

Keywords: Embryo transfer, Endometrial cancer, Hysteroscopy, Implantation failure, In vitro fertilization

Background

During the last decades, developments in ultrasound diagnostics and increased knowledge about the determinants of assisted reproduction's success have caused a downgrading of gynecological endoscopy's role in the assessment of female infertility. Hysteroscopy, for instance, in spite of being the undisputed gold standard for the examination of the uterine cavity, is controversial as a routine procedure [1]. However, growing evidence suggests a unique diagnostic and therapeutic role for hysteroscopy, especially in cases of repeated failures of assisted reproductive technology [2]. In such cases, abnormal hysteroscopic findings, such as endometrial polyps, submuscous fibroids, adhesions, and septa, are common [3–5], and hysteroscopy offers an opportunity for diagnosis and a convenient see-and-treat management [2, 6]. Endometrial malignancy, on the contrary, is unreported in large published series [3–5], and its impact on fertility, for obvious reasons, has not been studied.

We here present and discuss a case of unsuspected endometrial cancer which was accidentally diagnosed in a woman undergoing hysteroscopy because of repeated failure of in vitro fertilization (IVF) and embryo transfer (ET).

Methods

The data of this case report was obtained through retrospective chart review.

Results

A 38-year-old woman and her male partner had been under our care for primary infertility, at the Centre for Reproduction of Uppsala University Hospital, for 3 years. She had a normal body mass index (BMI; 22 kg/m^2) and regular ovulatory menstrual cycles. Previously, she had used combined oral contraceptives followed by an intrauterine device for 10 years. Baseline infertility investigations, including hormonal assessments for TSH and prolactin, pelvic ultrasonography, and semen analysis,

* Correspondence: gambadauro@gmail.com; pietro.gambadauro@ki.se
[1]Centre for Reproduction, Uppsala University Hospital, 751 85 Uppsala, Sweden
[2]Karolinska Institute, LIME/NASP-C7, 17177 Stockholm, Sweden
Full list of author information is available at the end of the article

were unremarkable. Tubal perviousness and no abnormalities were seen at hysterosalpingo-contrast sonography.

After the diagnosis of unexplained infertility, she had undergone three ovarian stimulations, one with clomiphene citrate, and the following two with low-dose follicle-stimulating hormone (FSH) followed by intrauterine insemination. No pregnancy had been obtained. The couple had then undergone two IVF treatments after conventional controlled ovarian stimulation, each one leading to one fresh elective single embryo transfer (SET) and to several frozen single or double embryo transfers (DET). Overall, eight embryo transfers (two fresh SET, four frozen SET, and two frozen DET) had been performed, but no intrauterine clinical pregnancy was ever achieved. A biochemical pregnancy occurred after the third transfer of the series (frozen). The fifth ET (frozen) resulted in a tubal pregnancy, which was managed by laparoscopic salpingectomy.

Prior to the start of a new controlled ovarian stimulation for IVF-ET, it was agreed to perform a hysteroscopy to rule out intrauterine abnormalities, in view of the several previous failures. At hysteroscopy, a small polypoid growth, having its base at the fundal region, was seen. Pathology of the resected specimen returned a diagnosis of endometrial atypia. After counseling, a conservative treatment with oral progestins (medroxyprogesterone acetate 10 mg daily) was commenced. However, an outpatient endometrial biopsy by pipelle at a 3-month follow-up showed endometrial cancer of endometrioid type. The patient was thoroughly counseled by fertility and oncology specialists about the possible therapeutic strategies, ranging from conservative treatments with progestins to the standard surgical staging for endometrial cancer. As a result of her informed choice to undergo surgery, a total hysterectomy with bilateral salpingectomy and preservation of the ovaries was performed by the gynecologic oncology surgeons. Surgery and the postoperative period were uneventful. The final pathology report described a highly differentiated, diploid, endometrioid adenocarcinoma of the endometrium which was classified as FIGO stage IA (G1). No adjuvant treatment was needed. At all planned follow-up visits, in accordance with local guidelines, she was always disease-free and reported a 100% score on quality-of-life measures. At our last contact, 5 years after the hysterectomy, she also reported having adopted a child and enjoying her motherhood.

Discussion

Hysteroscopy is not universally considered a routine procedure for the evaluation of the uterine cavity in subfertile women [1]. However, there is a high prevalence of previously undetected intrauterine abnormalities in IVF patients, particularly following to failed treatments [3–5]. This gives a pragmatic

measurement of the diagnostic potential of hysteroscopy, if we consider that women with failed treatments constitute a selected population which has obviously undergone several prior ultrasound exams. Besides, growing evidence, albeit of limited quality, suggests that hysteroscopic diagnosis and, when needed, treatment may improve IVF outcomes and also be cost-effective [2, 7].

Benign hysteroscopic findings are common among IVF patients, the majority of which being represented by endometrial polyps, submucous fibroids, adhesions, or uterine anomalies [3–5]. On the contrary, an endometrial malignancy is not an expected finding in these women. Endometrial cancer, in spite of an approximate lifetime risk of 2.8% women, is a rare occurrence before 40 years old [8, 9].

Our patient was 38 years old, and no intrauterine abnormality was ever diagnosed or suspected during 3 years of repeated fertility treatments. Hysteroscopy was only performed in view of the several failures and revealed a small polypoid growth that had not been seen at ultrasound. Polyps are an increasingly common finding [3, 10]; however, their association with malignancy is controversial in younger and asymptomatic women [11]. In our case, in spite of hysteroscopic resection and oral progestins treatment, the initially diagnosed atypia turned out to be an endometrial cancer at final diagnosis, which is a known possibility [12]. The cancer was also still present on the final specimen, meaning that it was not confined to the resected polypoid area, as often reported in the literature [12]. It seems therefore worth reminding that, although conservative treatment of early stage endometrial cancer by means of progestins and hysteroscopic resection has been proposed [9, 13], the gold standard includes a total hysterectomy [14]. In this case, following a patient-centered approach to care, the choice of undergoing hysterectomy was made by the patient after thorough information about different therapeutic alternatives. In spite of that, she could still fulfill her desire for motherhood through adoption.

Whether a link existed, in this case, between infertility and the malignancy is an intriguing albeit difficult question. Infertility does not seem to represent a strong risk factor for endometrial cancer, although some conditions such as chronic anovulation in PCOS patients imply unopposed estrogenic effect on the endometrium, hence a risk for abnormal proliferation [15]. Our patient had ovulatory cycles but had undergone various ovarian stimulations with gonadotrophins as well as hormonal replacement treatments for frozen embryo transfer. Her endometrial cancer was of endometrioid type, which is closely related to estrogens. Some studies have previously shown an increased risk for endometrial cancer in women receiving gonadotrophins and clomiphene for fertility treatment although a real causal relationship is far from demonstrated [16].

One could also wonder whether the neoplasia might have played a role in the several failed treatments experienced by our patient. While benign intrauterine conditions are thought to interfere with endometrial receptivity, the hypothesis of an association of endometrial cancer with implantation failure is suggestive but unverified. This possibility should however be kept in mind when counseling subfertile patients about conservative treatments of endometrial cancer, since much of the knowledge on fertility outcomes is based on experiences with fertile women.

Conclusions

Malignancy, albeit rare, is a possible occurrence in younger women undergoing fertility treatments. In the present case, an early diagnosis of endometrial cancer was facilitated by hysteroscopy, which was performed because of repeated IVF failures in a woman with no specific symptoms nor ultrasonographic signs of pathology. The possibility of repeatedly unsuccessful fertility treatments should be taken into account when counseling infertile women about conservative treatment of endometrial cancer.

Acknowledgements
None.

Authors' contributions
Both authors contributed to, read and approved the manuscript.

Competing interests
The authors declare that they have no competing interests.

Author details
[1]Centre for Reproduction, Uppsala University Hospital, 751 85 Uppsala, Sweden. [2]Karolinska Institute, LIME/NASP-C7, 17177 Stockholm, Sweden. [3]Department of Women's and Children's Health, Uppsala University, 751 85 Uppsala, Sweden.

References
1. National Institute for Health and Clinical Excellence (NICE) (2013) Fertility: assessment and treatment for people with fertility problems. Available at: http://guidance.nice.org.uk/CG156.
2. Pundir J, Pundir V, Omanwa K, Khalaf Y, El-Toukhy T (2014) Hysteroscopy prior to the first IVF cycle: a systematic review and meta-analysis. Reprod Biomed Online 28:151–161
3. Karayalcin R, Ozcan S, Moraloglu O, Ozyer S, Mollamahmutoglu L, Batıoglu S (2010) Results of 2500 office-based diagnostic hysteroscopies before IVF. Reprod Biomed Online 20:689–693
4. Makrakis E, Hassiakos D, Stathis D, Vaxevanoglou T, Orfanoudaki E, Pantos K (2009) Hysteroscopy in women with implantation failures after in vitro fertilization: findings and effect on subsequent pregnancy rates. J Minim Invasive Gynecol 16:181–187
5. Barri PN, Coroleu B, Clua E, Tur R, Boada M, Rodriguez I (2014) Investigations into implantation failure in oocyte-donation recipients. Reprod Biomed Online 28:99–105
6. Gambadauro P, Martínez-Maestre MA, Torrejón R (2014) When is see-and-treat hysteroscopic polypectomy successful? Eur J Obstet Gynecol Reprod Biol 178:70–73
7. Kasius JC, Eijkemans RJ, Mol BW, Fauser BC, Fatemi HM, Broekmans FJ (2013) Cost-effectiveness of hysteroscopy screening for infertile women. Reprod Biomed Online 26:619–626
8. Howlader N, Noone AM, Krapcho M, et al. (2015) SEER cancer statistics review, 1975-2012, National Cancer Institute. Bethesda, MD, based on November 2014 SEER data submission, posted to the SEER web site, April 2015; available from http://seer.cancer.gov/csr/1975_2012/.
9. Rodolakis A, Biliatis I, Morice P, Reed N, Mangler M, Kesic V, Denschlag D (2015) European Society of Gynecological Oncology Task Force for Fertility Preservation: clinical recommendations for fertility-sparing management in young endometrial cancer patients. Int J Gynecol Cancer 25:1258–1265
10. Gambadauro P, Torrejón R (2013) The relevance of endometrial polyps: a bibliometric study. Gynecol Surg 10(2):103–108
11. Gambadauro P, Martínez-Maestre MA, Schneider J, Torrejón R (2015) Endometrial polyp or neoplasia? A case-control study in women with polyps at ultrasound. Climacteric 18:399–404
12. Gambadauro P, Martínez-Maestre MA, Schneider J, Torrejón R (2014) Malignant and premalignant changes in the endometrium of women with an ultrasound diagnosis of endometrial polyp. J Obstet Gynaecol 34:611–615
13. Park JY, Nam JH (2015) Progestins in the fertility-sparing treatment and retreatment of patients with primary and recurrent endometrial cancer. Oncologist 20:270–278
14. Gurgan T, Bozdag G, Demirol A, Ayhan A (2007) Preserving fertility before assisted reproduction in women with endometrial carcinoma: case report and literature review. Reprod Biomed Online 15:561–565
15. Navaratnarajah R, Pillay OC, Hardiman P (2008) Polycystic ovary syndrome and endometrial cancer. Semin Reprod Med 26:62–71
16. Kessous R, Davidson E, Meirovitz M, Sergienko R, Sheiner E (2015) The risk of female malignancies after fertility treatments: a cohort study with 25-year follow-up. J Cancer Res Clin Oncol. DOI: 10.1007/s00432-015-2035-x

Dominant hand, non-dominant hand, or both? The effect of pre-training in hand-eye coordination upon the learning curve of laparoscopic intra-corporeal knot tying

Carlos Roger Molinas[1*], Maria Mercedes Binda[1] and Rudi Campo[2]

Abstract

Background: Training of basic laparoscopic psychomotor skills improves both acquisition and retention of more advanced laparoscopic tasks, such as laparoscopic intra-corporeal knot tying (LICK). This randomized controlled trial (RCT) was performed to evaluate the effect of different pre-training programs in hand-eye coordination (HEC) upon the learning curve of LICK.

Results: The study was performed in a private center in Asunción, Paraguay, by 60 residents/specialists in gynaecology with no experience in laparoscopic surgery. Participants were allocated in three groups. In phase $_1$, a baseline test was performed (T_1, three repetitions). In phase 2, participants underwent different training programs for HEC (60 repetitions): G1 with both the dominant hand (DH) and the non-dominant hand (NDH), G2 with the DH only, G3 none. In phase 3, a post HEC/pre LICK training test was performed (T_2, three repetitions). In phase 4, participants underwent a standardized training program for LICK (60 repetitions). In phase 5, a final test was performed (T_3, three repetitions). The score was based on the time taken for task completion system. The scores were plotted and non-linear regression models were used to fit the learning curves to one- and two-phase exponential decay models for each participant (individual curves) and for each group (group curves). For both HEC and LICK, the group learning curves fitted better to the two-phase exponential decay model. For HEC with the DH, G1 and G2 started from a similar point, but G1 reached a lower plateau at a higher speed. In G1, the DH curve started from a lower point than the NDH curve, but both curves reached a similar plateau at comparable speeds. For LICK, all groups started from a similar point, but immediately after HEC training and before LICK training, G1 scored better than the others. All groups reached a similar plateau but with a different decay, G1 reaching this plateau faster than the others groups.

Conclusions: This study demonstrates that pre-training in HEC with both the DH and the NDH shortens the LICK learning curve.

Keywords: Laparoscopy, Training, Intra-corporeal knot tying, Hand-eye coordination, Learning curve

* Correspondence: roger.molinas@neolife.com.py
[1]Neolife – Medicina y Cirugia Reproductiva, Avenida Brasilia 760, 1434
Asuncion, Paraguay
Full list of author information is available at the end of the article

Background

Today it is generally accepted that the traditional apprentice-tutor model is no longer valid for training all skills necessary for laparoscopic surgery [1]. This agreement is based upon the recognition that, in contrast with open surgery, laparoscopic surgery demands surgical skills and psychomotor skills that not necessarily should be trained together. Indeed, increasing evidences strongly suggests that psychomotor skills must be trained earlier and outside the operating room, and several models have been proposed for this aim [2–7].

Among these validated training models is the Laparoscopic Skills Training and Testing (LASTT) model, developed by The European Academy of Gynaecological Surgery, suitable for training basic laparoscopic psychomotor skills, such as laparoscopic camera navigation (LCN), hand-eye coordination (HEC), and bimanual coordination (BMC) [1, 8–13].

Several studies in these models, including the LASTT model, have sufficiently proved that training improves laparoscopic skills [8–10, 14], which also applies specifically to training in box models as recently reported in a meta-analysis [15]. The majority of the studies base this conclusion upon measurements performed at two or very few points (before and after training). The effect of training however can be better appreciated if several points are taken into consideration, allowing tracking the improvement in performance over time, which is defined as a learning curve [16]. Although learning curves have been observed for many health technologies [17], only recently, they have become regularly used and reported for laparoscopic procedures [10, 18–23].

Following the first system (few measurements before and after training), we have demonstrated in a randomized controlled trial (RCT) performed in a population of residents and specialist in OB&GYN that HEC training with both the dominant hand (DH) and non-dominant hand (NDH) facilitates the acquisition [9] and retention [24] of more complex laparoscopic tasks, such as intra-corporeal knot tying (LICK). The present study was performed to evaluate in detail the learning curves of LICK after different pre-training conditions (no HEC training, HEC training with the DH only, and HEC training with both the DH and the NDH) from non-reported data of the same RCT mentioned above [9].

Methods

Participants and venue

The study was carried out in the Centro Médico La Costa in Asunción, Paraguay, and included 60 specialists/residents in OB&GYN with experience in open surgery but with no experience in laparoscopic surgery.

Instruments, materials, and laparoscopic tasks

The tasks were performed in the LASTT model inserted in the Szabo trainer box with standard laparoscopic instruments (Karl Storz, Tuttlingen, Germany).

Task 1 (hand-eye coordination)

The ability to grasp and transport six objects to six specific targets with both the DH and NDH, while navigating a camera was evaluated in a validated model, as described previously [9]. Briefly, with forceps held with the hand being evaluated and the camera with the contra-lateral hand, the six different objects were grasped and transported to their targets in a fixed order. The time for each repetition was limited to 600 s. The task finished either when the last object was transported to its target or when the time limit expired. The task executed with the DH (task 1a) was scored separately than the task executed with the NDH (task 1b).

Task 2 (laparoscopic intra-corporeal knot tying)

The ability to perform a LICK was evaluated in a validated model, as described previously [9]. A soft pad with two pre-mounted sutures (vicryl 2-0, 20 cm length), 1 cm between entry and exit sites, and tails equally distributed at both sites was fitted in the Szabo trainer box in a horizontal position. The optic was introduced through a midline port and the needle holders through lower and lateral ports. With a camera fixed at a distance that allowed the visualization of the entire operating field and the needle holders held with the DH and NDH, the tip of the thread was grasped and the thread was pulled through the pad, leaving a 2 cm tail on the opposite side. Then, a double counter-clockwise knot was made, followed by a single clockwise knot, and finally, by a single counter-clockwise knot. The time for each repetition was limited to 600 s. The task finished either when the participant considered he/she completed the knot or when the time limit had expired. Then, the tutor performed a quality control, and only the flat and square knots were considered correctly performed.

Scoring system

The measurements were based on the time taken for task completion system [6, 15, 21, 25]. Thus, if the task was successfully accomplished within the time limit, the score was the time actually used to execute the task, ranging from 1 to 600. However, if the task was not successfully accomplished within the time limit, a penalty score of 1200 was given.

Experimental design

The data presented in this study were collected but not reported at the time of an already published RCT [9]. Participants were randomly allocated to three different groups (G1, G2, and G3; $n = 20$ per group). Within each group, they worked in fixed pairs throughout the study. Working sessions of 1–2 h were performed 2–3 times a week in order to optimize the results, as reported by other authors [26]. A supervisor was present at the working station in all sessions to ascertain the set up was correctly ensemble and to score the tasks. The study was carried out in five phases.

Phase 1. All participants received full explanation and video demonstrations of the different tasks and then performed a test (T_1) (three repetitions of each task) to evaluate the baseline skills before any training.
Phase 2. Participants performed different training programs for HEC, according to the group they belong to. G1 trained both the DH and the NDH (60 repetitions of each task in alternating order). G2 trained the DH only (60 repetitions). G3 did not train HEC at all.
Phase 3. All participants performed a second test (T_2), in the same manner than at T_1, to evaluate the skills acquired after HEC training but before LICK training.
Phase 4. All participants performed a standard training program for LICK (60 repetitions).
Phase 5. All participants performed a third test (T_3), in the same manner than at T_1 and T_2, to evaluate the post-training skills.

Statistics and curve fitting

All statistical comparisons were performed using the GraphPad Prism 6 (GraphPad Software, San Diego, California, USA).

Intergroup differences in age were evaluated with one-way ANOVA, whereas differences in gender, DH side and training status with chi-square tests.

The scores registered at all points were plotted to produce the learning curves for each student (individual learning curves) and for each group (group learning curves). Nonlinear regression models were used to fit the data to the one- and two-phase exponential decay models.

The one-phase exponential decay model is expressed as $Y = (Y_0 - \text{Plateau}) * \exp(-K*X) + \text{Plateau}$. The two-phase exponential decay model is expressed as $Y = \text{Plateau} + \text{SpanFast} * \exp(-KFast*X) + \text{SpanSlow} * \exp(-KSlow*X)$, where $\text{SpanFast} = (Y_0 - \text{Plateau}) * \text{PercentFast} * .01$, and $\text{SpanSlow} = (Y_0 - \text{Plateau}) * (100 - \text{PercentFast}) * .01$. Y is a dependent variable (score), and X is an independent variable (number of the repetition). Y_0 is the Y value when X is zero (the starting point before any training). Plateau is the Y value at infinite times, expressed in the same units as Y (the theoretical best score that a subject could achieve with infinite practice). K, $KFast$, and $KSlow$ are rate constant, expressed in reciprocal of the X units

and which measures the steepness of the curve (higher values of K indicates faster learning). Span is the difference between Y_0 and Plateau, expressed in the same units as Y values. PercentFast is the percentage of the Span accounted for by the faster of the two components. For LICK, the Y_3, which represents the Y extrapolated value from X_3 (the first point of the curve immediately after HEC training/before LICK training), was also calculated.

The extra sum-of-squares F test was used to evaluate curve fitting (one phase vs. two phase) and if one single curve adequately fits for all groups. The curve parameters (continuous variable normally distributed) are presented as means ± SEM, and parametric test were used for statistical comparisons. For HEC, differences in the DH learning curves between G1 and G2 were evaluated with unpaired t test (two groups), whereas differences between DH and NDH in G1 were evaluated with paired t test (one group with two curves). For LICK, differences in the learning curves between G1, G2, and G3 were evaluated with one-way ANOVA with Tukey's Multiple Comparison post-test (three groups). A two-tailed p value of $<.05$ was considered statistically significant.

Results

The demographics were already reported at the time of the first publication of this RCT [9]. The median age of the participants was 29 years (range 26–45 years), and gender was evenly distributed (50% males, 50% females, $n = 30$ each). The number of specialists ($n = 20$, 40%) was less than the number of residents ($n = 40$, 60%). As expected, the number of right-handed participants ($n = 55$, 92%) was greater than left-handed participants ($n = 5$, 8%). The demographics of the three groups are reported in Table 1. No intergroup differences were detected for any of the parameters.

Table 1 Participants' demographics

	Groups		
	G1 ($n = 20$)	G2 ($n = 20$)	G3 ($n = 20$)
Age (median and range in years)	29 (26–45)	29 (26–37)	32 (27–45)
Gender (%)			
▪ Male	12 (60%)	9 (45%)	9 (45%)
▪ Female	8 (40%)	11 (55%)	11 (55%)
Training status (%)			
▪ Residents	13 (65%)	16 (80%)	11 (55%)
▪ Specialists	7 (35%)	4 (20%)	9 (45%)
Dominant hand side			
▪ Right	19 (95%)	17 (85%)	19 (95%)
▪ Left	1 (5%)	3 (15%)	1 (5%)

Reproduced with permission from Molinas et al. [9]

For both HEC and LICK, the scores registered by each group at T_1, T_2, and T_3 were already reported in a previous study [9]. For the aims of the present study, the scores registered by each participant at all 69 repetitions (R0–R68) were plotted to evaluate the individual and the group learning curves.

HEC learning curves

The learning curves for the DH were evaluated in G1 and G2, whereas the learning curves for the NDH were evaluated in G1 only.

Most individual learning curves fitted better the one-phase model, whereas few of them fitted better to two-phase model or were ambiguous (did not fit to any model) (Fig. 1).

The group learning curves (G1-DH, G1-NDH, G2-DH) fitted better to the two-phase exponential decay model ($p < .0001$ for all comparisons). However, one single type of curve did not adequately fits for G1-DH and G2-DH ($p < .0001$), neither for G1-DH and G1-NDH ($p < .0001$). For the DH, G1 and G2 started from a similar Y_0 (NS), but G1 reached a lower Plateau ($p = .04$), with a higher PercentFast ($p = .01$) and lower KFast ($p = .02$) and KSlow ($p = .01$). In G1, the DH curve started from a lower Y_0 ($p < .0001$) than the NDH curve, but both curves reached a similar Plateau with comparable PercentFast (NS), KFast (NS), and KSlow (NS) (Fig. 2 and Table 2).

LICK learning curves

Most individual learning curves fitted better the one-phase model, whereas few of them fitted better to two-phase model or were ambiguous (did not fit to any model) (Fig. 3).

The group learning curves fitted better to a two-phase exponential decay model ($p < .0001$ for all groups) (Fig. 4 and Table 3). However, one single type of curve did not adequately fit for all groups ($p < .0001$). All groups started from a similar Y_0 (NS) and reached a similar Plateau (NS), but the curve decays were different. Indeed, as soon as at Y_3, which represents the extrapolated value from X_3 (the first point of the curve immediately after HEC training/before LICK training), the curve values were already significantly different, G1 scoring lower than G2 ($p < .05$) and G3 ($p < .05$). The Percent-Fast of G1 was higher than of G2 ($p < .05$) and G3 ($p < .05$), but the differences in KFast and KSlow were not statistically different (Table 3 and Fig. 4).

Discussion

This study was performed for insight assessment of the data gathered in the frame of an already published RCT [9] in which changes in the performance of HEC and LICK at three different time points were evaluated.

Indeed, in that study, the baseline scores before HEC training (T_1), after HEC training/before LICK training (T_2), and after LICK training (T_3) were evaluated, disregarding the scores registered at each of the 69 points of the study. In this study, the entire dataset was evaluated in order to characterize the learning curves of both HEC and LICK and, more specifically, to determine if pre-training HEC has an influence in the LICK learning curve.

For each task, the real scores of each individual participant were plotted, and obvious individual and group learning curves were observed, which were fitted to the one- and two-phase exponential decay models. An exponential decay equation models many chemical and biological processes. The one-phase model is used whenever the rate at which something happens is proportional to the amount that is left. The two-phase model is used when the outcome measured is the result of the sum of a fast and slow exponential decay, which is also called a double exponential decay. From these curves, the Y_0 (the starting point before any training), the Plateau (the theoretical best score that a subject could achieve with infinite practice), and the Span (the difference between Y_0 and the Plateau) were calculated. From the curves fitted to the one-phase exponential decay model the learning constant (K) was also calculated. From the curves fitted to the two-phase exponential decay model the learning constants (KFast and KSlow) and the PercentFast (the proportion of the Span accounting for the faster component of the decay) were also calculated.

The individual curves denoted a lot of variability between surgeons, specifically at the beginning of the curves, reflecting the natural heterogeneity in the population (Figs. 1 and 3). The variability, however, decreased significantly at the end of the curves, indicating the positive influence of training regardless the personal characteristics. For both HEC and LICK, some individual curves fitted better to the one-phase exponential decay model, whereas others fitted better to the two-phase exponential decay model regardless the training program.

The learning curves of HEC were characterized for the use of the DH in G1 and G2 and of the NDH in G1. All group curves fitted better to the two-phase exponential decay model. Differences between the DH and the NDH learning curves were evaluated in G1. Although no statistical significant differences were detected in the Plateau, the PercentFast and the learning constants, the NDH curve started from a higher Y_0. This is consistent with our previous report comparing the scores at three specific points, in which the DH scores were better (lower) than the NDH scores before any training (T_1), after HEC training/before LICK training (T_2), and after LICK training (T_3) [9]. We, therefore, hypothesized that

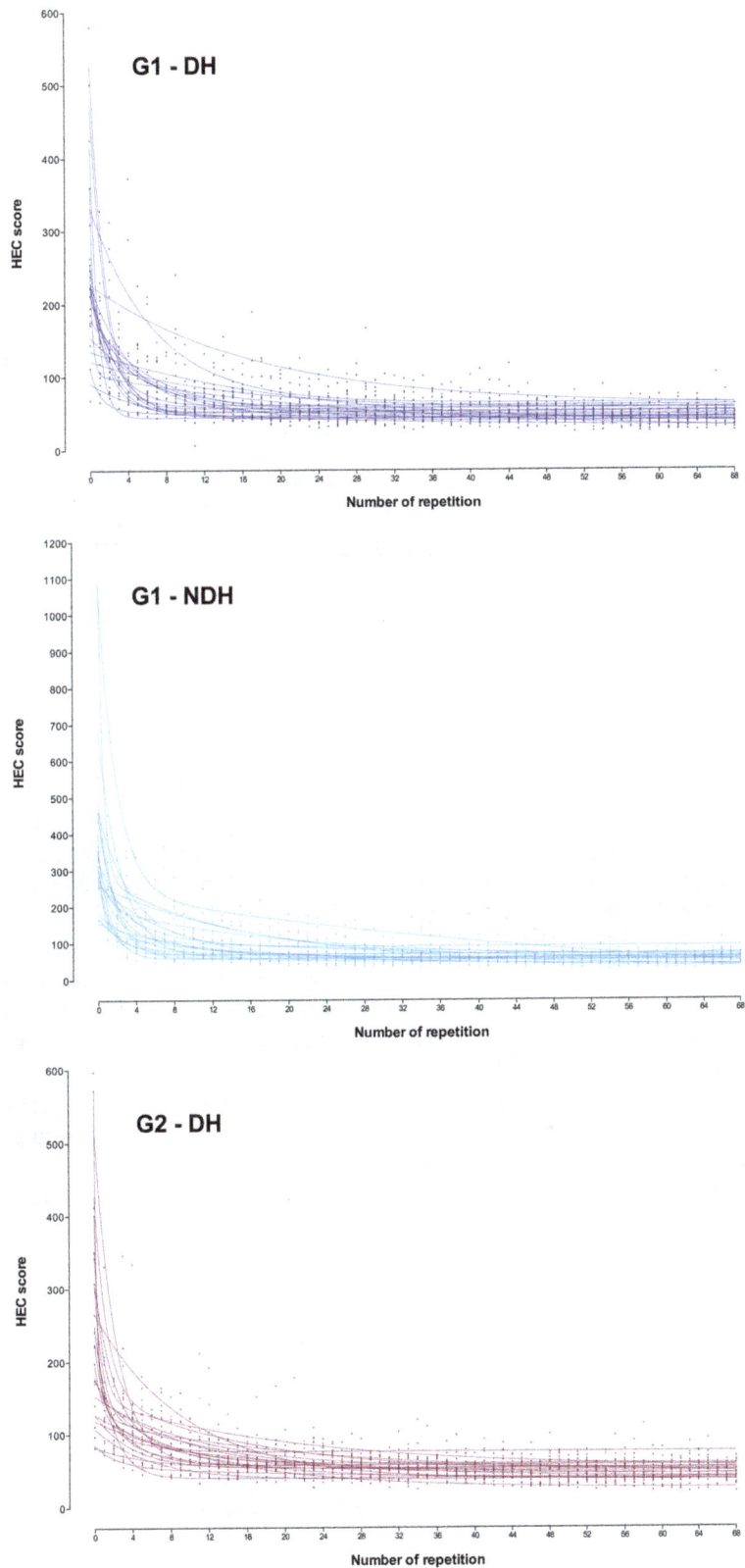

Fig. 1 Hand-eye coordination (HEC). Individual learning curves. Participants performed 69 consecutive repetitions (R0–R68) of the task (G1, with both the dominant hand and the non-dominant hand; G2, with the dominant hand only; G3, none). The scores were plotted and individual learning curves were observed, fitting to one- or two-phase exponential decay model according to participants' performance

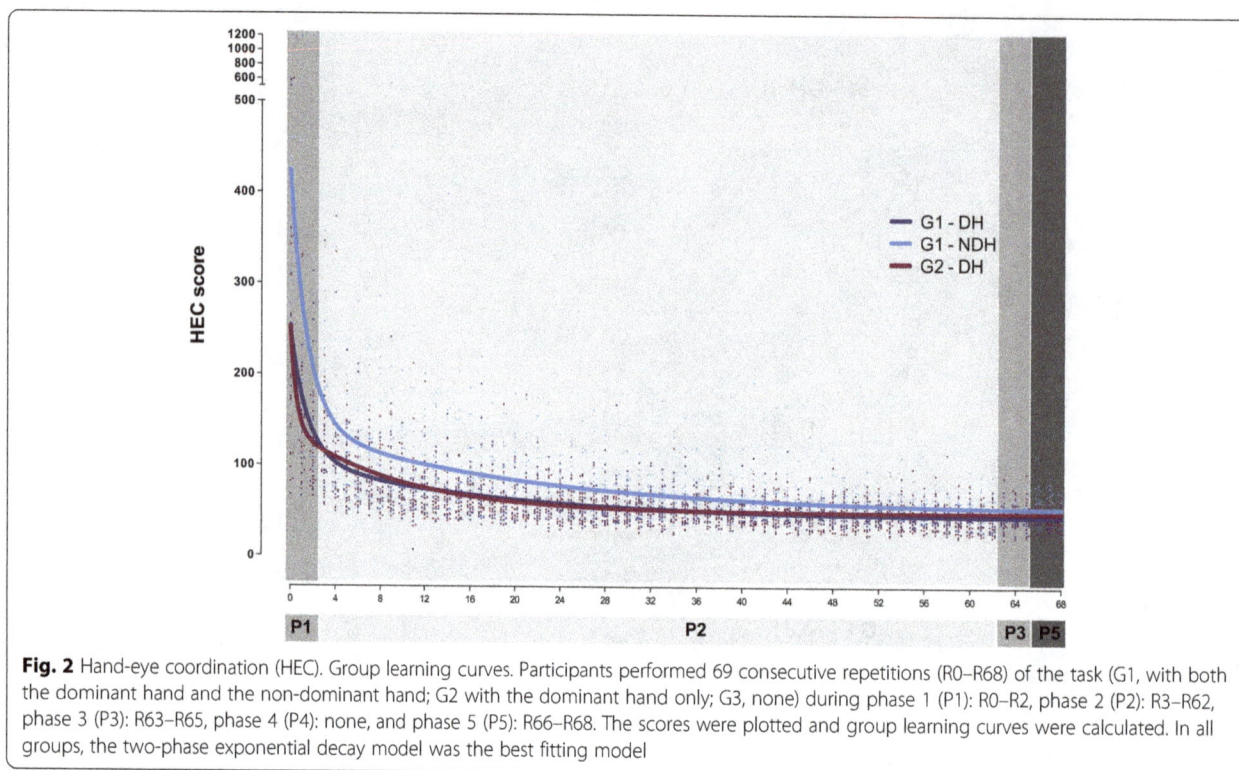

Fig. 2 Hand-eye coordination (HEC). Group learning curves. Participants performed 69 consecutive repetitions (R0–R68) of the task (G1, with both the dominant hand and the non-dominant hand; G2 with the dominant hand only; G3, none) during phase 1 (P1): R0–R2, phase 2 (P2): R3–R62, phase 3 (P3): R63–R65, phase 4 (P4): none, and phase 5 (P5): R66–R68. The scores were plotted and group learning curves were calculated. In all groups, the two-phase exponential decay model was the best fitting model

the DH curve would decay faster than the NDH curve. Surprisingly, however, the difference detected in this study was observed at the beginning of the curve and not at the Plateau, as would be expected, indicating that appropriate training counteracts the initial differences and that the NDH can achieve skills comparable than the DH. Differences in the DH learning curves of G1 and G2 were also evaluated. Although both curves started from a comparable Y_0, G1 reached a lower Plateau, with a higher PercentFast and lower KFast and KSlow. These better results in G1 can be explained by the fact that the training of the DH and the NDH were performed in alternate and not consecutive order, which could possibly influence positively the learning curve of

the DH. Moreover, this can also be explained by some experimental evidences saying that early in training when information about the movement was still spatially encoded and motor programs had not yet been formed, monkeys were able to transfer motor tasks learned with one limb to the opposite limb [27].

The learning curve of LICK was characterized in the control group with no previous training (G3), but because the most important aim of this study was to evaluate the effect of different pre-training conditions, the learning curve was also evaluated in the group that trained HEC with both DH and NDH (G1) and in the group that trained HEC with the DH only (G2). The curves of the three groups fitted better to the two-phase exponential decay model. As expected, all groups had comparable starting points (Y_0). All of them improved their scores at Y_3, which represents the calculated Y value at X_3 and which was included to evaluate specifically the impact of the previous HEC training. This improvement was observed in G3, but it was more pronounced in G2 and even more important in G1. In spite of these differences at the beginning of the curve, all groups reached a similar Plateau but again G1 depicted a faster decay, as demonstrated by its significantly higher PercentFast. Since G3 did not train HEC at all, the influence of repetition only cannot be neglected. Since G2 trained HEC with the DH only, the effect of this training is evident. However, the curve characteristics in G1 indicate the relevance of training HEC with both the DH

Table 2 Hand-eye coordination (HEC). Parameters of the learning curves

Parameter	Groups		
	G1 - DH	G1 - NDH	G2 - DH
Y_0	250 ± 6*	424 ± 13	253 ± 6
Plateau	44 ± 2#	51 ± 6	49 ± 1
PercentFast	70 ± 3#	76 ± 3	56 ± 4
KFast	0.67 ± 0.09#	0.67 ± 0.09	1.96 ± 0.52
KSlow	0.06 ± 0.01#	0.05 ± 0.01	0.10 ± 0.01

Mean ± SEM are presented
G1 trained both the DH and the NDH; G2 trained the DH only; G3 did not train HEC
*$p < .05$; G1 - DH vs. G1 - NDH
#$p < .05$; G1 - DH vs. G2 - DH

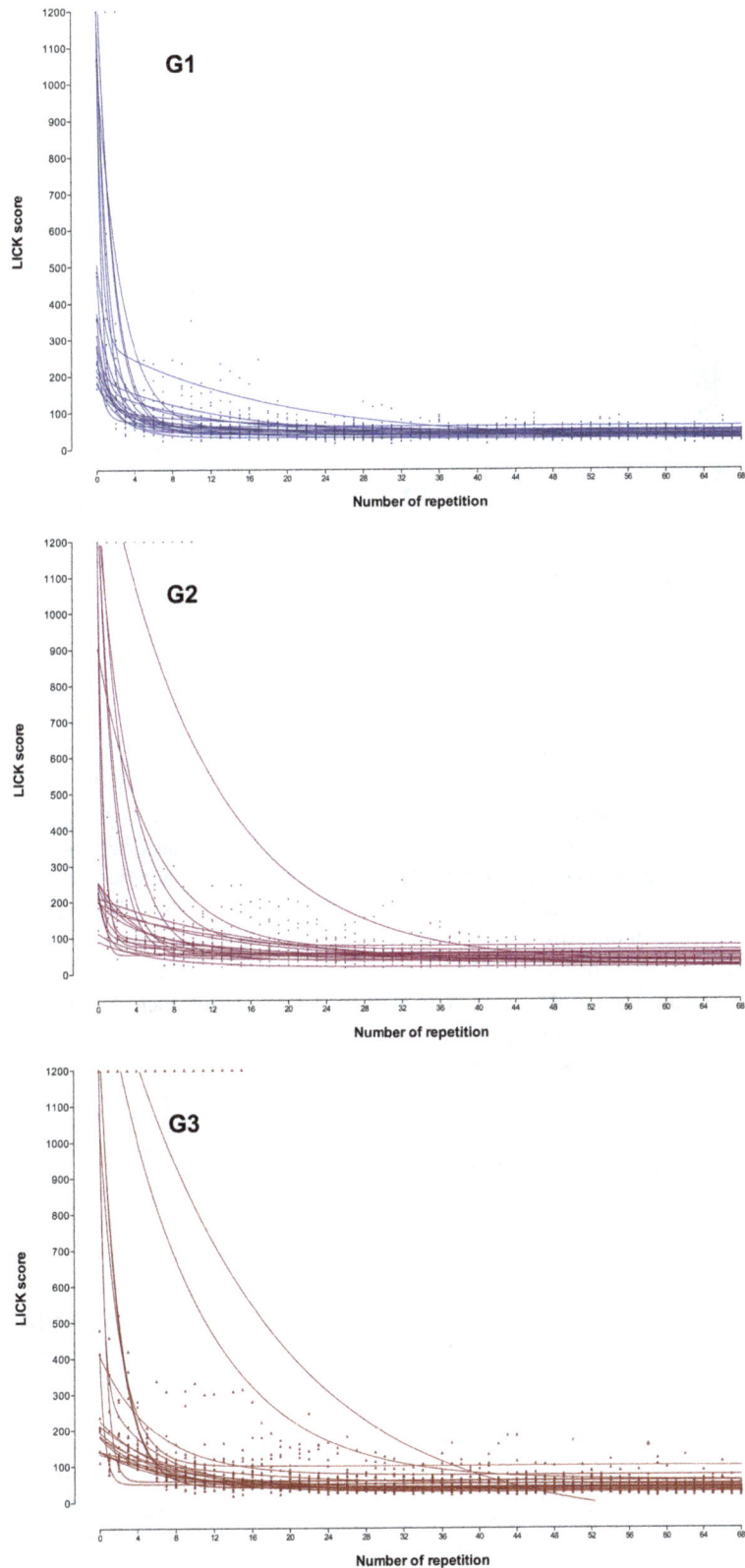

Fig. 3 Laparoscopic intra-corporeal knot tying (LICK). Individual learning curves. Participants of G1, G2, and G3 performed 69 consecutive repetitions (R0–R68) of the task. The scores were plotted and individual learning curves were observed, fitting to one- or two-phase exponential decay model according to participants' performance

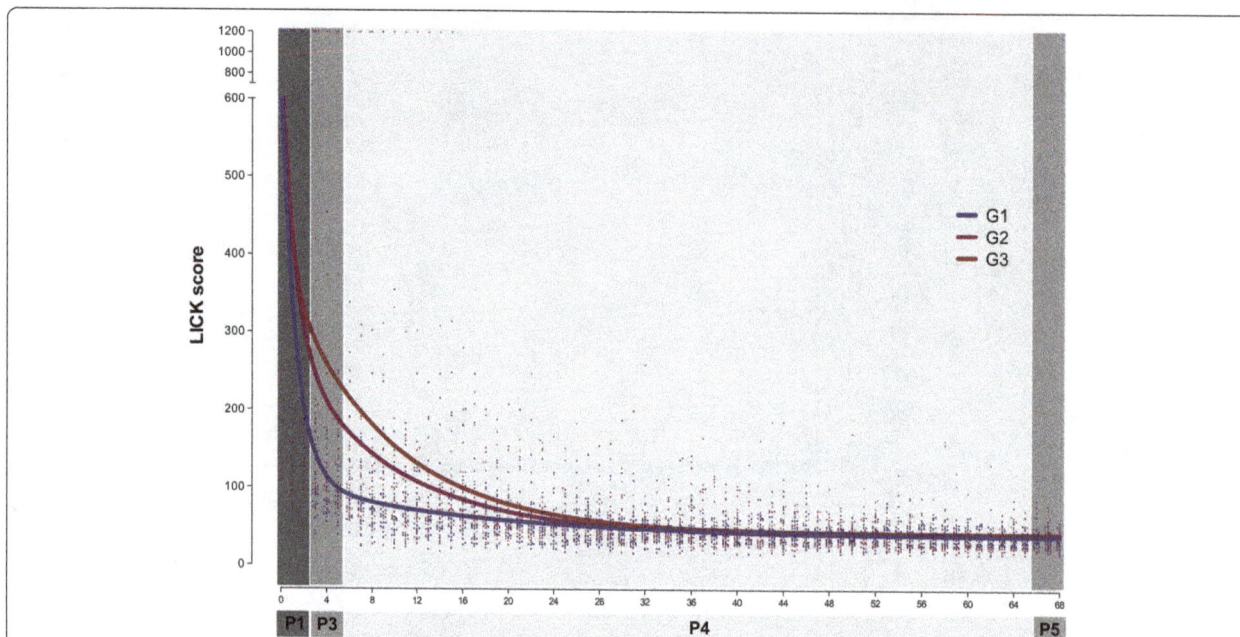

Fig. 4 Group laparoscopic intra-corporeal knot tying (LICK) learning curves. Participants of G1, G2, and G3 performed 69 consecutive repetitions (R0–R68) of the task during phase 1 (P1): R0–R2, phase 2 (P2): none, phase 3 (P3): R3–R62, phase 4 (P4): R63–R 65, and phase 5 (P5): R66–R68. The scores were plotted, and group learning curves were calculated. In all groups, the two-phase exponential decay model was the best fitting model

and the NDH in order not only to start the LICK training from a better point but also to achieve proficiency sooner. It is also important to consider an alternative hypothesis: the shorter learning curve observed in G1 was due to the different training volume (G1 performed 120 repetitions in total) and not necessarily due to the training of both hands. In order to define the cause of the positive effect, we would need another group training the DH only for 120 repetitions, but unfortunately, we did not consider such group in the study design.

Our data about HEC learning curves are consistent with previous studies about laparoscopic psychomotor skills in general. Indeed, we have described learning curves after 30 repetitions of HEC with the DH using the same model but with a different scoring system (i.e.,

Table 3 Laparoscopic intra-corporeal knot tying (LICK). Parameters of the learning curves

Score	Groups		
	G1	G2	G3
Y_0	615 ± 17	655 ± 29	622 ± 35
Y_3	143 ± 7*	246 ± 13	288 ± 17
Plateau	38 ± 5	39 ± 6	42 ± 6
PercentFast	88 ± 3*	62 ± 9	42 ± 9
KFast	0.79 ± 0.08	0.81 ± 0.22	1.26 ± 0.67
KSlow	0.06 ± 0.03	0.10 ± 0.03	0.11 ± 0.02

Mean ± SEM are presented
G1, G2, and G3 performed the same standard training program for LICK
*$p < .05$; G1 vs. G2 and G1 vs. G3

number of objects transported in 2 min) in 14 novices and 10 experts [10]. In that study, we reported that experts performed better than novices from the beginning till the end and that after some 20 repetitions, the scores remained similar, but the different parameters of a learning curve were not calculated. Brunner et al. have also described learning curves for 12 basic tasks using a virtual reality model in 12 medical students who performed 30 repetitions of each task in order to define how many repetitions would be necessary to reach the plateau. They reported their data fitted better to a spline model and that a lengthy learning curve existed for novices, which may be seen throughout 30 repetitions and possibly beyond [18].

Our data about LICK learning curves are also consistent with previous studies. Vossen et al. have reported in 29 trainee learning curves with one- or two-phase exponential decay model, the latter fitting their experimental points only marginally better [20]. Zhou et al. [28] and Thiyagarajan et al. [29] have also reported in 20 trainee learning curves with an exponential decay shape. Consistent with our results, the duration of the first knot varied with the previous laparoscopic experience being lower in more experienced trainees [20].

There are few studies evaluating the effect of previous HEC training upon LICK. Consistent with our study, Stefanidis et al. [30] demonstrated in 20 novices that training basic laparoscopic skills (bean drop, running string, block move, checkerboard, and endostitch), all of them representing different tasks for HEC, shortened the learning curve of a more complex laparoscopic task-like suturing. After completing basic skills training, this group achieved proficiency in laparoscopic suturing and knot tying considerably faster and after fewer repetitions (21 ± 8 repetitions) compared with the group with no previous training (50 ± 16 repetitions). They have also claimed the additional benefit of substantial cost savings because the trained group required significantly less active instruction and less overall costs of the suture material. In spite that learning curves were not reported, Fried et al. have also demonstrated in 215 surgeons that training a basic task (i.e., pegboard transfer), which is also a task for HEC, improves significantly the performance of LICK [31].

Although in this study, we did not evaluate effect of surgeon characteristics (age, gender, training status, and DH side) upon the results of the learning curves, in our previous study, we failed to demonstrate any influence of those factors upon the changes in scoring between T_1 and T_2, T_2 and T_3, and T_1 and T_3 [9], which is consistent with other studies showing that the learning curves are not substantially affected by previous exposure to surgery, either by assisting or by watching laparoscopic interventions, nor by personal characteristics, such as leisure activities, eye dysfunction, eye correction, dominant hand, personality, and gender [20, 22, 31]. For gender, however, Thorson et al. have claimed that among medical students, women had a worse performance than men [32], which might be explained by their smaller sample size than in our study ($n = 32$ vs. 60 participants).

It can be argued that one limitation of our study was the scoring system, which was based upon the widely used time taken for task completion system [6, 15, 21, 25]. We have to admit that time alone is not necessarily an accurate assessment of surgical skills and that accuracy and precision should be incorporated into the scoring system. In our system, however, these factors were implicitly incorporated because only objectives correctly achieved were scored. In relation to the basic tasks, this was obvious for both participant and tutor. In relation to LICK, however, knot's quality could be debatable and differences in participant and tutor validation should be considered. For the aim of this study, only tutor evaluation was considered valid. Unfortunately, we did not correlate both measurements to determine whether students' assessments improve over time.

On the other hand, we believe that the strength of this study is the measurement of each individual point during the entire training process, which have allowed us to evaluate the learning curves of both basic and advanced laparoscopic tasks. The characteristics of skills acquisition, reported in this study, and of skills retention, reported earlier [24] is consistent with other motor skills acquisition and retention characteristics. Indeed, compelling behavioral and neuro-imaging data suggest that the retention and perfection of skills reflects long-lasting experience-driven changes in the brain's organization (neural plasticity) [33]. Moreover, extensive motor skill training induces reorganization of movement representations and synaptogenesis within adult motor cortex [34]. Behavioral, functional imaging, electrophysiological, and cellular/molecular studies provide evidence that motor skill learning is a staged process [35]. From the neurological point of view, different mechanisms appear to be active at different times. During training, there is sequential demand for different circuitry. The acquisition phase is characterized by fast (within session) and slow learning (between sessions). Consolidation (i.e., stabilization of novel motor memory) occurs both during and after training. Task complexity may be an important determinant of how "staged" or segregated the process is. Complex motor tasks require several training sessions interspersed with periods of rest and sleep. For these tasks, acquisition and consolidation processes are interlocked, forming a complex sequence of events.

Conclusions

In conclusion, our study confirms that training improves both basic and advanced laparoscopic skills and demonstrates that the improvement (the decay of the curve) is different according to the individual characteristics, the task complexity, and the training program. This indicates that pre-training of HEC facilitates the acquisition of LICK skills and, moreover, that pre-training of HEC with both the DH and the NDH shortens the LICK learning curve. It remains to be elucidated the potential effect of continues tutoring during training, as suggested by some authors [36], and, moreover, the impact of all these factors upon real surgery in humans.

Acknowledgements
We would like to thank Alicia Amarilla and Rossana Paredes for their support in collecting the data, Centro Médico La Costa (Asunción, Paraguay) for offering its facilities for the study to be performed, Karl Storz (Tutlingen, Germany) for providing the instruments and materials, and specially to all gynaecologists who actively participated in the study. We thank Professors A. Karni, Y. Dubai, and N. Ofen for their comments and the suggested literature about motor skill acquisition and learning.

Funding
This study did not receive any funding and was funded by the authors' own resources.

Authors' contributions
CRM initiated the protocol/project development, data collection and management, data analysis, and manuscript writing/editing. MMB contributed to data analysis and manuscript writing/editing. RC developed the protocol/project development. All authors read and approved the final manuscript.

Competing interests

The authors declare that they have no competing interests.

Author details

[1]Neolife – Medicina y Cirugia Reproductiva, Avenida Brasilia 760, 1434 Asuncion, Paraguay. [2]European Academy of Gynaecological Surgery, Leuven, Belgium.

References

1. Campo R, Wattiez A, Tanos V, Di Spiezio SA, Grimbizis G, Wallwiener D, Brucker S, Puga M, Molinas R, O'Donovan P, Deprest J, Van BY, Lissens A, Herrmann A, Tahir M, Benedetto C, Siebert I, Rabischong B, De Wilde RL (2016) Gynaecological endoscopic surgical education and assessment. A diploma programme in gynaecological endoscopic surgery. Eur J Obstet Gynecol Reprod Biol 199:183–186

2. Diesen DL, Erhunmwunsee L, Bennett KM, Ben-David K, Yurcisin B, Ceppa EP, Omotosho PA, Perez A, Pryor A (2011) Effectiveness of laparoscopic computer simulator versus usage of box trainer for endoscopic surgery training of novices. J Surg Educ 68:282–289

3. Escamirosa FP, Flores RM, Garcia IO, Vidal CR, Martinez AM (2015) Face, content, and construct validity of the EndoViS training system for objective assessment of psychomotor skills of laparoscopic surgeons. Surg Endosc 29: 3392–3403

4. Hofstad EF, Vapenstad C, Chmarra MK, Lango T, Kuhry E, Marvik R (2013) A study of psychomotor skills in minimally invasive surgery: what differentiates expert and nonexpert performance. Surg Endosc 27:854–863

5. Munro MG (2012) Surgical simulation: where have we come from? Where are we now? Where are we going? J Minim Invasive Gynecol 19:272–283

6. Mulla M, Sharma D, Moghul M, Kailani O, Dockery J, Ayis S, Grange P (2012) Learning basic laparoscopic skills: a randomized controlled study comparing box trainer, virtual reality simulator, and mental training. J Surg Educ 69:190–195

7. Sroka G, Feldman LS, Vassiliou MC, Kaneva PA, Fayez R, Fried GM (2010) Fundamentals of laparoscopic surgery simulator training to proficiency improves laparoscopic performance in the operating room—a randomized controlled trial. Am J Surg 199:115–120

8. Campo R, Reising C, Van Belle Y, Nassif J, O'Donovan P, Molinas CR (2010) A valid model for testing and training laparoscopic psychomotor skills. Gynecol Surg 7:133–141

9. Molinas CR, Campo R (2010) Defining a structured training program for acquiring basic and advanced laparoscopic psychomotor skills in a simulator. Gynecol Surg 7:427–435

10. Molinas CR, De Win G, Ritter O, Keckstein J, Miserez M, Campo R (2008) Feasibility and construct validity of a novel laparoscopic skills testing and training model. Gynecol Surg 5:281–290

11. Campo R, Wattiez A, Tanos V, Di Spiezio SA, Grimbizis G, Wallwiener D, Brucker S, Puga M, Molinas CR, O'Donovan P, Deprest J, Van Belle Y, Lissens A, Herrmann A, Tahir M, Benedetto C, Siebert I, Rabischong B, De Wide RL (2016) Gynaecological endoscopic surgical education and assessment. A diploma programme in gynaecological endoscopic surgery. Gynecol Surg 13:133–137

12. Campo R, Molinas CR, De Wilde RL, Brolmann H, Brucker S, Mencaglia L, Odonovan P, Wallwiener D, Wattiez A (2012) Are you good enough for your patients? The European certification model in laparoscopic surgery. Facts Views Vis Obgyn 4:95–101

13. Campo R, Wattiez A, De Wilde RL, Molinas CR (2012) Training in laparoscopic surgery: from the lab to the OR. Zdrav Var 51:285–298

14. Torricelli FC, Barbosa JA, Marchini GS (2016) Impact of laparoscopic surgery training laboratory on surgeon's performance. World J Gastrointest Surg 8: 735–743

15. Nagendran M, Toon CD, Davidson BR, Gurusamy KS (2014) Laparoscopic surgical box model training for surgical trainees with no prior laparoscopic experience. Cochrane Database Syst Rev:CD010479

16. Cook JA, Ramsay CR, Fayers P (2007) Using the literature to quantify the learning curve: a case study. Int. J. Technol. Assess. Health Care, 23, 255–260

17. Ramsay CR, Grant AM, Wallace SA, Garthwaite PH, Monk AF, Russell IT (2001) Statistical assessment of the learning curves of health technologies. Health Technol Assess 5:1–79

18. Brunner WC, Korndorffer JR Jr, Sierra R, Massarweh NN, Dunne JB, Yau CL, Scott DJ (2004) Laparoscopic virtual reality training: are 30 repetitions enough? J Surg Res 122:150–156

19. Molinas CR, Binda MM, Mailova K, Koninckx PR (2004) The rabbit nephrectomy model for training in laparoscopic surgery. Hum Reprod 19: 185–190

20. Vossen C, Van Ballaer P, Shaw RW, Koninckx PR (1997) Effect of training on endoscopic intracorporeal knot tying. Hum Reprod 12:2658–2663

21. Rodriguez-Sanjuan JC, Manuel-Palazuelos C, Fernandez-Diez MJ, Gutierrez-Cabezas JM, Alonso-Martin J, Redondo-Figuero C, Herrera-Norena LA, Gomez-Fleitas M (2010) Assessment of resident training in laparoscopic surgery based on a digestive system anastomosis model in the laboratory. Cir Esp 87:20–25

22. Kolozsvari NO, Andalib A, Kaneva P, Cao J, Vassiliou MC, Fried GM, Feldman LS (2011) Sex is not everything: the role of gender in early performance of a fundamental laparoscopic skill. Surg Endosc 25:1037–1042

23. De Win G, Van Bruwaene S, Kulkarni J, Van Calster B, Aggarwal R, Allen C, Lissens A, De Ridder D, Miserez M (2016) An evidence-based laparoscopic simulation curriculum shortens the clinical learning curve and reduces surgical adverse events. Adv Med Educ Pract 7:357–370

24. Molinas CR, Campo R (2016) Retention of laparoscopic psychomotor skills after a structured training program depends on the quality of the training and on the complexity of the task. Gynecol Surg 13:962–964

25. Fransen SA, Mertens LS, Botden SM, Stassen LP, Bouvy ND (2012) Performance curve of basic skills in single-incision laparoscopy versus conventional laparoscopy: is it really more difficult for the novice? Surg Endosc 26:1231–1237

26. De Win G, Van Bruwaene S, De Ridder D, Miserez M (2013) The optimal frequency of endoscopic skill labs for training and skill retention on suturing: a randomized controlled trial. J Surg Educ 70:384–393

27. Hikosaka O, Nakahara H, Rand MK, Sakai K, Lu X, Nakamura K, Miyachi S, Doya K (1999) Parallel neural networks for learning sequential procedures. Trends Neurosci 22:464–471

28. Zhou M, Tse S, Derevianko A, Jones DB, Schwaitzberg SD, Cao CG (2012) Effect of haptic feedback in laparoscopic surgery skill acquisition. Surg Endosc 26:1128–1134

29. Thiyagarajan M, Ravindrakumar C (2016) A comparative study in learning curves of two different intracorporeal knot tying techniques. Minim Invasive Surg 2016:3059434

30. Stefanidis D, Hope WW, Korndorffer JR Jr, Markley S, Scott DJ (2010) Initial laparoscopic basic skills training shortens the learning curve of laparoscopic suturing and is cost-effective. J Am Coll Surg 210:436–440

31. Fried GM, Feldman LS, Vassiliou MC, Fraser SA, Stanbridge D, Ghitulescu G, Andrew CG (2004) Proving the value of simulation in laparoscopic surgery. Ann Surg 240:518–525

32. Thorson CM, Kelly JP, Forse RA, Turaga KK (2011) Can we continue to ignore gender differences in performance on simulation trainers? J Laparoendosc Adv Surg Tech A 21:329–333

33. Karni A & Korman M (2011) When and where in skill memory consolidation: neuro-behavioral constraints on the acquisition and generation of procedural knowledge. EDP Sciences. BIO Web of Conferences.

34. Kleim JA, Hogg TM, VandenBerg PM, Cooper NR, Bruneau R, Remple M (2004) Cortical synaptogenesis and motor map reorganization occur during late, but not early, phase of motor skill learning. J Neurosci 24:628–633

35. Luft AR, Buitrago MM (2005) Stages of motor skill learning. Mol Neurobiol 32:205–216

36. Van Bruwaene S, De Win G, Miserez M (2009) How much do we need experts during laparoscopic suturing training? Surg Endosc 23:2755–2761

Pregnancy following laparoscopic hysteropexy

Helen Jefferis* ⓘ, Natalia Price and Simon Jackson

Abstract

Background: Uterine-preserving prolapse surgery offers the chance to retain fertility; however, limited data is available for the safety of pregnancy following surgery and the effect of pregnancy on surgical outcome. Our operative technique involves mesh encircling the cervix and uterine arteries, which raises concerns that compromise of uterine blood flow during pregnancy may lead to foetal growth restriction. We also think this necessitates delivery by caesarean section. We report on six pregnancy outcomes following laparoscopic hysteropexy. Primary outcomes were live birth and birth weight. Secondary outcomes were integrity of mesh and immediate effect on prolapse.

Results: All patients had successful pregnancy outcomes with birth weights on or above the 10th centile. There was no effect on mesh integrity seen in any of the cases. There was no deterioration in apical prolapse when assessed post delivery, but two patients had new onset anterior vaginal wall prolapse.

Conclusions: We think our technique of hysteropexy is safe for those wishing to conceive. Larger numbers are needed to allow robust evidence-based guidance for patients and clinicians.

Keywords: Hysteropexy, Pregnancy, Fertility-preserving prolapse surgery

Background

Laparoscopic hysteropexy offers uterine preservation to patients with uterovaginal prolapse. It is the treatment of choice for patients wishing to retain fertility; however, limited data are available for pregnancy outcome following this surgery. Standard practice is to advise women to complete their family prior to any pelvic floor surgery, but in some cases, this may not be possible due to significant adverse effect on function and quality of life. In these cases, we need to be able to counsel women appropriately as to pregnancy outcome and whether further pregnancy is associated with recurrence of prolapse.

The technique previously reported from Oxford [1] entails complete cervical encirclage with polypropylene; a video describing this technique has been published [2]. A three or four port laparoscopic approach is used. The sacral promontory is dissected until a safe area of periosteum is identified. The peritoneum is then opened from this incision down to the right uterosacral ligament, keeping medial to the ureter. A flap of peritoneum is created at the level of the cervix to enable reperitonisation. The utero-vesical fold is opened and bilateral avascular windows were made in the broad ligament, lateral to the uterine arteries. Type 1 polypropylene mesh (ProleneTM mesh, Ethicon, Somerville, NJ, USA) is cut to a bifurcated shape; the arms are brought through the windows in the broad ligament, wrapped around the cervix and sutured to the cervix anteriorly. The mesh is completely reperitonised and transfixed to the sacral promontory using helical fasteners (ProtackTM, United States Surgical, Tyco Healthcare, Norwalk, CT, USA).The encirclage technique theoretically minimises the risk of mesh avulsing from the cervix, indeed we have not had a case of cervical avulsion in the 10 years we have been performing this surgery in Oxford (data not published). Complete encirclage as described above does, however, pose unique challenges in terms of future pregnancy. The mesh is placed lateral to the uterine arteries bilaterally. Compression of these could theoretically

* Correspondence: helenjefferis@doctors.org.uk
Department of Gynaecology, The Women's Centre 8 John Radcliffe Hospital, Oxford University Hospitals NHS Trust 9, Headley Way, Oxford OX3 9DU 10, UK

compromise blood flow to the utero-placental unit resulting in placental compromise and intrauterine growth restriction. It is also not known whether the mesh may inhibit or restrict formation of the lower uterine segment. In addition, the mesh encircles the cervix at the level of the internal os, preventing cervical dilatation and necessitating delivery by caesarean section. The impact of pregnancy on the mesh is also unknown—one concern would be the risk of a gravid uterus causing the mesh to avulse from the sacral promontory with subsequent recurrence of prolapse.

One case report has been published from our unit describing successful pregnancy outcome following this technique of laparoscopic hysteropexy [3]. Including this case, we now describe a series of six pregnancy outcomes, the largest data series in the literature to date. The primary outcome measures were live birth and birth weight. Secondary outcome measures were integrity of mesh and effect on prolapse.

Methods

Six patients have presented to our department following laparoscopic hysteropexy with spontaneous conceptions. These cases were discussed at a multidisciplinary meeting between the obstetric and urogynaecology teams to plan antenatal care and delivery. Patients underwent uterine artery Doppler assessment at 22–23 weeks to evaluate whether blood flow had been compromised. Growth scans with umbilical artery assessment were performed at 28, 32 and 36 weeks gestation. All patients were delivered by caesarean section with a member of the urogynaecology team present to assess for mesh avulsion from the promontory. Patients were then seen at 8 weeks post delivery by a member of the urogynaecology team and were asked to subjectively describe any vaginal symptoms. They were examined and the POP-Q system was used to objectively assess prolapse.

One patient was not seen antenatally as she was not referred for consultant led care and was delivered as an emergency. She also did not attend her postnatal review. Ethics approval was not sought for this article as it is a retrospective case report.

Results

All six cases resulted in live births with birth weight on or above the 10th centile (range 10–70th). The mesh remained attached to the sacral promontory in all cases. Follow-up took place at a median of 9 weeks post delivery (range 8–10 weeks). Two patients felt their prolapse was subjectively worse post delivery and objectively had developed new anterior compartment prolapse. No patient had any deterioration in apical support.

The six cases are described in detail below. Table 1 summarises pregnancy outcome data.

Patient 1

In a 41-year-old para 3, laparoscopic hysteropexy was performed due to uterovaginal prolapse (Ba −1 cm, Point C −1 cm pre-operatively, Ba −3 cm, Point C −6 cm post operatively). She had thought her family was complete; however, she conceived spontaneously 7 months post-surgery and decided to continue with the pregnancy. Pregnancy care was undertaken as described above. Her uterine artery Doppler at 23 weeks showed significant right angulation of both arteries at the level of the internal os, presumably due the mesh; however, pulsatility index (PI) and resistance index (RI) of the uterine arteries was normal. Serial growth scans showed a normally grown foetus but a persistently low lying posterior placenta. For this reason, delivery was brought forward to 38 weeks. At caesarean section, the lower segment was well formed. The mesh was seen under the peritoneum and below the lower segment, well away from the lower segment incision.

Exploration of the abdomen at section confirmed the mesh remained securely attached to the sacral promontory. Her baby boy was of normal birth weight at 3290 g (50th centile).

At postnatal review, she felt that her prolapse symptoms were a little worse than before. On examination, the cervix remained well supported (C −6) as did the posterior wall (Bp −3), but there was anterior wall prolapse (Ba 0) and she has subsequently gone on to have an anterior repair with good anatomical result.

Patient 2

A 42-year-old para 2 had a laparoscopic hysteropexy with posterior repair (Point C at 0 pre-operatively and −7 cm post operatively). She had a planned pregnancy with conception 1 year post surgery. Pregnancy care was as outlined above. Uterine artery Doppler and serial growth scans were normal. Caesarean section at 39 + 2 was uncomplicated, with a well-formed lower segment and no evidence of avulsion of the mesh. A baby girl was delivered with birth weight of 3520 g (70th centile). At postnatal review, she remained asymptomatic of prolapse, with the cervix remaining supported (C-7 cm).

Patient 3

A 42-year-old para 2 had required IVF to conceive previously due to unexplained infertility. Following her second delivery, she underwent laparoscopic hysteropexy (pre-operatively point C + 1 cm, post-operatively −7 cm). Within 4 months of surgery, she spontaneously conceived (no contraception was being used due to the prior history of infertility and pregnancy was a surprise).

Uterine artery Doppler and growth scans were normal. Caesarean section was carried out at 39 + 1, with a well-formed lower segment and no evidence of mesh avulsion. A girl was delivered weighing 3160 g (40th centile). At

Table 1 Summary of pregnancy and outcome

	Patient 1	Patient 2	Patient 3	Patient 4	Patient 5	Patient 6
Age	41	42	42	28	39	27
BMI	30.1	18.7	25.6	23.0	17.8	24.9
Parity	3	2	2	2	2	3
Interval between surgery and delivery (months)	14	21	13	33	31	10
Antenatal care	Angulated right uterine artery, nil else	No concerns	No concerns	Back pain	No concerns	Midwifery led care
Delivery	Placenta praevia	Uncomplicated	Uncomplicated	Uncomplicated	Mesh over lower segment	Uncomplicated
Birth weight (grams)	3290	3520	3160	3335	3520	2795
Postnatal—prolapse worse?	Yes (cystocoele)	No	No	Yes (cystocoele)	No	DNA review

postnatal review, no prolapse symptoms were reported and point C was at −6 cm.

Patient 4

A 28-year-old para 2 had a laparoscopic hysteropexy for symptomatic prolapse (pre-operatively point C at 0, post-operatively at −7 cm, Ba −3 cm). Two years later, she conceived spontaneously and decided to continue with pregnancy. Antenatal care was as outlined previously, with normal uterine artery Doppler and serial growth scans. She did experience lower back pain from 16 weeks and attended hospital on two occasions with this but was managed with analgesia and physiotherapy. Caesarean section at 39 weeks was uncomplicated, the lower segment was well formed and the mesh remained attached to the sacral promontory. A girl was delivered weighing 3335 g (50th centile).

At postnatal review, she did report increasing vaginal symptoms of prolapse. On assessment, there was no change in uterine prolapse (Point C −7 cm) but there was a cystocoele not previously described (Ba −1 cm). At present, this is being managed conservatively.

Patient 5

In a 39-year-old para 2, laparoscopic hysteropexy had been performed for uterine prolapse with point C + 2 cm (post-operatively −7 cm). The conception was 22 months following surgery and was planned. Antenatal care was as outlined above, with normal uterine artery Doppler and serial growth scans. During Caesarean section at 39 + 2 weeks, the mesh was felt over the lower segment and so a transverse hysterotomy was performed at the upper limit of the lower segment, resulting in a blood loss of 1000 mls. The mesh remained attached to the sacral promontory, and a baby girl weighing 3520 g (70th centile) was delivered.

At postnatal review, no prolapse symptoms were reported and point C remained −7 cm.

Patient 6

A 27-year-old para 3 underwent laparoscopic hysteropexy with pre-operative findings of point C + 1 cm; post-operatively, this was corrected to −6 cm. She conceived 1 month following but was a late booker in pregnancy, first seeing her midwife at 18 weeks. Her booking history stated a background of "prolapse surgery" but no referral to consultant led care was made, and she therefore followed a low risk, midwifery led pathway of antenatal care with no additional scans. She presented to labour ward at 39 + 4 with ruptured membranes and was draining thick meconium. She was reviewed by the obstetrician on call who discovered the history of hysteropexy and therefore proceeded to emergency caesarean section.

This was uncomplicated, with a well-formed lower segment and no mesh avulsion. A baby boy was delivered weighing 2795 g (10th centile). All three of her previous children had birth weights on the 10th centile.

Unfortunately, this patient has not attended for a postnatal review.

Discussion

Current advice to women is to complete their family prior to embarking on uterine-preserving prolapse surgery, due to the lack of knowledge about the impact of pregnancy on surgical outcome, and of any impact surgery may have on pregnancy. This series gives some limited data on the safety of encirclage mesh hysteropexy in women of childbearing age.

In the literature, two case reports of pregnancy following polypropylene mesh augmented sacrohysteropexy have been reported [4, 5]; however, this technique involved mesh transfixed to the posterior cervix only. The latter case experienced a recurrence of prolapse 2 years post delivery requiring repeat surgery. Pandeva et al. [6] report on eight pregnancy outcomes following a single sheet mesh sacrohysteropexy. Again, this technique does not encircle the cervix and so should not cause any alteration in uterine blood flow. One case report [7] describes a term vaginal delivery following an open sacrohysteropexy using a Y-shaped mesh transfixed anteriorly and posteriorly but not wrapping around the cervix.

The concerns regarding uterine artery compression with an encirclage technique appear to be unfounded; whilst one patient's uterine artery Doppler showed some angulation of the artery, there was no change to the PI or RI in any cases. Growth was normal for all foetuses, with all women delivering babies with birth weights on or above the 10th centile. No woman developed pregnancy-related hypertension. This suggests that (in this small cohort at least) placental development and perfusion is not compromised by the hysteropexy mesh.

The lower uterine segment develops from the isthmus of the uterus, above the level of the internal os. At caesarean section, all but one woman had a normally developed lower uterine segment, meaning caesarean delivery was straightforward. In one case where mesh was noted over the lower segment, it is possible that the original surgery had left the "wrap around" portion of the mesh too loose, meaning it slipped above its usual position at the internal os. Our usual practice is to transfix the arms of the mesh tightly around the cervix to prevent slippage. In all cases, the mesh had remained fixed to the sacral promontory.

At postnatal follow-up, none of the women had any deterioration in apical prolapse; however, two women developed new onset symptoms and prolapse of the anterior compartment. At 8 weeks post-partum, the uterus has involuted to its usual size; however, patients may not have resumed full activity, making it harder to assess symptomatology. One patient has had further prolapse surgery in the form of an anterior colporrhaphy since her delivery. None of the other patients have re-presented with troublesome prolapse symptoms.

The main limitation of this study is the small sample size, meaning it is not possible to draw general conclusions about either foetal or maternal outcome. It is, however, the largest series to date and so offers some information for women and clinicians considering fertility-preserving prolapse surgery.

One concern for women undergoing pregnancy post hysteropexy is the question of how to manage pregnancy loss. Our belief is that in the first trimester, miscarriage could be managed as per usual protocols, as the cervical canal should admit a small suction curette. However, mid trimester and third trimester losses would result in the need for hysterotomy with the associated morbidity and impact on any future pregnancy.

The majority of women undergoing prolapse surgery will be past childbearing age. Our advice for the younger patients remains that they complete their family prior to reconstructive surgery. However, this will not always be possible; some younger women have significant prolapse impacting negatively on quality of life, and we need to be able to counsel them appropriately. All fertile women undergoing uterine preservation surgery in our unit are advised of the possible impact of pregnancy and if pregnancy is not desired should be offered reliable contraception at the time of surgery (in the form of a coil or salpingectomy). Those who are considering pregnancy should be advised that a caesarean section seems mandatory and that they should inform their GP or midwife at booking of the need for consultant led antenatal care.

Conclusions

This study suggests that the Oxford Hysteropexy is suitable for women who wish to conceive. The hysteropexy does not appear to have an adverse effect on foetal growth, and delivery by caesarean is feasible. Furthermore, pregnancy does not appear to compromise long-term hysteropexy uterine support. In two out of the five patients assessed in the post-partum, there was de novo anterio vaginal wall prolapse. However, the study is small and further patient numbers are required before we can give patients robust evidence-based guidance as to the safety of pregnancy following hysteropexy. As these cases are uncommon, it would be sensible for units to pool any outcome data in the form of a national registry and database.

Competing interests
The authors declare that they have no competing interests.

Authors' contributions
HJ contributed to the data collection and manuscript writing. NP contributed to the manuscript editing. SJ contributed to the project development and manuscript editing. All authors read and approved the final manuscript.

References
1. Rahmanou P, White B, Price N, Jackson S (2014) Laparoscopic hysteropexy: 1- to 4-year follow-up of women postoperatively. Int Urogynecol J 25(1): 131–138. doi:10.1007/s00192-013-2209-5
2. Rahmanou P, Price N, Jackson S (2014) Laparoscopic hysteropexy: a novel technique for uterine preservation surgery. Int Urogynecol J 25:139–140
3. Rahmanou P, Price N, Black R, Jackson S (2015) Pregnancy post-laparoscopic hysteropexy. J Obstet Gynaecol 35(3):303–304
4. Busby G, Broome J (2010) Successful pregnancy outcome following laparoscopic sacrohysteropexy for second degree uterine prolapse. Gynecol Surg 7:271–273
5. Lewis CM, Culligan P (2012) Sacrohysteropexy followed by successful pregnancy and eventual reoperation for prolapse. Int Urogynecol J 23:957–959
6. Pandeva I, Mistry M, Fayyad A (2017) Efficacy and pregnancy outcomes of laparoscopic single sheet mesh sacrohysteropexy. Neurourol Urodynam 36:787–793. doi:10.1002/nau.23026
7. Balsak D, Eser A, Erol O, Deniz Altıntaş D, Aksin Ş (2015) Pregnancy and vaginal delivery after sacrohysteropexy. Case Rep Obstet Gynecol 2015:3. doi:10.1155/2015/305107

6

Oophoropexy for ovarian torsion: a new easier technique

Tamer A. Hosny

Abstract

Background: Oophoropexy for ovarian torsion is easy to be done by many tools either suturing to the lateral pelvic wall, plication of the ovarian ligament or even fixation to the back of the uterus, but it is little bit difficult to do it for pregnant women with less manipulation.

Objective: We propose that using trocar site closure needle can be easier and faster technique to do this. To assess the feasibility of using the trocar site closure needle to do oophoropexy in ovarian torsion and its possible applicability.

Patients: Seven patients presented with ovarian torsion; four of them were pregnant at 7, 15, 19 and 20 weeks of gestation, two patients with ovarian hyperstimulation in IVF cycles and one adolescent patient with hemorrhagic cyst. They were diagnosed by clinical presentation and ultrasound with Doppler analysis, and confirmed by laparoscopy where they underwent detorsion and fixation of the ovary using the trocar site closure needle.

Results: Follow up of all the cases after one week showed improvement of the symptoms and normal Doppler flow of the target ovary then after three weeks by ultrasonography which revealed normal Doppler flow in the previously torsioned ovary. Two pregnant women underwent cesarean delivery where the operated ovary was observed during the delivery and was normal in shape and freely mobile with no adhesions.

Conclusion: We propose that this technique is easier, faster and more comfortable especially in ovarian torsion in pregnant women and torsion in hyperstimulated ovaries.

Keywords: Ovarian torsion, Oophoropexy, Laparoscopy, Ovarian hyperstimulation syndrome, Trocar site closure needle

Background

Ovarian torsion occurs when the ovary rotates around the infundibulopelvic ligament and the ovarian ligament interfering with its blood supply, which may be partial or complete. It is one of the most common gynecologic emergencies in all age groups [1]. The primary risk factor for the ovarian torsion is the presence of a mass which may be either a physiologic cyst or a neoplasm [2–4].

The frequent presenting symptoms are acute onset of pelvic pain, nausea, vomiting, fever, and adnexal mass with or without abnormal genital tract bleeding [4, 5]. A high index of suspicion is required to make the diagnosis especially if there is a history of ovulation induction for treatment of infertility [6] or during pregnancy. Pelvic ultrasound is still the first-line image study for diagnosing a patient with suspected ovarian torsion. The sonographic findings that are associated with ovarian torsion are described in many studies [7, 8]. Diminished or absent ovarian vessel flow on two-dimensional, color, and three-dimensional Doppler ultrasound has been proposed as a test for ovarian torsion [9–12]. Direct visualization of the rotated ovary remains the confirmatory way to diagnose the torsion, and the laparoscopic approach is typically used also to evaluate the ovarian viability [13].

Ovarian conservation is the preferred approach for premenopausal women, and most ovaries should be considered potentially viable unless there is a high degree of certainty that the ovary is not viable due to

Correspondence: dr_tamer_hosny@yahoo.com
Department of Obstetrics and Gynecology, Alexandria University Hospital,
16A Mohamed Said Pasha street, San Stefano, Alexandria 21411, Egypt

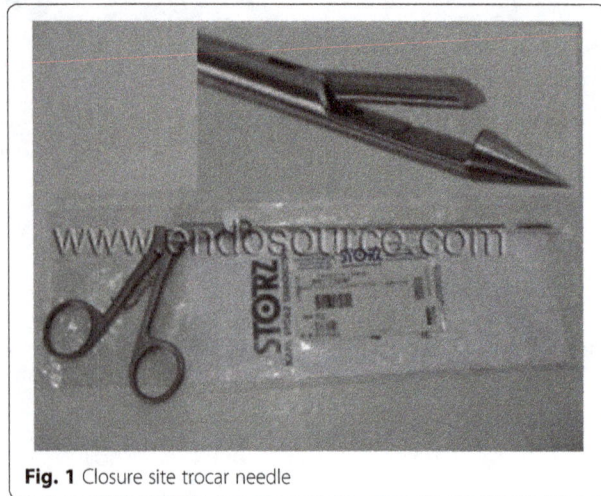

Fig. 1 Closure site trocar needle

Patients and methods

Seven patients presented with unilateral ovarian torsion to the emergency room in Alexandria University Hospital between November 2014 and May 2015; four of them were pregnant at 7, 15, 19, and 20 weeks of gestation; the torsioned ovaries were hyperstimulated in those pregnant women at 7, 15, and 20 weeks of gestation while there was an ovarian cyst in the pregnant woman at 19 weeks of gestation. Two patients had ovarian hyperstimulation in IVF cycles and one adolescent patient had a hemorrhagic cyst. They were diagnosed by clinical presentation and ultrasound with Doppler analysis and confirmed by conventional laparoscopy (Additional file 1: Video 1), where they underwent detorsion and fixation of the ovary using the trocar site closure needle (Fig. 1) at the same setting.

the presence of necrotic tissue. The conservative management consists of detorsion of the ovary followed by cystectomy if a mass is present. As ovarian torsion may recur after detorsion [14, 15], unilateral or bilateral oophoropexy following detorsion may be performed to prevent recurrence [16].

Technique

This idea is mainly to present an easy technique for emergency procedure.

➤ Laparoscopic entry after pneumoperitoneum insufflation via Veress needle at the umbilicus or Palmer point for the pregnant women. The camera

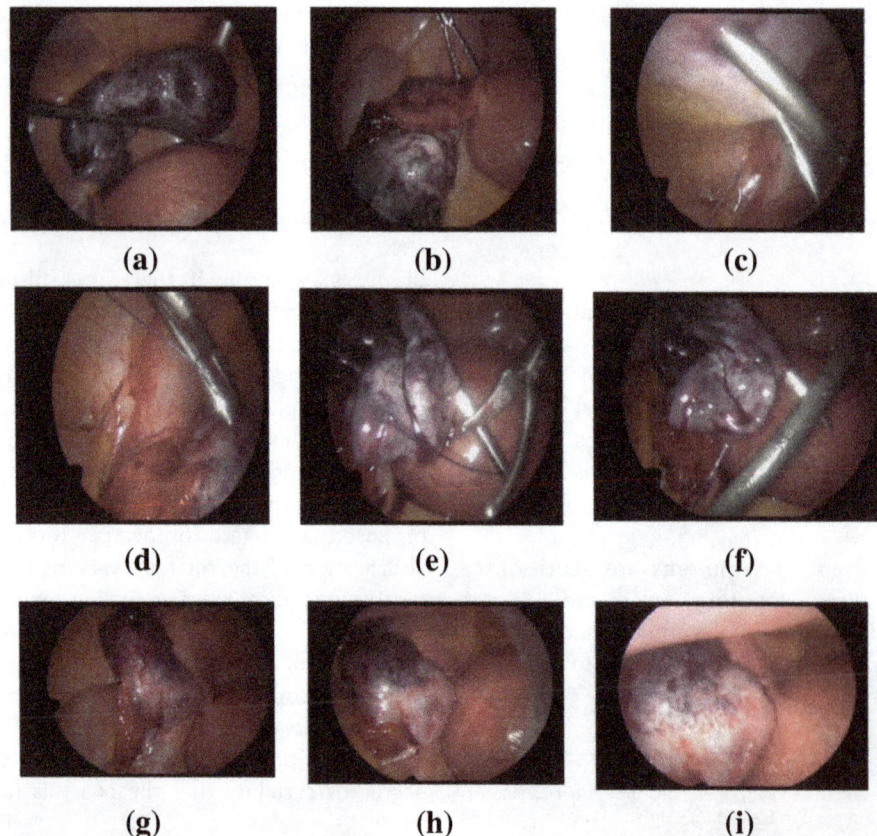

(a)　　　　　　(b)　　　　　　(c)

(d)　　　　　　(e)　　　　　　(f)

(g)　　　　　　(h)　　　　　　(i)

Fig. 2 a Twisted right ovary. **b** Detorsion. **c** Site of entrance for trocar site needle. **d** Entry through the ovary. **e** Holding threads after transfixing the ovary. **f** Second entry. **g** Fixing the ovary to the abdominal wall. **h** During deflation. **i** After complete deflation was placed in a 10-mm trocar at the umbilicus or in a 5-mm trocar at the Palmer point for the pregnant women at 19 and 20 weeks of gestation.

➤ Using two ancillary trocars, detorsion was performed followed by ovarian bivalving or cystectomy in cases of ovarian cysts

➤ Fixation of the ovary by transfixing the trocar site closure needle with absorbable vicryl 2-0 suture through the ovary then picking the suture from another transfixing point through the ovary then tying the suture around the sheath (Additional file 2: Video 2).

➤ The technique is illustrated in Fig. 2.

Results

Follow-up of all the cases after 1 week showed improvement of the symptoms and then normal Doppler flow of the target ovary after 3 weeks by ultrasonography which revealed normal Doppler flow in the previously torsioned ovary. Two pregnant women underwent cesarean delivery where the operated ovary was observed during the delivery and was normal in shape and freely mobile with no adhesions (Fig. 3).

Discussion

Although oophoropexy for ovarian torsion is debatable situation, retorsion may occur [14, 15]. Oophoropexy for ovarian torsion is emergency procedure, if we compare the most accepted way of oophoropexy by ovarian ligament placation I think it needs more training for suturing by laparscopy and it will be very difficult in cases of pregnant uterus, so we propose that this technique may be helpful although comparative study must be done between ovarian ligament placation and this technique illustrated, but limited number of cases of ovarian torsion, as it is one of the rare emergency situation.

Conclusions

We propose that this technique is easier, faster, and more comfortable especially in ovarian torsion in pregnant women and torsion in hyperstimulated ovaries.

Competing interests
The author declares that he has no competing interests.

References
1. McWilliams GD, Hill MJ, Dietrich CS 3rd (2008) Gynecologic emergencies. Surg Clin North Am 88:265
2. Varras M, Tsikini A, Polyzos D et al (2004) Uterine adnexal torsion: pathologic and gray-scale ultrasonographic findings. Clin Exp Obstet Gynecol 31:34
3. Houry D, Abbott JT (2001) Ovarian torsion: a fifteen-year review. Ann Emerg Med 38:156
4. White M, Stella J (2005) Ovarian torsion: 10-year perspective. Emerg Med Australas 17:231
5. Huchon C, Panel P, Kayem G et al (2012) Does this woman have adnexal torsion? Hum Reprod 27:2359
6. Gorkemli H, Camus M, Clasen K (2002) Adnexal torsion after gonadotrophin ovulation induction for IVF or ICSI and its conservative treatment. Arch Gynecol Obstet 267:4
7. Anthony EY, Caserta MP, Singh J, Chen MY (2012) Adnexal masses in female pediatric patients. AJR Am J Roentgenol 198:W426
8. Wilkinson C, Sanderson A (2012) Adnexal torsion—a multimodality imaging review. Clin Radiol 67:476
9. Albayram F, Hamper UM (2001) Ovarian and adnexal torsion: spectrum of sonographic findings with pathologic correlation. J Ultrasound Med 20:1083
10. Vijayaraghavan SB (2004) Sonographic whirlpool sign in ovarian torsion. J Ultrasound Med 23:1643
11. Yaman C, Ebner T, Jesacher K (2002) Three-dimensional power Doppler in the diagnosis of ovarian torsion. Ultrasound Obstet Gynecol 20:513
12. Lee EJ, Kwon HC, Joo HJ et al (1998) Diagnosis of ovarian torsion with color Doppler sonography: depiction of twisted vascular pedicle. J Ultrasound Med 17:83
13. Oelsner G, Cohen SB, Soriano D et al (2003) Minimal surgery for the twisted ischaemic adnexa can preserve ovarian function. Hum Reprod 18:2599
14. Pansky M, Smorgick N, Herman A et al (2007) Torsion of normal adnexa in postmenarchal women and risk of recurrence. Obstet Gynecol 109:355
15. Grunewald B, Keating J, Brown S (1993) Asynchronous ovarian torsion—the case for prophylactic oophoropexy. Postgrad Med J 69:318
16. Abeş M, Sarihan H (2004) Oophoropexy in children with ovarian torsion. Eur J Pediatr Surg 14:168

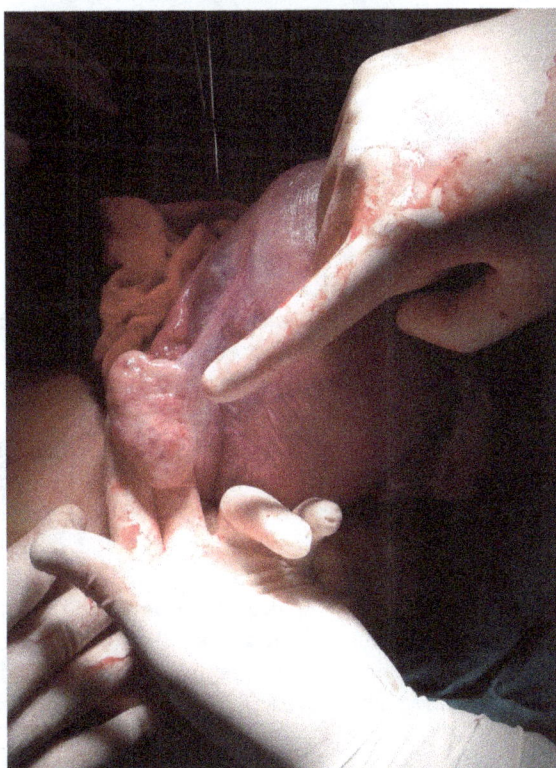

Fig. 3 Picture of ovary during cesarean section

7

Face and content validity of the virtual reality simulator 'ScanTrainer®'

Amal Alsalamah[1*], Rudi Campo[2], Vasilios Tanos[3], Gregoris Grimbizis[4], Yves Van Belle[2], Kerenza Hood[5], Neil Pugh[6] and Nazar Amso[1]

Abstract

Background: Ultrasonography is a first-line imaging in the investigation of women's irregular bleeding and other gynaecological pathologies, e.g. ovarian cysts and early pregnancy problems. However, teaching ultrasound, especially transvaginal scanning, remains a challenge for health professionals. New technology such as simulation may potentially facilitate and expedite the process of learning ultrasound. Simulation may prove to be realistic, very close to real patient scanning experience for the sonographer and objectively able to assist the development of basic skills such as image manipulation, hand-eye coordination and examination technique.

Objective: The aim of this study was to determine the face and content validity of a virtual reality simulator (ScanTrainer®, MedaPhor plc, Cardiff, Wales, UK) as reflective of real transvaginal ultrasound (TVUS) scanning.

Method: A questionnaire with 14 simulator-related statements was distributed to a number of participants with differing levels of sonography experience in order to determine the level of agreement between the use of the simulator in training and real practice.

Results: There were 36 participants: novices ($n = 25$) and experts ($n = 11$) who rated the simulator. Median scores of face validity statements between experts and non-experts using a 10-point visual analogue scale (VAS) ratings ranged between 7.5 and 9.0 ($p > 0.05$) indicated a high level of agreement. Experts' median scores of content validity statements ranged from 8.4 to 9.0.

Conclusions: The findings confirm that the simulator has the feel and look of real-time scanning with high face validity. Similarly, its tutorial structures and learning steps confirm the content validity.

Keywords: Ultrasound, Validation, Virtual reality simulation, Medical education, Transvaginal ultrasonography, ScanTrainer

Background

Simulation tools are either simplistic models or complex applications, and regardless of the technology used, a simulator must demonstrate validity to be an effective education tool [1]. This entails gathering evidence from multiple sources to show that the interpretation of image, examination or assessment is sound and sensible [1, 2]. At the outset, validation will usually attempt to confirm the fundamental reasons that these tools need to exist for learning [3–6]. From an educational perspective, a simulated performance should appear realistic when creating a cognitive-sensory mechanism known as 'sense of presence' because it allows the trainee/operator to interact with the remote environment as if s/he were present within the environment [7]. With regard to the role of simulation in developing ultrasound knowledge and skills, the validity and reliability of a simulator system for educational goals must be proven, through structured face, content and construct validity studies [1, 8–10].

Face validity is defined as the extent of a simulator's realism and appropriateness when compared to the actual task [11–13], whereas content validity is defined as the extent to which a simulator's content is representative of the knowledge or skills that have to be learnt in the real environment. This is based on detailed examination of the learning resources, tutorials and tasks [3, 14–16]. Hence, in the context of ultrasound, face validity addresses the question of how realistic is the simulator, for example, in

* Correspondence: alsalamahA@icloud.com
[1]School of Medicine, College of Biomedical and Life Sciences, Cardiff University, Office 220, 45 Salisbury road, Cathays, Cardiff CF24 4AB, UK
Full list of author information is available at the end of the article

examining the female pelvis and how realistic is the simulated feel (haptic sensation) experienced during the examination. Similarly, content validity addresses the question of how useful is the ultrasound simulator in learning relevant skills such as measuring endometrial thickness and foetal biometry [13, 17, 18].

According to McDougall and colleagues [4], Kenney and colleagues [19] and Xiao and colleagues [16], face validity is expressed as the assessment of virtual realism by novices, while content validity refers to experts' assessment of the suitability of a simulator as a teaching tool. However, reports in the literature are diverse and some authors undertake face validity of a simulator by seeking the opinion of any user including expert and non-expert subjects [12, 13, 15, 20–22]. Others have argued that subjects' experience is required for face validity of any educational instrument [18, 23–26]. With regard to content validity, it widely refers to experts' judgement towards the learning content and tasks of a simulator [14, 17, 27–29]. Nevertheless, many published studies rely on subjects with different levels of experience in evaluating content validity of a simulator [12, 13, 22, 30–32].

The ultrasound simulator [33] enables the student to acquire transabdominal (TAS) or transvaginal ultrasound scanning (TVUS) skills through a series of simulation tutorials, each with one or more assignments that include specified tasks reflecting real ultrasound practice. Upon completion of the tasks, the simulator provides computer-generated individualised student/trainee feedback. The hypotheses were that the simulator was (1) realistic for the purpose of developing ultrasound skills and reflects real-life scanning and (2) the content of its structured learning approach represents the knowledge and psychomotor skills that must be learnt when scanning patients.

The aim of this study was to determine face and content validity of TVUS ScanTrainer. The objectives were (1) to recruit practitioners with varying levels of ultrasound experience from attendees of an international conference and (2) instruct study volunteers to undertake relevant simulator tutorials and complete a structured questionnaire including statements on face and content validity.

Methods

Subjects were voluntarily recruited from delegates visiting the 'ESGE Simulation Island' during the 23rd European Congress of Obstetrics and Gynaecology (2014) in Glasgow, Scotland, UK. Each delegate was given a brief, general introduction on the purpose of the study and instructions on how to use the simulator and the relevant tutorials. They gave verbal consent to participate and proceeded to explore specific tasks in three tutorials with the TVUS ScanTrainer (Fig. 1). These were (1) core

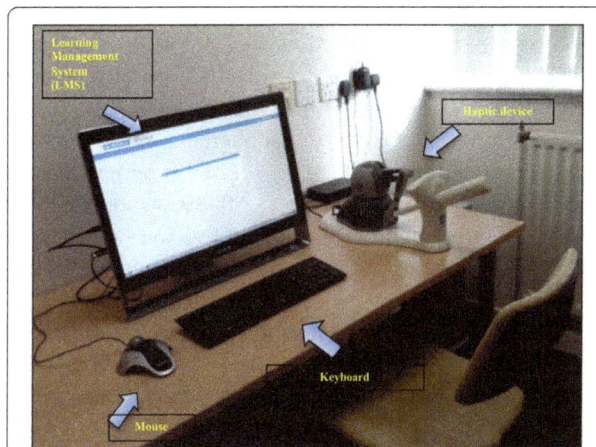

Fig. 1 Ultrasound simulator ScanTrainer consists of (1) a monitor which represents learning contents as programmed by specific learning software, and the monitor connects to (2) a haptic device, (3) mouse and (4) keyboard

skills gynaecology which has assignments on assessing the uterus, ovaries and adnexa and measuring the endometrial thickness, (2) core skills early pregnancy which has assignments on assessing the gestational sac, yolk sac as well as evaluating foetal viability and measurements and (3) advanced skills that consisted of several case studies, e.g. ovarian cyst, ectopic pregnancy and twin pregnancy. At the conclusion of the session, subjects completed a short questionnaire. Participants took between 10 and 15 min to complete the three tutorials.

The structured questionnaire (Additional file 1) consisted of two sections: one detailed subjects' demographic information, previous ultrasound experience and any previous experience with VR simulation or ultrasound mannequins. The other section included simulation-related statements. An expert was defined as a subject who had ultrasonography experience of nearly 2 years or more, conducted daily scanning sessions and considered her/himself as an independent practitioner. Some experts with many years of independent ultrasound experience had less than daily or weekly sessions due to other commitments. A non-expert was defined as having limited experience with ultrasound, had less than 2 years TVUS experience, with occasional or very limited scanning sessions, e.g. once/month, or considered her/himself as a trainee under supervision, newly qualified or not yet competent in TVUS scanning.

Fourteen simulation-related statements/parameters were subjectively scored along a 10-cm visual analogue scale (VAS) line by marking the point that subjects felt most appropriate, with (0) at one end (very bad) and (10) at the other (very good). Statements 1 to 6 assessed face validity, 7 to 12 evaluated the simulator's learning content and 13 and 14 were general statements on the value of the simulator as training tool (for practical skill acquisition purpose) and testing tool (for assessment purpose). Ratings on the scale were defined in 'mm' as 0–9 (very strongly disagree), 10–19 (strongly disagree), 20–29 (disagree), 30–39 (moderately disagree), 40–49 (mildly disagree), 50 (undecided), 51–59 (mildly agree), 60–69 (moderately agree), 70–79 (agree), 80–89 (strongly agree), 90–100 (very strongly agree). Millimetres were considered for accurate readings of subjects' marking on scale and later converted to centimetres for final analysis.

The study was conducted in accordance with the general terms and conditions of the South East Wales Research Ethics Committee SEWREC (NHS REC Reference 10/WSE02/75) approval and approval of the study protocol by the congress organising committee.

Statistical data analysis

IBM SPSS Statistics software version 20.0 was used for statistical analysis. Median values were chosen in preference to mean values as the data were not normally distributed. Median scores and box plots were constructed for each statement as rated by non-experts and experts. Box plots and whiskers represented the median, first and third quartiles, minimum, maximum and outliers of scores obtained by expert and non-expert ratings of the 13 statements. Face validity and general statement items were stratified by expert and non-expert status, while content validity data were reported for experts only. Differences between experts and non-expert ratings were analysed using the Mann-Whitney U test using a p value ≤ 0.05 to indicate significance.

Results

Demographic: Thirty-six subjects, 24 females (67%) and 12 males (33%), participated in this pilot study. Nine were UK-based and 27 were based in other European countries. Eleven subjects (31% expert group) rated themselves as skilled with more than 2 years of experience and practiced independently ($n = 10$) or with 1 to 2 years of experience and had daily ultrasound sessions ($n = 1$). Twenty-five subjects (69% non-expert group) were trainees under supervision and included two subjects with more than 2 years TAS experience and limited TVUS scanning. Median age for the expert group was 51 years (range 32–67) and 31 years (range 25–39) for the non-expert group. The median ultrasound experience for experts was more than 2 years and for non-experts was 6 to 11 months. Further breakdown of demographics and years of ultrasound experience is detailed in Table 1.

Face validity: Median scores of face validity statements are detailed in Table 2. In summary, experts' and non-experts' ratings ranged between 7.5 and 9.0 and were slightly higher than those by experts in two statements (2 and 6) relating to 'realism of the simulator to simulate

Table 1 Participants' demographics and ultrasonography experience

	Non-expert	Expert
No. of participants ($n = 36$)	25 (69%)	11 (31%)
Gender		
Female	17 (68%)	7 (64%)
Male	8 (32%)	4 (36%)
Country of practice		
Within UK	6 (24%)	3 (27%)
Outside UK	19 (75%)	8 (73%)
Speciality		
Consultant	–	3 (27%)
Obs/Gyn specialist	2 (8%)	4 (36%)
Specialist trainee	20 (80%)	3 (27%)
Medical student	1 (4%)	–
Radiographer	–	1 (10%)
Other (midwives)	2 (8%)	–
Median age	31 (25–39)	51 (32–67)
Years of ultrasound experience		
Never	3 (12%)	–
< 6 months	5 (20%)	–
6–11 months	9 (36%)	–
1–2 years	6 (24%)	1 (10%)
> 2 years	2 (8%)	10 (90%)
Transvaginal ultrasound experience		
Independent practitioner	2 (8%)	11 (100%)
Trainee under supervision	23 (92%)	–
Ultrasound sessions		
Never	4 (16%)	–
Daily	1 (4%)	5 (46%)
Once/week	9 (36%)	–
Once/month	3 (12%)	2 (18%)
Occasionally	5 (20%)	2 (18%)
Other	3 (12%)	2 (18%)
Previous experience with the ScanTrainer®		
Yes	3 (12%)	3 (27%)
No	22 (88%)	8 (73%)
Previous experience with ultrasound model, i.e. blue Phantom™		
Yes	4 (16%)	4 (36%)
No	21 (84%)	7 (64%)

the TVUS scan of female pelvis and realism of the simulator to provide actual action of all buttons provided in the control panel'. Two statements (1 and 3) were rated lower by experts and related to 'relevance of the simulator for actual TVUS scanning and the realism of the simulator to simulate the movements possibly required

Table 2 Face validity 'median scores' ratings by experts and non-experts (n = 36)

Face validity statements	Median score (range)			p value
	Expert (n = 11)	Non-expert (n = 25)	Overall	
Statement 1: Relevance of the simulator for actual transvaginal ultrasound scanning	7.5 (5.0–10)	9.0 (7.0–10)	8.7 (5.0–10)	0.1
Statement 2: Realism of the simulator to simulate the transvaginal scan of female pelvis	8.3 (5.0–10)	8.0 (5.9–10)	8.1 (5.0–10)	0.9
Statement 3: Realism of the simulator to simulate the movements possibly required to perform in the female pelvic anatomy (uterus, ovaries/adnexa, POD)	7.7 (1.0–10)	9.0 (5.0–10)	9.0 (1.0–10)	0.1
Statement 4: Realism of the ultrasound image generated during the performance	9.0 (1.3–9.8)	9.0 (6.0–10)	9.0 (1.3–10)	0.2
Statement 5: Force feedback provided on the operator's hand to simulate real scan	7.5 (3.0–9.5)	7.5 (2.7–10)	7.5 (2.7–10)	0.4
Statement 6: Realism of simulator to provide actual action of all buttons provided in the control panel	9.0 (1.0–10)	8.7 (3.0–10)	9.0 (1.0–10)	0.5
General statements				
Statement 13: Overall value of the simulator as a training tool	9.0 (5.0–10)	9.3 (6.0–10)	9.0 (5.0–10)	0.2
Statement 14: Overall value of the simulator as a testing tool	9.0 (5.0–10)	9.5 (5.6–10)	9.3 (5.0–10)	0.2

to perform in the female pelvic anatomy (uterus, ovaries/adnexa, Pouch of Douglas POD)'. The remaining two statements (4 and 5) referring to 'realism of the ultrasound image generated during the performance and force feedback provided on the operator's hand to simulate real scan' were equally rated. Two general statements (13 and 14) were also rated lower by experts. However, there were no statistically significant differences between the two groups' ratings in all statements (Table 1). Median values and box plots of the eight statements in the two groups are shown in Figs. 2 and 3.

Content validity: Experts' median scores of content validity statements ranged from 8.4 to 9.0 and are detailed in Table 3. Median values and box plots of the six statements are shown in Fig. 4.

Discussion
In this study, the ScanTrainer® simulator demonstrated high face and content validity and its overall value as a

training and testing tool received high ratings as well. To accurately measure participants' level of agreement with relevant statements, VAS method was used in the questionnaire [34]. Higher ratings were given by non-experts than experts with regard to 'relevance of the simulator to actual TVUS' and 'its realism to simulate the movements required to perform in the examination of the female pelvis' (statements 1 and 3) highlighting the fact that such realism is crucial for non-experts for several reasons. This may be because experts need to develop greater understanding of the strengths and limitations of the simulator compared to trainees [35]. Alternatively, beginners in the early stages of learning ultrasound skills are able to address their learning needs through simulated learning compared to the experts who expect variety and advanced or more complex performance rather than basic tutorials [12].

There are no comparable 'face and content' validity studies addressing virtual reality simulators for TVUS in obstetrics and gynaecology have been published in the

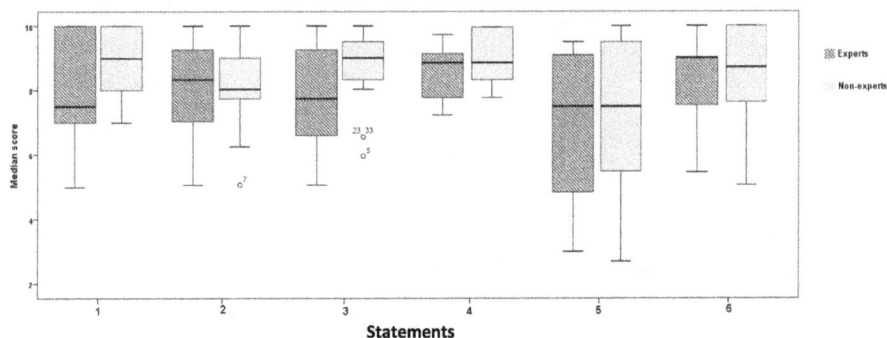

Fig. 2 Box plots represented the median, first and third quartiles, minimum, maximum and outliers of scores obtained by expert and non-expert ratings of the six face validity statements. Dots (outliers) represented those experts who scored lower than others and the number referred to participant's code number in data analysis and that did not relate to score value

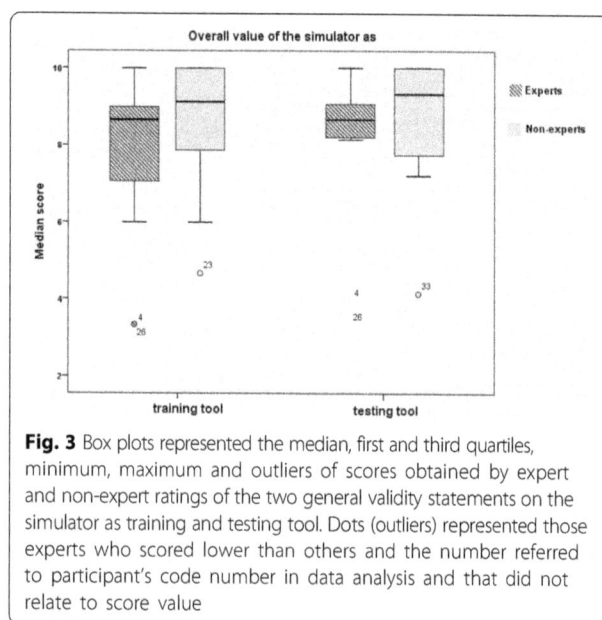

Fig. 3 Box plots represented the median, first and third quartiles, minimum, maximum and outliers of scores obtained by expert and non-expert ratings of the two general validity statements on the simulator as training and testing tool. Dots (outliers) represented those experts who scored lower than others and the number referred to participant's code number in data analysis and that did not relate to score value

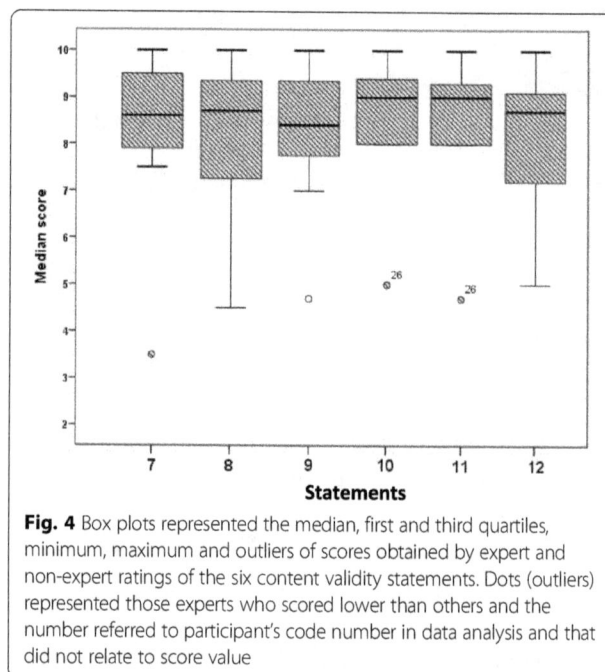

Fig. 4 Box plots represented the median, first and third quartiles, minimum, maximum and outliers of scores obtained by expert and non-expert ratings of the six content validity statements. Dots (outliers) represented those experts who scored lower than others and the number referred to participant's code number in data analysis and that did not relate to score value

literature. In a face validity study of the dVT robotic surgery simulator, experts rated the simulator as less useful for training experts than for students/juniors and pointed out to the experts' need for more critical and advanced procedures in gynaecological surgery and that simulators specifically designed for learning basic skills are less preferable to experts [32]. Creating simulated scenarios to correspond to real ones is always a challenge [3, 29, 36, 37].

Experts' ratings were higher for two statements relating to the realism of the simulator to simulate the TVUS scan of a female pelvis and in providing actual action of all buttons in the control panel (statements 2 and 6) This may stem from non-experts' limited knowledge and experience, or they might not be familiar with the measurement possibilities of virtual simulators [20, 23]. Similarly, Weidenbach and colleagues [1] argued that experts gave a better grading for the realism of the EchoCom echocardiography simulator because they were not distracted to drawbacks such as mannequin size and its surface properties, which were harder and more slippery than the human skin, and that experts scanned more

instinctively. The author noted that this mental flexibility seemed to be as yet underdeveloped in beginners.

Non-experts' and experts' ratings were similar when evaluating the realism of the ultrasound image generated during the performance and the force feedback provided onto the operator's hand (statements 4 and 5). Force feedback (haptics) scored 7.5 out of 10, the lowest score in this study. Similar to this study, Chalasani and colleagues [38] reported low face validity ratings for the haptic force-feedback device of a transrectal ultrasound TRUS-guided prostatic biopsy virtual reality simulator (experts' lifelike rating 64% and novices' 67%) even though the author pointed out that haptics, often very difficult to replicate in a simulator environment, were realistic. Haptics will not replace the real-patient scan experience but should enhance the learning approach and improve self-confidence. A further factor is that the ScanTrainer's haptic device can be tailored to three force feedback levels: normal resistance (most realistic), reduced and minimal (lowest) designed to avoid overheating during heavy use, and it is likely that a lower force

Table 3 Content validity 'median scores' ratings by experts (*n* = 11)

Content validity statements	Expert median (range)
Statement 7: Realism of the simulator to provide the endometrial thickness measurement in gynaecology task	8.6 (3.5–10)
Statement 8: Realism of the simulator to provide measurements of the ovary in gynaecology task	8.7 (4.5–10)
Statement 9: Ability to test normal gynaecological anatomy: uterus, adnexa and Pouch of Douglas	8.4 (4.7–10)
Statement 10: Ability to test early pregnancy structures: fetus, viability and placenta	9.0 (5.0–10)
Statement 11: Realism of the simulator to provide the CRL measurement in early pregnancy task	9.0 (4.7–10)
Statement 12: Relevance of the simulator's learning resource, videos and ScanTutor function	8.7 (5.0–10)

feedback setting might have contributed to the lower scores.

The role of force feedback in laparoscopic surgery is not clear [20]. Improving the realism of the simulator and its anatomical structures increases costs considerably due to increased demands for more complex hardware and software. In contrast, Lin and colleagues [39] encouraged learning of bone-sawing skills with simulators that provide force feedback rather than not, confirming the importance of force feedback when seeking to enhance hand-eye coordination. With regard to Scan-Trainer, virtual ultrasound and haptics are used instead of a mannequin allowing measurement of the force applied to the probe and provide a somewhat realistic force-feedback during scanning. However, it still has the limitation of allowing a lower range of movements to the probe while lacking a simulated environment exemplified by the absence of a physical mannequin [40].

There are numerous simulator systems in usage particularly in the fields of laparoscopy and endoscopy, and several authors emphasised the importance of evaluating their content, including reviewing each learning task and assessing its overall value to determine whether it is appropriate for the test and whether the test contains several steps and skills for practice [12, 17, 31, 38]. In this study, experts' data were used to assess content validity. They had adequate time to review the simulator's learning resources, help functionality 'ScanTutor', read the task-specific instructions and undertake specified tasks before going on to the next step in the same tutorial. In addition, participants had the opportunity to review feedback on their performance in the respective tasks. The results of this study demonstrated that the simulator's content and metrics were appropriate and relevant for ultrasound practice.

There are a number of published content validity studies in ultrasound simulation, such as the educational curriculum for ultrasonic propulsion to treat urinary tract calculi [41], web-based assessment of the extended focused assessment sonography in trauma (EFAST) [2] and validation of the objective structured assessment of technical skills for duplex assessment of arterial stenosis (DUOSATS) [42] which is not based on virtual reality simulator devices. Shumard and colleagues [43] reported on face and content validity of a novel second trimester uterine evacuation task trainer designed to train doctors to perform simulated dilatation and evacuation under ultrasound guidance. Although all respondents were residents with limited ultrasound experience, they rated the task trainer as excellent.

Other studies evaluated the effectiveness of simulation-based training in obstetrics and gynaecology ultrasound, whether to investigate the construct validity of a simulator system [9, 40, 44, 45] or to compare simulation training to conventional methods such as theoretical lectures and hands-on training on patients [10, 46].

Feedback that is automatically generated immediately after a practical simulator session should enhance trainees' knowledge and ability to reflect critically on their performance and improve their skills [47]. However, the big challenge is to determine how accurate, realistic and trusted the feedback is and, thus, should also be validated appropriately.

Validation studies at national scientific meetings have been reported previously [25, 48]. They offer researchers a rich environment where subjects from different backgrounds and levels of experience are present in one place at the same time. A potential limitation of the study is that it did not determine in advance the sample size required to obtain a reliable result for face and content validation. There is no agreement on the adequacy of sample size in such studies [12, 13]. The number of subjects in this study was higher, and the findings are consistent with others [18, 22, 31, 49]. In addition, many face and content validity studies of simulators were based on smaller sample size compared to the current study [13, 19, 30, 36, 50, 51]. A larger number of participants in this study might have improved the confidence in the results [2]. Participants in this study were from different UK and European institutions unlike others who were from single academic institution [41]; thus, it may be more widely generalizable.

Conclusions

In summary, this study confirms that ScanTrainer simulator has the feel and look (face validity) and tutorial structure (content validity) to be realistic and relevant for actual TVUS scanning. This study also concurs with the notion that advancing computer technologies have been able to incorporate virtual reality into training to facilitate the practice of basic skills as well as complex procedures that leave little room for error or mistake [3, 10, 24, 20]. Equally, such simulators should be part of the skill training labs in teaching hospitals as it is recommended for endoscopic surgery [52, 53]. It should be subject to an ongoing validation to address trainees' learning needs, provide a structured training path and provide validated test procedures with the global and final aim to improve patient care and safety [30, 31, 36, 52].

Acknowledgements
This study was funded by the Ministry of Higher Education, Riyadh, Saudi Arabia. Portions of this research were presented in the UK and international. Special thanks to the European Academy for Gynaecological Surgery and the

European Society for Gynaecological Endoscopy for their support and for providing the facilities at simulation island during the 23rd European Congress of Obstetrics and Gynaecology (2014) in Glasgow, Scotland, UK. We are thankful to all the participants for sharing their experience and valuable feedback.

Authors' contributions

AA and NA are the principal investigators and conceived the study. NA and NP were the co-supervisors of the PhD thesis. AA, NA, RC, VT, GG, and YvB designed the study and questionnaire. AA undertook the study and carried out the statistical analysis under the supervision of KH. All authors critically reviewed the manuscript and approved it before submission.

Competing interests

Amal Alsalamah was a PhD student funded by the Government of Saudi Arabia. Nazar Amso is a founder of, owns stocks in and is a board member of MedaPhor, a spin-off company of Cardiff University. He is a co-inventor of a patent for ultrasound simulation training system.

Author details

[1]School of Medicine, College of Biomedical and Life Sciences, Cardiff University, Office 220, 45 Salisbury road, Cathays, Cardiff CF24 4AB, UK. [2]European Academy of Gynaecological Surgery, Leuven, Belgium. [3]Aretaeion Medical Center, Nicosia, Cyprus. [4]First Department Obstetrics/Gynecology, Aristotle University of Thessaloniki, Thessaloniki, Greece. [5]Centre for Trials Research, College of Biomedical & Life Sciences, Cardiff University, Cardiff, UK. [6]Department of Medical Physics and Radiology, University Hospital of Wales, Cardiff and Vale University Health Board, Cardiff, UK.

References

1. Weidenbach M, Rázek V, Wild F, Khambadkone S, Berlage T, Janousek J, Marek J (2009) Simulation of congenital heart defects: a novel way of training in echocardiography. Heart 95(8):636–641
2. Markowitz JE, Hwang JQ, Moore CL (2011) Development and validation of a web-based assessment tool for the extended focused assessment with sonography in trauma examination. J Ultrasound Med 30(3):371–375
3. Carter FJ, Schijven MP, Aggarwal R, Grantcharov T, Francis NK, Hanna GB, Jakimowicz JJ (2005) Consensus guidelines for validation of virtual reality surgical simulators. Surg Endosc 19:1523–1532
4. McDougall M, Corica FA, Boker JR, Sala LG, Stoliar G, Borin JF, Chu FT, Clayman RV (2006) Construct validity testing of a laparoscopic surgical simulator. J Am Coll Surg 202(5):779–787
5. Gilliam AD, Acton ST (2007) Echocardiographic simulation for validation of automated segmentation methods. Image Processing, ICIP 2007. IEEE Int Conf 5:529–532
6. Wilfong DN, Falsetti DJ, McKinnon JL, Daniel LH, Wan QC (2011) The effects of virtual intravenous and patient simulator training compared to the traditional approach of teaching nurses: a research project on peripheral i.v. catheter insertion. J Infus Nurs 34(1):55–62
7. Aiello P, D'Elia F, Di Tore S, Sibilio M (2012) A constructivist approach to virtual reality for experiential learning. E-Lear Digital Media 9(3):317–324
8. Wright MC, Segall N, Hobbs G, Phillips-Bute B, Maynard L, Taekman JM (2013) Standardized assessment for evaluation of team skills: validity and feasibility. Soc Simul Healthc 8:292–303
9. Madsen ME, Konge L, Norgaard LN, Tabor A, Ringsted C, Klemmensen A, Ottesen B, Tolsgaard M (2014) Assessment of performance and learning curves on a virtual reality ultrasound simulator. Ultrasound Obstet Gynecol 44(6):693–699
10. Tolsgaard M, Ringsted C, Dreisler E, Nørgaard LN, Petersen JH, Madsen ME, Freiesleben NL, Sørensen JL, Tabor A (2015) Sustained effect of simulation-based ultrasound training on clinical performance: a randomized trial. Ultrasound Obstet Gynecol 46(3):312–318
11. Byrne A, Greaves J (2001) Assessment instruments used during anaesthetic simulation: review of published studies. Br J Anaesth 86(3):445–450
12. Hung AJ, Zehnder P, Patil MB, Cai J, Ng CK, Aron M, Gill IS, Desai MM (2011) Face, content and construct validity of a novel robotic surgery simulator. J Urol 186(3):1019–1024
13. Alzahrani T, Haddad R, Alkhayal A, Delisle J, Drudi L, Gotlieb W, Fraser S, Bergman S, Bladou F, Andonian S, Anidjar M (2013) Validation of the da Vinci surgical skill simulator across three surgical disciplines. Can Urol Assoc J 7(7–8):520–529
14. Nicholson W, Patel A, Niazi K, Palmer S, Helmy T, Gallagher A (2006) Face and content validation of virtual reality simulation for carotid angiography. Simul Healthc 1(3):147–150
15. Schreuder HW, van Dongen KW, Roeleveld SJ, Schijven MP, Broeders IA (2009) Face and construct validity of virtual reality simulation of laparoscopic gynecologic surgery. Am J Obstet Gynecol 200(5):540 e541–540 e548
16. Xiao D, Jakimowicz JJ, Albayrak A, Buzink SN, Botden SM, Goossens RH (2014) Face, content, and construct validity of a novel portable ergonomic simulator for basic laparoscopic skills. J Surg Educ 71(1):65–72
17. Seixas-Mikelus S, Stegemann AP, Kesavadas T, Srimathveeravalli G, Sathyaseelan G, Chandrasekhar R, Wilding GE, Peabody JO, Guru KA (2011) Content validation of a novel robotic surgical simulator. BJU Int 107(7):1130–1135
18. Dulan G, Rege RV, Hogg DC, Gilberg-Fisher KK, Tesfay ST, Scott DJ (2012) Content and face validity of a comprehensive robotic skills training program for general surgery, urology, and gynecology. Am J Surg 203(4):535–539
19. Kenney PA, Wszolek MF, Gould JJ, Lobertino JA, Moinzadeh A (2009) Face, content, and construct validity of dV-trainer, a novel virtual reality simulator for robotic surgery. Urology 73(6):1288–1292
20. Verdaasdonk EG, Stassen LP, Monteny LJ, Dankelman J (2006) Validation of a new basic virtual reality simulator for training of basic endoscopic skills: the SIMENDO. Surg Endosc 20(3):511–518
21. Seixas-Mikelus S, Kesavadas T, Srimathveeravalli G, Chandrasekhar R, Wilding GE, Guru KA (2010) Face validation of a novel robotic surgical simulator. Urology 76(2):357–360
22. Kelly D, Margules AC, Kundavaram CR, Narins H, Gomella LG, Trabulsi EJ, Lallas CD (2012) Face, content, and construct validity of the da Vinci skills simulator. Urology 79(5):1068–1072
23. Schijven M, Jakimowicz J (2002) Face-, expert, and referent validity of the Xitact LS500 laparoscopy simulator. Surg Endosc 16(12):1764–1770
24. Sweet R, Kowalewski T, Oppenheimer P, Weghorst S, Satava R (2004) Face, content and construct validity of the University of Washington virtual reality transurethral prostate resection trainer. J Urol 172(5):1953–1957
25. Maithel S, Sierra R, Korndorffer J, Neumann P, Dawson S, Callery M, Jones D, Scott D (2006) Construct and face validity of MIST-VR, Endotower, and CELTS, are we ready for skills assessment using simulators? Surg Endosc 20:104–112
26. Aydin A, Ahmed K, Brewin J, Khan MS, Dasgupta P, Aho T (2014) Face and content validation of the prostatic hyperplasia model and holmium laser surgery simulator. J Surg Educ 71(3):339–344
27. Fisher J, Binenbaum G, Tapino P, Volpe NJ (2006) Development and face and content validity of an eye surgical skills assessment test for ophthalmology residents. Ophthalmology 113(12):2364–2370
28. Scott DJ, Cendan JC, Pugh CM, Minter RM, Dunnington GL, Kozar RA (2008) The changing face of surgical education: simulation as the new paradigm. J Surg Res 147(2):189–193
29. Gould D (2010) Using simulation for interventional radiology training. Br J Radiol 83:546–553
30. Vick LR, Vick KD, Borman KR, Salameh JR (2007) Face, content, and construct validities of inanimate intestinal anastomoses simulation. J Surg Educ 64(6):365–368
31. Gavazzi A, Bahsoun A, Haute W, Ahmed K, Elhage O, Jaye P, Khan M, Dasgupta P (2011) Face, content and construct validity of a virtual reality simulator for robotic surgery (SEP Robot). Ann R Coll Surg Engl 93(2):152–156
32. Schreuder HR, Persson JE, Wolswijk RG, Ihse I, Schijven MP, Verheijen RH (2014) Validation of a novel virtual reality simulator for robotic surgery. Sci World J 2014:30
33. Medaphor® Plc, The ScanTrainer (2016) [online] Available at http://www.medaphor.com/scantrainer/ [Accessed 30 June 2016]
34. Jensen MP, Chen C, Brugger AM (2003) Interpretation of visual analog scale ratings and change scores: a reanalysis of two clinical trials of postoperative pain. J Pain 4(7):407–414
35. Shanmugan S, Leblanc F, Senagore AJ, Ellis CN, Stein SL, Khan S, Delaney CP, Champagne BJ (2014) Virtual reality simulator training for laparoscopic

colectomy: what metrics have construct validity? Dis Colon rectum 57(2): 210–214

36. O'Leary SJ, Hutchins MA, Stevenson DR, Gunn C, Krumpholz A, Kennedy G, Tykocinski M, Dahm M, Pyman B (2008) Validation of a networked virtual reality simulation of temporal bone surgery. Laryngoscope 118(6):1040–1046

37. de Vries AH, van Genugten HG, Hendrikx AJ, Koldewijn EL, Schout BM, Tjiam IM, van Merriënboer JJ, Muijtjens AM, Wagner C (2016) The Simbla TURBT simulator in urological residency training: from needs analysis to validation. J Endourol 30(5):580–587

38. Chalasani V, Cool DW, Sherebrin S, Fenster A, Chin J, Izawa JI (2011) Development and validation of a virtual reality transrectal ultrasound guided prostatic biopsy simulator. Can Urol Assoc J 5(1):19–26

39. Lin Y, Wang X, Wu F, Chen X, Wang C, Shen G (2014) Development and validation of a surgical training simulator with haptic feedback for learning bone-sawing skill. J Biomed Inform 48:122–129

40. Chalouhi GE, Bernardi V, Gueneuc A, Houssin I, Stirnemann JJ, Ville Y (2015) Evaluation of trainees' ability to perform obstetrical ultrasound using simulation: challenges and opportunities. Am J Obstet Gynecol 214(4):525.e1–525.e8

41. Hsi RS, Dunmire B, Cunitz BW, He X, Sorensen MD, Harper JD, Bailey MR, Lendvay TS (2014) Content and face validation of a curriculum for ultrasonic propulsion of calculi in a human renal model. J Endourol 28(4):459–463

42. Jaffer U, Singh P, Pandey VA, Aslam M, Standfield NJ (2014) Validation of a novel duplex ultrasound objective structured assessment of technical skills (DUOSATS) for arterial stenosis detection. Heart Lung Vessel 6(2):92–104

43. Shumard KM, Akoma UN, Street LM, Brost BC, Nitsche JF (2015) Development of a novel task trainer for second trimester ultrasound-guided uterine evacuation. Simul Healthc 10(1):49–53

44. Maul H, Scharf A, Baier P, Wüstemann M, Günter HH, Gebauer G, Sohn C (2004) Ultrasound simulators: experience with the SonoTrainer and comparative review of other training systems. Ultrasound Obstet Gynecol 24(5):581–585

45. Merz E (2006) Ultrasound simulator—an ideal supplemental tool for mastering the diagnostics of fetal malformations or an illusion? Ultraschall in Med 27(4):321–323

46. Williams CJ, Edie JC, Mulloy B, Flinton DM, Harrison G (2013) Transvaginal ultrasound simulation and its effect on trainee confidence levels: a replacement for initial clinical training? Ultrasound 21(2):50–56

47. Cline BC, Badejo AO, Rivest II, Scanlon JR, Taylor WC, Gerling GJ (2008) Human performance metrics for a virtual reality simulator to train chest tube insertion. IEEE Systems Inf Eng Des Symp:168–173 doi:10.1109/SIEDS. 2008.4559705

48. Stefanidis D, Korndorffer JR, Markley S, Sierra R, Heniford BT, Scott DJ (2007) Closing the gap in operative performance between novices and experts: does harder mean better for laparoscopic simulator training? J Am Coll Surg 205(2):307–313

49. White MA, Dehaan AP, Stephens DD, Maes AA, Maatman TJ (2010) Validation of a high fidelity adult ureteroscopy and renoscopy simulator. J Urol 183(2):673–677

50. Bright E, Vine S, Wilson MR, Masters RS, McGrath JS (2012) Face validity, construct validity and training benefits of a virtual reality turp simulator. Int J Surg 10(3):163–166

51. Shetty S, Panait L, Baranoski J, Dudrick SJ, Bell RL, Roberts KE, Duffy AJ (2012) Construct and face validity of a virtual reality-based camera navigation curriculum. J Surg Res 177(2):191–195

52. Campo R, Puga M, Meier Furst R, Wattiez A, De Wilde RL (2014) Excellence needs training "Certified programme in endoscopic surgery". Facts Views Vis Obgyn 6(4):240–244

53. Campo R, Wattiez A, Tanos V, Di Spiezio SA, Grimbizis G, Wallwiener D, Brucker S, Puga M, Molinas R, O'Donovan P, Deprest J, Van Belle Y, Lissens A, Herrmann A, Tahir M, Benedetto C, Siebert I, Rabischong B, De Wilde RL (2016) Gynaecological endoscopic surgical education and assessment. A diploma programme in gynaecological endoscopic surgery. Gynecol Surg 13:133–137

8

The effect of music in gynaecological office procedures on pain, anxiety and satisfaction: a randomized controlled trial

N. Mak[1*], I. M. A. Reinders[2,4], S. A. Slockers[1], E. H. M. N. Westen[3], J. W. M. Maas[1] and M. Y. Bongers[1,4]

Abstract

Background: Pain can interfere with office procedures in gynaecology. The aim of this study is to measure the positive effect of music in gynaecological office procedures.

Methods: A randomized controlled trial was performed between October 2014 and January 2016. Women scheduled for an office hysteroscopy or colposcopy were eligible for randomization in the music group or control group. Stratification for hysteroscopy and colposcopy took place. The primary outcome is patients' level of pain during the procedure measured by the visual analogue scale (VAS). Secondary outcomes include patients' level of pain after the procedure, anxiety and satisfaction of patient and doctor.

Results: No positive effect of music on patients' perception of pain during the procedure was measured, neither for the hysteroscopy group (57 mm vs. 52 mm) nor for the colposcopy group (32 mm vs. 32 mm). Secondary outcomes were also similar for both groups.

Conclusions: This study showed no positive effect of music on patients' level of pain, anxiety or satisfaction of patient or doctor for office hysteroscopy and colposcopy. We believe a multimodal approach has to be used to decrease patient distress in terms of pain and anxiety, with or without music.

Keywords: Pain, Anxiety, Music, Office procedures, Hysteroscopy, Colposcopy

Background

Today, office procedures in gynaecology are widely used to diagnose and directly treat gynaecological abnormalities [1–3]. However, pain and anxiety remain problems that may impede the procedure and can contribute to a negative experience for the patient [4–8].

Listening to music could be an easy and non-invasive way to decrease pain and anxiety. However, the literature is not clear about the efficacy of music therapy. Music for pain relief of any type was previously examined in a review including 31 studies. The studies showed a high variation in the results. Pooled data

demonstrated a significant reduction of 0.4 points on a 0–10 scale, which is of doubtful clinical importance [9]. Research on this topic in gynaecology is also not conclusive. The meta-analysis of Wang et al. suggested a positive effect of music regarding pain, anxiety and satisfaction for patients undergoing endoscopic surgery. For patients undergoing colposcopy, no effect was found [10]. This result is the sum of two randomized controlled trials with contradictory results regarding the impact of music in office colposcopy, with no effect versus an almost 2 point decrease in pain measured by the VAS (0–10) in favour of music therapy [7, 11, 12]. Only one article could be found on the effect of music during office hysteroscopy. Angioli et al. showed a positive effect of the use of music with a reduction of pain and anxiety [13].

The effect of music in gynaecological office procedures on satisfaction of patients is less frequently examined.

---

* Correspondence: N.mak@alumni.maastrichtuniversity.nl
[1]Department of Obstetrics and Gynaecology, Máxima Medical Centre, Veldhoven, The Netherlands
Full list of author information is available at the end of the article

Danhauer et al. found no effect [11]. Other studies in office gynaecology did not examine the efficacy of music on satisfaction of patients [12, 13]. The satisfaction of the doctor is not described in any of these articles [11–13]. However, music can have a negative influence on task performance and level of irritation of the surgeon in laparoscopic surgery [14, 15]. Therefore, this satisfaction of the doctor should not be ignored.

Previous research on the effect of music in gynaecological office procedures was not blinded for patients or doctors, meaning there was a risk of bias [11–13]. Moreover, other interventions to decrease the patient's discomfort, such as verbal communication between patient and doctor or nurse, are not mentioned or are excluded in previous studies [11–13]. Positive interactions between patient and doctor or nurse may interact with pain and anxiety and such interaction is often used in daily practice. The use of local anaesthetics, the use of information leaflets and the use of videoscopy are all methods used to improve patients' experience [3, 6, 7, 16].

We can conclude from previous research that a large discrepancy exists in the efficacy of music in the reduction of pain and anxiety. Research on the effect of music on the satisfaction of patient and doctor is rare. Previous research is possibly biased and does not answer the question of whether music is beneficial for patients and doctors in daily practice. The aim of this study is to demonstrate the complementary value of music in gynaecological office procedures on patients' level of pain, anxiety and satisfaction during and after the procedure in daily practice. The experience of the doctor will be evaluated as well.

Methods

Trial design

Between October 2014 and July 2016, a single-blind prospective randomized controlled superiority trial was performed at the Department of Obstetrics and Gynaecology in the Máxima Medical Centre in Veldhoven, the Netherlands. The trial was approved by the Medical Ethics Committee of the hospital (Study number 2014–28) and was registered in the Dutch Trial Register under trial ID number NTR4924.

Participants

All patients who referred to the outpatient clinic for a hysteroscopy or colposcopy were considered for inclusion. Inclusion criteria were Dutch-speaking women, of at least 18 years of age, planned for an office hysteroscopy or colposcopy with biopsy or large loop excision of the transformation zone (LLETZ). Exclusion criteria were hearing impairments, blindness and known anatomical characteristics that may make performing the office procedure more difficult (e.g., cervical conization, Manchester Fothergill).

Outcomes

The primary outcome was the experience of pain during the procedure, measured with the VAS on a 0–100 mm scale. The measurement took place during biopsy or LLETZ in the group of women undergoing colposcopy or during the passage of the internal ostium in the group of women undergoing hysteroscopy. Secondary outcomes were heart rate and anxiety during the procedure, pain after the procedure and satisfaction of patient and doctor. The heart rate was measured by using a pulse oximeter. The highest heart rate was used which was measured at the same time as the VAS during the procedure.

Anxiety of the patient was measured using the validated Dutch version of the State-Trait Anxiety Inventory (STAI) before and after the procedure. State anxiety and trait anxiety were both assessed by 20 items with scores ranging from 20 to 80, with higher scores indicating greater levels of anxiety. Satisfaction of patient and doctor was described using a scale of 1 to 5. In addition, the participants were asked if they would recommend the procedure in this setting to a friend. The doctor was asked if he or she would like to repeat the procedure in the same setting. Further, if applicable, the doctor was asked for the level of irritation regarding the music. Data and scores were reported in a case report form (CRF) and subsequently imported in the database by one person and controlled by another person. Excel was used as database.

Procedure

The researchers informed the patients who met the inclusion criteria in advance of their hospital visit. The eligible participants were told that they would participate in a study of pain relief during office procedures. In order to perform single-blind testing, they were not informed about the role of music. After giving informed consent, the following information was collected from all participants before the procedure: age, height, weight, drug use, use of painkillers before the procedure, parity, intensity of dysmenorrhoea and expected pain of the procedure both measured by the VAS. Participants were asked to arrive 15 min before their appointment to fill out the questionnaire with baseline characteristics and the STAI. Furthermore, the participant's heart rate was measured before the procedure.

The researchers randomized participants to the music group or control group. Stratification for hysteroscopy and colposcopy took place. Sealed numbered opaque envelopes were used for randomization. Participants who were randomized for the music group could choose between three types of music: pop, classical music and spa music. An iPod with speakers was used to play the music instead of headphones to maintain a good communication. The volume of the speakers could be adjusted by the doctor or researchers in a way so that the music was audible without disturbing the interaction between the participant and doctor or nurse. A gynaecologist or a resident performed the procedure. The experience of pain in VAS and participant's heart rate were measured during the procedure.

To determine whether or not music is beneficial for patients and doctors in daily practice, other contemporary interventions to decrease patients' discomfort remained unchanged with respect to the standard procedure. These include the use of information leaflets, the advice to use a painkiller before the procedure, the communication between patient and doctor, the emotional support by a nurse and the use of videoscopy during the procedure. A cervical block for patients undergoing a colposcopy was used if indicated according to the doctor.

After the procedure, participants were asked again to fill out a questionnaire regarding their level of satisfaction and the STAI. The doctor was asked for the degree of difficulty of the procedure. To achieve a smooth implementation of the study without influencing the standard procedure, a pilot study with ten participants was conducted before the start of this study to train the staff.

Statistical methods

Based on the previous research, a decrease of 20 mm on the VAS scale was expected when using music during the procedure [12, 13]. A sample size of 38 participants for each arm was calculated for both hysteroscopy and colposcopy based on the power analysis with a power of 0.90, a 5% significance level and an expected loss to follow-up of 5%.

The Shapiro-Wilk test was used to test the normality of the data. Depending on this result, the t test or the Mann-Whitney U test was used. Categorical data were tested using the chi-square test. If there was a statistical significant difference in base characteristics between the music group and the control group, linear regression was used to test for confounding. In case of confounding, the primary outcome was calculated with correction of these variables by linear regression. For all outcomes, the intention-to-

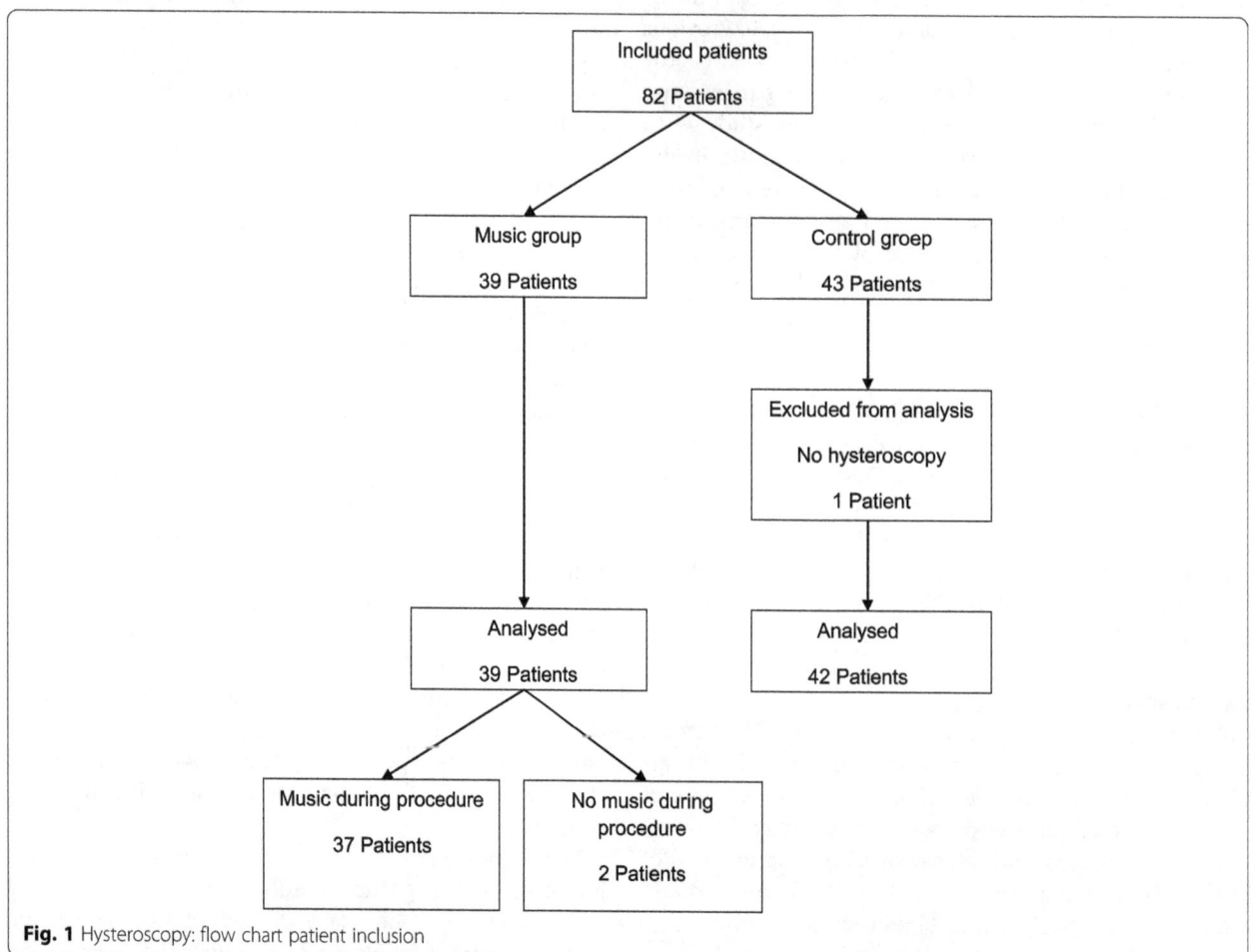

Fig. 1 Hysteroscopy: flow chart patient inclusion

treat analysis was used. In addition, a per-protocol analysis was performed for the primary outcome. All statistical analyses were performed using IBM SPSS Statistics for Windows (version 21.0, Armonk: NY, IBM Corp).

Results

Hysteroscopy

Eighty-two participants were included, 39 participants in the music group and 43 participants in the control group. One participant in the control group received a saline infusion sonohysterography (SIS) only and was excluded from further analyses. Thus, 81 participants (39 in the music group and 42 in the control group) were considered for the statistical analyses. Two participants from the music group did not receive music during the passage of the internal ostium of the cervix, due to a technical problem with the iPod (Fig. 1).

Baseline characteristics are shown in Table 1. These characteristics were similar for both groups. No statistical significance was found for pain during the procedure between the music group and the control group (57.1 (25.7) mm vs. 51.6 (27.1) mm, $p = .382$). Secondary outcomes were also similar, including heart rate and

anxiety during the procedure, pain after the procedure and satisfaction of patient and doctor ($p > .05$) (Table 2). No complications occurred.

In three cases (8%) in the music group, the doctor was (very) dissatisfied. One doctor reported that this was caused by the music, which was not a genre he or she enjoys. In another procedure, the doctor mentioned the dissatisfaction was correlated with the difficulty of the procedure. The reason for the last case was not reported. In two cases (5%), the doctor in the music group mentioned that he or she did not want to repeat the procedure in the same setting. The disturbing music was the reason for one of these two cases. The most popular music choice in the music group was pop music (58%), followed by classical music (21%) and spa music (21%).

Besides an intention-to-treat analysis, a per-protocol analysis was performed only for the primary outcome because two participants from the control group did not receive music during the passage of the internal ostium. Again, no difference was found (59.2 (24.3) mm vs. 50.0 (27.7) mm, $p = .154$).

Table 1 Hysteroscopy: patient characteristics

	Music group N = 39	Control group N = 42
Age (y)	45.4 (13.2)	45.2 (15.0)
Height (m)	1.67 (0.07)	1.66 (0.07)
Weight (kg)	77.3 (20.7)	73.2 (14.5)
Body mass index	27.6 (7.6)	26.7 (6.4)
Dysmenorrhea (mm VAS)	38.7 (31.4)	41.0 (26.7)
Expected pain (mm VAS)	51.2 (21.3)	54.6 (22.9)
Heart rate before procedure (bpm)	80.4 (11.1)	78.6 (13.2)
Use of a painkiller (%)	82	88
Difficulty of procedure (%)		
Very easy	27	37
Easy	40	23
Normal	19	34
Difficult	11	3
Very difficult	3	3
Intervention (%)		
Diagnostic	23	31
Biopsies	23	21
Therapeutic	54	48
Diameter 5.5 mm Hysteroscope (%)	67	74
STAI 1 score before procedure	40.7 (13.0)	42.6 (12.5)
STAI 2 score	34.0 (8.0)	36.0 (10.5)

Data are expressed as mean (SD) or percentage

Table 2 Hysteroscopy: results

	Music group N = 39	Control group N = 42	P value
Pain during procedure (mm VAS)	57.1 (25.7)	51.6 (27.1)	0.382
Pain after procedure (mm VAS)	29.2 (25.9)	32.2 (27.8)	0.715
Heart rate during procedure (bpm)	82.6 (14.0)	83.3 (13.7)	0.833
Patient recommend a friend (%)	97	93	0.617
Patient satisfaction (%)			0.958
Very satisfied	59	62	
Satisfied	31	31	
Normal	8	5	
Dissatisfied	2	2	
Very dissatisfied	0	0	
Doctor refuses same procedure in same setting for this patient (%)	5	2	0.610
Satisfaction doctor (%)			0.165
Very satisfied	50	60	
Satisfied	29	20	
Normal	13	5	
Dissatisfied	0	10	
Very dissatisfied	8	5	
Complications (%)	0	0	NS
STAI 1 score after procedure	34.1 (8.6)	35.9 (9.6)	0.491
STAI 1 score difference	6.3 (12.8)	5.7 (10.9)	0.820

Data are expressed as mean (SD) or percentage
NS not significant

Colposcopy

Eighty participants were included, 42 participants in the music group and 38 participants in the control group. In each group, 3 participants did not meet the inclusion criteria because no biopsy or LLETZ was performed during colposcopy. These participants were excluded from further analyses. Therefore, 74 participants (39 music group and 35 control group) were considered for statistical analyses. One participant of the music group refused music during the procedure (Fig. 2).

Baseline characteristics are shown in Table 3. A significant difference between the groups was found for dysmenorrhoea (24.1 (24.8) mm vs. 38.2 (22.9) mm, $p = .013$) and the performance of a cervical block (72 vs. 47%, $p = .031$). For all other characteristics, no difference was found ($p > .05$). No significant difference was found for pain during the procedure between the music group and control group (32.4 (24.3) mm vs. 31.6 (27.3) mm, $p = .826$). Secondary outcomes were also similar, including heart rate and anxiety during the procedure, pain after the procedure and satisfaction of the

patient and doctor ($p > .05$) (Table 4). No complications occurred.

In five cases in the music group (12%), the doctor noticed he or she was disturbed by the music during the procedure. In three of these cases, the volume of the music was too loud; in one case, the music was not of the genre preferred by the doctor; and in the last case, no explanation was given. In one case in the music group, the doctor was dissatisfied without mentioning a reason (3%). The most popular music genre chosen in the music group was pop music (67%), followed by classical music (18%) and spa music (15%).

In addition to the intention-to-treat analysis, a per-protocol analysis was performed only for the primary outcome because one participant refused music. Still no difference was found in pain between the groups (33.3 (24.0) mm vs. 30.7 (27.4) mm, $p = .579$). Dysmenorrhoea and performance of a cervical block were both different between the groups (Table 3). After performing a linear regression, we concluded that both variables are confounders for the primary outcome. Correction of these

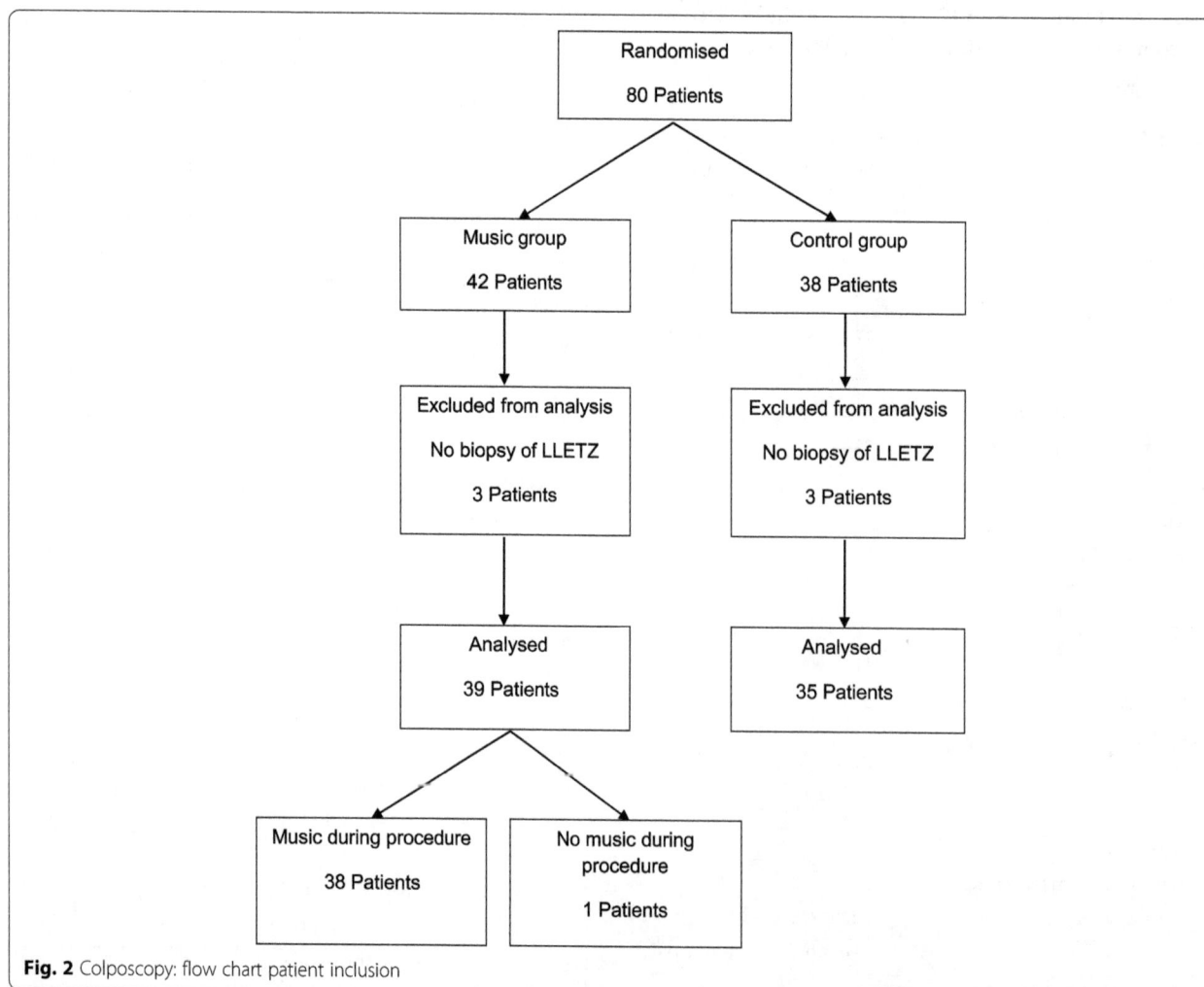

Fig. 2 Colposcopy: flow chart patient inclusion

Table 3 Colposcopy: patient characteristics

	Music group N = 39	Control group N = 35
Age (y)	38.8 (8.3)	38.9 (10.7)
Height (m)	1.69 (0.06)	1.70 (0.06)
Weight (kg)	69.0 (13.3)	69.6 (17.8)
Body mass index	24.0 (4.1)	24.1 (6.1)
Dysmenorrhea (mm VAS)	24.1 (24.8)	38.2 (22.9)
Expected pain (mm VAS)	43.1 (23.9)	49.4 (22.1)
Heart rate before procedure (bpm)	78.2 (15.1)	82.1 (14.8)
Use of a painkiller (%)	8	9
Use of cervical block (%)	72	47
Pap smear score (PAP) (%)		
PAP 2	29	26
PAP 3a	48	48
PAP 3b	23	26
Colposcopic impression (%)		
Normal	6	7
Low grade	47	64
High grade	44	29
Carcinoma	3	0
Difficulty of procedure (%)		
Very easy	47	65
Easy	29	26
Normal	18	0
Difficult	3	6
Very difficult	3	3
Intervention (%)		
Cold biopsy	28	54
Hot biopsy	3	0
LLETZ	69	46
STAI 1 score before procedure	42.1 (12.3)	42.6 (8.7)
STAI 2 score	34.9 (10.1)	34.3 (7.9)

Data are expressed as mean (SD) or percentage

Table 4 Colposcopy: results

	Music group N = 39	Control group N = 35	P value
Pain during procedure (mm VAS)	32.4 (24.3)	31.6 (27.3)	0.826
Pain after procedure (mm VAS)	23.6 (21.5)	27.6 (25.6)	0.637
Heart rate during procedure (bpm)	82.4 (16.1)	82.7 (15.1)	0.929
Patient recommends a friend (%)	95	88	0.408
Patient satisfaction (%)			0.571
Very satisfied	77	79	
Satisfied	15	15	
Normal	3	3	
Dissatisfied	5	0	
Very dissatisfied	0	3	
Doctor refuses same procedure in same setting for this patient (%)	5	3	1.000
Satisfaction doctor (%)			0.769
Very satisfied	74	79	
Satisfied	18	15	
Normal	5	6	
Dissatisfied	3	0	
Very dissatisfied	0	0	
Complications (%)	0	0	NS
STAI 1 score after procedure	38.4 (15.3)	35.5 (9.6)	0.584
STAI 1 score difference	3.8 (14.4)	7.5 (10.2)	0.463

Data are expressed as mean (SD) or percentage
NS not significant

variables for pain during the procedure resulted in the same conclusion, i.e. no statistical significance between the two groups (p = .806). A per-protocol analysis with correction for these two confounders showed the same result (p = .563).

Discussion
Main findings
The aim of this study was to measure the additional effect of music in gynaecological office procedures on patients' level of pain, anxiety and satisfaction during and after the procedure in daily practice. The experience of the doctor was evaluated as well. We found no positive effect of music, neither in hysteroscopy nor in colposcopy.

Strength and limitations
To our knowledge, this is the first randomized controlled trial investigating the effect of music in gynaecological office procedures taking into account the opinion of the doctor. Moreover, we explored the additional effect of music in daily practice. Methods that were already used to improve patients' experience remained unchanged with respect to the standard procedure to increase external validity. Another asset of this study is its use of single-blind testing. The participants in this study were not informed about the role of music in this study; they were only informed about the goal to improve patients' experience during office procedures in a non-invasive manner with a controlled trial. This is unique in comparison to other studies.

A limitation of this study is that waiting time and duration of the procedure were not examined. Waiting time can possibly change the anxiety and pain level of the patient and prolonged duration of the procedure can increase the dissatisfaction of the patient and the doctor. Another limitation is the difference in experience between the doctors. In both groups, hysteroscopy and colposcopy, the doctors consisted of both gynaecologists and residents. According to the literature, pain scores can be lower when an experienced doctor performs the procedure [17]. iPod speakers were used to play the music which prevented double-blind testing. However, during the pilot study, headphones turned out to impede the interaction between patient and doctor. For this reason, headphones were waived.

Interpretation

Despite randomization, we found a difference between dysmenorrhoea and the use of a cervical block between the groups in the patients receiving a colposcopy. The women in the music group had less dysmenorrhoea, but more of them received cervical anaesthesia (Table 3). Significantly, less dysmenorrhoea could imply a higher pain threshold in that group which may confound the primary outcome. The difference in cervical anaesthesia could be explained by the difference in intervention between the groups (p = .056). Women who underwent cold biopsies did not receive a cervical block in contrast with electrical biopsies and LLETZ. The cervical block given in this trial consists of an anaesthetic (articaine) and a vasoconstrictor (epinephrine). According to Gajjar et al., receiving local anaesthetics and a vasoconstrictor could possibly reduce pain experience in women undergoing colposcopy. Therefore, the difference in dysmenorrhoea and the use of a cervical block between the groups is relevant. For this reason, a correction was performed for these confounders. Still, no difference was found between the music group and control group. Thus, the result remained unchanged.

Previous research in music for pain relief showed a large difference in results with high heterogeneity in studies as described in the systematic review of Cepeda et al. A positive effect of music in gynaecological office procedures was found in randomized controlled trials performed by Angioli et al. and Chan et al. However, another randomized controlled trial by Danhauer et al. found no difference between the music group and the control group for pain, anxiety or satisfaction. These results are similar to the results in this current trial. Danhauer et al. suggest that their results are probably different from the results of the two previously mentioned trials because of the limited choice of five music genres, the number of physicians and the difficulty in hearing what the doctor was saying because of the headphones. However, according to a systematic review, the decline in pain intensity is similar in studies wherein patients selected the type of music and in those wherein patients did not select their music [9]. Instead of the headphones used in the trial

of Danhauer et al., iPods with speakers were used in our study, giving the same result.

The potential positive effect of music may have been overpowered by the multimodal approach in our study. The use of information leaflets, analgesics, the interaction between patient and doctor, a nurse to offer emotional support and the use of videoscopy are all used in daily practice. For that reason, they remained unchanged with respect to the standard procedure in this trial. Information leaflets increase the patient's knowledge and therefore could improve the patient's experience [7]. The value of oral analgesics is limited [3, 18], but local anaesthesia could be effective at achieving pain relief [3]. A monitor for videocolposcopy, allowing the patient to view the procedure, reduces patient anxiety and pain during routine colposcopic examination [16]. Finally, active emotional support can reduce pain [19].

Another explanation for our results, which is possibly associated with the multimodal approach described above, is the relatively low pain score in our trial. The control group in the colposcopy group showed lower scores in comparison with the trials of Chan et al. and Danhauer et al., namely 31.6 in this trial versus 50.3 and 51.7 in the other trials. The power analysis and expected pain reduction in this trial were based on these results from previous trials. Moreover, a score of VAS 40 is frequently used in the literature as a pain threshold [17, 20, 21]. Therefore, with an initial pain score lower than 40, the clinical relevance of pain relief is doubtful. Thus, we believe that our multimodal approach already greatly improves patients' experience and possibly hereby camouflages the potential effect of music.

We found no difference in the satisfaction of the doctors between the music group and the control group for both hysteroscopy and colposcopy. However, some doctors mentioned that they were disturbed by the music; one case in the hysteroscopy group (3%) and five cases in the colposcopy group (12%). The difference between the two groups can be explained by the different doctors performing a hysteroscopy or a colposcopy. Despite the fact that the volume could be adjusted, the reasons they mentioned for their irritation were the volume of the music and the fact that it was not the kind of music they enjoy. Therefore, perhaps the use of more neutral music set at a lower volume would satisfy these doctors. Unfortunately, we did not examine the music preferences of the doctors.

Conclusion

In conclusion, our study showed no positive effect of music regarding pain, anxiety or satisfaction for office hysteroscopy and colposcopy. We believe a multimodal approach should be used to decrease patient distress in terms of pain and anxiety, with or without music.

Funding

This study did not receive any funding.

Authors' contributions

NM contributed to the protocol development, data collection, data analysis and manuscript writing. IMAR contributed to the data collection and manuscript writing. SAS contributed to the protocol development and data collection. EHMNW contributed to the protocol development, data collection and manuscript writing. JWMM contributed to the manuscript writing. MYB contributed to the protocol development and manuscript writing. All authors read and approved the final manuscript.

Competing interests

The authors declare that they have no competing interests.

Author details

[1]Department of Obstetrics and Gynaecology, Máxima Medical Centre, Veldhoven, The Netherlands. [2]Department of Obstetrics and Gynaecology, VieCuri Medical Centre, Venlo, The Netherlands. [3]Department of Obstetrics and Gynaecology, Rode Kruis Hospital, Beverwijk, The Netherlands. [4]Department of Obstetrics and Gynaecology, GROW—School for Oncology and Developmental Biology, Maastricht University Medical Centre, Maastricht, The Netherlands.

References

1. Bettocchi S, Nappi L, Ceci O, Selvaggi L (2004) Office hysteroscopy. Obstet Gynecol Clin N Am 31:641–654
2. Nagele F, OÇonnor H, Davies A, et al (1996) 2500 Outpatient diagnostic hysteroscopies. Obstet Gynecol 88(1):87–92
3. Gajjar K, Martin-Hirsch PPL, Bryant A, Owens GL (2016) Pain relief for women with cervical intraepithelial neoplasia undergoing colposcopy treatment. Cochrane Database Syst Rev 18;7:CD006120.doi:10.1002/14651858.CD006120
4. Marteau TM, Walker P, Giles J et al (1990) Anxieties in women undergoing colposcopy. BJOG 97:859–861
5. Gambadauro P, Navaratnarajah R, Carli V (2015) Anxiety at outpatient hysteroscopy. Gynec Surg 12(3):189–196
6. Ahmad G, O'Flynn H, Attarbashi S, et al (2010) Pain relief for outpatient hysteroscopy. Cochrane Database Syst Rev 10;(11):CD007710. doi: 10.1002/14651858.CD007710
7. Galaal K, Bryant A, Deane KHO et al (2011) Interventions for reducing anxiety in women undergoing colposcopy. Cochrane Database Syst Rev 7(12):CD006013. doi:10.1002/14651858.CD006013
8. De Carvalho Schettini JA, Ramos de Amorim MM, Ribeiro Costa AA, Albuquerque Neto LC et al (2007) Pain evaluation in outpatients undergoing diagnostic anesthesia-free hysteroscopy in a teaching hospital: a cohort study. J Minim Invasive Gynecol 14(6):729–735
9. Cepeda MS, Carr DB, Lau J, Alvarez H (2006) Music for pain relief. Cochrane Database Syst Rev 19;(2):CD004843
10. Wang MW, Zhang LY, Zhang YL, et al (2014) Effect of music in endoscopy procedures: systematic review and meta-analysis of randomized controlled trials. Pain Med 15(10):1786–1794. doi:10.1111/pme.12514
11. Danhauer SC, Marler B, Rutherford CA et al (2007) Music or guided imagery for women undergoing colposcopy: a randomized controlled study of effects on anxiety, perceived pain, and patient satisfaction. J Low Genit Tract Dis 11(1):39–45
12. Chan YM, Lee PW, NG TY, et al (2003) The use of music to reduce anxiety for patients undergoing colposcopy: a randomised trial. Gynecol Oncol 91(1):213–217
13. Angioli R, De Cicco Nardone C, Plotti F, et al. (2014) Use of music to reduce anxiety during office hysteroscopy: prospective randomized trial. J Minim Invasive Gynecol 21(3):454–459. doi:10.1016/j.jmig.2013.07.020
14. Pluyter JR, Buzink SN, Rutkowski AF, Jakimowics JJ (2010) Do absorption and realistic distraction influence performance of component task surgical procedure? Surg Endosc 24(4):902–907. doi:10.1007/s00464-009-0689-7
15. Way TJ, Long A, Weihing J, et al (2013) Effect of noise on auditory processing in the operating room. J Am Coll Surg 216(5):933–938. doi:10.1016/j.jamcollsurg.2012.12.048
16. Walsh JC, Curtis R, Mylotte M (2004) Anxiety levels in women attending a colposcopy clinic: a randomised trial of an educational intervention using video colposcopy. Patient Educ Couns 55(2):247–251
17. Campo R, Molinas CR, Rombouts L et al (2005) Prospective multicentre randomized controlled trial to evaluate factors influencing the success rate of office diagnostic hysteroscopy. Hum Reprod 20(1):258–263
18. Tam WH, Yuen PM (2001) Use of diclofenac as an analgesic in outpatient hysteroscopy: a randomized, double-blind, placebo-controlled study. Fertil Steril 76(5):1070–1072
19. Ireland LD, Allen RH (2016) Pain management for gynecologic procedures in the office. Obstet Gynecol Surv 71(2):89–98. doi:10.1097/OGX.0000000000000272
20. Cepeda MS, Africano JM, Polo R et al (2003) What decline in pain intensity is meaningful to patients with acute pain? Pain 105(1–2):151–157
21. Litta P, Cosmi E, Saccardi C et al (2008) Outpatient operative polypectomy using a 5 mm-hysteroscope without anaesthesia and/or analgesia: advantages and limits. Eur J Obstet Gynecol Reprod Biol 139(2):210–214. doi: 10.1016/j.ejogrb.2007.11.008

9

Applying a statistical method in transvaginal ultrasound training: lessons from the learning curve cumulative summation test (LC-CUSUM) for endometriosis mapping

Vered H. Eisenberg[1*], Juan L. Alcazar[2], Nissim Arbib[1], Eyal Schiff[1], Reuven Achiron[1], Motti Goldenberg[1] and David Soriano[1]

Abstract

Background: Methods available for assessing the learning curve, such as a predefined number of procedures or direct mentoring are lacking. Our aim was to describe the use of a statistical method to identify the minimal training length of an experienced sonographer, newly trained in deep infiltrating endometriosis (DIE) mapping by evaluating the learning curve of transvaginal ultrasound (TVUS) in the preoperative assessment of endometriosis.

Methods: A retrospective study in a tertiary referral center for endometriosis. Reports and stored data from TVUS scans performed by one operator with training in general gynecological ultrasound, but not in endometriosis mapping, were analyzed retrospectively for patients who subsequently underwent laparoscopy, which served as a reference standard. The performance of TVUS was assessed for the following sites: endometriomas, bladder, vagina, pouch of Douglas, bowel and uterosacral ligaments, and correlated with laparoscopic findings. Sensitivity, specificity, PPV, NPV, and accuracy were calculated, and the operator's diagnostic performance was assessed using the learning curve cumulative summation test (LC-CUSUM).

Results: Data from 94 women were available for analysis. The learning curve using the LC-CUSUM graph showed that the sonographer reached the predefined level of proficiency in detecting endometriosis lesions after 20, 26, 32, 31, 38, and 44 examinations for endometriomas, bladder nodules, vaginal nodules, pouch of Douglas obliteration, bowel nodules, and uterosacral ligament nodules, respectively.

Conclusions: LC-CUSUM allows monitoring of individual performance during the learning process of new methodologies. This study shows that a sonographer trained in general gynecologic ultrasonography, who devotes time to learn TVUS for DIE mapping, can achieve proficiency for diagnosing the major types of endometriotic lesions after examining less than 50 patients who subsequently undergo surgery in a training setting.

Keywords: Transvaginal ultrasound, Endometriomas, Deep infiltrative endometriosis, Learning curve, LC-CUSUM, Individualized assessment

* Correspondence: veredeis@bezeqint.net
[1]Department of Obstetrics and Gynecology, Sheba Medical Center, Tel-Hashomer, Tel-Aviv University, 52621 Ramat Gan, Israel
Full list of author information is available at the end of the article

Background

Endometriosis is a common benign gynecological condition with a prevalence rate of up to 15% [1] in reproductive age women. It is defined as the presence of endometrial tissue, glands and stroma outside the endometrial cavity. The clinical manifestations of endometriosis vary widely and may include secondary dysmenorrhea, chronic pelvic pain, dyspareunia, dyschezia, intermittent diarrhea and constipation, hematochezia, dysuria, pain on urination, irritable bladder, and hematuria. The mean age at diagnosis of endometriosis is 25–29 years and may be higher in women who present with infertility rather than pelvic pain [2]. Deep infiltrating endometriosis (DIE) is defined as endometriotic lesions that penetrate more than 5 mm from under the peritoneum [1]. These may be multifocal and are most commonly found in the uterosacral ligaments, posterior vaginal fornix, retro cervical region, rectovaginal septum, vesicouterine pouch, bladder, and anterior wall of the recto sigmoid.

The available pre-operative diagnostic tools include the patient's history, pelvic examination, transvaginal ultrasonography (TVUS), and magnetic resonance imaging (MRI) [3, 4]. A negative imaging workup does not exclude endometriosis. An average diagnostic delay from symptom onset till definitive diagnosis can be up to 12 years [5, 6]. Chronic pelvic pain and infertility significantly affect the patient's quality of life and carry a high economic burden [7]. It is imperative that a prompt and accurate diagnosis is reached in order to bypass the diagnostic delay and refer patients for adequate care by endometriosis specialists in dedicated centers [8], to improve counseling and preoperative preparation and to determine the multidisciplinary team to be present in order to allow definitive surgical treatment.

While it is recognized that TVS should be the first-line imaging examination for the preoperative work-up of patients [9], its performance for diagnosing endometriosis and more specifically endometriomas, has been shown to be accurate only in the hands of experienced sonographers [3, 10–14]. Most experienced sonographers will easily identify endometriotic cysts [4, 12, 13], whereas sonographic diagnosis of DIE lesions requires skill and dedication, after which reported accuracy can be as high as 99% [3, 4, 8–11, 14]. The determination of how much experience is required to reach proficiency in the diagnosis of DIE is extremely important for planning training programs, and is not sufficiently known [4, 8].

Biau et al. introduced the learning curve cumulative summation test (LC-CUSUM) that was specifically designed to determine when a level of proficiency has been reached. The LC-CUSUM is a statistical tool which is performed in order to indicate when a process has reached a predefined level of performance [15–17]. The importance of establishing a learning curve is significant for quality assurance, patient safety, and cost analysis, and has been previously described for varied procedures, in surgery and in obstetrics and gynecology.

The purpose of this study was to determine the learning curve of TVUS in the preoperative assessment of endometriosis and in particular DIE by an experienced sonographer, newly trained in endometriosis mapping.

Methods

This study evaluated the performance of dedicated TVUS for the diagnosis of endometriosis and DIE. All the examinations were performed by the same sonographer with previous experience in gynecological ultrasound but without previous experience in DIE mapping expect for an introductory course. She had previously performed more than 10,000 gynecological general examinations over the years but had not performed dedicated endometriosis scanning apart from the incidental endometriomas and no specific DIE scanning. She had undergone training and learning DIE mapping as described by previous authors [3, 8–11, 14] during 2010–2011. Starting from May 2011, all patients referred to our endometriosis center underwent TVS as preoperative assessment. Out of 250 patients who were examined during the study period, the 94 who underwent surgery at our institution were included in the analysis. The remaining women either did not qualify for surgery or were operated on at another institution. The indications for surgery were intractable pain or infertility. The patient's clinical history and symptoms were obtained from the electronic hospital records. These data included patient's age, body mass index (BMI, kg/m^2), parity, previous cesarean sections, smoking history, dysmenorrhea, dyspareunia, urinary and gastrointestinal symptoms, infertility history, fertility treatment and type, and number of previous IVF cycles.

The TVUS were carried out using a transvaginal 5–9 MHz probe with 2D/3D capabilities (Voluson 730 or E6, GE Medical Systems). Images were interpreted in real-time and were stored for later analysis. The examination was performed in a standardized way for all patients. This included a thorough evaluation of all pelvic viscerae, for lesions consistent with endometriosis: endometriomas, tubal adhesions, vagina, posterior and lateral vaginal fornices, the retro cervical area with torus uterinum, the parametria laterally, the rectovaginal septum, the bowel, peritoneal surfaces, bladder and vesicouterine pouch, and uterosacral ligaments, as previously described by other authors [18–20]. Organ mobility was evaluated in the anterior and posterior compartment. Movement of the posterior surface of the uterus, cervix or vagina in relation to the bowel was examined in order to determine pouch of Douglas obliteration, previously described as the "sliding sign" [21, 22]. For a more thorough description of the methodology, please refer to the Appendix.

The reference standard for diagnosis was defined as surgical findings during laparoscopy. Success of the ultrasound procedure was defined as agreement between TVUS findings and surgical findings. All of the patients underwent laparoscopic surgery by trained endoscopic surgeons in a multidisciplinary team which included also urological and colorectal surgeons as required. Pelvic endometriosis was diagnosed based on any of the following: presence of endometrial tissue (endometrial glands and stroma) in pathological examination in at least one resected lesion, direct visualization of deep pelvic lesions of endometriosis associated with only fibrosis at biopsy, direct visualization of deep pelvic lesions of endometriosis which could not be resected, or complete cul-de-sac obliteration secondary to endometriosis which was deemed unresectable, because of a significant surgical risk to adjacent structures. The severity of endometriosis at surgery was evaluated retrospectively by one of the co-authors who were blinded to the ultrasound report, based on the Revised American Society for Reproductive Medicine (ASRM) Classification [23] and the histopathological reports were reviewed. The findings at TVUS were compared with the descriptive visual findings at surgery. Pathological confirmation of the presence of endometriosis in resected lesions was obtained later but was not a prerequisite for inclusion as surgical findings are those that determine severity.

Statistical analysis

Statistical analysis was performed using SPSS software (SPSS, IBM Corporation, Chicago, IL, USA). Continuous variables were expressed as means ± SD or medians, while categorical variables were expressed as frequencies and percentages. Sensitivity, specificity, positive predictive value (PPV), negative predictive value (NPV), and accuracy were calculated for the diagnosis of endometriomas, bladder nodules, vaginal nodules, pouch of Douglas obliteration, bowel nodules (including rectum, sigma, and Douglas pouch), and uterosacral ligament nodules with the results of laparoscopic surgery as the reference standard for diagnosis. The analysis was performed by anatomic location. Statistical significance was set at $P < 0.05$.

A standard CUSUM test monitors a sequential procedure with ability to reject the null hypothesis H_0 that the process is in control [15], while the alternative hypothesis H_1 is that the process is out of control. The process is deemed acceptable as long as the CUSUM score remains below a limit known as h. The learning curve summation (LC-CUSUM) test was used to assess whether the process has reached a predefined level of performance by signaling when the process can be considered to be in control [16, 17]. The LC-CUSUM

sequentially tests the inverted hypotheses, the null hypothesis, namely, inadequate performance (H_0), against the alternative hypothesis, namely, adequate performance (H_1). It computes a score, from the successive outcomes, with successes yielding an increase in the score and failures yielding a decrease in the score, i.e., negative scores for correct interventions and positive scores for incorrect results are calculated as previously reported by Biau et al. [16, 17]. Once the summation score reaches a predefined level (h), the test rejects the null hypothesis in favor of the alternative hypothesis, which indicates an adequate performance level. The LU-CUSUM remains responsive at all times, so that as performance improves the trainee do not need to compensate unnecessarily for previous failures. Acceptable (P_1) and unacceptable (P_0) failure rates, the required level of performance and the properties of the test have to be set. Acceptable and unacceptable failure rates for this study were set at 10% ($P_1 = 0.10$) and 25% ($P_0 = 0.25$), respectively. These limits were chosen assuming that the pooled failure rates for an expert examiner could be around 10–25%, taking into account both false positive and false negative results. The failure rates were chosen based on the accuracy of TVUS for diagnosing endometriomas and DIE in experienced hands [24–26]. Type I (α) and type II (β) error rates were set at 0.1. A limit $h = 2.0$ was chosen from computer simulations which means that the risk of declaring a trainee proficient when his or her performance is inadequate was limited to 10% over 100 procedures. CUSUM values are plotted on the y-axis, and the number of examinations is plotted on the x-axis. Horizontal lines are plotted at regular intervals on the y-axis, defining $h0$ and $h1$ for the spacing between acceptable and unacceptable boundary lines, respectively. Competence is declared when the plot falls below two consecutive boundary lines.

Ethical approval was given from our local research ethics committee. Informed consent was not required as the ultrasound assessment was offered as part of standard clinical care at our center.

Results

Ninety-four women were included in the analysis, all of whom underwent TVUS and subsequent laparoscopic surgery over the study period. Demographic data and patient symptoms are presented in Table 1. The median disease severity (ASRM) score at surgery was 43 (range 1–148), and the median ASRM stage was 4 (range 1–4): 15 (16%) patients had stage I, 4 (4.3%) stage II, 19 (20.2%) stage III and 56 (59.6%) had stage IV disease. All of the patients described long standing symptoms before being referred to our center. 49 (52%) women had had previous surgery for endometriosis.

Table 1 Demographic data and symptoms in 94 patients who underwent transvaginal sonography (TVUS) and subsequent laparoscopic surgery for endometriosis

Variable	Value (n = 94)
Age, mean ± SD, years (range)	34.1 ± 6.0 (20–47)
BMI, mean ± SD, kg/m² (range)	23.6 ± 4.8 (16.9–40.2)
Parity, median (range)	0 (0–6)
Previous cesarean section (%)	12 (12.8)
Smoker (%)	28 (29.8)
Dysmenorrhea (%)	87 (92.6)
Dyspareunia (%)	60 (63.8)
Urinary complaints (%)	27 (28.7)
Gastrointestinal complaints (%)	51 (55.3)
Infertility (%)	34 (36.1)
Previous IVF treatments (%)	24 (25.5)
Number of IVF cycles, median (range)	5 (0–16)

Based on the gold standard of findings during surgery, 57 (60.6%) of women had endometriomas, 11 (11.7%) had bladder nodules, 39 (41.5%) had vaginal nodules, 48 (51.1%) had pouch of Douglas obliteration, 20 (21.3%) had bowel nodules (rectum, bowel, and pouch of Douglas), and 50 (53.2%) had uterosacral ligament involvement. Surgical findings in the 94 patients with pelvic endometriosis along with the sensitivity, specificity, PPV, NPV, and accuracy for TVUS findings and agreement with endometriosis findings at laparoscopy are presented in Table 2.

LC-CUSUM analysis

The cumulative summation test for the learning curve (LC-CUSUM) graphs for TVUS for endometriomas and DIE in our study is presented in Fig. 1.

Endometriomas

There were 57 endometriomas at surgery. The sonographer diagnosed all of the endometriomas correctly. There were also other lesions including one borderline serous tumor, one peritoneal cyst, one corpus luteum cyst, and one multicystic benign mesothelioma with decidual changes. None of these lesions was mistaken for an endometrioma, and they were all recognized as other lesions. Based on the LU-CUSUM curve it, takes the sonographer 20 examinations to become proficient at diagnosing endometriomas correctly.

Bladder lesions

Eleven patients had bladder lesions at laparoscopy with penetration of the bladder wall and detrusor involvement (Fig. 2). The accuracy for their diagnosis was 99%. Based on the LU-CUSUM curve, it takes 26 examinations to become proficient at diagnosing bladder nodules correctly. There was one failed diagnosis by the sonographer in the fifth case from study start, the lesion was very small and was not resected by the surgeon due to lack of symptoms.

Vaginal lesions

Thirty-nine women had vaginal nodules located in the vaginal fornix or rectovaginal septum. There was one false positive diagnosis by the sonographer and three false negatives. The false negatives were found to be lesions in the border between the rectovaginal and recto sigmoid area, which the surgeon described as rectovaginal lesions but which the sonographer classified as recto sigmoid bowel lesions. In all of these cases, the main symptom was infertility rather than posterior compartment complaints. The adhesions were so severe that the lesions were left in place in order to prevent causing extensive damage since there were no associated symptoms. The sonographer diagnosed the lesions accurately in 96% of the patients. Based on the LU-CUSUM curve, it takes 32 examinations to become proficient at diagnosing vaginal lesions (Fig. 3).

Pouch of Douglas obliteration

Forty-eight (51.1%) of women had pouch of Douglas obliteration. The graphs for vaginal nodules and pouch of Douglas obliteration are very similar. There were three false negative diagnoses, which were the same cases

Table 2 Surgical findings in 94 patients with pelvic endometriosis. Sensitivity, specificity, PPV, NPV, and accuracy for TVUS findings and agreement with endometriosis findings at laparoscopy

Disease location	Cases (n = 94)	Sensitivity (%)	Specificity (%)	PPV (%)	NPV (%)	Accuracy (%)
Endometriomas	57 (60.6%)	100	100	100	100	100
Bladder nodules	11 (11.7%)	90.9	100	100	98.8	98.9
Vaginal nodules	39 (41.5%)	92.3	98.2	97.3	94.7	95.7
Pouch of Douglas obliteration	48 (51.1%)	93.8	91.3	91.8	93.3	92.5
Bowel lesions (rectum, sigma, POD)	20 (21.3%)	80	98.6	94.1	94.8	94.7
Uterosacral ligaments	50 (53.2%)	60	70.5	69.8	60.8	64.9

PPV positive predictive value, *NPV* negative predictive value, *TVUS* transvaginal ultrasound

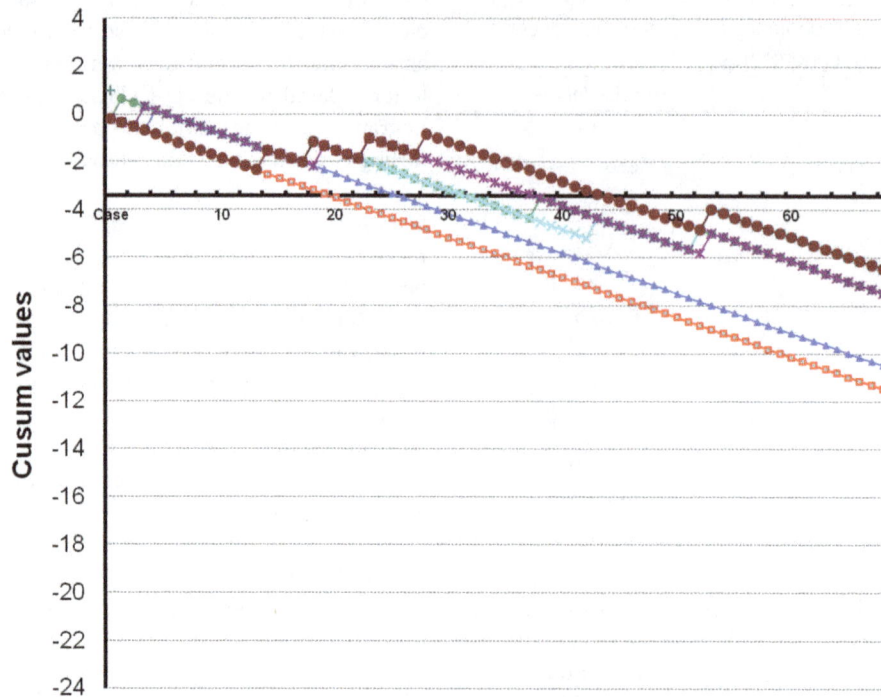

Fig. 1 Cumulative summation test for the learning curve (LC-CUSUM) graphs for TVUS for endometriomas and deep infiltrative endometriosis. The vertical axis shows the CUSUM values, the horizontal axis shows the case number. Dotted horizontal lines show acceptable/unacceptable boundary lines of the CUSUM score. As long as the score remains over the limit h (dotted line), the operator is not considered as proficient, whereas when the LC-CUSUM score crosses this limit, he is considered to have become proficient. As long as the score remains under the limit, the operator is considered to maintain an acceptable performance. Performance was reached after 20 exams for endometriomas (red line), 26 exams for bladder nodules (blue), 32 exams for vaginal nodules (green), 31 exams for pouch of Douglas obliteration (turquoise), 38 exams for bowel nodules (purple), and 44 exams for uterosacral ligament nodules (dark red)

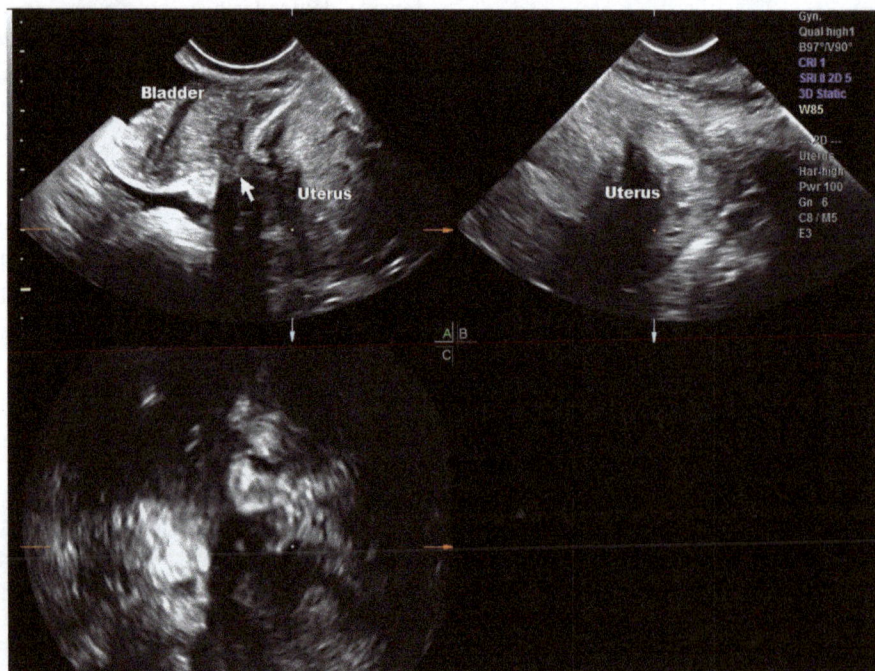

Fig. 2 Multiplanar 3D image of TVUS of bladder detrusor endometriosis penetrating from the anterior uterine wall. See hourglass appearance of nodule penetration (arrow). The uterus is affected by adenomyosis

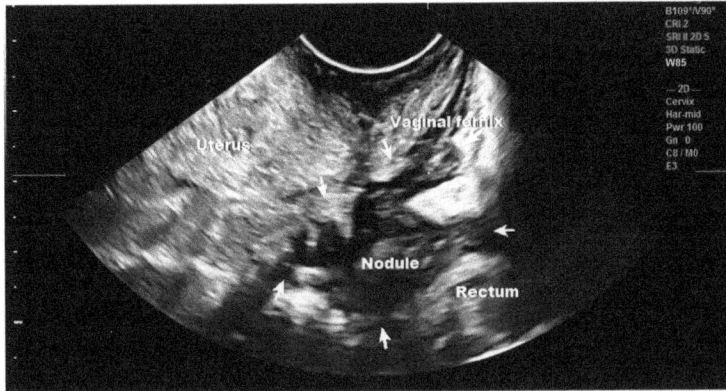

Fig. 3 TVUS of a large vaginal nodule extending to the rectosigmoid. The sonographer interpreted this lesion as a rectosigmoid bowel lesion while the surgeon described it as a vaginal lesion. Arrows show extent of lesion

described above. There were four false positives by the sonographer. Based on the LU-CUSUM curve, it takes the sonographer 31 examinations to become proficient at diagnosing pouch of Douglas obliteration correctly.

Bowel lesions
There were 20 lesions located in the rectum, sigmoid colon or higher pouch of Douglas. Four high lesions were missed by the sonographer, and these were located diffusely in the bowel far from the pouch of Douglas and were not accessed by the transducer. There was one false positive diagnosis by the sonographer early on in the

learning procedure in case four. Based on the LU-CUSUM, curve it takes the sonographer 38 examinations to become proficient at diagnosing bowel lesions correctly (Fig. 4).

Uterosacral ligaments
Fifty patients had lesions in at least one of the uterosacral ligaments, which the sonographer diagnosed correctly in 65% of the patients. There were 20 false negative diagnosis by the sonographer were the lesions were deep in adhesions so that the uterosacral ligament was poorly visualized. Not all were resectable and were

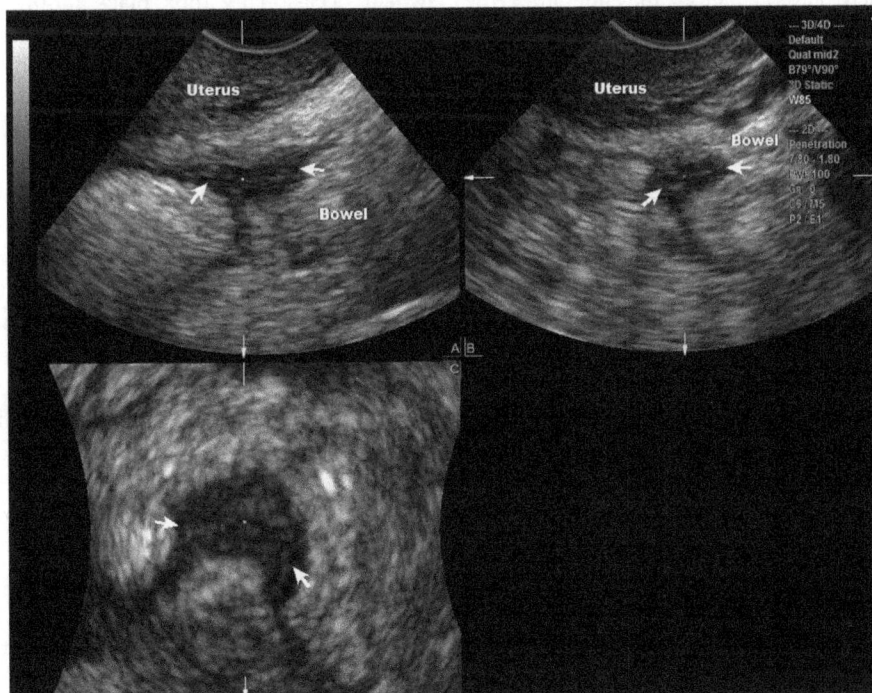

Fig. 4 Multiplanar 3D image of TVUS of a bowel nodule behind the cervix. Nodule is shown in arrows

thus determined based on visualization during surgery. There were 13 false positives where lesions were assumed to occur in large conglomerates of adhesions but were not found after the adhesions were dissolved. In both of these situations, this did not affect the actual surgical procedure which was determined by the presence of vaginal, bowel nodules or pouch of Douglas obliteration. Based on the LU-CUSUM curve, it takes the sonographer 44 examinations to become proficient at diagnosing uterosacral ligament lesions correctly.

Discussion

TVUS is increasingly utilized in the many developing subspecialties of gynecological imaging. Some of these fields entail specialized and structured training programs. Ultrasound diagnosis of endometriosis is such a developing field and is now considered to be the first-line imaging modality for disease mapping [9]. Despite this, it is not widely known up to this time how many clinical examinations are required in order to train an experienced ultrasonographer to be proficient in endometriosis imaging. This study shows that a sonographer trained in general gynecological ultrasound, who devotes time to learn TVUS for DIE mapping, can apparently achieve proficiency for diagnosing the varied types of endometriotic lesions within 44 examinations provided that the patient subsequently undergoes surgery and that feedback is available.

Learning a new procedure carries the risk of unacceptable standards, therefore continuous supervision and monitoring is required until an acceptable level of performance is reached. Several factors may influence the learning process, these being the procedure, the trainee, the mentor, the setting, all of which will affect the time and number of procedures required to complete the learning process [17].

Tammaa et al. [8] recently described the length of time required to become proficient in diagnosing pouch of Douglas obliteration and deep infiltrating endometriosis of the rectum with TVUS. However, their study defined the expert sonographer as the reference standard rather than laparoscopic surgery [8]. Bazot et al. [4] described their results of the learning curve of four inexperienced trainees in the diagnosis of endometriomas, finding LC-CUSUM to be adequate for this purpose, but their reference standard was also the expert sonographer rather than surgery [4]. Saba et al. [27] described the learning curve in the detection of ovarian and deep endometriosis by using MRI findings and by comparing them with surgical results. In this retrospective study, datasets were analyzed by the same performer before surgery and re-analyzed 12 and 24 months later to determine proficiency and results were compared between the analyses. They found that the performer's expertise over time increased diagnostic accuracy, but that it takes at least

1 year of intensive training and at least 100 exams of patients with endometriosis, in order to acquire adequate experience. Alcazar et al. [28] evaluated an intensive training program for ultrasound diagnosis of adnexal masses using LC-CUSUM graph analyses. They found that this methodology can be used in the evaluation of the feasibility of a training program [28].

Recently, Piessens et al. [29] described their experience with a sonographer learning endometriosis screening in just 1 week of specialized training. Using the LU-CUSUM, this sonographer achieved competency within 38 scans for POD obliteration and 36 scans for bowel lesions. The study was also performed by an experienced gynecological sonographer, who had not previously performed DIE mapping. Overall, more than 100 examinations were performed [29]. Our findings also lend support to their findings, while we additionally described uterosacral ligament evaluation.

Our study has several strengths and limitations which should be acknowledged: a significant strength is the use of a validated statistical model for assessing the learning curve, the LU-CUSUM, which was described [17]. However, the acceptable and unacceptable failures were chosen arbitrarily based on previous reports. These values can be modified according to recommendations which are applicable to the specified procedure [17].

A significant strength of the present study is the fact that the analysis was performed against the reference standard of surgery with histo-pathological confirmation. The definitive diagnosis was only reached after surgery, which occasionally took place months after the ultrasound exam. The performance of these recommended 44 exams, with adequate surgical feedback, can take time depending on how many endometriosis surgeries are performed each week. In our study, this took well over a year and approximately 250 scans overall.

The accuracy of TVUS in diagnosis of endometriomas and DIE in our study is in concordance with previous reports [12–14] and with two recent meta-analyses [25, 26]. This provides further confirmation that TVUS remains the first-line imaging technique for suspected DIE. A sonographer with general gynecological experience is expected to diagnose all ovarian endometriomas correctly, as indeed was the case in our study. The present study also had a very good sensitivity for diagnosing bladder nodules, which were identified with the standardized approach. The preoperative diagnosis of bowel involvement and pouch of Douglas obliteration greatly impacts decision-making [9]. While competency is achieved reasonably fast, any missed diagnosis may be harmful. It is therefore imperative to ensure that the trainee and the surgeon speak the same language, as most inaccuracies may be the result of a different terminology. The surgeon was not blinded to the ultrasound report in this study, because he was expected to plan surgery based upon it. Furthermore, despite the high proficiency of our surgeons, some very deep lesions may not have been seen on laparoscopy and could have been missed [7]. The poorer performance which was obtained in the diagnosis of uterosacral ligament lesions is also in concordance with previous reports, and is in fact somewhat better in our study.

An additional limitation of our study is that all of the patients had TVUS because of suspected DIE, which may have caused a diagnostic bias. The analysis was performed in a tertiary referral center with a high number of advanced cases of severe endometriosis with multiple lesions, which does not reflect the standard patient population. Therefore, we analyzed more locations of endometriosis in an attempt to overcome this potential bias.

All of the TVUS examinations were performed by a single operator with training in general gynecological sonography, who had previously not been exposed to DIE scanning. This limits the generalization of our data to other potential operators, with a different degree of expertise in general gynecological imaging, who may in practice have a different learning curve. At the time of the study, this was the only trained sonographer at our center dedicated to endometriosis mapping, thus inter-observer comparisons cannot be discussed. Furthermore, the sonographer in question received tertiary referrals from other centers where eventually the surgery was undertaken. This may have affected the learning curve as well. Similar studies are necessary in order to learn more about the learning curve for different performance and competency levels. A trainee should ideally show evidence of satisfactory performance, before he or she can be encouraged to perform the procedure without supervision [17].

While the LC-CUSUM has been used here to assess the performance of a single individual, it may prove useful for monitoring the introduction of a new procedure in any setting where feedback is available and corrective actions can be implemented, or in monitoring new trainees, who have the advantage of being trained by an experienced DIE sonographer. It may also prove useful for professional societies that are responsible for developing guidelines for good practice [17]. It is clear that any general gynecologic sonographer could benefit from such training, provided that feedback on diagnosis is available. We believe that our experience may serve as a guiding point to other operators who aim to learn endometriosis mapping. With the new consensus opinion recently published by Guerriero et al. [30], better standardization and education is becoming feasible.

Conclusions

This study shows that a sonographer trained in general gynecologic ultrasonography, who devotes time to learn TVUS for DIE mapping, can achieve proficiency for diagnosing the major types of endometriotic lesions after examining less than 50 patients who subsequently undergo surgery in a training setting. This goal can be accomplished within a reasonable time frame in many tertiary referral centers involved in the care of endometriosis patients. Diagnostic accuracy may be further advanced in these centers by improving agreement on terminology and feedback between surgeons and imaging specialists. Determining the learning curve for DIE TVUS mapping can aid training programs in dedicated endometriosis centers and may be of value to general gynecology TVUS education programs as well. Improving training for new ultrasound performers may in the future enable earlier non-invasive diagnosis of endometriosis which will have a favorable impact on the healthcare of women. Despite the fact that we have described the experience of a single operator, we believe that this may encourage other gynecological ultrasound experts to further their expertise into the field of endometriosis mapping.

Appendix

The TVUS were carried out using a transvaginal 5–9 MHz probe with 2D/3D capabilities (Voluson 730 or E6, GE Medical Systems). Images were interpreted in real-time and were stored for later analysis. The examination was performed in a standardized way for all patients, which included a thorough evaluation of all pelvic viscera, in search of endometriosis findings. The examination was performed at any time of the menstrual cycle regardless of hormonal therapy. Bowel preparation was not utilized and is not standard practice at our center. The probe covering is filled generously with ultrasound gel to act as acoustic window. The uterus was studied in a midsagittal plane identifying the uterine cavity and cervical canal, moving to the right and left in order to encompass the entire uterine cavity. The probe was then rotated 90 ° to the left to view the uterus in the transverse plane. The myometrium was thoroughly evaluated for any abnormalities in all planes. The operator then evaluated the adnexae for lesions consistent with endometriomas, tubal adhesions, DIE, pouch of Douglas obliteration, the parametria, recto sigmoid, vagina and retro cervical area, and organ movement.

On B-mode ultrasound, endometriomas were defined as uni- or multilocular cysts with ground glass echogenicity of the cyst fluid and no papillation with detectable blood flow [18]. When the B-mode was inconclusive, power Doppler imaging was performed to exclude corpus luteum cysts [19]. The location (bilateral, right, or left) and size of each endometrioma were evaluated. In the presence of multifocal or bilateral endometriomas, the largest endometrial cyst was taken into account and measured.

The peritoneal surfaces of the anterior compartment were visualized. Bladder nodules were seen as hypo-echoic lesions in the vesicouterine pouch or bladder wall, with or without cystic areas and regular or irregular margins, bulging towards the lumen. The distal ureters were also seen. Bladder adhesions of the vesicouterine pouch were evaluated by the presence or absence of movement between the uterus and the bladder. Infiltration of the bladder wall was noted [20].

Posterior compartment lesions were evaluated in the vagina, posterior and lateral vaginal fornices, the retro cervical area with torus uterinum, the parametria laterally, the rectovaginal septum, and bowel. Vaginal nodules were visualized as hypo-echoic lesions in the vaginal fornix. Bowel involvement was visualized as a hypo-echoic lesion adhering to the bowel wall and bowel layers were examined for penetration. The number of lesions, their size in three dimensions and location from the anus were described. Uterosacral ligaments involvement was searched for in the parametria in the paracervical area and was seen as an infiltrating irregular hypoechogenic tissue [20]. When there were multiple adhesions in the area of the uterosacral ligaments, they were interpreted as involved with DIE. Organ mobility was evaluated in the anterior and posterior compartment. Movement of the posterior surface of the uterus, cervix, or vagina in relation to the bowel was examined in order to determine pouch of Douglas obliteration, previously described as the sliding sign [21, 22].

Acknowledgements
Prof. Daniel S. Seidman and Prof. Gideon Koren for manuscript review and corrections.

Funding
None received.

Authors' contributions
VHE contributed to the project development, research design, data collection, data analysis, and manuscript writing. JLA contributed to the research design, data analysis, and critical manuscript reading. NA contributed to the data collection and critical manuscript reading. ES contributed to the critical manuscript reading. RA contributed to the critical manuscript reading. MG contributed to the data collection and critical manuscript reading. DS contributed to the data collection, data analysis, and critical manuscript reading. All authors read and approved the final manuscript.

Competing interests
On behalf of all authors, the corresponding author states that there is no competing interest.

Author details
[1]Department of Obstetrics and Gynecology, Sheba Medical Center, Tel-Hashomer, Tel-Aviv University, 52621 Ramat Gan, Israel. [2]Department of Obstetrics and Gynecology, Clinica Universidad de Navarra, University of Navarra, Pamplona, Spain.

References
1. Melis GB, Ajossa S, Guerriero S et al (1994) Epidemiology and diagnosis of endometriosis. Ann N Y Acad Sci 734:352–357
2. Dmowski WP, Lesniewicz R, Rana N, Pepping P, Noursalehi M (1997) Changing trends in the diagnosis of endometriosis: a comparative study of women with pelvic endometriosis presenting with chronic pelvic pain or infertility. Fertil Steril 67:238–243
3. Bazot M, Thomassin I, Hourani R, Cortez A, Darai E (2004) Diagnostic accuracy of transvaginal sonography for deep pelvic endometriosis. Ultrasound Obstet Gynecol 24:180–185
4. Bazot M, Darai E, Biau DJ, Ballester M, Dessolle L (2011) Learning curve of transvaginal ultrasound for the diagnosis of endometriomas assessed by the cumulative summation test (LC-CUSUM). Fertil Steril 95:301–303
5. Ballard K, Lowton K, Wright J (2006) What's the delay? A qualitative study of women's experiences of reaching a diagnosis of endometriosis. Fertil Steril and agreement with endometriosis findings at laparoscopyand agreement with endometriosis findings at laparoscopy 86:1296–1301
6. Hudelist G, Fritzer N, Thomas A et al (2012) Diagnostic delay for endometriosis in Austria and Germany: causes and possible consequences. Hum Reprod 27:3412–3416
7. Nnoaham KE, Hummelshoj L, Webster P et al (2011) World Endometriosis Research Foundation Global Study of Women's Health consortium. Impact of endometriosis on quality of life and work productivity: a multicenter study across ten countries. Fertil Steril 96:366–373
8. Tammaa A, Fritzer N, Strunk G, Krell A, Salzer H, Hudelist G (2014) Learning curve for the detection of pouch of Douglas obliteration and deep infiltrating endometriosis of the rectum. Hum Reprod 29:1199–1204
9. Piketty M, Chopin N, Dousset B et al (2009) Preoperative work-up for patients with deeply infiltrating endometriosis: transvaginal ultrasonography must definitely be the first-line imaging examination. Hum Reprod 24:602–607
10. Hudelist G, Ballard K, English J et al (2011) Transvaginal sonography vs. clinical examination in the preoperative diagnosis of deep infiltrating endometriosis. Ultrasound Obstet Gynecol 37:480–487
11. Hudelist G, English J, Thomas A, Tinelli A, Singer CF, Keckstein J (2011) Diagnostic accuracy of transvaginal ultrasound for non-invasive diagnosis of bowel endometriosis: systematic review and meta-analysis. Ultrasound Obstet Gynecol 37:257–263
12. Alcazar JL, Laparte C, Jurado M, Lopez-Garcia G (1997) The role of transvaginal ultrasonography combined with color velocity imaging and pulse Doppler in the diagnosis of endometrioma. Fertil Steril 67:487–491
13. Van Holsbeke C, Van Calster B, Guerriero M et al (2009) Imaging in gynaecology: how good are we in identifying endometriomas? Facts Views Vis ObGyn 1:7–17
14. Abrao MS, Gonçalves MO, Dias JA Jr, Podgaec S, Chamie LP, Blasbalg R (2007) Comparison between clinical examination, transvaginal sonography and magnetic resonance imaging for the diagnosis of deep endometriosis. Hum Reprod 22:3092–3097
15. Wohl H (1977) The cusum plot: Its' utility in the analysis of clinical data. N Engl J Med 296:1044–1045
16. Biau DJ, Porcher R, Salomon LJ (2008) CUSUM: a tool for ongoing assessment of performance. Ultrasound Obstet Gynecol 31:252–255
17. Biau DJ, Williams SM, Schlup MM, Nizard RS, Porcher R (2008) Quantitative and individualized assessment of the learning curve using LC-CUSUM. Br J Surg 95:925 929
18. Van Holsbeke C, Van Calster B, Guerriero S et al (2010) Endometriomas: their ultrasound characteristics. Ultrasound Obstet Gynecol 35:730–740
19. Guerriero S, Ajossa S, Mais V, Risalvato A, Lai MP, Melis GB (1998) The diagnosis of endometriomas using colour Doppler energy imaging. Hum Reprod 13:1691–1695

20. Exacoustos C, Malzoni M, Di Giovanni A et al (2014) Ultrasound mapping system for the surgical management of deep infiltrating endometriosis. Fertil Steril 102:143–150

21. Hudelist G, Fritzer N, Staettner S et al (2013) Uterine sliding sign: a simple sonographic predictor for presence of deep infiltrating endometriosis of the rectum. Ultrasound Obstet Gynecol 41:692–695

22. Reid S, Lu C, Casikar I et al (2013) Prediction of pouch of Douglas obliteration in women with suspected endometriosis using a new real-time dynamic transvaginal ultrasound technique: the sliding sign. Ultrasound Obstet Gynecol 41:685–691

23. American Society for Reproductive Medicine (1997) Revised American Society for Reproductive Medicine Classification of endometriosis. Am Soc Reprod Med 5:817–821

24. Alcázar JL, Guerriero S, Laparte C, Ajossa S, Ruiz-Zambrana A, Melis GB (2011) Diagnostic performance of transvaginal gray-scale ultrasound for specific diagnosis of benign ovarian cysts in relation to menopausal status. Maturitas 68:182–188

25. Guerriero S, Ajossa S, Minguez JA et al (2015) Accuracy of transvaginal ultrasound for diagnosis of deep endometriosis in uterosacral ligaments, rectovaginal septum, vagina and bladder: systematic review and meta-analysis. Ultrasound Obstet Gynecol 46:534–545

26. Guerriero S, Ajossa S, Orozco R et al (2015) Accuracy of transvaginal ultrasound for diagnosis of deep endometriosis in the rectosigmoid: systematic review and meta-analysis. Ultrasound Obstet Gynecol 47:281–289

27. Saba L, Guerriero S, Sulis R et al (2011) Learning curve in the detection of ovarian and deep endometriosis by using Magnetic Resonance comparison with surgical results. Eur J Radiol 79:237–244

28. Alcazar JL, Diaz L, Florez P, Guerriero S, Jurado M (2013) Intensive training program for ultrasound diagnosis of adnexal masses: protocol and preliminary results. Ultrasound Obstet Gynecol 42:218–223

29. Piessens S, Healey M, Maher P, Tsaltas J, Rombauts L (2014) Can anyone screen for deep infiltrating endometriosis with transvaginal ultrasound? Aust N Z J Obstet Gynaecol 54:462–468

30. Guerriero S, Condous G, Van Den Bosch T et al (2016) Systematic approach to sonographic evaluation of the pelvis in women with suspected endometriosis, including terms, definitions and measurements: a consensus opinion from the International Deep Endometriosis Analysis (IDEA) group. Ultrasound Obstet Gynecol. https://doi.org/10.1002/uog.15955

10

Spigelian hernia in gynaecology

Anastasia Ussia[1,2], Fabio Imperato[1], Larissa Schindler[3], Arnaud Wattiez[3] and Philippe R. Koninckx[4*]

Abstract

Background: A Spigelian hernia is a rare hernia through the Spigelian fascia between the rectus muscle and the semilunar line. This hernia is well known in surgery. Symptoms vary from insidious to localised pain, an intermittent mass and/or a bowel obstruction.

Results: The Spigelian hernia is poorly known in gynaecology. Spigelian hernias may be causally related to secondary trocar insertion. This review is written to increase awareness in gynaecology and is illustrated by a case report in which the diagnosis was missed for 4 years even by laparoscopy. Smaller hernias risk not to be diagnosed and will thus not be treated. Even larger Spigelian hernias might not be recognised and treated appropriately.

Conclusions: The gynaecologist should consider a Spigelian hernia in women with localised pain in the abdominal wall lateral of the rectus muscle some 5 cm below the umbilicus. Smaller hernias can be closed by laparoscopy without a mesh. Larger hernias require a mesh repair.

Keywords: Endometriosis, Spigelian hernia, Pelvic pain, Deep endometriosis

Background

Spigelian hernia or Spiegel hernia was recognised by Josef T. Klinkosh in 1764, and named after Adriaan van der Spieghel, a Flemish anatomist who described the semilunar line in 1645 [1]. The Spigelian fascia is the aponeurotic layer between the rectus abdominis muscle medially and the semilunar line laterally. This hernia can present as a localised pain, as an intermittent mass or as a bowel obstruction [2]. Symptoms however can also be insidious and non-specific. Spigelian hernia carries a risk of bowel incarceration and should therefore be repaired [3]. For smaller Spigelian hernias, a mesh-free laparoscopic suture repair is feasible [4, 5].

Spigelian hernia is rare, representing 1 to 2% of all abdominal hernias. It occurs mostly in women over 60 years of age [6] but can occur at a younger age [7], even in neonates [8, 9]. The aetiology is unclear; obesity with rapid weight loss, multiple pregnancies and chronic obstructive pulmonary disease (COPD) are considered predisposing factors. Recently, it was suggested that Spigelian hernia could be caused by a previous trocar insertion [10–13].

* Correspondence: pkoninckx@gmail.com
[4]Department of Obstetrics and Gynecology, Catholic University Leuven, University Hospital, Gasthuisberg, B-3000 Leuven, Belgium. Vuilenbos 2 3360, Bierbeek, Belgium
Full list of author information is available at the end of the article

A missed diagnosis for 4 years in a woman operated 4 years previously for (deep) endometriosis, and the potential causal relationship with trocar insertion prompted us to review the literature.

Methods
Literature review

PubMed was screened for 'Spigelian hernia' generating 486 articles of which 126 since 1 January 2010, of which only three in a gynaecological journal [10, 13]. Most articles are case reports—the first publication in gynaecological literature was in 1992 [14]—or small series, the largest describing 40 cases [4]. Considering that five reviews were published since 11 January 2015 [15–20] and that articles before 1 January 2010 were almost exclusively case reports adding little to ethology, diagnosis or treatment, the review was limited to the last 6 years.

Results
Symptoms of a Spigelian hernia

Spigelian hernias can present as acute small bowel obstructions [15, 21] even of the colon [22]. Most Spigelian hernias present a localised hernia, or as local pain with or without a hernia sac [15–20]. Symptoms however can also be insidious and vague. A Spigelian hernia can harbour an endometrioma [23], even an acute appendicitis [8, 24] or an incarceration of omentum [25].

Diagnosis of a Spigelian hernia

According to the surgical literature, dealing with larger and symptomatic hernias, the diagnosis is based on clinical examination helped by ultrasound or computed tomography [16]. Since most hernias reduce spontaneously in a supine position, the diagnosis, especially of smaller hernias, remains difficult and ultrasound diagnosis has been suggested to be performed in a standing position [8]. Diagnosis remains a diagnostic challenge [26] and requires a high index of suspicion given the lack of consistent symptoms and signs [27]. Larger or symptomatic Spigelian hernia's can be suspected by CAT scan [28].

Treatment of a Spigelian hernia

The laparoscopic repair is effective but used in few reference centres. A recent systematic review of the laparoscopic repair of a Spigelian hernia [15] identified 55 articles and concluded that laparoscopic repair of the Spigelian hernia is a safe and acceptable method. Although intraperitoneal mesh technique is the most popular repair method, various techniques were used in these 237 repairs without a single randomised trial.

An extra peritoneal mesh repair remains the gold standard [16]. Also during these repairs, laparoscopy is a useful aid as discussed in two recent case reports [29, 30].

Recurrences are around 3%. No predictive factors were identified [6].

Case report

Our patient, who was 35 years of age, underwent laparoscopic surgery for excision of superficial/deep/ovarian endometriosis. A week after laparoscopy she suddenly developed pain in the right fossa which severely limited physical activity. She had difficulty to elevate the right leg, difficulty to walk, and felt severe pain when getting up from a chair by a rotating movement of the body. Intercourse was reported to be almost impossible because of this pain. In the absence of a positive finding during clinical exams, ultrasound, MRI and CAT scans, a tentative non-specific diagnosis was made that a nerve lesion must have occurred during the previous surgery either the genito-femoralis or the pudendal nerve. The local pain in the wall was considered a nerve entrapment or pain in the scar of the trocar, and local infiltrations with cortisone were made. Because of persisting severe complaints in the absence of a clinical finding, she was subsequently thought to exaggerate her symptoms and anti-depressive drugs were given. Although a triathlon runner before, she could not do any exercise and gained more than 20 kg. Two years later, a second laparoscopy was performed to exclude progression of the endometriosis but only a few spots of superficial endometriosis were reported. She then conceived by IVF (3 cycles), and

during the Caesarean section, 'pelvic endometriosis' and adherences were reported but not treated. Subsequently, medical therapy with oral contraception was started. For the local pain, repetitive infiltrations in the wall were given, without a positive result.

When the patient visited us, 4 years after the first laparoscopy, she still had severe pain with difficulty to walk, to do physical activity, to have intercourse and to get up from a chair. Other symptoms were vague and not specific. Clinical exam revealed a severe localised pain in the right fossa upon palpation also with contracted abdominal muscles. The gynaecological exam and a transvaginal ultrasound and a MRI were normal, except some vague pain in the right vaginal fornix on deep palpation, some tenderness over the right Alcock canal and a small cystic ovarian endometriosis in both ovaries. Since the patient insisted, we accepted to perform a (third) diagnostic laparoscopy and we hoped to find a cause and solution for this persisting severe pain preventing physical activity. The cystic ovarian endometriosis was not considered sufficient to explain the pain. Also an Alcock syndrome, persistent deep endometriosis with perineal pain, or pain from the appendix seemed remote possibilities.

The main finding during laparoscopy was a Spigelian hernia under the rectus muscle (Fig. 1) exactly where the pain was found by abdominal palpation. This hernia was excised and repaired with interrupted stitches of vicryl 0. Two small ovarian endometriosis cysts of less than 1 cm in diameter were excised from the left and right ovaries. A superficial plaque of endometriosis overlying the right ischial spine up to the bowel was excised. Because of the suspicion of Alcock syndrome, a dissection of the lateral side wall was performed exposing the right ischial spine, but no endometriosis was found. Because of the symptoms and despite having a normal appearance, an appendectomy was performed. To our surprise, the morning after surgery, the patient reported to be pain free and she was able to walk normally. A few

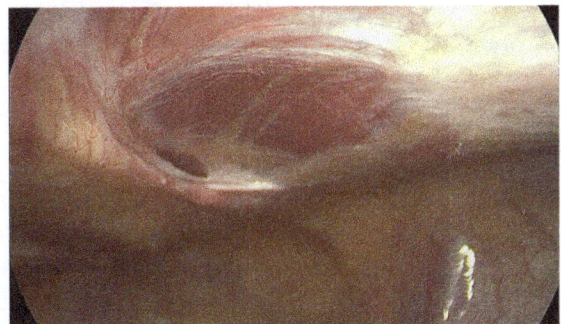

Fig. 1 Spigelian hernia under rectus muscle causing severe pain limiting physical activity

days later she resumed normal physical activity, something that had not been possible for over 4 years.

The pathology of the hernia wall and of the appendix was reported as hernia lipoma and chronic appendicitis respectively. Pathology also confirmed the superficial pelvic and the cystic ovarian endometriosis.

Discussion

Although we did not recognise this hernia as a Spigelian hernia, a hernia repair was performed since AU had seen many years before a similar hernia when assisting her brother who is a general surgeon. We were surprised and confused by the discrepancy between the severe pain symptoms, the minor surgery performed for endometriosis and the appendectomy and the immediate pain relief after surgery. Weeks later, after discussing this observation with other endoscopists, we realised that the hernia had been a Spigelian hernia. Since we consider that the endometriosis surgery performed and the appendectomy could not explain the immediate and complete pain relief within 24 h, we suspect that the Spigelian hernia had been the cause of the pain. This prompted us to review the literature to find that awareness of Spigelian hernia among gynaecological surgeons seems limited and that it might be caused by trocar insertion. Having been misled by the symptoms, we considered that reporting our lack of knowledge could increase awareness of Spigelian hernia.

Spigelian hernias generally present as an acute abdomen secondary to bowel strangulation or as a mass protruding from the wall. The prevalence and symptoms of smaller Spigelian hernias are unclear, since they risk not to be diagnosed, at least not by gynaecological laparoscopists. We indeed do not recognise what we do not know. Moreover, in gynaecology a localised hypogastric pain lateral to the rectus muscle which can be reproduced during contraction of the rectus muscle risks to be diagnosed as a nerve entrapment—as we did—and thus treated by local infiltration—as was done repetitively in this patient. An endometriosis lesion in the abdominal wall can be considered especially when the pain is cyclical and in the absence of a palpable lesion treatment will be conservative. Anyway, most of these women will not undergo a laparoscopy and the diagnosis risks not to be made.

A Spiegel hernia with such severe debilitating pain limiting physical activity is rare. The severe pain with difficulty to walk, work, move the right leg and have intercourse were erroneously considered for 4 years as the consequence of a nerve trauma while the local pain was considered a nerve entrapment in the wall. Only afterwards after making the diagnosis, we realised that this had been an antalgic reaction. Illustrative was the comment of the husband the morning of the day after surgery: 'The problem is solved: my wife gets up straight from the bed whereas before she made a rotating movement.' It also illustrates how confusing the history of a previous deep endometriosis surgery can be. Indeed an extensive dissection for deep endometriosis with afterwards still pain and difficulties to elevate or cross the right leg and to walk, raises suspicion of incomplete surgery and/or pelvic nerve damage. For this, repeat surgery will rarely be proposed and medical treatment will be given. Also in this case, we would not have performed a laparoscopy and thus would have missed the diagnosis without the insistent request of the patient.

The Spigelian hernia is suggested to be the cause of the pain since the pain symptoms, both the spontaneous pain and the pain during palpation of the wall had disappeared immediately after surgery. The small endometriotic cysts in the ovaries, and the superficial endometriosis were not painful during clinical exam before surgery and are unlikely to have caused the severe pain symptoms limiting physical activity nor the local pain in the wall. This also applies to the appendix. The fibrosis around the ischial spine may have given some Alcock-like symptoms, but does not explain the pain symptoms. It remains unclear why this Spigelian hernia caused such severe pain, since no bowel or omentum entrapment, or local inflammation was found.

Important is that a Spigelian hernia might be caused by a previous trocar insertion. This was suggested [10] and also in this woman the pain started acutely 1 week after the first surgery. It would therefore not be surprising that (smaller) Spigelian hernias are much more frequent than suspected since in the absence of severe symptoms they risk to remain undiagnosed. We gynaecological endoscopists should consider a Spigelian hernia in women with localised pain lateral to the rectus muscle 5 cm below the umbilicus mimicking a nerve entrapment especially after previous laparoscopy. The causal relationship with trocar insertion might be an argument to use secondary trocars with an atraumatic round instead of a triangular tip in order to decrease the muscular and fascial trauma [31]. The suggestion to use round tip trocars can moreover be generalised since incisional hernias also occur after 5-mm trocar insertion especially following extensive manipulation [32].

The specific location of the Spigelian hernia moreover suggests that it might be wise to avoid the angle between the semilunar line and the rectus abdominis muscle when inserting a secondary trocar. In a gynaecological surgery, a larger 10-mm secondary trocar is generally used on the left side. Most Spigelian hernias occur on the right side possibly related to appendectomies. The number of recent publications indeed suggests an increase in the occurrence;

Conclusions

In conclusion, this case report intends to increase awareness among gynaecological laparoscopists of Spigelian hernia. It is suggested that previous trocar insertion might be causally related. It is speculated that the prevalence of smaller Spigelian hernias could be higher than believed today. It is suggested that it might be wise to perform a diagnostic laparoscopy in women with spontaneous pain and pain on palpation, in the angle between the rectus abdominis muscle and the semilunar line, especially after a previous laparoscopy or with an acute onset of pain thereafter. This case report also illustrates how misleading deep endometriosis can be. It also is a lesson in humility. Indeed we must admit that if in this woman a deep endometriosis nodule would have been found during surgery, compatible with her complaints, we might not have treated this Spigelian hernia since it was unknown to us at that moment.

Acknowledgements
We do thank Prof Victor Gomel, Vancouver, Canada, for reviewing this manuscript. We do thank Prof Baki Topal for initiating us to the Spiegel hernia.

Funding
The authors did not have any funding.

Authors' contributions
Surgery was performed by PK, AU and FI. LS reviewed the literature and the manuscript was finalised with the help of AW. All authors read and approved the final manuscript.

Competing interests
Koninck is a shareholder of Endosat. The rest of the authors declare that they have no competing interests.

Author details
[1]Villa Del Rosario, Rome, Italy. [2]Gemelli Hospitals, Università Cattolica, Rome, Italy. [3]Latifa Hospital, Dubai, United Arab Emirates. [4]Department of Obstetrics and Gynecology, Catholic University Leuven, University Hospital, Gasthuisberg, B-3000 Leuven, Belgium. Vuilenbos 2 3360, Bierbeek, Belgium.

References
1. Ghosh SK, Sharma S, Biswas S, Chakraborty S (2014) Adriaan van den Spiegel (1578–1625): anatomist, physician, and botanist. Clin Anat 27:952–957
2. Larson DW, Farley DR (2002) Spigelian hernias: repair and outcome for 81 patients. World J Surg 26:1277–1281
3. Vos DI, Scheltinga MR (2004) Incidence and outcome of surgical repair of Spigelian hernia. Br J Surg 91:640–644
4. Kelly ME, Courtney D, McDermott FD, Heeney A, Maguire D, Geoghegan JG et al (2015) Laparoscopic spigelian hernia repair: a series of 40 patients. Surg Laparosc Endosc Percutan Tech 25:e86–e89
5. Moreno-Egea A, Campillo-Soto A, Morales-Cuenca G (2015) Which should be the gold standard laparoscopic technique for handling Spigelian hernias? Surg Endosc 29:856–862
6. Polistina FA, Garbo G, Trevisan P, Frego M (2015) Twelve years of experience treating Spigelian hernia. Surgery 157:547–550
7. Spinelli C, Strambi S, Pucci V, Liserre J, Spinelli G, Palombo C (2014) Spigelian hernia in a 14-year-old girl: a case report and review of the literature. European J Pediatr Surg Rep 2:58–62
8. Smereczynski A, Kolaczyk K, Lubinski J, Bojko S, Galdynska M, Bernatowicz E (2012) Sonographic imaging of Spigelian hernias. J Ultrason 12:269–275
9. Fascetti-Leon F, Gobbi D, Gamba P, Cecchetto G (2010) Neonatal bilateral Spigelian hernia associated with undescended testes and scalp aplasia cutis. Eur J Pediatr Surg 20:123–125
10. Bassi A, Tulandi T (2013) Small bowel herniation through a Spigelian defect within 48 hours after laparoscopy. J Minim Invasive Gynecol 20:392–393
11. Tsu JH, Ng AT, Wong JK, Wong EM, Ho KL, Yiu MK (2014) Trocar-site hernia at the 8-mm robotic port after robot-assisted laparoscopic prostatectomy: a case report and review of the literature. J Robot Surg 8:89–91
12. Slakey DR, Teplitsky S, Cheng SS (2002) Incarcerated Spigelian hernia following laparoscopic living-donor nephrectomy. JSLS 6:217–219
13. Kamel A, Abdallah N, El-Sandabesee D (2012) Spigelian hernia following laparoscopy. J Obstet Gynaecol 32:310–311
14. Carter JE, Mizes C (1992) Laparoscopic diagnosis and repair of Spigelian hernia: report of a case and technique. Am J Obstet Gynecol 167:77–78
15. Barnes TG, McWhinnie DL (2016) Laparoscopic Spigelian hernia repair: a systematic review. Surg Laparosc Endosc Percutan Tech 26:265–270
16. Pinna A, Cossu ML, Paliogiannis P, Ginesu GC, Fancellu A, Porcu A (2016) Spigelian hernia. A series of cases and literature review. Ann Ital Chir 87:306–311
17. Bhardwaj A, Kalhan S, Bhatia P, Khetan M, John S, Bindal V et al (2015) Topic: abdominal wall hernia—Spigelian hernia, anatomy, incidence, repair. Hernia 19(1):S344
18. Campanella AM, Licheri S, Barbarossa M, Saba A, Pinna E, Reccia I et al (2015) Topic: abdominal wall hernia—Spigelian hernia, anatomy, incidence, repair. Hernia 19(1):S215
19. Foster D, Nagarajan S, Panait L (2015) Richter-type Spigelian hernia: a case report and review of the literature. Int J Surg Case Rep 6C:160–162
20. Jones BC, Hutson JM (2015) The syndrome of Spigelian hernia and cryptorchidism: a review of paediatric literature. J Pediatr Surg 50:325–330
21. John RJ, Ulahannan SE, Kurien JS, Joseph A, Kurien AS, Varghese SA et al (2016) Rare hernias presenting as acute abdomen—a case series. J Clin Diagn Res 10:R01–R04
22. Velimezis G, Vassos N, Kapogiannatos G, Koronakis D, Salpiggidis C, Perrakis E et al (2016) Strangulation and necrosis of right hemicolon as an extremely rare complication of Spigelian hernia. Arch Med Sci 12:469–472
23. Moris D, Michalinos A, Vernadakis S (2015) Endometriosis in a Spigelian hernia sac: an unexpected finding. Int Surg 100:109–111
24. Deshmukh S, Ghanouni P, Mindelzun R, Roos J (2010) Computed tomographic diagnosis of appendicitis within a Spigelian hernia. J Comput Assist Tomogr 34:199–200
25. Mederos R, Lamas JR, Alvarado J, Matos M, Padron I, Ramos A (2017) Laparoscopic diagnosis and repair of Spigelian hernia: a case report and literature review. Int J Surg Case Rep 31:184–187
26. Srivastava KN, Agarwal A (2015) Spigelian hernia: a diagnostic dilemma and laparoscopic management. Indian J Surg 77:35–37
27. Cinar H, Polat AK, Caglayan K, Ozbalci GS, Topgul HK, Polat C (2013) Spigelian hernia: our experience and review of the literature. Ann Ital Chir 84:649–653
28. Bittner JG, Edwards MA, Shah MB, MacFadyen BV Jr, Mellinger JD (2008) Mesh-free laparoscopic Spigelian hernia repair. Am Surg 74:713–720
29. Matsui S, Nitori N, Kato A, Ikeda Y, Kiatagwa Y, Hasegawa H et al (2016) Laparoscopic totally extra-peritoneal hernia repair for bilateral Spigelian hernias and coincident inguinal hernia: a case report. Int J Surg Case Rep 28:169–172
30. Patterson AL, Thomas B, Franklin A, Connor C, Pullatt R (2016) Transabdominal preperitoneal repair of Spigelian hernia. Am Surg 82:E18–E19
31. Tarnay CM, Glass KB, Munro MG (1999) Incision characteristics associated with six laparoscopic trocar-cannula systems: a randomized, observer-blinded comparison. Obstet Gynecol 94:89–93
32. Nezhat C, Nezhat F, Seidman DS, Nezhat C (1997) Incisional hernias after operative laparoscopy. J LaparoendoscAdvSurgTechA 7(2):111–115

11

Laparoscopic uterovaginal prolapse surgery in the elderly: feasibility and outcomes

Samuel W. King[1,2,3,4*], Helen Jefferis[1,3], Simon Jackson[1,3], Alexander G. Marfin[3] and Natalia Price[1,3]

Abstract

Background: Uterovaginal prolapse in very elderly women is a growing problem due to increased life expectancy. Surgeons and anaesthetists may be wary of performing quality of life surgery on this higher risk group. Where surgery is undertaken, it is commonly performed vaginally; there is a perception that this is better tolerated than abdominal surgery. Little data is published about laparoscopic prolapse surgery tolerability in this population, and laparoscopic surgery is perceived within the urogynaecological community as complex and lengthy and hence inherently unsuitable for the very elderly.

In Oxford, UK, laparoscopic abdominal surgical techniques are routinely employed for urogynaecological reconstructive surgery. The authors offer abdominal laparoscopic prolapse surgery to patients suitable for general anaesthesia with apical vaginal prolapse, irrespective of age. We here report outcomes in this elderly patient cohort and hypothesise these to be acceptable.

This is a retrospective case note review of all patients aged 79 years old and above undergoing laparoscopic prolapse surgery (hysteropexy or sacrocolpopexy) in two centres in Oxford, UK, over a 5-year period ($n = 55$). Data were collected on length of surgery, length of stay, intraoperative complications, early and late post-operative complications and surgical outcome.

Results: Mean age was 82.6 years (range 79–96). There were no deaths. Minor post-operative complications such as UTI and constipation were frequent, but there were no serious (Clavien-Dindo grade III or above) complications; 80% achieved objective good anatomical outcome.

Conclusions: Laparoscopic prolapse surgery appears well tolerated in the elderly with low operative morbidity and mortality.

Keywords: Elderly, Hysteropexy, Laparoscopic, Prolapse, Sacrocolpopexy

Background

Older women are disproportionately affected by pelvic prolapse compared with their younger counterparts. Those in their eighth decade generate ten times as many consultation hours regarding pelvic prolapse as those in their fourth [1]. "Elderly" is frequently defined in the literature as over 65 years of age, and the safety and effectiveness of vaginal prolapse surgery has been analysed in this group previously. Indeed, some papers define "elderly" at an even younger age [2]. However, few clinicians would now regard a 66-year-old as elderly. For the purposes of this study, "elderly" is defined as those patients in their

80th year and beyond. This age cut-off is arbitrary, and clearly, "biological age", reflecting concomitant disease, is of more relevance for many than chronological age. However, whilst many surgeons have few qualms operating on patients in their 70s, those over 80 are often viewed with more concern.

The population of people age over 75 in the UK is expected to double and that of those over 85 nearly treble in the next 30 years [3]. With a higher proportion of elderly people being women [4], vaginal prolapse is a significant and growing burden on health services. Prolapse significantly impacts quality of life in this population, causing discomfort, urinary symptoms, and psychosexual issues. However, surgeons and anaesthetists may be wary of operating on this age group as surgery is life-enhancing rather than life-saving. Traditionally, vaginal repair surgery

* Correspondence: sam.king@doctors.org.uk
[1]Department of Urogynaecology, Oxford University Hospitals, Oxford, UK
[2]Oxford Medical School, John Radcliffe Hospital, University of Oxford, Oxford, UK
Full list of author information is available at the end of the article

performed includes vaginal hysterectomy, anterior/posterior colporrhaphy and sacrospinous fixation. All of these carry a significant morbidity, such as secondary haemorrhage, infection and exacerbation of pre-existing medical problems. These risks increase in the very elderly. We hypothesise that reconstructive laparoscopic surgery, with low infection risk and little risk of significant blood loss, is an acceptable alternative option for this age group.

Data were collected for patients aged 79 and above who underwent laparoscopic hysteropexy or sacrocolpopexy, with or without additional procedures, as operated on by or under direct supervision of the two consultant gynaecological surgeon authors across two centres in Oxford. The primary aim was to evaluate morbidity and mortality in this cohort.

Methods

Approval was granted by the regional audit committee to retrospectively analyse the records of patients aged 79 years of age and over undergoing laparoscopic sacrocolpopexy or hysteropexy over a period of 5 years. Ethics approval was not required as this was a retrospective case note review.

The inclusion criteria were as follows: patients of 79 years and older at the time of procedure, undergoing either laparoscopic sacrocolpopexy or hysteropexy, and with or without additional procedures. When seen in clinic, patients with symptomatic vaginal apical prolapse are counselled regarding both conservative and surgical management options. If surgery is chosen, and they are suitable for general anaesthesia, both vaginal and laparoscopic surgery is discussed. Our preference is laparoscopic abdominal surgery as our experience suggests this is well tolerated and effective. However, if not suitable for general anaesthesia, then abdominal laparoscopic surgery is contraindicated.

Notes were reviewed retrospectively for all patients fitting the inclusion criteria over a period of 5 years (2010–2015). Both paper notes and electronic records were reviewed, including pre-operative assessments, intraoperative notes, anaesthetic notes, post-operative in-patient notes, discharge summaries and follow-up clinic letters.

Prolapse was objectively assessed in clinic pre-operatively by measuring and graded using the pelvic organ prolapse quantification (POP-Q). American Society of Anaesthesiologists (ASA) grades were calculated by a consultant anaesthetist and used as a proxy for pre-operative morbidity of patients. ASA grade is scored from 1 to 6, where 1 is a healthy person, 2 corresponds to mild systemic disease, and 3 to severe systemic disease. None of the included patients had a score of 4 (severe disease which is a constant threat to life) or above.

Surgical technique was as previously described [5, 6]. Antibiotic prophylaxis was used in all cases as per local

trust surgical site infection guidelines. Venous thromboembolism risk assessment was performed for all cases, and all were prescribed post-operative low molecular weight heparin until discharge.

Data collected included length of surgery, intraoperative complications, early post-operative complications (defined as from end of surgery to discharge from hospital) and late post-operative complications (defined as from discharge to outpatient follow-up). Complications were classified using the Clavien-Dindo surgical complication classification system [7].

Results

Fifty-five women aged 79 and over were operated on during the 5-year study period. They had a mean age of 83 (range, 79–96 years) on the day of procedure. One woman underwent laparoscopic hysteropexy twice over the time period, and so this was counted as two procedures, resulting in 56 procedures in total; 26 were laparoscopic hysteropexy, and 30 were laparoscopic sacrocolpopexy. During the same time period, only nine patients aged 79 and over underwent vaginal procedures for apical prolapse (vaginal hysterectomy, sacrospinous fixation or both).

There were seven (12.5%) patients with an ASA grade of 1, 40 (71.4%) with a grade of 2 and eight (14.3%) with a grade of 3. One patient did not have an ASA grade or co-morbidities reported in their notes. There were no patients with POP-Q stage of 1, eight (14.3%) with a grade of 2, 26 (46.4%) with a stage of 3 and 19 (34%) with a stage of 4.

Twenty-eight patients (50%) had concomitant additional procedures which included anterior and/or posterior colporrhaphy and oophorectomy. For those without additional procedures, mean duration of laparoscopic surgery was 76 min (range, 35–145 min), whilst mean duration of surgery with additional procedures was 82 min (range, 35–205). Three of the procedures were performed by a urogynaecology subspecialty registrar under the supervision of a consultant urogynaecologist, whilst the rest were performed by one of the two consultant co-authors (NP and SJ).

One patient sustained a bladder injury intraoperatively which was repaired during the procedure, and did not affect the operative outcome. There were no other intraoperative complications. Blood loss was not formally measured but estimated at less than 100 ml in all cases; no patient had clinical indication for a post-operative full blood count measurement, and no patient required a blood transfusion.

In the early post-operative period, there were ten grade I and nine grade II complications. In the late post-operative period, there were nine grade I and four grade II complications. This is summarised in Table 1. There were no grade III or higher complications.

The mean length of stay was 2.3 days (range, 1–15 days). With the exception of one particularly complex patient

Table 1 Frequency of early and late post-operative complications

Clavien-Dindo complications	Early (theatre to discharge)	Late (discharge to follow-up)
Grade I		
Constipation	6	7
Diarrhoea	1	0
Voiding difficulty	1	2
Faecal incontinence	1	0
Grade II		
UTI	3	3
Hypertension	2	0
Vaginal infection	1	1
Fall	1	0
Pneumonia	1	0
Altered ECG	1	0

Clavien-Dindo scoring system used: grade I is any deviation from the normal post-operative course without the need for pharmacological treatment or surgical, endoscopic and radiological interventions. Grade II are those requiring pharmacological treatment with drug other than such allowed for grade I complications. No higher category complications occurred

with a large number of comorbidities and very large prolapse protruding 20 cm beyond the introitus (POP-Q stage IV), mean length of stay was 2.0 days (range, 1–5 days). There was a weak positive correlation between ASA grade and length of stay ($r = 0.35$) and none between age and length of stay ($r = 0.08$).

Six patients did not attend follow-up clinic. All six were still living at time of data collection according to their electronic patient records, and had not been admitted or referred back by their general practitioner for complications relating to their procedure, or attended hospital for complications related to their procedure. The rest attended with follow-up taking place at a mean period of 73 days post-operatively (range, 20–186 days). Forty-five (80%) patients had objective evidence of good anatomical results with no remaining or recurring prolapse. Five (9%) had prolapse requiring further surgery whilst six (11%) had minor residual prolapse with minimal symptoms.

Discussion

Stepp et al. [8] investigated the outcomes of urogynaecological surgery in 267 women over 75 years old. They found that the overall perioperative morbidity rate in elderly women who underwent urogynaecological surgery was low. However, the vast majority of procedures were solely via a vaginal approach, and those approached laparoscopically were not separated out on analysis.

Friedman et al. [9] compared 120 women over the age of 79 undergoing non-laparoscopic gynaecological surgery with 1497 younger women. Although length of stay for the elderly was slightly increased, mortality and complication rates were comparable to that of younger patients. They concluded that age need not be the sole determinant in the decision to undergo major elective gynaecological surgery.

Laparoscopic hysteropexy and sacrocolpopexy are reported as safe and effective for the treatment of prolapse in younger populations [10, 11]. These procedures are, however, regarded by many as complex major surgery that should consequently be avoided in the elderly. However, laparoscopic surgery has been evaluated in the elderly population in general surgery in cholecystectomy and ventral rectopexy, with the conclusion that it is well tolerated [12, 13]. Little has been published specific to laparoscopic prolapse surgery in older patients, and that which has been published has mixed conclusions. Elneil et al. described a series of 19 patients aged over 76 undergoing laparoscopic prolapse surgery and concluded it offered a good alternative to the vaginal approach [14]. Turner et al. however compared patients over and under the age of 65 undergoing laparoscopic sacrocolpopexy and found that the older group had higher rates of complications, concluding that age was a significant predictor of post-operative morbidity [15]. Our own data suggest age does not preclude surgery, and specifically laparoscopic abdominal surgery is not contraindicated. Indeed, during this study period, the majority of our elderly patients were treated with this approach; only nine other over 79 years old were treated surgically within our unit (vaginal hysterectomy or sacrospinous fixation) during the study period.

There was one intraoperative complication; this was not age related: a bladder injury was treated intraoperatively without impacting on the planned procedure, and she made an uneventful post-surgical recovery. No patient experienced a grade III or higher post-operative complication. Whilst grade I and II complications were relatively common, none of these resulted in major harm or long-term detriment to the patient. The most frequent complications, both early and late, were constipation and urinary tract infection with cumulative rates of 8.9 and 19.6%, respectively. These are both common complications of prolapse surgery, as shown in a younger cohort undergoing hysteropexy where rates were 12.9% for constipation and 2.9% for UTI are reported [10]. Whilst the incidences of both of these complications were increased in our more elderly cohort, elderly patients in general have a greater frequency of constipation and UTI. There was no statistically significant difference in the rate of Clavien-Dindo grade II complications in the early post-operative period in our patients compared with that in laparoscopic rectopexies in patients over 80 years of age ($p = 0.98$) [13]. The overall objective cure rate of this surgery was 80%. In a previous study of laparoscopic sacrocolpopexy in younger women by our group, the objective cure rate was 88% [5], perhaps suggesting a reduction in the quality of connective tissue in older women.

Urogynaecologists have traditionally favoured vaginal surgery over abdominal, because the vaginal approach has been considered less invasive, with shorter post-operative recovery, and lower morbidity as compared with a laparotomy. However, this is now changing as minimally invasive laparoscopic techniques allow an abdominal approach without laparotomy. There is a perception that laparoscopic surgery is not suitable for the elderly, because general anaesthesia is mandatory, and the surgery can be prolonged and complex. Our data indicate this is not valid.

The results from our series indicate a laparoscopic abdominal approach is safe in this age group. However, the surgery was performed in a centre with a high laparoscopic urogynaecology workload, and the surgeons are very familiar with laparoscopic techniques and operate relatively swiftly. Sacrocolpopexy operation duration varies considerably in differing studies [16, 17]; whether surgery in the elderly would be well tolerated if operations took 2–3 h to perform is debatable and has not been tested by our study.

A limitation of this study is a relatively short follow-up time post-operatively; it would be desirable to assess satisfaction with outcome and incidence of surgery-associated complications over a longer time period. However, the purpose of this study was to investigate safety in the elderly; we have previously published on laparoscopic efficacy [10]. Perioperative and post-operative complications associated with elderly patients would be expected to occur within 6 weeks of surgery, and our study captures this data. A further limitation is the use of ASA score, as this does not fully capture the frailty of elderly patients. However, our literature search has confirmed that there is no specific perioperative risk scoring system for the elderly, and so this widely used scoring system was used as the best approximation.

Conclusions

This series suggests that contrary to popular belief, laparoscopic prolapse surgery is well tolerated in an ageing population. Laparoscopic prolapse surgery in experienced hands has comparable operative times to open surgery, and the avoidance of laparotomy reduces the risk of infection, haematoma, wound dehiscence and hernia formation, none of which were seen in this study. It allows the advantages of abdominal mesh to be conferred to the elderly. In other studies, this has reduced recurrence rates compared with non-mesh surgery and extrusion rates when compared with vaginal mesh surgery. We conclude that laparoscopic prolapse surgery is an acceptable approach for the very elderly.

Abbreviations
ASA: American Society of Anaesthesiologists; POP-Q: Pelvic organ prolapse quantification

Funding
No funding was provided for this research.

Authors' contributions
SWK participated in the data collection, manuscript writing and data analysis. HJ carried out the manuscript writing and data analysis. SJ contributed to the project development and manuscript editing. AGM carried out the data analysis. NP contributed to the project development and manuscript writing. All authors approved the manuscript for submission.

Authors' information
SWK is a foundation doctor at Harrogate District Hospital and was a medical student at Oxford University at the time of this research.
HJ is an obstetrics and gynaecology trainee at Oxford University Hospitals NHS Foundation Trust.
AGM is a consultant anaesthetist at Oxford University Hospitals NHS Foundation Trust.
SJ and NP are consultant gynaecologists at Oxford University Hospitals NHS Foundation Trust.

Competing interests
The authors declare that they have no competing interests.

Author details
[1]Department of Urogynaecology, Oxford University Hospitals, Oxford, UK. [2]Oxford Medical School, John Radcliffe Hospital, University of Oxford, Oxford, UK. [3]John Radcliffe Hospital, Oxford University Hospitals NHS Foundation Trust, Oxford, UK. [4]Harrogate District Hospital, Lancaster Park Rd, Harrogate, UK.

References
1. Luber KM, Boero S, Choe JY (2001) The demographics of pelvic floor disorders: current observations and future projections. Am J Obstet Gynecol 184: 1496–1501, discussion 1501–1503
2. Hefni M, El-Toukhy T, Bhaumik J, Katsimanis E (2003) Sacrospinous cervicocolpopexy with uterine conservation for uterovaginal prolapse in elderly women: an evolving concept. Am J Obstet Gynecol 188:645–650
3. Age UK (2016) Later life in the United Kingdom. Age UK. http://www.ageuk.org.uk/Documents/EN-GB/Factsheets/Later_Life_UK_factsheet.pdf?dtrk=true. Accessed 2 July 2016
4. ONS (2015) Statistical bulletin: Population Estimates for UK, England and Wales, Scotland and Northern Ireland: mid-2015. Office of National Statistics. https://www.ons.gov.uk/peoplepopulationandcommunity/populationandmigration/populationestimates/bulletins/annualmidyearpopulationestimates/mid2015. Accessed 1 Apr 2017
5. Price N, Slack A, Jackson SR (2011) Laparoscopic sacrocolpopexy: an observational study of functional and anatomical outcomes. Int Urogynecology J 22:77–82. doi:10.1007/s00192-010-1241-y
6. Rahmanou P, Price N, Jackson S (2014) Laparoscopic hysteropexy: a novel technique for uterine preservation surgery. Int Urogynecology J 25:139–140. doi:10.1007/s00192-013-2129-4
7. Dindo D, Demartines N, Clavien P-A (2004) Classification of surgical complications: a new proposal with evaluation in a cohort of 6336 patients and results of a survey. Ann Surg 240:205–213
8. Stepp KJ, Barber MD, Yoo E-H et al (2005) Incidence of perioperative complications of urogynecologic surgery in elderly women. Am J Obstet Gynecol 192:1630–1636. doi:10.1016/j.ajog.2004.11.026

9.   Friedman WH, Gallup DG, Burke JJ et al (2006) Outcomes of octogenarians and nonagenarians in elective major gynecologic surgery. Am J Obstet Gynecol 195:547–552. doi:10.1016/j.ajog.2006.03.085, discussion 552–553

10. Rahmanou P, White B, Price N, Jackson S (2014) Laparoscopic hysteropexy: 1- to 4-year follow-up of women postoperatively. Int Urogynecology J 25: 131–138. doi:10.1007/s00192-013-2209-5

11. Maher C, Feiner B, Baessler K, Schmid C (2013) Surgical management of pelvic organ prolapse in women. Cochrane Database Syst Rev 4:CD004014. doi:10.1002/14651858.CD004014.pub5

12. Caglià P, Costa S, Tracia A et al (2012) Can laparoscopic cholecystectomy be safety performed in the elderly? Ann Ital Chir 83:21–24

13. Wijffels N, Cunningham C, Dixon A et al (2011) Laparoscopic ventral rectopexy for external rectal prolapse is safe and effective in the elderly. Does this make perineal procedures obsolete? Colorectal Dis Off J Assoc Coloproctology G B Irel 13:561–566. doi:10.1111/j.1463-1318.2010.02242.x

14. Elneil S, Cutner A, Remy M, et al (2003) Laparoscopic prolapse surgery in the elderly. International Continence Society. http://www.ics.org/Abstracts/Publish/41/000554.pdf. Accessed 17 July 2016

15. Turner LC, Kantartzis K, Lowder JL, Shepherd JP (2014) The effect of age on complications in women undergoing minimally invasive sacral colpopexy. Int Urogynecology J 25:1251–1256. doi:10.1007/s00192-014-2391-0

16. Mustafa S, Amit A, Filmar S et al (2012) Implementation of laparoscopic sacrocolpopexy: establishment of a learning curve and short-term outcomes. Arch Gynecol Obstet 286:983–988. doi:10.1007/s00404-012-2391-6

17. Park Y-H, Yang SC, Park ST et al (2014) Laparoscopic reconstructive surgery is superior to vaginal reconstruction in the pelvic organ prolapse. Int J Med Sci 11:1082–1088. doi:10.7150/ijms.9027

12

Essure® present controversies and 5 years' learned lessons: a retrospective study with short- and long-term follow-up

Sara Câmara* ⓘ, Filipa de Castro Coelho, Cláudia Freitas and Lilia Remesso

Abstract

Background: The risk-benefit of contraception with Essure® is being readdressed due to an increase of reports of adverse effects with this device. Our aim was to proceed to an internal quality evaluation and to identify opportunities for protocol improvement.

We proceeded to a one-center, retrospective consecutive case series of women admitted for Essure® placement, from 1 January 2012 until 31 December 2016 (5 years).

Results: In a total of 274 women, technical difficulties were mainly unilateral, with no acute or short-term severe complications. The procedure was brief (median 3.2 min, IQR 2.5–5.2) and moderately painful (median of 4 in a 0–10 scale; IQR 3–5). At 3 months, the failure rate was 2%, with no pregnancies. Second surgery indication (< 1%) resumed to a case of nickel hypersensitivity. At 1 year, pregnancy rate was 1%. Ninety-eight percent of the patients would recommend the method.

Conclusions: We identified high patient satisfaction and low failure rates, both at short and long term. Investigation about whether some women still have patent tubes at the 3-month follow-up could lead to protocol improvement. It is important that clinicians look for second causes for adverse effects related to Essure® and avoid the erroneous indication for implant removal. Long follow-up allowed for both internal quality evaluation and clarification of misconception; it could possibly also have contributed to patient satisfaction.

Keywords: Hysteroscopy, Sterilization, Counseling, Patient satisfaction, Pelvic pain

Background

Office hysteroscopic sterilization is more cost-effective than laparoscopic sterilization and is a better option in high-operative-risk women [1]. Its success depends on careful patient selection, surgeon's experience, reliable compliance of back-up contraception, and observance of the 3-month follow-up [2]. Recently, there has been an imperative urge to survey Essure® risk-benefit profile during its life cycle, due to an intensification of adverse effect report [2, 3].

While being a highly satisfactory permanent contraception method, pelvic pain (related or not to menses) and irregular bleeding or heavy menstruation are among the most frequent late complications related to the procedure [2]. However, these symptoms are not always related to the micro-inserts itself but to other underlying gynecologic conditions (endometriosis, adenomyosis, or others), which could erroneously indicate the implant surgical removal [2, 4].

Several studies have been reported which describe long-term follow-ups (from 1 to 5 years) of patients submitted to sterilization with Essure® [5–7]. In this study, the authors have proceeded to a retrospective consecutive case series analysis of *one-center* (*two hysteroscopists*), 5 years' experience with Essure®. The authors' aim was first to evaluate internal quality (procedure-associated surgical difficulties; patient acute complications; failure and pregnancy rates; adverse effects; and satisfaction at long follow-up) and second, to identify opportunities for protocol improvement.

* Correspondence: sara.cam.camara@gmail.com
Department of Obstetrics and Gynecology, Hospital Dr. Nélio Mendonça,
Avenida Luís de Camões nº 57, Funchal 9004-514, Portugal

Methods

A retrospective case series analysis of women admitted to hysteroscopy with intention to treat for Essure® placement, at our center, from 1 January 2012 until 31 December 2016, was done.

Patient selection always included a previous standardized initial appreciation and information on this permanent contraception method (Table 1). All women received contraceptive counseling and were clinically evaluated by one of the two hysteroscopists, who would realize the procedure. Premedication with paracetamol or with non-steroidal anti-inflammatory was used at patient discretion, and this information could not be retrospectively confirmed. At all times, the placement of the micro-inserts was accomplished by vaginoscopy, without anesthesia or cervical dilatation. Women who were not using contraception at this moment or who were using barrier methods would be advised to start a hormonal contraceptive pill for back-up contraception, except if contraindicated.

Collected variables were:

- demographic characteristics (age, gravidity, parity, contraceptive method in use);
- procedure description (surgeon's perceived difficulty; duration of the procedure from the hysteroscope entrance until its exit from the uterine cervix external ostium; patient reported pain immediately after the procedure, in a numeric scale of 1–10);
- follow-up at 3 months (consisting of an appointment with the hysteroscopist of reference to monitor early complications; confirm correct localization of the micro-inserts either by X-ray, gynecological ultrasound, hysterosalpingography, or hysterosonography; and inform the patient if the back-up contraception should be prolonged or abandoned);

Table 1 Previous counseling included items

• Full gynecological evaluation (clinical history, gynecological observation, transvaginal ultrasound, and cervical and breast cancer screening if indicated)
• Confirming the motivation to permanent contraception
• Evaluation of nickel or metal allergy
• Full information on the procedure (anatomical and technical details)
• Full information on possible complications and restrictions — *Early*: infection, acute pain, perforation/migration/expulsion *Late*: chronic pain or irregular/heavy bleeding *Restrictions*: ✓ Magnetic resonance—safe if using a 1.5 T magnet; artifact possibility ✓ Electrosurgical procedures—should be avoided if near the micro-inserts

- and follow-up after the first completed year (women were contacted by phone by the same medically trained operator and were asked to classify their satisfaction with the method as "very unsatisfied," "unsatisfied," "satisfied," or "completely satisfied" to state reasons in case they were not completely satisfied and if they would likely recommend this method).

Finally, failure (defined by incorrect micro-implant localization or tubal permeability) rates and pregnancy rates at 3 months and 1 year were calculated, and second surgery requirement and indication were explored.

Results
Essure® delivery
During 5 years, 274 women were admitted to hysteroscopy with intention to treat for Essure® delivery (Table 2).

This was not achieved bilaterally in 7.3% of the patients mainly because of obstruction to the delivery catheter progression but also because of non-identified ostium or ostia (Table 3). The minority of patients with non-identified ostium or ostia were using continuous hormonal contraception (either a combined estroprogestative or a progestative-only pill). Device (manufacturer)-related difficulties were not identified. Women who could not be successfully sterilized with Essure® underwent either laparoscopic tubal ligation or salpingectomy (according to the woman's informed choice). There were no severe acute complications. The only acute complication was one case of vagal reaction, immediately after successful implant delivery (with complete satisfaction at long follow-up).

Early (3 months) follow-up (n = 254)
For the 3-month follow-up, we considered the 254 women with successful delivered micro-inserts. No loss of follow-up or pregnancy was registered. In 2% (n = 4), the confirmatory exams revealed that the procedure was

Table 2 Demographic characteristics of patients submitted to hysteroscopy for Essure® delivery

Age (years)	mean = 38 (SD = 4; range 27–46)
Gravidity	median = mode = 2 (IQR 2–3; range 0–7)
Parity	median = mode = 2 (IQR 2–3; range 0–6)
Previous contraceptive method	• SARC users: 65% (n = 178), of which 96% (n = 171) were using a contraceptive pill • LARC users 15% (n = 42) • Others (barrier or natural method of contraception) 20% (n = 54)

SARC short-acting reversible contraception, *LARC* long-acting reversible contraception

Table 3 Procedure description

Surgical difficulties	• Surgeon's perceived difficulty in inserts delivery 11% ($n = 31$), of which 65% ($n = 20$) unilateral • Successful placement not achieved in 7.3% ($n = 20$): ✓ tube obstruction because of spasm/stenosis ($n = 16$) ✓ non-identified ostium/ostia ($n = 4$)
Hysteroscopy duration (minutes)	Δt median 3.2 (IQR 2.5–5.2; range 1–15)
Patient reported pain (0–10 scale)	median score = 4 (IQR 3–5; range 0–8); mode = 3

ineffective (two cases of contrast leakage; one case of leakage in the post-salpingectomy side, with confirmed contralateral obstruction; and one case of insert unilateral expulsion, brought in hand by the patient and confirmed by imaging). This last patient underwent subsequent placement of a new micro-insert which she again noticed to deliver per the vagina some days afterwards (with correct number of coils trailing in uterine cavity, namely three, bilaterally and without perceived surgical difficulty during its placement).

During this first trimester, there were no cases of fever, documented infection, or pelvic pain requiring further care.

One allergic reaction to nickel manifested shortly after the 3-month follow-up with a generalized dyshidrotic eczema, and this was confirmed by immunoallergology patch test. This woman had no history of allergy to metals, and the situation resolved completely after hysterectomy (which was the decision taken together with patient, considering the surgical risks of a more conservator approach, including that of incomplete device removal).

Late (≥ 1 year) follow-up, complications, and satisfaction (n = 249)

Considering the patients with a 3-month follow-up which confirmed correct Essure® placement, a total of 249 patients had the implants for more than 1 year before. Not all these patients could be contacted by telephone at several attempts. At the end, 72% of them ($n = 179$) answered to the satisfaction survey; 88% ($n = 158$) were completely satisfied and 9% ($n = 17$) were very satisfied but reported abnormal menstrual bleeding and/or pelvic pain (related or not to menstruation). Two percent ($n = 4$) were unsatisfied or very unsatisfied and were the only who would not recommend this method of contraception (two of these women had the same symptoms than the other patients but more severe, requiring the reintroduction of hormonal therapy; the other two women had correct micro-insert placement documented by either X-ray and ultrasound or by hysterosalpingography but reported a pregnancy diagnosed

at their private medical assistance). Assuming these two cases of pregnancy, the pregnancy rate at 1 year was 1%.

In this satisfaction survey, two women pointed out that they had been denied magnetic resonance. This question was readdressed and clarified during the satisfaction survey. Some women revealed misconceptions about the procedure (relating it to the posterior appearance of an adnexal mass or to abnormal cervical smear), which was elucidated at that moment.

Discussion

Although there are presently many controversies about Essure®, evidence about long-term follow-up of patients submitted to this type of definitive contraception is scarce. The importance to proceed to an extended survey of patients' satisfaction has been unanimously strengthened by previous studies [5–9]. In what concerns the demographic findings in our population, they are similar to what has been described by others [5–9].

Surgical difficulty and unsuccessful procedure

In our experience, the surgeon perceived the procedure as difficult in 11% of the cases (mainly unilateral difficulty), with an unsuccessful micro-insert delivery (either with or without attempt), comparable to the results found in the literature (7.3 versus 1.5% [9], 2.8% [7], 8% [6], 12% [10]). Systematic use of a non-steroidal anti-inflammatory or a spasmolytic before the procedure (except if contraindicated) could possibly contribute to diminish tubal spasm and subsequent obstruction, but this is yet to be probed. Although we had no event of perforation or abdominal migration, these events could be related to tubal cannulation attempts and, therefore, also benefit from tubal spasm prevention. In what concerns continuous hormonal contraception, it is thought to improve visibility and therefore facilitate the implant delivery. Theoretically, continuous progestins, instead of combined hormonal contraception, may be more favorable due to a higher atrophic effect of the endometrium, but this is not evidence-based. In our sample, however, all women with non-identified ostium/ostia were using continuous hormonal contraception.

Patient acute complications

Besides acute pain and one self-limited vagal reaction, we had no other incidents like perforation, syncope, or infection. In the literature, there is no evidence about acute complication incidence, but our findings and of others support that this procedure is moderately painful even if brief [5–8]. An incidence of 4.2% of pain chronification (lasting more than 3 months after the procedure) has been estimated [10]. Because our study is retrospective, we could not identify our incidence of chronic pain.

Failure and pregnancy rates

A good adherence to the 3-month confirmatory tests and back-up birth control after hysteroscopic sterilization is important to avoid unintended pregnancies. Remarkably, we had no loss to follow-up or pregnancy events at 3 months, with a correct placement confirmed in 99% of the tests which is analogous to previous publications (99.5% [7] and 99.6% [9]; even if in these series a lower first control compliance rate is reported 90.8 and 96.8%, respectively). Our 3-month follow-up detected failures were due to contrast leakage or micro-insert expulsion. In the second case, we would now opt for another type of sterilization instead of a second attempt. In view of the fact that the implant expulsed had been delivered with no difficulty, that a correct number of coils trailed in the cavity, and the facility at which it was asymptomatically expulsed, we can imagine that there can be a sort of tubal incompetency.

At 1-year follow-up, we had two pregnancies reported (corresponding to a failure rate of 1%), after documented correct micro-inserts localization. Both, incorrect interpretation of those tests or correct interpretation of localization tests but without obstruction confirmation, are plausible explanations. However, it may also be hypothesized that some women may produce less or slower reaction to the implant, accounting for cases of migration or expulsion, or even for cases of pregnancy after the 3-month correct follow-up. In agreement with this hypothesis, higher than expected tubal patency at intervals less than 1 year [11] and cases of pregnancy after the 3-month ideal follow-up have been published [2, 7]. Failure rates of all types of sterilization failures are estimated in 0.9% [12] but there is uncertainty about specific failure rates for Essure® due to either short follow-up studies, discrepancy between study results, or lack of information on follow-up or on accomplished protocol [13, 14].

Adverse effects and satisfaction at long follow-up

Complication rate for laparoscopic sterilization has been estimated in 1.6% [15]. In our study, we had no case of infection, perforation, embolus, or death. Considering the case of nickel hypersensitivity, our post-procedure second surgery was 0.4%. We consider that the suspicion of nickel allergy should contraindicate the procedure even if since 2011 this is no longer contraindicated by the Food and Drug Administration and if some authors would recommend further evaluation but nevertheless consider the procedure [7]. In the manufacturer's official site, it can be read that *no* test can reliably predict this adverse effect [16].

Like in our study, studies evaluating women satisfaction have constantly found high levels of early and late satisfaction with levels of moderate or lower pain [6–8]. The most frequent reported secondary adverse effects are pelvic pain (with or without dysmenorrhea) and increased menses bleeding or irregularity [2]. Unfortunately, we could not assess "de novo" pain cases because most of these women were previously under hormonal contraception, which could have masked previous symptoms. Resuming hormonal therapy ameliorated the symptoms, avoiding the need for second surgery for implant removal (guaranteeing a more effective contraception). Others have enlightened the importance to clearly evaluate the complaints that patients relate to Essure®, at the risk of removing the implants without improvement [2, 4]. With reported second surgery rates of 0.4% [7] to 4.3% [4], according to a recent retrospective cohort study, more than half of surgeries post-Essure® placement were related to pain complaints and the majority of them related to subjacent gynecological conditions [4]. We believe that this finding is of great relevance for clinicians who evaluate women with Essure®.

Final considerations

The most important weakness of our study is its retrospective nature. With our findings, we now look forward to proceed in our investigation in a prospective way and to a longer interval of follow-up.

Finally, we believe that the possibility to inform women about misconceptions of long-term effects of the method contributes to a higher patient satisfaction, though this has not been previously studied. Further investigation is needed to identify which benefits can be obtained by premedication and if a different first follow-up control could have higher sensitivity in the detection of the method failure.

Conclusions

From 5 years of experience with Essure®, we identified very high rates of satisfaction with this extremely effective and accessible method, associated to moderate pain in a fast procedure, with a low need for second surgery. The unsatisfaction related to the method is usually due to misconceptions about it, which is why we attribute great relevance to prior candidate selection and specific counseling. Long follow-up allows for both further identification of method failure and for a second chance for misconception clarification. It can probably also contribute to a higher patient satisfaction.

Abbreviations
LARC: Long-acting reversible contraception; SARC: Short-acting reversible contraception

Acknowledgements
Nothing to declare.

Funding
Not applicable.

Authors' contributions

All the designated authors have contributed to this article conception and production. All authors read and approved the final manuscript.

Authors' information

Nothing to declare.

Competing interests

The authors declare that they have no competing interests.

References

1. Carney PI, Yao J, Lin J, Law A (2017) Comparison of healthcare costs among commercially insured women in the United States who underwent hysteroscopic sterilization versus laparoscopic bilateral tubal ligation sterilization. J Women's Health (Larchmt) 26(5):483–490. doi:10.1089/jwh.2016.6035

2. American Association of Gynecologic Laparoscopists (AAGL). Advancing Minimally Invasive Gynecology Worldwide. AAGL Advisory Statement: Essure Hysteroscopic Sterilization. J Minim Invasive Gynecol. 2016;23(5):658–59. doi:10.1016/j.jmig.2016.06.005

3. Walter JR, Ghobadi CW, Hayman E, Xu S (2017) Hysteroscopic sterilization with Essure: summary of the U.S. Food and Drug Administration actions and policy implications for postmarketing surveillance. Obstet Gynecol 129(1): 10–19. doi:10.1097/AOG.0000000000001796

4. Kamencic H, Thiel L, Karreman E, Thiel J (2016) Does Essure cause significant de novo pain? A retrospective review of indications for second surgeries after Essure placement. J Minim Invasive Gynecol 23(7):1158–1162. doi:10.1016/j.jmig.2016.08.823

5. Gibon E, Lopès P, Linet T, Martigny H, Orieux C, Philippe H-J (2006) Stérilisation tubaire par voie hystéroscopique : faisabilité et évaluation à un an. Gynécologie Obs Fertil 34(3):202–208. doi:10.1016/j.gyobfe.2006.01.029

6. Chudnoff SG, Nichols JE, Levie M (2015) Hysteroscopic Essure inserts for permanent contraception: extended follow-up results of a phase III multicenter international study. J Minim Invasive Gynecol 22(6):951–960. doi:10.1016/j.jmig.2015.04.017

7. Franchini M, Zizolfi B, Coppola C et al (2017) Essure permanent birth control, effectiveness and safety: an Italian 11-year survey. J Minim Invasive Gynecol 24(4):640–645. doi:10.1016/j.jmig.2017.02.004

8. Arjona JE, Miño M, Cordón J, Povedano B, Pelegrin B, Castelo-Branco C (2008) Satisfaction and tolerance with office hysteroscopic tubal sterilization. Fertil Steril 90(4):1182–1186. doi:10.1016/j.fertnstert.2007.08.007

9. Povedano B, Arjona J, Velasco E, Monserrat J, Lorente J, Castelo-Branco C (2012) Complications of hysteroscopic Essure® sterilisation: report on 4306 procedures performed in a single centre. BJOG 119:795–799. doi:10.1111/j.1471-0528.2012.03292

10. Yunker AC, Ritch JM, Robinson EFGC (2015) Incidence and risk factors for chronic pelvic pain after hysteroscopic sterilization. J Minim Invasive Gynecol 22(3):390–394. doi:10.1016/j.jmig.2014.06.007

11. Rodriguez AM, Kilic GS, Vu TP, Kuo Y-F, Breitkopf D, Snyder RR Analysis of tubal patency after essure placement. J Minim Invasive Gynecol 20(4):468–472. doi:10.1016/j.jmig.2013.01.013

12. Trussell J, Guilbert E, Hedley A (2003) Sterilization failure, sterilization reversal, and pregnancy after sterilization reversal in Quebec. Obstet Gynecol 101(4):677–684 http://www.ncbi.nlm.nih.gov/pubmed/12681870

13. Cleary TP, Tepper NK, Cwiak C et al (2013) Pregnancies after hysteroscopic sterilization: a systematic review. Contraception 87(5):539–548. doi:10.1016/j.contraception.2012.08.006

14. la Chapelle CF, Veersema S, Brölmann HAM, Jansen FW (2015) Effectiveness and feasibility of hysteroscopic sterilization techniques: a systematic review and meta-analysis. Fertil Steril 103(6):1516-25-3. doi:10.1016/j.fertnstert.2015.03.009

15. Jamieson DJ, Hillis SD, Duerr A, Marchbanks PA, Costello C, Peterson HB (2000) Complications of interval laparoscopic tubal sterilization: findings from the United States Collaborative Review of Sterilization. Obstet Gynecol 96(6):997–1002 http://www.ncbi.nlm.nih.gov/pubmed/11084192

16. http://www.hcp.essure-us.com/index.php. Accessed 16 Apr 2017

13

Treating symptomatic uterine fibroids with myomectomy: current practice and views of UK consultants

R. Fusun Sirkeci[1] (iD), Anna Maria Belli[2] and Isaac T. Manyonda[3*]

Abstract

Background: The demand for uterus-sparing treatments is increasing as more women postpone childbirth to their 30–40s, when fibroids are more symptomatic. With an increasing choice of treatment options and changing care-provider profiles, now is an opportune time to survey current practices and opinions. Using a 25-stem questionnaire, a web-based survey was used to capture the practices and opinions of UK consultant gynecologists on the treatment of symptomatic fibroids, including the types of procedure most frequently used, methods used to reduce blood loss, and awareness and acceptability of treatment options, and to assess the impact of gender and experience of the treating gynecologist.

Results: The response rate was 22%. Laparascopic myomectomy is used least frequently, with 80% of the respondents using GnRHa preoperatively to minimize blood loss and correct anemia, while vasopressin is most frequently used to reduce intraoperative blood loss. Female consultants operate significantly less frequently than males. Those with more than 10 years consultant experience are more likely to perform an open myomectomy compared to those with less than 10 years experience.

Conclusions: Compared to a similar survey performed 10 years ago, surgical methods remain to be the most common treatments, but use of less invasive treatments such as UAE has increased. Consultants' attitudes appear to be responding to the patient demand for less radical treatments. However, it is yet to be seen if the changing consultant demographics will keep up with this demand. The low response rate warrants cautious interpretation of the results, but they provide an interesting snapshot of current views and practices.

Keywords: Fibroids, Myomectomy, UAE, GnRHa, Vasopressin, Consultant practices

Background

Fibroids are the most common tumor in women of reproductive age [1, 2]. Recent years have seen a demographic shift in childbirth trends, with many women delaying starting their families until they reach their third or fourth decade [3, 4]. This is the age when fibroids are more prevalent and symptomatic [5, 6]. The old adage "children then fibroids and then hysterectomy" therefore no longer applies to many a modern woman, and there is likely to be an increasing demand for fertility-preserving treatments for symptomatic uterine fibroids.

The repertoire of uterus-preserving treatments for symptomatic fibroids has increased in recent years. Just over 20 years ago, the use of uterine artery embolization (UAE) was first reported [7]. The National Institute for Health and Clinical Excellence (NICE) has reviewed its efficacy and recommends UAE as an alternative treatment to hysterectomy and myomectomy [8]. Magnetic resonance (MR)-guided focused ultrasound (MRgFUS) [9] is another new technique, but its adoption has been slow, partly due to the high infrastructure costs of setting up such a service, and because of its limitations in treating large and/or numerous fibroids [10, 11]. Pharmaceutical agents continue to be developed. While it was originally introduced as a pre-myomectomy treatment [12], ulipristal acetate has recently acquired a license for use as a stand-alone treatment for symptomatic fibroids [13] and is regarded by many as the

* Correspondence: imanyond@gmail.com; imanyond@sgul.ac.uk
[3]Department of Obstetrics and Gynecology, St George's Healthcare NHS Foundation Trust, St George's, University of London, Blackshaw Road, Tooting, SW17 0QT London, UK
Full list of author information is available at the end of the article

"first-in-class" medical therapy for fibroids [14]. Despite the emergence of these new and exciting treatments for managing symptomatic uterine fibroids, in reality, when the uterus is to be preserved, myomectomy, especially the open abdominal approach, remains the treatment of choice of many gynecologists.

Surveys can be a useful tool in the evaluation of healthcare, whether by the recipients of healthcare or the healthcare professionals themselves. Historically, surveys were predominantly paper based, but the advent of the Internet and the development of dedicated software such as SurveyMonkey have made surveys much more efficient and powerful tools. With the new treatment modalities now embedding, and the changing demographics of both the profile of gynecological consultants and the population they serve, we considered it an opportune time to survey the views and practices of current UK consultant gynecologists on uterus-sparing techniques. We conducted an online survey and present and compare our findings to a similar paper-based survey conducted 10 years ago [15].

Methods

Using a web-based survey system (SurveyMonkey, Inc.) a 25-item questionnaire was designed that included questions on the respondents' gender, current place of work (i.e., district general hospital or tertiary center), how long they had been in a consultant role, and current clinical interests and subspecialty. The questionnaire further sought the respondents views and practices on the three types of myomectomy (open, laparoscopic, and hysteroscopic) and methods used to reduce blood loss both pre- and perioperatively. Additional questions were enquired about the respondents' access to, and use of, cell salvage, and their views on UAE and ulipristal acetate (UPA). To refine and reduce ambiguity, the questionnaire was piloted among local gynecology consultants before invitations to participate were sent out nationally. A copy of the final version of the questionnaire is included in the Additional file 1.

The questionnaires were completed anonymously. The survey was active between November 2014 and April 2015. To maximize the response rate, the survey was advertised in the Royal College of Obstetricians and Gynecologists (RCOG) monthly electronic newsletter, the Scanner, which is e-mailed to all RCOG members. Two months after, the survey opened an invitation to participate and the link to the survey was also e-mailed to members of the British Society for Gynecological Endoscopy (BSGE).

As the study did not involve patients or their data, ethical approval was not required.

Statistical analysis was performed using SPSS software (IBM SPSS Statistics V22, Chicago, IL). The results are expressed in percentages (%) and absolute values (n). A p value equal to or less than 0.05 was considered significant.

Results
Response rate
Of the 1375 consultants invited to participate in the survey, 299 responded, a response rate of 22%.[1] Among the respondents, a minority did not answer every question applicable to them. Therefore, for some questions discussed below, the total numbers are smaller than 299.

Demographics
Thirty-six percent ($n = 108$) of respondents were female and 51% ($n = 152$) were male while 13% ($n = 39$) did not to disclose their gender. This correlates well with the actual gender distribution of current consultants in practice and gives some credence that the responses in our survey are representative of the workforce as a whole: as of 2013, 47% of the consultant workforce in the UK was female and 53% male [16]. Just under half of the respondents (48%, $n = 143$) were based in district general hospitals, 36% ($n = 106$) were working in university teaching hospitals, 4% ($n = 11$) worked exclusively in the private sector and 12% ($n = 36$) did not indicate the sector in which they worked. Since doctors enter into the specialty at varying ages, we did not record our respondents' age, but rather how many years they have been at the consultant grade. We found that male respondents had practiced for more years than their female colleagues. While 60% of female consultants had less than 10 years experience, 72% of males had 10 years or more experience. This is also in line with the experience status of the current consultant cohort [16].

Thirty-nine percent ($n = 117$) described themselves as generalists in Obstetrics and Gynecology, and 15% ($n = 44$) responded that they were sub-specialists in Minimal Access Surgery (MAS) (Table 1.).

Performance of myomectomy for symptomatic fibroids
With regard to performing myomectomy, 81% ($n = 243$) stated that they performed some type of myomectomy. Open myomectomy was the procedure performed by the vast majority (74%, $n = 221$). Hysteroscopic procedures were performed by 56% ($n = 166$), and 32% of the

Table 1 How the respondents defined themselves

	%	Total number of responses (N)
Generalist	39	117
Minimal access surgeon	15	44
Urogynecologist	8	25
Reproductive medicine specialist	8	25
Gynecological oncologist	5	15
Non subspecialist obstetrician	2	7
Non subspecialist gynecologist	6	19
Missing response	12	36
Total	100	299

respondents ($n = 95$) stated that they perform laparoscopic myomectomy, while 29% ($n = 86$) of our respondents reported that they perform all three types of myomectomy.

Three fifths (46%, $n = 138$) of respondents reported that the size of the uterus would not influence their decision whether or not to perform open myomectomy. There is no limit on the number of fibroids removed laparoscopically by 18% ($n = 54$) and hysteroscopically by 31% ($n = 93$). Only 43% ($n = 127$) aim to remove all fibroids during an open myomectomy.

Male consultants are significantly more likely to perform a myomectomy compared to their female counterparts (90%, $n = 137$ males versus 69%, $n = 74$ females). Logistic regression modeling confirmed that this association was significant. Binary logistic regression modeling also showed that the experience and subspecialty/special interests of the consultants had a significant impact on their choice of performing or not performing myomectomy (Table 2).

Consultants with more experience are significantly more likely to perform myomectomy than their colleagues with less than 10 years' experience at consultant level (OR = 0.312, $p = 0.012$). Similarly, male consultants are also significantly more likely to operate compared to their female counterparts (OR = 0.232, $p = 0.01$). Perhaps unsurprisingly, respondents who described themselves as fetal medicine specialists operate significantly less than those in other subspecialties. The majority of respondents (89%, $n = 194$) agreed that complex fibroid surgery should only be performed by experienced gynecologists who frequently perform this operation.

Attitudes towards myomectomy and women's wishes

Fifty-four percent ($n = 160$) of our respondents said that they would offer a myomectomy to a woman whose family is complete, but who simply wishes to retain her uterus because she feels a more "complete woman".

Similarly, 175 respondents (59%) stated that they would perform a repeat myomectomy on a woman who wished to retain her fertility.

Preventing and minimizing blood loss, the use of GnRH analogues (GnRHa), uterine artery embolization (UAE), and ulipristal acetate (UPA)

Although used in women undergoing all three types of myomectomy, the responses to our survey show that 86% ($n = 257$) of consultants use GnRHa prior to open myomectomy. Twenty-one percent ($n = 62$) used GnRHa prior to laparoscopic myomectomy while 44% ($n = 131$) use GnRHa prior to hysteroscopic myomectomy. The indications stated for GnRHa use were to correct anemia prior to surgery (50%, $n = 148$) and to reduce fibroid size to allow a lower transverse incision rather than a midline one (51%, $n = 151$). Interestingly, 41% ($n = 122$) stated that they use them despite knowing that GnRHa destroy tissue planes, thus rendering surgery more difficult.

Thirty percent ($n = 91$) of our respondents reported that they cross match blood for every open myomectomy they perform. Vasopressin was used by 29% ($n = 86$), while tourniquets/clamps were used by 20% ($n = 57$) to minimize blood loss during open myomectomy. Fifteen percent reported that they do not use any specific technique, and 44% ($n = 132$) have access to a cell salvage facility (Table 3).

Sixty-two percent ($n = 184$) of the respondents have access to UAE for the treatment of symptomatic uterine fibroids. When asked whether they would offer UAE to women wishing to conceive, 43% ($n = 127$) replied that they would. Forty-nine percent ($n = 146$) have read the joint guidelines published by The Royal College of Obstetrics and Gynecologists/Royal College of Radiologists [17] on the use of UAE for the treatment of uterine fibroids.

Table 2 Key drivers for not performing myomectomy

Variables	SE	Sig.	OR
Female (compared to male)	*.459*	*.001*	*.232*
Experience 0–9 years (compared to 10 years+)	*.464*	*.012*	*.312*
Obstetrics and Gynecology (compared to Generalist)		*.001*	
Obstetrics (non-subspecialist) only	14,129.622	.999	.000
Gynecology (non-subspecialist) only	.672	.078	.306
Subspecialist/special interest in Gynecological Oncology	.861	.496	.556
Subspecialist/special interest in Urogynecology	*.645*	*.003*	*.146*
Subspecialist/special interest in Reproductive Medicine	.835	.975	1.027
Subspecialist/special interest in Fetal Maternal Medicine	*.842*	*.000*	*.035*
Subspecialist/special interest in Minimal Access Surgery	1.066	.108	5.554
Constant	.533	.000	32.073

Coefficients significantly different from zero at the 0.05 level or better are shown in italics
SE Standard error, *Sig* Significance, *OR* odds ratio

Table 3 Methods used to reduce intraoperative blood loss

Methods used to minimize blood loss	N	%
Vasopressin	86	29
Tourniquets/clamps	57	19
Tranexamic acid	37	12
Oxytocin	3	1.0
Misoprostol	1	0.3
No method used	43	14
Missing	72	24
Total	299	100

Seventy-three percent ($n = 218$) reported that they were aware of UPA, and 32% ($n = 96$) had used it pre-myomectomy. On the other hand, 29% ($n = 87$) respondents had never used UPA, while a mere 10% ($n = 29$) had used UPA for treating conditions other than symptomatic uterine fibroids, such as emergency contraception.

Discussion

With a response rate of 22%, we are acutely aware of the need to interpret our findings with caution. However, the correlation between the results obtained in our survey with published gender breakdown of current consultants suggests that our respondents reflect the make up of consultants in the UK [16], and therefore, our findings provide a useful snapshot of current views and practices in the management of fibroids.

Although surveys are an important tool in the evaluation of health services, it would appear that response rates to most surveys have been declining over the years. Historically, surveys were conducted via the post, with apparently good responses. Thus, a postal survey on the same issue of myomectomy conducted by Taylor et al. [15] 10 years ago yielded a response rate of 54%. One would have assumed that the advent of the internet, with access to online surveys and the advantages of instant survey delivery, real-time data collection, ease of access for respondents, and increased respondent anonymity would increase the response rates for surveys. This does not appear to be the case, and it is reported that response rates differ among various specialties [18]. The ease of use of e-surveys may in fact be a factor contributing to the decline in response rates, as people are bombarded with a multitude of surveys, and it is so easy to delete the e-mail without even opening it. In a meta-analysis of 68 web-based health surveys, the mean response rate reported in 49 studies was 39.6% [19]. However, our own recent experience of a 28% response rate from a postal survey [20] would suggest that there is indeed a general decline in response rates, and this is mirrored in the experience of other colleagues (Sultan et al., personal communication). Thus, many factors probably

contribute to the declining response rates, and it is unlikely that this trend can be improved significantly.

Despite the emergence of minimally invasive techniques, including UAE, and the pharmacological agent UPA, our work suggests that surgery is still the most common form of fibroid treatment offered in the UK, a finding supported by work published by the Health and Social Care Information Centre, Hospital Episode Statistics (HES) [21].

From their postal survey published 10 years ago, Taylor et al. [15] reported that 64% of their respondents performed at least one open myomectomy per year; with around half (51%) performing between one and five procedures annually. Our own survey suggests that the number of surgeons reporting that they performed between one and ten myomectomies per year has increased to 62%. Similarly, the rate of laparoscopic myomectomy has risen from 11 to 32%. Whether this is a reflection of the increased demand for uterine sparing procedures or has resulted from surgeons having a higher caseload or both remains to be answered.

The use of pre-myomectomy GnRHa use has not changed in the intervening 10 years: Taylor et al. [15] reported that 85% of their respondents use GnRHa pre-myomectomy, and our own survey yielded a similar result of 86%. Interestingly, 41% of our respondents stated that GnRHa destroy tissue planes and thus render the surgery more difficult. The Cochrane review on the preoperative use of GnRH comments that "fibroid capsule will become less evident and may be missed, tumours will not "shell out" cleanly and the excision may be more difficult" [22]. The literature also reports that the use of GnRHa is not cost-effective [23], delays surgery, and is associated with significant side effects and bone demineralization, and there are much cheaper alternatives such as progestogens to prevent menstruation while correcting anemia [24]. Further evidence is emerging regarding the preoperative use of UPA which could be a better alternative to GnRH: a recent study from Canada investigated the surgical experience of patients that underwent laparoscopic or robotic myomectomy following UPA treatment and found no difference compared to non-treated patients [25]. On a similar note, Sancho et al. described a case series where no difficulty was observed during hysteroscopic fibroid resection following UPA treatment [26].

Only one in five of the respondents to our survey reported that they used tourniquets or clamps. This is despite reports that the application of tourniquets is more effective than GnRHa in minimizing blood loss [27]. Our survey found that perioperatively, 29% ($n = 86$) of gynecologists use vasopressin to minimize blood loss. This relatively low rate may reflect concerns that have been raised recently concerning the safety of vasopressin [28].

Taylor et al. [15] reported that only 28% of their respondents were prepared to perform a myomectomy on a 50-year-old woman, presumably on the assumption that they no longer needed their uterus. While we did not ask this exact same question, 54% of respondents to our survey replied that they would perform a myomectomy on a woman who has completed her family, and 59% would perform a repeat myomectomy. These responses may reflect an increasing awareness and acceptance of women's autonomy, as well as being driven by the changing demography of many women delaying childbirth until later in life.

Transformed attitudes may also be reflected in the increased awareness and acceptance of UAE seen in our survey. Taylor et al. [15] reported that only around half of their respondents had ready access to UAE. Our work suggests that this figure has risen to 62%. In the past, it was a common opinion that UAE should not be offered to women wishing to conceive, and this is reflected in 26% of the participants in Taylor et al.'s study who agreed that they would offer UAE to such women. With ever increasing reports of women having successful pregnancies following UAE, guidance is no longer quite so didactic, and in our survey, 43% of all our respondents would offer UAE to women planning conception. It is interesting to note that the advent of UAE and other uterus-sparing treatments have not reduced the number of myomectomies being carried out, perhaps another reflection that women have been demanding more uterine saving procedures compared to a decade ago.

According to the Centre for Workforce Intelligence's latest report [16], the number of women in the Obstetrics and Gynecology workforce has increased more than fourfold, from around 200 in 1998 to over 893 in 2013. In the last few years, over four fifths (81%) of specialist trainees in Obstetrics and Gynecology are female. In our survey, three fifths (59%) of respondents were male. Of the male respondents, 90% reported that they performed some type of myomectomy, while the figure is significantly lower among females. The percentage of male consultants performing myomectomy with 10 years or more experience is 90% whereas the corresponding figure for females is 74% ($p = 0.003$). Among those with less than 10 years experience, the contrast is even starker as only 64% of females perform myomectomy compared to 91% of male consultants ($p = 0.016$). This raises an important question: is the lower surgery rate seen in women in our survey a result of their relative inexperience, or does this signify a paradigm shift away from surgery that female gynecologists deem unnecessary and towards the use of other primary treatments for symptomatic uterine fibroids? If the former, then our survey raises an important issue, which has major implications for training and workforce planning, namely, who will perform the myomectomies of tomorrow?

If we are to offer our patients the best outcomes, then any treatment of significant complexity should be delivered by a highly trained individual who administers that treatment on a frequent basis. Our specialty has seen a move away from "generalists" and towards dedicated sub-specialists such as those treating gynecological cancers, women with urinary disorders, and high-risk pregnancies. Fibroid surgery can be challenging, and it is informative that 89% of all our respondents agreed that only experienced gynecologists who perform these operations frequently should undertake complex fibroid surgery. Increasing rates of both open and minimally access surgery rates support our views that there is a demand for a subspecialist competent in all forms of myomectomy. As fibroids present in a wide range of sizes and locations with variety of symptoms, and patients may wish to have a selection of treatments; we believe that there simply is no single ideal treatment. Case-by-case assessment of each individual patient is therefore necessary to optimize the treatment where the role of experienced benign gynecological surgeon is indisputable.

Conclusions

The changing demography of childbirth, with women increasingly postponing pregnancy to an age when fibroids are more numerous and symptomatic, poses a variety of challenges. There is a need to research and optimize the treatment options available, a cadre of highly skilled surgeons will be required, and this has major implications for the training of gynecologists, and new treatments must be sought that enhance fertility potential and symptom relief with minimal risk to the woman. Surveys such as the one presented here provide crucial snapshots of current practices and views and hopefully help to shape those practices and future directions.

Endnote

[1] There were 2225 consultants employed in 154 NHS units as of 2013. https://www.rcog.org.uk/globalassets/documents/careers-and-training/census-workforce-planning/census-report-2013.pdf.

Abbreviations
GnRHa: Gonadotrophin-releasing hormone analogue; UAE: Uterine artery embolization; UPA: Ulipristal acetate

Acknowledgements
The authors would like to thank Royal College of Obstetricians and Gynecologists (RCOG) and British Society for Gynecological Endoscopy (BSGE) for advertising the link to our survey to their members.

Funding
The authors obtained no specific funding for this study.

Authors' contributions

ITM and FS had the original idea. FS and ITM prepared the questionnaire. FS collected and analyzed the data. ITM, AMB, and FS wrote the manuscript. ITM and AMB supervised FS. All authors read and approved the final manuscript.

Competing interests

The authors declare that they have no competing interests.

Author details

[1]St George's, University of London, London, UK. [2]Department of Radiology, St George's Healthcare NHS Foundation Trust, St George's, University of London, London, UK. [3]Department of Obstetrics and Gynecology, St George's Healthcare NHS Foundation Trust, St George's, University of London, Blackshaw Road, Tooting, SW17 0QT London, UK.

References

1. Baird DD, Dunson DB, Hill MC, Cousins D, Schectman JM (2003) High cumulative incidence of uterine leiomyoma in black and white women: ultrasound evidence. Am J Obstet Gynecol 188:100–7
2. Laughlin SK, Schroeder JC, Baird DD (2010) New directions in the epidemiology of uterine fibroids. Semin Reprod Med 28(3):204–17
3. Schmidt L, Sobotka T, Bentzen JG, Nyboe Andersen A, ESHRE Reproduction and Society Task Force (2012) Demographic and medical consequences of the postponement of parenthood. Hum Reprod Update 18(1):29–43
4. Office for National Statistics, Births in England and Wales 2015. Available online at: https://www.ons.gov.uk/peoplepopulationandcommunity/births deathsandmarriages/livebirths/bulletins/birthsummarytablesengland andwales/2015. (Accessed 23 June 2017)
5. Marshall LM, Spiegelman D, Barbieri RL, Goldman MB, Manson JE, Colditz GA et al (1997) Variation in the incidence of uterine leiomyoma among premenopausal women by age and race. Obstet Gynecol 90(6):967–73
6. Okolo S (2008) Incidence, aetiology and epidemiology of uterine fibroids. Best Pract Res Clin Obstet Gynaecol 22(4):571–88
7. Ravina JH, Herbreteau D, Ciraru-Vigneron N et al (1995) Arterial embolisation to treat uterine myomata. Lancet 346:671–672
8. The National Institute for Health and Care Excellence: Uterine artery embolisation for fibroids, NICE interventional procedure guidance [IPG367]. Available online at: https://www.nice.org.uk/guidance/ipg367. (Accessed 25 Nov 2015)
9. Stewart EA, Gedroyc WM, Tempany CM, Quade BJ, Inbar Y, Ehrenstein T et al (2003) Focused ultrasound treatment of uterine fibroid tumors: safety and feasibility of a noninvasive thermoablative technique. Am J Obstet Gynecol 189(1):48–54
10. Schlesinger D, Benedict S, Diederich C, Gedroyc W, Klibanov A, Larner J (2013) MR-guided focused ultrasound surgery, present and future. Med Phys 40(8):080901
11. Gizzo S, Saccardi C, Patrelli TS, Ancona E, Noventa M, Fagherazzi S et al (2014) Magnetic Resonance-Guided Focused Ultrasound Myomectomy: Safety, Efficacy, Subsequent Fertility and Quality-of-Life Improvements, A Systematic Review. Reprod Sci 21(4):465–76.2013
12. Donnez J, Tatarchuk TF, Bouchard P, Puscasiu L, Zakharenko NF, Ivanova T et al (2012) Ulipristal acetate versus placebo for fibroid treatment before surgery. N Engl J Med 366:409–420
13. Donnez J, Donnez O, Matule D, Ahrendt HJ, Hudecek R, Zatik J et al (2016) Long-term medical management of uterine fibroids with ulipristal acetate. Fertil Steril 105(1):165–173, e4
14. Levens ED, Potlog-Nahari C, Armstrong AY et al (2008) CDB-2914 for uterine leio- myomata treatment: a randomized controlled trial. Obstet Gynecol 111:1129–36
15. Taylor A, Sharma M, Tsirkas P, Di Spiezio SA, Mastrogamvrakis G et al (2005) Surgical and radiological management of uterine fibroids – a UK survey of current consultant practice. Acta Obstet Gynecol Scand 84:478–482
16. Centre for Workforce Intelligence (CfWI); Securing the future workforce supply: Obstetrics and Gynaecology stock take. Available online at: http://webarchive. nationalarchives.gov.uk/20161007101116/http://www.cfwi.org.uk/publications/ obstetrics-and-gynaecology-stocktake. (Accessed 23 June 2017)
17. The Royal College of Obstetricians and Gynaecologists and The Royal College of Radiologists (2013) Clinical recommendations on the use of UAE in the management of fibroids, Thirdth edn. RCOG and RCR, London, Ref No. BFCR(13)
18. Delnevo CD, Abatemarco DJ, Steinberg MB (2004) Physician response rates to a mail survey by specialty and timing of incentive. Am J Prev Med 26(3):234–6
19. Cook C, Health F, Thompson RL (2000) Meta-Analysis of Response Rates in Web- or Internet-Based Survey. Educ Psychol Measurement 60(6):821–36
20. Gupta S, Onwude J, Stasi R, Manyonda I (2012) Refusal of blood transfusion by Jehovah's Witness women: a survey of current management in obstetric and gynaecological practice in the U.K. Blood Transfus 10(4):462–70
21. Health and Social Care Information Centre, Hospital Episode Statistics (HES), Hospital Episode Statistics Excel spreadsheets years 2013–2014. Admitted patient care 2013-2014. Available online at: http://content.digital.nhs.uk/ searchcatalogue?productid=17192&topics=2%2fHospital+care%2fAdmissions +and+attendances%2fElective+admissions&covdate=%2c2014%2c%2c 2013&sort=Relevance&size=10&page=2#top. (Accessed 23 June 2017)
22. Lethaby A, Vollenhoven B, Sowter M (2001) Pre-operative GnRH analogue therapy before hysterectomy or myomectomy for uterine fibroids. Cochrane Database Syst Rev 2:CD000547
23. Farquhar C, Brown PM, Furness S (2002) Cost effectiveness of pre-operative gonadotrophin releasing analogues for women with uterine fibroids undergoing hysterectomy or myomectomy. BJOG 109(11):1273–80
24. Talaulikar V, Belli AM, Manyonda I (2012) GnRH agonists: do they have a place in the modern management of fibroid disease? J Obstet Gynaecol India 62(5):506–10
25. Luketic L, Shirreff L, Kives S, Liu G, El Sugy R, Leyland N, Solnik MJ, Murji AJ (2017) Does Ulipristal Acetate Affect Surgical Experience at Laparoscopic Myomectomy? Minim Invasive Gynecol (17):30227–3
26. Sancho JM, Delgado VS, Valero MJ, Soteras MG, Amate VP, Carrascosa AA (2016) Hysteroscopic myomectomy outcomes after 3-month treatment with either Ulipristal Acetate or GnRH analogues: a retrospective comparative study. Eur J Obstet Gynecol Reprod Biol 198:127–30
27. Al-Shabibi N, Chapman L, Madari S, Papadimitriou A, Papalampros P, Magos A (2009) Prospective randomised trial comparing gonadotrophin-releasing hormone analogues with triple tourniquets at open myomectomy. BJOG 116(5):681–7
28. Chudnoff S, Glazer S, Levie M (2012) Review of vasopressin use in gynecologic surgery. J Minim Invasive Gynecol 19(4):422–33

14

Vaginal McCall culdoplasty versus laparoscopic uterosacral plication to prophylactically address vaginal vault prolapse

Kathy Niblock[1*], Emily Bailie[2], Geoff McCracken[1] and Keith Johnston[2]

Abstract

Background: Studies have shown that vaginal vault prolapse can affect up to 43% of women following hysterectomy for pelvic organ prolapse. Many techniques have been described to prevent and treat vaginal vault prolapse. The primary objective of our study was to compare McCall's culdoplasty (when performed along side vaginal hysterectomy) with laparoscopic uterosacral plication (when performed along side total laparoscopic hysterectomy) for prevention of vaginal vault prolapse. Secondary outcomes included inpatient stay and perioperative complications.

A retrospective comparison study comparing 73 patients who underwent 'laparoscopic hysterectomy and uterosacral plication' against 70 patients who underwent 'vaginal hysterectomy and McCall culdoplasty'. All operations were carried out by two trained surgeons.

Results: There was no significant difference between BMI or parity. There were statistically significantly more patients presenting with post hysterectomy vault prolapse (PHVP) in the group of patients who had undergone uterosacral plication (12 out of 73) compared with McCalls culdoplasty (0 out of 70) $P = 0.000394$. Inpatient stay in the uterosacral plication group was significantly shorter mean 1.8 compared to 3.6 for McCall group (P-Value is <0.00001). There was no significance in the perioperative complications between both groups ($P = 0.41$).

Conclusions: McCalls is a superior operation to prevent PHVP compared to uterosacral plication with no difference in terms of perioperative complications.

Keywords: Vault prolapse, McCall culdoplasty, Uterosacral plication

Background

The International Continence Society defines post-hysterectomy vault prolapse (PHVP) as descent of the vaginal cuff scar below a point that is 2 cm less than the total vaginal length above the plane of the hymen [1]. The incidence of PHVP has been reported to affect up to 43% of hysterectomies. The risk of prolapse following hysterectomy is 5.5 times more common in women whose initial hysterectomy was for pelvic organ prolapse as opposed to other reasons [1].

Preventative techniques can be used at the time of a hysterectomy to prevent PHVP. McCall culdoplasty and sacrospinous fixation can be carried out at vaginal hysterectomy [2]. Suturing the cardinal and uterosacral ligaments to the vaginal cuff at the time of abdominal or laparoscopic hysterectomy is effective in preventing post-hysterectomy vaginal prolapse [3].

Recommended management for PHVP can be largely divided into surgical and non-surgical. Methods of treatment offered depend on severity of prolapse but also takes into consideration patient wishes and expectations

* Correspondence: kathyniblock@doctors.org.uk
[1]Craigavon Area Hospital, 68 Lurgan Rd, Portadown, Craigavon, BT63 5QQ, Northern Ireland
Full list of author information is available at the end of the article

and suitability for surgery. Conservative management includes weight loss, treatment of constipation and avoidance of heavy lifting. Patients may also avail of physiotherapy and ring pessaries [4].

Techniques available to manage PHVP aim to ultimately suspend the vaginal vault. Approaches include vaginal, e.g. uterosacral ligament suspension, sacrospinous ligament fixation, open procedures and more recently laparoscopic, e.g. sacrocolpopexy and uterosacral plication [2, 5]. The decision-making process for managing these patients is similar to that of any prolapse, namely the response to conservative management, the effect on the quality of life and fitness for surgery [1].

Methods

Patients were identified who underwent 'laparoscopic hysterectomy with uterosacral plication' and 'vaginal hysterectomy with McCall culdoplasty' for pelvic organ prolapse performed by two consultant gynaecologists in Northern Ireland between January 2008 and January 2014. One surgeon performed each of the described procedures.

All patients had presented with subjective symptoms of pelvic organ prolapse, and objectively, this was confirmed on objective Pelvic Organ Prolapse Quantification (POP-Q) examination.

The technique used for vaginal hysterectomy and McCall culdoplasty is described by Raymond Lee of The Mayo Clinic [6]. Following vaginal hysterectomy, one to two internal McCall sutures are placed using a zero monofilament absorbable suture. Each McCall suture is placed deeply into the left pararectal fascia then across the front of the sigmoid colon and deep into the right pararectal fascia. An external McCall suture is subsequently placed, more cephalad to the internal McCall suture. A 1-0 delayed absorbable suture is passed through the posterior vaginal wall incorporating the peritoneum. The same suture is then placed deep through the left pararectal fascia, across the sigmoid colon and deep through the right pararectal fascia. The same external McCall suture is then placed back through the vaginal wall. Depending on anterior and posterior compartment prolapse, the patients may have also undergone an anterior and/or posterior colporrhaphy. All patients underwent routine cystoscopy with indigo carmine.

In the patients undergoing uterosacral plication, following total laparoscopic hysterectomy, the ureters were re-identified. A non-absorbable, zero monofilament suture was used to place three helical sutures full thickness in each uterosacral ligament, beginning in the distal third of the ligament and incorporating the posterior vagina. The ends of the suture were tied with an extra-corporeal knot-tying technique, thus shortening the uterosacral ligaments.

Both groups of patients had their charts reviewed retrospectively and were followed up on a regional electronic care record to see if they attended anywhere in the province for subsequent pelvic organ prolapse repairs.

A total of 143 patients were identified including 73 who had undergone total laparoscopic hysterectomy and uterosacral plication and 70 who had vaginal hysterectomy and McCall culdoplasty.

Mean follow-up was 36 months (range 5–84) in the uterosacral plication group and 41 months (range 5–71) in the McCall culdoplasty group.

The notes were reviewed for parity, age, BMI, indication for surgery, the surgical procedure performed, perioperative or post-operative complications, duration of inpatient stay and findings at their 6-month post-operative review where a POP-Q was performed along with any subsequent attendances.

Results

Demographics

The demographics for the uterosacral plication and the McCall culdoplasty groups are summarized in Table 1.

The mean parity and BMI in both groups were comparable with P values of 0.21 and 0.09 respectively. (P values were calculated using Student's t test.) The mean parity in patients who underwent uterosacral plication was 3.1 compared with 3.0 in the McCall culdoplasty group. The mean BMI in patients who underwent uterosacral plication was 26.5 compared with 28.0 in the McCall culdoplasty group.

There was a statistical significance in the age difference of both groups of patients ($P = 0.00024$). The McCall patient group had a mean age of 59 (range 37–82) while the patients undergoing uterosacral plication had a mean age of 52.3 (range 31–72)

Inpatient stay

The mean inpatient stay for patients in the laparoscopic hysterectomy and uterosacral plication group was 1.8 days (range 1–5 days). The mean inpatient stay for patients in the vaginal hysterectomy and McCall culdoplasty group was 3.6 days (range 2–7 days). There was a statistically significant difference in the duration of

Table 1 Demographics for the uterosacral plication and the McCall culdoplasty patient groups

	USP	McCall's	P value
Mean age (range)	52.3 (31–72)	59 (37–82)	0.00024
Mean parity (range)	3.1 (1–6)	3.0 (1–8)	0.21
Mean BMI (range)	26.5 (16.7–41)	28.0 (20–36)	0.09

hospital stay in the two groups; *P* value is <0.00001 using Student's *t* test.

Indication

In both groups, the indication for surgery in all patients was vaginal prolapse. In patients who had objective associated anterior or posterior vaginal wall prolapse, additional procedures were carried out to address this. These procedures included anterior colporrhaphy, posterior colporrhaphy and laparoscopic paravaginal repair. Laparoscopic paravaginal repair is a procedure using a delayed absorbable suture to attach the lateral aspects of the front vaginal wall back to the arcus tendinous. It is a procedure used to address anterior lateral vaginal wall defects.

In the patients undergoing vaginal hysterectomy and McCall culdoplasty, four patients also complained of heavy menstrual bleeding. In the patients undergoing laparoscopic hysterectomy and uterosacral ligament plication, three patients also complained of heavy menstrual bleeding.

Procedure

Details of the procedures performed for utero-vaginal prolapse are summarized in Tables 2 and 3.

Complications

Seventeen patients in total had reported complications. This included ten patients in the McCall culdoplasty group and seven patients in the uterosacral plication group. See Tables 4 and 5 for details.

In the patients undergoing laparoscopic hysterectomy and uterosacral plication, three patients require antibiotics for port site wound infections. Two patients had post-operative urinary retention, one that was managed conservatively and one that required release of sutures at the bladder neck following paravaginal repair. One patient re-attended with port

Table 2 Details of laparoscopic procedure

Procedure	Number of patients
Total laparoscopic hysterectomy (±BSO) and uterosacral plication	32
Total laparoscopic hysterectomy (±BSO) and uterosacral plication and posterior colporrhaphy	21
Total laparoscopic hysterectomy (±BSO) and uterosacral plication and laparoscopic paravaginal repair	9
Total laparoscopic hysterectomy (±BSO) and uterosacral plication and posterior colporrhaphy and laparoscopic paravaginal repair	5
Total laparoscopic hysterectomy (±BSO) and uterosacral plication and anterior colporrhaphy	5
Total laparoscopic hysterectomy (±BSO) and uterosacral plication and anterior colporrhaphy and posterior colporrhaphy	1
Total	73

Table 3 Details of vaginal procedure

Procedure	Number of patients
Vaginal hysterectomy (±BSO) and McCall culdoplasty and anterior colporrhaphy and posterior colporrhaphy	60
Vaginal hysterectomy (±BSO) and McCall culdoplasty and anterior colporrhaphy	4
Vaginal hysterectomy (±BSO) and McCall culdoplasty	3
Vaginal hysterectomy (±BSO) and McCall culdoplasty and posterior colporrhaphy	3
Total	70

site herniation, 2 weeks after surgery, that required surgical management. One patient had a vault haematoma, which was managed conservatively with antibiotics.

One patient undergoing McCall culdoplasty required intraoperative release of the McCall due to evidence of ureteric obstruction at routine cystoscopy performed during the procedure. Six patients in the McCall culdoplasty group had post-operative urinary retention. All of these were successfully managed conservatively with a period of intermittent self-catheterization. Two patients returned to theatre for a laparotomy for post-operative intra-abdominal bleeding in the first 24 h post-operatively. One patient required a subsequent Blair Bell (Fenton's) procedure for post-operative dyspareunia which failed to respond to conservative measures.

Post-operative findings

Mean follow-up time was 36 months in the uterosacral plication group and 41 months in the McCall culdoplasty group. All patients were assessed 6 months post-

Table 4 Complications in uterosacral plication patient group

Complication	Operation	Management
Wound infection	Laparoscopic hysterectomy and uterosacral plication and posterior colporrhaphy	Oral antibiotics
Wound infection	Laparoscopic hysterectomy and uterosacral plication	Oral antibiotics
Wound infection	Laparoscopic hysterectomy and uterosacral plication	IV antibiotics
Urinary retention	Laparoscopic hysterectomy and uterosacral plication and posterior colporrhaphy and paravaginal repair	Conservative —ISC
Urinary retention	Laparoscopic hysterectomy and uterosacral plication and paravaginal repair	Revision of sutures at bladder neck following paravaginal repair
Vault haematoma	Laparoscopic hysterectomy and uterosacral plication	IV antibiotics
Port site herniation	Laparoscopic hysterectomy and uterosacral plication	Surgically managed

Table 5 Complications in the McCall culdoplasty patient group

Complication	Operation	Management
Urinary retention	Vaginal hysterectomy and McCall culdoplasty and anterior colporrhaphy and posterior colporrhaphy	Conservative—ISC
Urinary retention	Vaginal hysterectomy and McCall culdoplasty and anterior colporrhaphy and posterior colporrhaphy	Conservative—ISC
Urinary retention	Vaginal hysterectomy and McCall culdoplasty and anterior colporrhaphy and posterior colporrhaphy	Conservative—ISC
Urinary retention	Vaginal hysterectomy and McCall culdoplasty and anterior colporrhaphy and posterior colporrhaphy	Conservative—ISC
Urinary retention	Vaginal hysterectomy and McCall culdoplasty and anterior colporrhaphy and posterior colporrhaphy	Conservative—ISC
Urinary retention	Vaginal hysterectomy and McCall culdoplasty and anterior colporrhaphy and posterior colporrhaphy	Conservative—ISC
Post-operative bleeding	Vaginal hysterectomy and McCall culdoplasty and anterior colporrhaphy and posterior colporrhaphy	Return to theatre; laparotomy
Post-operative bleeding	Vaginal hysterectomy and McCall culdoplasty and anterior colporrhaphy and posterior colporrhaphy	Return to theatre; laparotomy
Post-operative dyspareunia	Vaginal hysterectomy and McCall culdoplasty and anterior colporrhaphy and posterior colporrhaphy	Blair Bell/Fenton's procedure
Ureteric obstruction seen at cystoscopy	Vaginal hysterectomy and McCall culdoplasty and anterior colporrhaphy and posterior colporrhaphy	Release of McCall culdoplasty intraoperatively

There was no significance in the perioperative complications between both groups ($P = 0.41$)

operatively where subjective and objective (POP-Q) assessments of subsequent prolapse symptoms were ascertained by the same two surgeons.

Uterosacral plication

In the uterosacral plication group, 53 out of 73 (72.6%) patients had no further pelvic organ prolapse.

Twelve patients (16.4%) have had PHVP. Eight patients have opted for surgical repair. Of the eight patients undergoing surgical repair for PHVP, four patients had a subsequent laparoscopic sacrocolpopexy, one patient had a laparoscopic sacrocolpopexy that was converted to an open procedure intraoperatively due to

dense adhesions, one patient had a sacrospinous ligament fixation and two patients had repeat uterosacral ligament plications performed. Four patients opted for insertion of vaginal pessary. See Table 6.

Seven patients (9.5%) have had de novo anterior compartment prolapse. Four patients (5.4%) had recurrence of anterior wall prolapse. Seven patients opted for surgical repair, two patients opted for vaginal pessary insertion and two patients have chosen conservative management. See Table 7.

McCall culdoplasty

In the McCall culdoplasty group, there have been no patients with PHVP. Four patients have represented with

Table 6 Vaginal vault prolapse following laparoscopic hysterectomy and uterosacral plication

Original operation	Repair of PHVP
Laparoscopic hysterectomy and uterosacral plication	Laparoscopic sacrocolpopexy
Laparoscopic hysterectomy and uterosacral plication and paravaginal repair	Laparoscopic sacrocolpopexy
Laparoscopic hysterectomy and uterosacral plication	Laparoscopic sacrocolpopexy
Laparoscopic hysterectomy and uterosacral plication and paravaginal repair	Laparoscopic sacrocolpopexy
Laparoscopic hysterectomy and uterosacral plication and paravaginal repair	Laparoscopic sacrocolpopexy converted to open sacrospinous ligament fixation
Laparoscopic hysterectomy and uterosacral plication	Vaginal sacrospinous ligament fixation
Laparoscopic hysterectomy and uterosacral plication	Laparoscopic uterosacral ligament plication
Laparoscopic hysterectomy and uterosacral plication and paravaginal repair	Laparoscopic uterosacral ligament plication
Laparoscopic hysterectomy and uterosacral plication and anterior colporrhaphy	Pessary
Laparoscopic hysterectomy and uterosacral plication	Pessary
Laparoscopic hysterectomy and uterosacral plication and posterior colporrhaphy	Pessary
Laparoscopic hysterectomy and uterosacral plication	Pessary

Table 7 Anterior compartment prolapse following laparoscopic hysterectomy and uterosacral plication

Original operation	Management
Laparoscopic hysterectomy and uterosacral plication and posterior colporrhaphy	Anterior colporrhaphy
Laparoscopic hysterectomy and uterosacral plication	Anterior colporrhaphy
Laparoscopic hysterectomy and uterosacral plication	Anterior colporrhaphy
Laparoscopic hysterectomy and uterosacral plication and anterior colporrhaphy	Anterior colporrhaphy
Laparoscopic hysterectomy and uterosacral plication and paravaginal repair	Laparoscopic paravaginal repair
Laparoscopic hysterectomy and uterosacral plication	Laparoscopic paravaginal repair
Laparoscopic hysterectomy and uterosacral plication and anterior colporrhaphy	Vaginal Elevate mesh
Laparoscopic hysterectomy and uterosacral plication	Conservative—no treatment
Laparoscopic hysterectomy and uterosacral plication and paravaginal repair	Conservative—no treatment
Laparoscopic hysterectomy and uterosacral plication	Pessary
Laparoscopic hysterectomy and uterosacral plication	Pessary

Four patients (5.4%) have had de novo posterior compartment prolapse; three have opted for surgical repair

posterior compartment prolapse (Table 8), and two patients have represented with anterior compartment prolapse. Two of these patients have required surgical management for their symptoms. One patient underwent a subsequent anterior colporrhaphy, and one patient has undergone a subsequent posterior colporrhaphy. See Tables 9 and 10.

Discussion and conclusions

The aetiology of PHVP is multifactorial; however, damage to the level one supports of the vagina during hysterectomy are thought to be a major contributing factor. The risk of this is thought to be greatest when the hysterectomy is performed for the indication of pelvic organ prolapse [7].

Table 8 Posterior compartment prolapse following laparoscopic hysterectomy and uterosacral plication

Original operation	Management
Laparoscopic hysterectomy and uterosacral plication	Posterior colporrhaphy
Laparoscopic hysterectomy and uterosacral plication and paravaginal repair	Posterior colporrhaphy
Laparoscopic hysterectomy and uterosacral plication	Posterior colporrhaphy
Laparoscopic hysterectomy and uterosacral plication and anterior colporrhaphy	Conservative—no treatment

Table 9 Anterior compartment prolapse following vaginal hysterectomy and McCall culdoplasty

Original operation	Management
Vaginal hysterectomy and McCall culdoplasty and anterior colporrhaphy and posterior colporrhaphy	Anterior colporrhaphy
Vaginal hysterectomy and McCall culdoplasty and anterior colporrhaphy and posterior colporrhaphy	Conservative

There are very few studies comparing vaginal McCall culdoplasty to laparoscopic uterosacral plication for prevention of subsequent prolapse.

In 1957, McCall described attaching the uterosacral ligaments to the posterior vaginal cuff and the cul de sac peritoneum in order to close off the cul de sac and prevent subsequent prolapse [8].

Uterosacral plication does not obliterate the cul de sac. It involves placing sutures distally on the uterosacral ligaments and tying them in the midline under tension away from their attachment into the vagina. The support this provides for the vagina has so far been unclear [9]. One of the theoretical advantages of laparoscopic over vaginal technique is the ability to identify the ureters, thus reducing the chance of inadvertent ureteric injury. Our study shows that in trained hands and with the prudent employment of indigo carmine and routine cystoscopy, the rate of ureteric injury is not significantly higher in the vaginal McCall group.

This study has retrospectively evaluated the McCall culdoplasty and the laparoscopic uterosacral plication when performed alongside hysterectomies in order to prevent PHVP. It has found them comparable in terms of complications encountered. Laparoscopic uterosacral plication has a statistically significant shorter hospital admission; however, McCall culdoplasty has proven to be superior to laparoscopic uterosacral plication in terms of patients representing with subsequent pelvic organ prolapse.

While both groups had a low rate of PHVP, in this study, McCall culdoplasty was a more successful operation compared to uterosacral plication with no difference in terms of perioperative complications.

Table 10 Posterior compartment prolapse following vaginal hysterectomy and McCall culdoplasty

Original operation	Management
Vaginal hysterectomy and McCall culdoplasty and anterior colporrhaphy and posterior colporrhaphy	Posterior colporrhaphy
Vaginal hysterectomy and McCall culdoplasty and anterior colporrhaphy and posterior colporrhaphy	Conservative
Vaginal hysterectomy and McCall culdoplasty and anterior colporrhaphy and posterior colporrhaphy	Conservative
Vaginal hysterectomy and McCall culdoplasty and anterior colporrhaphy and posterior colporrhaphy	Conservative

Abbreviations
BMI: Body mass index; BSO: Bilateral salpingo-oophorectomy;
ISC: Intermittent self-catheterization; PHVP: Post-hysterectomy vault prolapse;
POP-Q: Pelvic Organ Prolapse Quantification

Authors' contributions
KN handled project development, data collecting and manuscript writing. EB
handled data collecting and manuscript writing. GMC and KJ handled
project development. All authors read and approved the final manuscript.

Competing interests
The authors declare that they have no competing interests.

Author details
[1]Craigavon Area Hospital, 68 Lurgan Rd, Portadown, Craigavon, BT63 5QQ,
Northern Ireland. [2]Antrim Area Hospital, 45 Bush Rd, Antrim BT41 2RL,
Northern Ireland.

References
1. RCOG and BSUG joint guideline 2015. Green top guideline no 46—post
   hysterectomy vaginal vault prolapse, published 24/07/2015. https://www.
   rcog.org.uk/globalassets/documents/guidelines/gtg-46.pdf
2. NICE. Sacrocolpopexy using mesh for vaginal vault prolapse repair—NICE
   interventional procedure guideline IPG283 January 2009. https://www.nice.
   org.uk/guidance/ipg283/chapter/1-Guidance
3. Reda A, Sayed AT (2005) Post-hysterectomy vaginal vault prolapse. TOG 7:89–97
4. Azubuike U, Farag KA (2009) Vaginal vault prolapse. Int Obstet Gynecol
   2009:275621
5. Chene G (2007) Anatomical and functional results of McCall culdoplasty in
   the prevention of enteroceles and vault prolapse after vaginal
   hysterectomy. Int Urogynaecol J 19:1007–1011
6. Lee R (2003) Vaginal hysterectomy with repair of enterocele, cystocele and
   rectocele. Clin Obstet Gynecol 36(4):967–975
7. Altman D, Falconer C, Cnattingius S, Granath F (2008) Pelvic organ prolapse
   surgery following prolapse for benign indications. Am J Obstet Gynecol
   198(5):572
8. AAGL Advancing Minimally Invasive Gynecology Worldwide (2014) AAGL
   practice guidelines on the prevention of apical prolapse at the time of
   benign hysterectomy. J Minim Invasive Gynecol 21(5):715–722
9. O'Donovan P, Downes E (2002) Advances in gynaecological surgery, 1st
   edn. Greenwich Medical Media, London, pp 82–83, Chapter 7. Vault
   prolapse can it be prevented

15

The role of the multidisciplinary team in the management of deep infiltrating endometriosis

Lilian Ugwumadu*⬤, Rima Chakrabarti, Elaine Williams-Brown, John Rendle, Ian Swift, Babbin John, Heather Allen-Coward and Emmanuel Ofuasia

Abstract

The multidisciplinary team (MDT) is considered good practice in the management of chronic conditions and is now a well-established part of clinical care in the NHS. There has been a recent drive to have MDTs in the management of women with severe endometriosis requiring complex surgery as a result of recommendations from the European Society for Human Reproduction and Embryology (ESHRE) and British Society for Gynaecological Endoscopy (BSGE). The multidisciplinary approach to the management of patients with endometriosis leads to better results in patient outcomes; however, there are potentially a number of barriers to its implementation and maintenance. This paper aims to review the potential benefits, disadvantages and barriers of the multidisciplinary team in the management of severe endometriosis.

Keywords: Multidisciplinary team, Multidisciplinary care, Multidisciplinary meetings, Deep infiltrating endometriosis, Rectovaginal endometriosis

Introduction

Endometriosis is a common non-malignant multi-organ disease characterised by the presence of endometrial glands and stroma outside the uterus. Three clinical presentations of this condition have been described: peritoneal endometriosis, ovarian endometrioma and deep infiltrating endometriosis [1]. Deep infiltrating endometriosis (DIE) is the most aggressive form, defined as endometriosis located more than 5 mm beneath the peritoneal surface [2]. It affects the bowel and urinary tract in 5–40% and 1–4% of women with pelvic endometriosis respectively [3, 4]. When the bowel or urinary tract is involved, a combined approach with the colorectal surgeon, urologist and gynaecological surgeon is mandatory. Due to the complexity of this condition, there is greater demand on healthcare services to provide high-quality multidisciplinary care across related specialties for women with severe endometriosis. In 1995, the Calman-Hine report outlined reforms of the UK's cancer services with the aim of reducing

inequalities and improving clinical outcomes in NHS cancer care. Its main recommendation which was endorsed by the UK Department of Health was the use of multidisciplinary teams (MDT) as the core model for managing chronic conditions which is now an established part of NHS clinical care and service provisions [5]. This has also been highlighted in the European Society for Human Reproduction and Embryology (ESHRE) Guideline on the Diagnosis and Management of Endometriosis, which emphasised the complexity of the management of deep infiltrating endometriosis and the need to refer to tertiary centres with the appropriate expertise to offer all available treatments in a multidisciplinary approach [6]. The British Society for Gynaecological Endoscopy has also established criteria for these centres carrying out complex endometriosis surgery before accreditation. One of the criteria includes working in a multi-disciplinary team with a named colorectal surgeon and nurse specialist [7].

Methods

This aim of this paper is to evaluate the role, benefits, and drawback of multidisciplinary team management of

* Correspondence: lilian.ugwumadu@nhs.net
Croydon Endometriosis Centre, Croydon University Hospital, 530 London Road, Croydon CR7 7YE, UK

women with deep infiltrating endometriosis. A literature search was performed using the following databases: PubMed, Medline, Ovid and Cochrane for English-language articles published from 1987 till date. The search terms used were various combinations of "multidisciplinary team", "multidisciplinary approach", "multidisciplinary care", "multidisciplinary treatment", "multidisciplinary meetings", and deep infiltrating endometriosis. All papers and references were reviewed by the authors and relevant papers identified.

Benefits

Multidisciplinary team work involves coordinated efforts between specialists with expertise in their disciplines in the management of a patient. These MDT meetings ensure higher quality decision-making, reduced incidence of questionable practices, standardised patient care and improved outcomes [8–10]. Endometriosis is a chronic condition and an integrated approach involving a multidisciplinary team is essential in optimising patient management. It ensures that a full range of therapeutic options are considered early so patients receive appropriate and timely treatments. The MDT led by an experienced gynaecological surgeon working together with a urologist, colorectal surgeon, specialist nurse, specialist gynaecology radiologist, pain specialist, counsellors/psychologist and patient support organisations is essential in managing complex cases [11]. They all play an important role in providing adequate treatment as well as increasing the likelihood of providing consistent, evidence based and cost effective care [12]. Patient support groups and organisations work closely and collaborate with endometriosis specialists, researchers and policy makers to increase awareness of endometriosis and drive research forward. Women also benefit from these support groups as they can share the emotional aspect of this disease, effects on their lives and families and coping strategies.

Preoperative work-up

Preoperative work-up is important in planning a multidisciplinary surgical treatment. Reliably detecting deep infiltrating endometriosis especially in posterior compartment endometriosis could inform surgeons of the need for bowel preparation before surgery and a colorectal surgeon presence at the time of surgery. For the evaluation of bowel endometriosis, physical examination has a limited capacity to diagnose deep infiltrating endometriosis [13]. Several imaging modalities have been used to evaluate deep infiltrating endometriosis in the preoperative setting including transvaginal ultrasound and MRI of the pelvis [14]. Transvaginal ultrasound is the most studied imaging technique for deep infiltrating endometriosis, showing a pooled estimate of sensitivities

and specificities of 91 and 98%, respectively [15]. Transvaginal ultrasound is operator dependent with higher accuracy obtained when performed by more experienced operators. In our practice, transvaginal ultrasound scan is recommended and performed by an experienced gynaecologist for the initial assessment of patients with suspected endometriosis and it may be useful to triage patients appropriately.

Currently, MRI is not routinely recommended in women with suspected endometriosis but could be particularly useful in detecting rectovaginal and bowel endometriosis [16–18]. Abrao et al. [19] found that MRI had a sensitivity and specificity of 83 and 98% and a recent Cochrane review [16] showed a sensitivity and specificity of 79 and 94% respectively for rectovaginal endometriosis.

A recent systematic review on ureteral endometriosis found that abdominopelvic ultrasound and/or MRI or CT-scan were routinely performed in the initial evaluation. In some studies cystoscopy was also performed when bladder infiltration was suspected [20].

These investigations aims to (1) determine disease location; (2) extent of the disease; (3) planning multidisciplinary team meetings; (4) discuss postoperative care and complications. In our referral centre, all patients with suspected DIE or rectovaginal endometriosis are discussed in our monthly multidisciplinary team meeting attended by the gynaecologist, radiologist, urologist, colorectal surgeon, and the endometriosis nurse specialist where the patient's history, clinical examination findings and preferences are discussed, images reviewed and a recommendation is made.

Operative treatment

Laparoscopy is the gold standard used to diagnose and to classify endometriosis [21]. The aim of endometriosis surgery is to reduce pain, reoccurrence rate, and improve fertility without compromising ovarian function. With this in mind, a multidisciplinary surgical treatment approach involving the gynaecologist, urologist and colorectal surgeon with complete excision of all endometriotic lesions is paramount to achieve better long-term outcomes [6]. Observational studies have shown that laparotomy and laparoscopy are equally effective in the treatment of endometriosis-associated pain [22]. However, laparoscopy is preferred to laparotomy because it is associated with a better postoperative recovery, shorter hospital stay, and better cosmesis [23]. Women with deep infiltrating endometriosis should be managed in a tertiary referral centre that offers advanced laparoscopic treatment in a multidisciplinary context [24]. We perform a four-step surgical procedure for these women: (1) the urologist performs a cystoscopy, inspects the bladder wall and inserts ureteric stents; (2) the gynaecologist excises all endometriosis to restore normal pelvic anatomy; (3) the urologist excises any bladder endometriosis; lastly (4) the colorectal surgeon excises bowel disease. However, if deep infiltrating endometriosis is found incidentally during laparoscopy, we will only perform what was agreed and documented on the consent form. We will inform the patient of the laparoscopy findings, discuss treatment options allowing her to make an informed decision. If the indication for laparoscopy is to manage a life threatening condition such as a ruptured ectopic pregnancy then it is in the best interest of the patient to do what is required surgically to allow adequate access to remove the ectopic pregnancy.

Benefits to the clinician

Healthcare professionals also benefit from the multidisciplinary approach for the management of patients. Several studies have shown that it provides a framework for the understanding of the disease process thereby enabling better decision making and providing support for more complex cases [25]. Moreover, greater job satisfaction and psychological wellbeing has being demonstrated by engineering a team approach [8]. Clinicians working together in a MDT learn from each other across disciplines through active discussions, review of cases and how combined treatments can improve patient outcomes. Collaborative research is also encouraged within MDTs, which promotes greater participations in clinical trials, which helps to improve the understanding of this condition, diagnosis and ensure effective treatment options [25]. It also offers educational opportunities for trainees and medical students who can gain greater insight into the importance of multidisciplinary team work in the management of patients with chronic conditions.

Disadvantages

One of the disadvantages of MDT discussions is the lack of patient involvement since patients are not present at these meetings. If patient preferences or social circumstances are not taken into account, team decisions may be inappropriate or rejected. However, patient attendance at these meetings may not be beneficial because of their limited understanding of medical terminology, which may restrict the free flow of information and in addition lead to ineffective input from patients. This may be potentially overcome by the use of questionnaires in the clinic which could guide the MDT in recommending a particular treatment plan best suited to the patient. The effective functioning of an MDT requires constructive input from all team members. A lack of clear roles, objectives and also enthusiasm from its members can hinder the development of constructive management.

This does not only have implications for patient care and safety but also has medicolegal implications. All professionals who attend team meetings have a duty of care for decisions made [26]. Clear documentation is important to improve communication between team members and also with the patient. In our centre, the gynaecologist is the primary clinician who takes responsibility for patient care with input from other related specialties. All recommendations following MDT meetings are documented in patients' notes for reference.

Barriers

Although it has been established that multidisciplinary team management improves patient outcome, there are a number of barriers that prevent the full realisation of these benefits. Such barriers include cost, time constraints, and poor interprofessional relationships. The estimated total monthly cost of gynaecological cancer MDTs in the UK is £101,880 [27]. This prompts the debate of the cost-effectiveness of MDTs when used for routine benign cases. The cost should be balanced with the cost of reduced economic productivity from patients with severe endometriosis. The WERF EndoCost study has shown that the costs of productivity loss of €6298 per woman were double the health care costs of €3113 per woman suffering from endometriosis-associated symptoms and treated in referral centres [12]. In 2005, the UK Endometriosis All Party Parliamentary Group (EAPPG) carried out a survey on pain and quality of life. They showed that 78% of symptomatic women with endometriosis lose a mean of 5.3 days of work a month because of their symptoms, with a potential cost of €30 billion across Europe [28]. Additionally, there is a diagnostic delay of over 8 years with 65% of women with endometriosis initially misdiagnosed and almost 50% having to see five doctors or more before a correct diagnosis is made. This is likely to increase the cost to the woman if she is unable to work and the cost to the healthcare system [28]. The indirect cost of infertility treatment, drugs and surgery in women with chronic pelvic pain is estimated at £24 million in the UK [29].

Therefore, early referral to a tertiary centre where the appropriate skills and expertise exist to make the correct diagnosis and implement effective management of endometriosis will significantly reduce time to diagnosis and costs.

As a minimum, time required to facilitate MDT meetings and treatment plans should be included in job plans to allow an effective high quality service. Poor interprofessional relationship can also affect teamwork and hinder shared responsibility.

Conclusions

Although informal discussions already exist in many hospitals, a formalised multidisciplinary preoperative work up and surgical treatment in an endometriosis referral centre is necessary to plan patients counselling and treatment plan implementation which assures improved outcomes. This should be carried out in collaboration with the MDT including a gynaecologist, urologist, colorectal surgeon, specialist nurse, radiologist, pain specialist, counsellors/psychologist and patient support organisations. The success of MDT's in cancer care should encourage its uptake in benign but chronic conditions such as endometriosis. In future, research should focus on the effect of MDT's on patient long-term outcomes, cost effectiveness and perception amongst clinicians.

Authors' contributions
All authors read and approved the final manuscript.

Competing interests
The authors declare that they have no competing interests.

References

1. Koninckx PR, Meuleman C, Demeyere S et al (1991) Suggestive evidence that pelvic endometriosis is a progressive disease, whereas deeply infiltrating endometriosis is associated with pelvic pain. Fertil Steril 55:759–765
2. Cornillie FJ, Oosterlynck D, Lauwerys JM, Koninckx PR (1990) Deeply infiltrating pelvic endometriosis: histology and clinical significance. Fertil Steril 53:978–983
3. Jubanyik KJ, Comite F (1997) Extrapelvic endometriosis. Obstet Gynecol Clin N Am 24(2):411–440
4. Fleisch MC, Xafis D, De Bruyne F et al (2005) Radical resection of invasive endometriosis with bowel or bladder involvement long-term results. Eur J Obstet Gynecol Reprod Biol 123:224–229
5. Calman–Hine Report (1995) A policy framework for commissioning cancer services: a report by the Expert Advisory Group on cancer to the Chief Medical Officers of England and Wales. Department of Health, London
6. Kennedy S, Bergqvist A, Chapron C, D'Hooghe T, Dunselman G, Greb R, Hummelshoj L, Prentice A, Saridogan E (2005) ESHRE guideline for the diagnosis and management of endometriosis. Hum Reprod 20:2698–2704
7. British Society for Gynaecological Endoscopy (BSGE) 'Criteria for a BSGE recognised centre for laparoscopic treatment of women with recto-vaginal endometriosis'. http://www.bsge.org.uk. Accessed 2 Jan 2017
8. Haward R, Amir Z, Borrill C, Dawson J, Scully J, West M et al (2003) Breast cancer teams: the impact of constitution, new cancer workload, and methods of operation on their effectiveness. Br J Cancer 89:15–22
9. Wagner E (2004) Effective teamwork and quality of care. Med Care 42:1037–1039
10. Mickan SM (2005) Evaluating the effectiveness of health care teams. Aust Health Rev 29:211–217
11. D'Hooghe T (2006) Hummelshoj L (2006) multi-disciplinary centres/networks of excellence for endometriosis management and research: a proposal. Hum Reprod 21(11):2743–2748
12. Simoens S, Dunselman G et al (2012) The burden of endometriosis: costs and quality of life of women with endometriosis and treated in referral centres. Hum Reprod 27(5):1292–1299
13. Chapron C, Dubuisson JB, Pansini V, Vieira M, Fauconnier A, Barakat H, Dousset B (2002) Routine clinical examination is not sufficient for diagnosing and locating deeply infiltrating endometriosis. J Am Assoc Gynecol Laparosc 9:115–119
14. Bazot M, Detchev R, Cortez A, Amouyal P, Uzan S, Darai E (2003) Transvaginal sonography and rectal endoscopic sonography for the assessment of pelvic endometriosis: a preliminary comparison. Hum Reprod 18:1686–1692
15. Hudelist G, English J, Thomas AE et al (2011) Diagnostic accuracy of transvaginal ultrasound for noninvasive diagnosis of bowel endometriosis: systematic review and meta-analysis. Ultrasound Obstet Gynecol 37:257
16. Nisenblat V, Bossuyt PMM, Farquhar C, Johnson N, Hull ML (2016) Imaging modalities for the non-invasive diagnosis of endometriosis. Cochrane Database Syst Rev Issue 2. doi:10.1002/14651858
17. Kinkel K, Frei KA, Balleyguier C, Chapron C (2006) Diagnosis of endometriosis with imaging: a review. Eur Radiol 16:285–298
18. Saba L, Sulcis R, Melis GB, de Cecco CN, Laghi A, Piga M et al (2014) Endometriosis: the role of magnetic resonance imaging. Acta Radiol 56(3):355–367
19. Abrao MS, Gonc alves MO, Dias JA Jr, Podgaec S, Chamie LP, Blasbalg R (2007) Comparison between clinical examination, transvaginal sonography and magnetic resonance imaging for the diagnosis of deep endometriosis. Hum Reprod 22:3092–3097
20. Cavaco-Gomes J et al (2017) Laparoscopic management of ureteral endometriosis: a systematic review. Eur J Obstet Gynecol Reprod Biol 210:94–101
21. American Society for Reproductive Medicine (1997) Revised American Society for Reproductive Medicine classification of endometriosis. Fertil Steril 67(5):817–21.
22. Crosignani PG, Vercellini P, Biffignandi F, Costantini W, Cortesi I, Imparato E (1996) Laparoscopy versus laparotomy in conservative surgical treatment for severe endometriosis. Fertil Steril 66:706–711
23. Wolthuis AM, Meuleman C, Tomassetti C, D'Hooghe T, de Buck van Overstraeten A, D'Hoore A (2014) Bowel endometriosis: colorectal surgeon's perspective in a multidisciplinary surgical team. World J Gastroenterol 20(42):15616–15623
24. Dunselman GA, Vermeulen N, Becker C, Calhaz-Jorge C, D'Hooghe T, De Bie B, Heikinheimo O, Horne AW, Kiesel L, Nap A, Prentice A, Saridogan E, Soriano D, Nelen W (2014) ESHRE guideline: management of women with endometriosis. Hum Reprod 29:400–412
25. Fleissig A, Jenkins V, Catt S, Fallowfield L (2006) Multidisciplinary teams in cancer care: are they effective in the UK? Lancet Oncol 7:935–943
26. Sidhom MA, Paulsen MG (2006) Multidisciplinary care in oncology: medicolegal implications of group decisions. Lancet 7:951–954
27. Leso PB, Coward JI, Letsa U et al (2013) A study of the decision outcomes and financial costs of multidisciplinary team meetings (MDMs) in oncology. Br J Cancer 109:2295–2300
28. Hummelshoj L, Prentice A, Groothuis P (2006) Update on endometriosis. Womens Health 2:53–56
29. Stones RW, Selfe S (2000) Psychosocial and economic impact of chronic pelvic pain. Baillieres Clin Obstet Gynaecol 14:415–431

16

Perioperative surgical outcome of conventional and robot-assisted total laparoscopic hysterectomy

W. J. van Weelden[1,2*], B. B. M. Gordon[2], E. A. Roovers[1], A. A. Kraayenbrink[1], C. I. M. Aalders[1], F. Hartog[1] and F. P. H. L. J. Dijkhuizen[1]

Abstract

Background: To evaluate surgical outcome in a consecutive series of patients with conventional and robot assisted total laparoscopic hysterectomy.

Methods: A retrospective cohort study was performed among patients with benign and malignant indications for a laparoscopic hysterectomy. Main surgical outcomes were operation room time and skin to skin operating time, complications, conversions, rehospitalisation and reoperation, estimated blood loss and length of hospital stay.

Results: A total of 294 patients were evaluated: 123 in the conventional total laparoscopic hysterectomy (TLH) group and 171 in the robot TLH group. After correction for differences in basic demographics with a multivariate linear regression analysis, the skin to skin operating time was a significant 18 minutes shorter in robot assisted TLH compared to conventional TLH (robot assisted TLH 92m, conventional TLH 110m, p0.001). The presence or absence of previous abdominal surgery had a significant influence on the skin to skin operating time as did the body mass index and the weight of the uterus.
Complications were not significantly different. The robot TLH group had significantly less blood loss and lower rehospitalisation and reoperation rates.

Conclusions: This study compares conventional TLH with robot assisted TLH and shows shorter operating times, less blood loss and lower rehospitalisation and reoperation rates in the robot TLH group.

Keywords: Total laparoscopic hysterectomy, Robot, Complication, Operating time

Background

In recent years, it has become clear that laparoscopic hysterectomy offers a safe and feasible alternative to abdominal hysterectomy [1]. Patients with a laparoscopic hysterectomy have less complications, shorter hospital stays, and faster return to normal activities compared to abdominal hysterectomy [2]. When vaginal hysterectomy is not possible or not indicated, laparoscopic hysterectomy is the preferred alternative [2]. Despite the benefits of laparoscopic hysterectomy, abdominal hysterectomy remains the most common surgical approach, possibly

because of the long learning curve and high-level laparoscopic skills necessary for a total laparoscopic hysterectomy [3–8]. Robotic surgery could overcome these difficulties, making laparoscopic surgery possible for more patients. The da Vinci system is the only registered robotic surgery system. It offers a three-dimensional vision, EndoWrist instruments, that mimics the human wrist and optimal ergonomics.

Up till now, the role of robotic surgery in total laparoscopic hysterectomy remains unclear. Studies comparing surgical outcome in conventional and robot-assisted total laparoscopic hysterectomy have shown mixed results [7, 9–11].

We performed the present study to evaluate the perioperative surgical outcome in a consecutive series of

* Correspondence: willemjanvanweelden@hotmail.com
[1]Department of Obstetrics and Gynecology, Rijnstate hospital, Wagnerlaan 55, 6815 AD Arnhem, The Netherlands
[2]Department of Obstetrics and Gynecology, Radboud University Nijmegen Medical Center, Geert Grooteplein-Zuid 22, 6525 GA Nijmegen, The Netherlands

patients with conventional and robot-assisted total laparoscopic hysterectomy.

Methods

Design and setting

We conducted a retrospective cohort study comparing conventional total laparoscopic hysterectomy (TLH) with robot-assisted TLH. The study was performed between 2002 and 2014 in Rijnstate hospital Arnhem, a large teaching hospital in The Netherlands.

Participants

All patients undergoing conventional or robot-assisted TLH with or without bilateral salpingo-oophorectomy were included in the study. We included all patients from the introduction of both techniques in our hospital onwards.

Patients with benign as well as malignant indications were eligible. Benign indications included fibroids, dysfunctional blood loss, and adenomyosis. Malignant indications included only low-grade endometrioid endometrial carcinoma. Patients with other subtypes of endometrial cancer and cervical cancer or patients who needed surgical staging procedures were not included [12]. Whenever a vaginal hysterectomy was deemed possible, that operation was preferred to a conventional or robot-assisted TLH in benign indications. These patients were also not included in this study.

Follow-up was performed in the outpatient clinic 6 weeks after operation. Further follow-up visits were planned if complaints or complications arose. In case of a malignancy, follow-up was planned according to the national guideline [12].

The institutional research board approved the present study. All patients gave informed consent for being included in the study.

Procedure

All patients had general anesthesia and received preoperative antibiotics (cefazolin and metronidazole). Conventional TLH was performed using one 10-mm port at the umbilicus or in the midline 1.5 cm above the umbilicus, one assistant 5-mm port, and one assistant 12-mm port. For robot-assisted TLH, one 10-mm port in the midline 1.5 cm above the umbilicus and two 8-mm and one 12-mm assistant ports were inserted. Closed and open introduction techniques were used according to the discretion of the gynecologist. The surgical technique for both procedures was similar and is published elsewhere [13]. For the conventional TLH, we used the Gyrus bipolar system (Gyrus ACMI, Southborough, MA, USA); for the robot-assisted TLH, we used the da Vinci system with bipolar and monopolar currency (Intuitive Surgical Inc., Sunnyvale CA, USA). For vaginal manipulation of the uterus, we used the

Clermont-Ferrand uterine manipulator (Karl Storz GmbH & Co., Tuttlingen, Germany). The vaginal cuff was closed laparoscopically in the same way for both procedures using a Quill or V-Lock running suture or knotted Vicryl 0 sutures.

Four laparoscopic gynecologists performed all conventional and robot-assisted TLH procedures. All were experienced in other gynecological laparoscopic operations, most notably laparoscopic supracervical hysterectomies before starting with conventional total laparoscopic hysterectomies.

Gynecologists performing robot-assisted TLH were trained according to the guideline for implementation of a new surgical technique from the Dutch Society of Endoscopic Surgery [14] and completed robotic training provided by Intuitive Surgical.

Outcome

Demographic data including age, body mass index (BMI), indication for surgery (benign or malignant), and previous abdominal surgery was recorded.

Surgical outcomes were as follows:

- Operation room (OR) time: from patient arrival to departure of the OR.
- Skin to skin time: total operating time from skin incision to closure of the skin wounds.
- Complications: scored as a major or minor complication [15] (Table 1).
- Rehospitalisations and reoperations in case of a complication, estimated blood loss (EBL), and length of hospital stay (LHS, hospital stay started on the day of operation).

Statistics

Comparisons of group characteristics were made using chi-square or Fisher's exact test for differences in

Table 1 Description of complications: major and minor [15]

Major	Minor
Hemorrhage requiring transfusion	Hemorrhage not requiring transfusion
Hematoma requiring surgical drainage	Hematoma: spontaneous drainage
Bowel injury	Infection: chest, urinary, wound, pelvic
Bladder injury	Deep vein thrombosis
Ureteric injury	Others
Pulmonary embolus	
Conversion to laparotomy	
Wound dehiscence	
Fistula	

proportions and Mann-Whitney U test for non-parametric distributed variables.

To correct for baseline differences between the two groups, multivariate linear regression analysis was performed in which type of robot-assisted TLH, conventional TLH, BMI, uterus weight, previous abdominal surgery, and indication for surgery (benign or malignant) were entered as independent variables. Operation room time and skin to skin operating time were entered as dependent variables. To get meaningful regression parameters, BMI and uterus weight were centered at 20 kg/m^2 and 80 g, respectively. A p value of 0.05 was considered statistically significant. Statistical analysis was performed using IBM SPSS Statistics (version 21).

Results

Patient characteristics

Two hundred ninety-four patients were included in the study: 123 in the conventional TLH group and 171 in the robot TLH group. BMI and positive history of abdominal surgery did not differ significantly between the two groups. Age, uterus weight, and indication did differ significantly. Patients in the conventional TLH group were significantly younger (conventional TLH median age 49 years, robot-assisted TLH median age 57 years, p 0.03), had significantly higher uterus weights (conventional TLH 145 g, robot-assisted TLH 114 g, p 0.04), and were operated for malignant indications less frequently (conventional TLH 45%, robot-assisted TLH 58%, p 0.04) (Table 2).

Operation room time

The median OR time was 173 min in the robot TLH group and 190 min in the conventional TLH group ($p = 0.14$ not significant) (Table 3).

In the multivariate linear regression analysis of the OR time, robot-assisted TLH was 9 min shorter compared to conventional TLH (141 min versus 150 m versus p 0.10, not significant). Furthermore, previous abdominal surgery, BMI, and uterus weight all had significant influences on the OR time. Patients with previous abdominal surgery had an increased OR time of 12.5 min (p 0.02). If the BMI was higher than 20 kg/m^2, 2.1 min for every extra point of BMI was added ($p < 0.001$) to the OR time. If the uterus weight was higher than 80 g, 0.2 min for every gram of uterus weight was added to the OR time ($p < 0.001$). Benign or malignant indication for surgery had no significant influence on the OR time.

For example, a patient with a BMI of 20, a uterus weight of 80 g, and no previous abdominal surgery would have an OR time of 141 min if a robot-assisted TLH was performed or 150 min if a conventional TLH was performed.

The average patient in this study had a BMI of 27, a uterus weight of 128 g, and no previous abdominal surgery. The OR time in this patient would have been 165 min in the case of a robot-assisted TLH or 174 min in a conventional TLH. If that same patient would have a prior abdominal operation, an extra 12.5 min would have to be added to the OR times in both robot-assisted and conventional TLH.

Skin to skin operating time

The median skin to skin time was significantly shorter in the robot group compared to the conventional group (120 versus 145 min $p < 0.001$) (Table 3).

A multivariate linear regression analysis of the skin to skin time showed a significant 18-min difference favoring the robot TLH group (robot-assisted TLH 92 m, conventional TLH 110 m, p 0.001). The skin to skin time increased 11.8 min for patients with previous abdominal surgery (p 0.02), 1.8 min for each point of BMI above 20 ($p < 0.001$), and 0.2 min for each extra gram of weight of the uterus over 80 g ($p < 0.001$).

Hence, a patient with a BMI of 27, a uterus weight of 128 g, and no previous abdominal surgery would have a skin to skin operating time of 114 min in the robot group or 132 min in the conventional group.

Table 2 Baseline characteristics of conventional and robot TLH patients

	Conventional TLH (n 123)	Robot TLH (n 171)	p value
Age, median, years (range)	49 (29–89)	57 (27–88)	0.03
BMI, median, kg/m^2 (range)	27 (17–52)	28 (18–59)	0.12
Uterus weight, grams (range)	145 (20–470)	114 (37–1009)	0.04
Indication for surgery, n (%)			
Benign	67 (55%)	72 (42%)	0.04
Malignant	56 (45%)	99 (58%)	
History of abdominal surgery, n (%)			
Positive	42 (34%)	77 (45%)	0.07
Negative	80 (66%)	94 (55%)	

Table 3 Perioperative surgical outcome

	Conventional	Robot	p value
Operation room time (min), median (range)	190 (102–303)	173 (116–393)	0.14
Skin to skin time (min), median (range)	145 (43–250)	120 (72–302)	<0.001
Complications, n (%)			
Major	9 (7.3%)	7 (4.1%)	0.48
Minor	14 (11.4%)	19 (11.1%)	
No	100 (81.3%)	145 (84.8%)	
Conversion, n (%)	4 (3.3%)	3 (1.8%)	0.46
Rehospitalisation, n (%)	13 (10.6%)	7 (4.1%)	0.04
Reoperation, n (%)	7 (5.7%)	2 (1.2%)	0.04
Blood loss (ml), median (range)	100 (0–800)	25 (0–600)	<0.001
Blood transfusion, n	0	0	1.0
Length of hospital stay (days), median (range)	4 (2–41)	3 (2–8)	<0.001

If that the same patient has a BMI of 35, the skin to skin operating time would have been 129 min in the robot group or 147 min in the conventional group.

Complications, conversions, rehospitalisations, and reoperations

No significant differences could be found in complications or conversions (Tables 3 and 4). There were 16 major complications: seven in the robot group and nine in the conventional TLH group (Table 4). In the robot group, there were three conversions to laparotomy, one hemorrhage requiring transfusion, one bladder injury, one pulmonary embolus, and one would dehiscence. In the conventional group, there were four conversions to laparotomy, two postoperative fistulas, one bowel and one bladder injury, and one hemorrhage requiring transfusion. All conversions were performed for strategic reasons. The minor complications did not differ significantly as well (conventional group 14 (11.4%) versus robot group 19 (11.1%)) (Table 4).

Rehospitalisations and reoperations were significantly more prevalent in the conventional TLH group. Rehospitalisation occurred in 13 cases (10.6%) in the conventional group compared to seven cases (4.1%) in the robot group (p 0.04). Reoperation was necessary in seven cases in the conventional TLH group (5.7%) and two cases in the robot TLH group (1.2%) (p 0.04).

Estimated blood loss

The median EBL was 100 ml in the conventional TLH group compared to 25 ml in the robot TLH group (p < 0.001) (Table 3). After correction for differences in BMI, weight of the uterus, indication, and previous abdominal surgery, there was 70 ml more

blood loss in the conventional TLH than in the robot TLH group (p < 0.001).

Length of hospital stay

The median LHS was 4 days in the conventional TLH group and 3 days in the robot TLH group (p < 0.001). After correction for differences in BMI, weight of the uterus, indication, previous abdominal surgery, and age, the LHS was 0.74 day longer in the conventional TLH group compared to the robot TLH group (p < 0.001).

Discussion

We conducted a retrospective cohort study to evaluate the perioperative surgical outcomes of conventional and robot-assisted total laparoscopic hysterectomy. This study shows that patients in the robot TLH group have faster skin to skin operating times, less blood loss, and

Table 4 Encountered complications

	Conventional TLH	Robot TLH
Major complication	9	7
Hemorrhage requiring transfusion	1	1
Bowel injury	1	0
Bladder injury	1	1
Pulmonary embolus	0	1
Unintented conversion to laparotomy	4	3
Wound dehiscence	0	1
Vesicovaginal fistula	2	0
Minor complication	14	19
Hemorrhage not requiring transfusion	0	1
Infection: chest, urinary, wound, pelvic	12	12
Hematoma: spontaneous drainage	0	2
Deep vein thrombosis	0	0
Others	2	4

lower rehospitalisation and reoperation rates. After correction for BMI, uterus weight, indication, and history of previous abdominal surgery, the advantages in operating time, estimated blood loss, and length of hospital stay persisted.

Although the skin to skin time was faster, the OR time did not differ significantly. This difference might be explained by more extensive preoperative positioning in the robot group. The positioning needs to be more precise in robot patients because of the impossibility to adjust the position of the patient after connection of the operating ports to the robot. In conventional TLH, small adjustments in positioning are possible during the operation. We hypothesized that the OR time in the robot TLH group would become shorter when less time was necessary for positioning in a more experienced operation team. Indeed, a comparison of conventional and robot TLH groups without the first 25 cases of robot-assisted TLH procedures showed a significant 15 min shorter OR time in the robot group (p 0.009).

Our analysis clearly shows how OR time and skin to skin operating time in conventional and robot-assisted TLH are influenced by BMI, weight of the uterus, and previous abdominal surgery. To our knowledge, no previous study has demonstrated this so clearly in robot-assisted TLH.

With this knowledge, one could hypothesize that advantages of robot-assisted TLH are more outspoken in a specific subset of patients. Unfortunately, this study was too small to allow any comparison of complications and operation times in more complicated cases like patients with a BMI above 40 kg/m^2 or with multiple previous abdominal operations. Further research is necessary to identify specific populations that profit specifically from a robot-assisted TLH.

The operating times in our study correspond well with the literature [10, 11, 16]. Shorter operating times are reported as well, but they originate mostly from early adopters of robotic surgery or centers with more experience in laparoscopic hysterectomies [17–19].

When comparing operating times between conventional and robot-assisted TLH, most studies have found shorter operating times in conventional TLH [10, 16–18, 20]. A Cochrane review conducted by Liu et al. concluded that moderate quality evidence exists for longer operating times in robot-assisted TLH [21]. This finding is based on two randomized controlled trials with in total 148 patients, which is half the population of our study [17, 19]. Other studies have also found shorter operating times in robot-assisted TLH [11, 16].

The present study, among many others, was not powered to show differences in the complication rate. Major complications like bladder injury and vaginal cuff dehiscence occur in about 2 and 1% of conventional total laparoscopic hysterectomies [6, 15]. A prospective trial with enough patients to show significant differences in these complications has to our knowledge never been performed. Our results however do give some indications for safer surgery in the robot TLH group. First, the estimated blood loss is 70 ml lower in the robot TLH group compared to the conventional TLH group. One could argue that 70 ml hardly has any clinical significance, but on the other hand, it might mean that robot-assisted TLH confers lower operation risks [16]. Also, the lower rehospitalisation and reoperation rates in the robot TLH group suggest that a robot-assisted TLH might convey a lower risk of complications than a conventional TLH.

Strengths of this study include the high number of cases included, the correction for relevant confounders, and the fact that the two operations are compared in one hospital performed by the same group of gynecologists. Two important limitations need to be addressed. First, the demographics differed between the conventional and robot TLH groups. By using a multivariate linear regression analysis, we corrected for these differences. Second, there are limitations inherent to the retrospective design of this study. In our experience, the operation itself has not changed dramatically from 2002 to 2014. The length of hospital stay however has decreased for all patients in our hospital. The difference in length of hospital stay that we found in this study therefore has to be interpreted with care.

Conclusions

In conclusion, this study compares conventional TLH with robot-assisted TLH and shows that patients with a robot-assisted TLH have shorter skin to skin operation times and blood loss. Complications are not significantly lower in robot-assisted TLH, but when a complication arises, chances of rehospitalisation and reoperation are lower in the robot TLH group.

Acknowledgements
None.

Funding
None.

Authors' contributions
WW and FD participated in the project development, data collection, and manuscript writing. BG and AK carried out the project development and data collection. ER contributed to the data collection and management. CA and FH carried out the data collection. All authors read and approved the final manuscript.

Competing interests
The authors declare that they have no competing interests.

References

1. Spaner SJ, Warnock GL (1997) A brief history of endoscopy, laparoscopy and laparoscopic surgery. J laparoendosc Adv Surg Tech A 7(6):369–373

2. Nieboer TE, Johnson N, Lethaby A, Tavender E, Curr E, Garry R, van Voorst S, Mol BWJ, Kluivers KB (2009) Surgical approach to hysterectomy for benign gynaecological disease. Cochrane Database of Syst Rev Issue 3. Art. No.: CD003677. doi:10.1002/14651858.CD003677.pub4

3. ACOG (2015) Committee opinion no. 628: robotic surgery in gynecology. Obstet Gynecol 125(3):760–767

4. Wu JM, Wechter ME, Geller EJ, Nguyen TV, Visco AG (2007) Hysterectomy rates in the United States, 2003. Obstet Gynecol 110(5):1091–1095

5. Twijnstra ARH, Kolkman W, Trimbos-Kemper GC, Jansen FW (2010) Implementation of advanced laparoscopic surgery in gynecology: national overview of trends. J Minim Invasive Gyncol 17(4):487–492

6. Twijnstra AR, Blikkendaal MD, van Zwet EW, van Kesteren PJM, de Kroon CD, Jansen FW (2012) Predictors of successful surgical outcome in laparoscopic hysterectomy. Obstet Gynecol 119:700–708

7. Wright JD, Ananth CV, Lewin SN, Bruke WM, Lu YS, Al N, Herzog TJ, Hershman DL (2013) Robotically assisted vs laparoscopic hysterectomy among women with benign gynaecologic disease. JAMA 309(7):689–698

8. Driessen SR, Baden NL, van Zwet EW, Twijnstra AR, Jansen FW (2015) Trends in the implementation of advanced minimally invasive gynecologic surgical procedures in the Netherlands. J Minim Invasive Gynecol 22(4):642–647

9. Rosero EB, Kho KA, Joshi GP, Giesecke M, Schaffer JL (2014) Comparison of robotic and laparoscopic hysterectomy for benign gynecologic disease. Obstet Gynecol 123:255–262

10. Pasic RP, Rizzo JA, Fang H, Ross S, Moore M, Gunnarsson C (2010) Comparing robot-assisted with conventional laparoscopic hysterectomy: impact on cost and clinical outcomes. J Minim Invasive Gynecol 17:730–738

11. Lönnerfors C, Reynisson P, Persson J (2015) A randomized trial comparing vaginal and laparoscopic hysterectomy vs robot-assisted hysterectomy. J Minim Invasive Gynecol 22:78–86

12. Integraal Kankercentrum Nederland (2011) Endometriumcarcinoom landelijke richtlijn met regionale toevoegingen versie 3.0. http://www.oncoline.nl/endometriumcarcinoom

13. Kluivers KB, Hendriks JCM, Mol BWJ, Bongers MY, Bremer GL, de Vet HCW, Vierhout ME, Brolmann HAM (2007) Quality of life and surgical outcome after total laparoscopic hysterectomy versus total abdominal hysterectomy for benign disease: a randomized, controlled trial. J Minim Invasive Gynecol 14:145–152

14. Nederlandse Vereniging voor Endoscopische Chirurgie (2008) Plan van aanpak en beleid minimal invasieve chirurgie: eisen aan locale gebruiksgroepen. http://www.oncoline.nl/uploaded/docs/Revisie%20oesofagusca/PLan%20van%20Aanpak%20Optimalisering%20MIC%20traject%20NVEC.pdf

15. Garry R, Fountain J, Mason S, Hawe J, Napp V, Abbot J et al (2004) The eVALuate study: two parallel randomized trials, one comparing laparoscopic with abdominal hysterectomy, the other comparing laparoscopic with vaginal hysterectomy. BMJ 328:1229–1236

16. Orady M, Hrynewych A, Nawfal AK, Wegienka G (2012) Comparison of robotic-assisted hysterectomy to other minimally invasive approaches. JSLS 16(4):542–548

17. Sarlos D, Kots L, Stevanovic N, Schaer G (2010) Robotic hysterectomy versus conventional laparoscopic hysterectomy: outcome and cost analyses of a matched case-control study. Eur J Obstet Gynecol Reprod Biol 150(1):92–96

18. Sarlos D, Kots L, Stevanovic N, von Felten S, Schär G (2012) Robotic compared with conventional laparoscopic hysterectomy: a randomized controlled trial. Obstet Gynecol 120:604–11

19. Paraiso MF, Ridgeway B, Park AJ, Jelovsek JE, Barber MD, Falcone T, Einarsson JL (2013) A randomized trial comparing conventional and robotically assisted total laparoscopic hysterectomy. Am J Obstet Gynecol 368:e1–e7

20. Payne TN, Dauterive FR (2008) A comparison of total laparoscopic hysterectomy to robotically assisted hysterectomy: surgical outcomes in a community practice. J Minim Invasive Gynecol 15(3):286–291

21. Liu H, Lawrie TA, Lu D, Song H, Wang L, Shi G (2014) Robot-assisted surgery in gynaecology. Cochrane Database of Syst Rev Issue 12. Art. No.: CD011422. doi:10.1002/14651858.CD011422

17

N$_2$O strongly prevents adhesion formation and postoperative pain in open surgery through a drug-like effect

Roberta Corona[1,2], Maria Mercedes Binda[1], Leila Adamyan[3], Victor Gomel[4] and Philippe R. Koninckx[1,5*]

Abstract

Background: Microsurgical tenets and peritoneal conditioning during laparoscopic surgery (LS) decrease postoperative adhesions and pain. For a trial in human, the strong beneficial effects of N$_2$O needed to be confirmed in open surgery (OS).

Results: In a mouse model for OS, the effect of the gas environment upon adhesions was evaluated. Experiment I evaluated desiccation and the duration of exposure to CO$_2$, N$_2$O or CO$_2$ + 4%O$_2$. Experiment II evaluated the dose-response curve of adding N$_2$O to CO$_2$. Experiment III compared humidified CO$_2$ + 10% N$_2$O during LS and OS.

In OS, 30- and 60-min exposure to non-humidified CO$_2$ caused mortality of 33 and 100%, respectively. Mortality was prevented by humidification, by dry N$_2$O or dry CO$_2$ + 4%O$_2$. Adhesions increased with the duration of exposure to CO$_2$ ($p < 0.0001$) and decreased slightly by humidification or by the addition of 4% O$_2$. N$_2$O strongly decreased adhesions at concentrations of 5% or greater. With humidified CO$_2$ + 10% N$_2$O, adhesion formation was similar in OS and LS.

Conclusions: The drug-like and strong beneficial effect of low concentrations of N$_2$O is confirmed in OS.

Keywords: Postoperative adhesions, N$_2$O, Conditioning, Humidification, Microsurgery, Microsurgical principle

Background

The peritoneal cavity with its peritoneal fluid is a specific environment different from that of plasma. The mesothelial cell lining of the peritoneal cavity and its organs facilitates the gliding of the bowels and actively regulates homeostasis and transport of fluids, molecules and cells. In males, the volume of peritoneal fluid is small. In women of reproductive age, follicular exudation increases the volume and adds high concentrations of steroid hormones. The peritoneal cavity is not vascularised and constitutes a sterile cavity that does not belong to the body homeostasis. Any trauma in the peritoneal cavity causes an inflammatory reaction and a mesothelial cell retraction, exposing the basal membrane. This abolishes the blood-peritoneal fluid barrier and permits the entry of immunocompetent cells and facilitates diffusion of larger molecules as immunoglobins, which is an efficient defence mechanism to intruders [1, 2].

The large and flat mesothelial cells react within seconds to any trauma by retraction and bulging [1, 2] causing an acute inflammation [3] which increases with the duration and severity of the trauma. Identified traumas are surgical manipulation, mesothelial cell hypoxia by CO$_2$ pneumoperitoneum, deeper ischaemia at an intraperitoneal pressure of more than 8 mmHg and ischaemia-reperfusion at desufflation [4], oxidative stress [5] or reactive oxygen species (ROS) induced by exposure to air with 20% of oxygen, desiccation and saline as irrigation liquid. The severity and the duration of this acute inflammation of the entire peritoneal cavity create an inversely proportional reduction of fibrinolysis. This, in turn, increases the potential of adhesion formation through a reduction in tissue plasminogen activator (tPA) and an increase in plasminogen activator

* Correspondence: pkoninckx@gmail.com
[1]Department of Obstetrics and Gynaecology, KU Leuven – Catholic University of Leuven, 3000 Leuven, Belgium
[5]KU Leuven, Vuilenbosstraat 2, 3360 Bierbeek, Belgium
Full list of author information is available at the end of the article

inhibitor (PAI) [6, 7]. During laparoscopic surgery, the retraction and bulging of mesothelial cells cause a progressive increase in CO_2 resorption. The acute peritoneal inflammation increases postoperative C-reactive protein concentrations (CRP) and causes postoperative pain [2].

During laparoscopic surgery, prevention of the mesothelial cell retraction and the subsequent acute inflammation effectively prevents or decreases the associated consequences including postoperative adhesion formation and postoperative pain. In addition, it accelerates recovery and in animal experiments decreases tumour metastasis. The most effective preventive factors are the addition of more than 5% of nitrous oxygen to the CO_2 pneumoperitoneum, cooling of the peritoneal cavity below 31 °C, minimalising mechanical trauma and ROS production, using Ringer's lactate instead of saline and administering one or two doses dexamethasone postoperatively [2]. If used together with a barrier [8], this approach results in virtually adhesion free surgery [9].

The similarity between our current knowledge derived largely from animal experiments, and the microsurgical tenets developed in the early 1970s empirically, but controlled by systematic second-look laparoscopy, 8–12 weeks after the initial operation, is striking. These principles were developed for open surgery and soon after applied in laparoscopic surgery [10]. These microsurgical principles indeed are a combination of gentle tissue handling, judicious use of electrical and/or laser energy, use of inert sutures, continuous irrigation with Ringer's lactate at room temperature during the procedure to avoid desiccation, shielding the bowels from the ambient air, thorough lavage of the peritoneal cavity at the end of the procedure, instillation of Ringer's lactate solution containing a minimum of 500 mg of hydrocortisone succinate into the peritoneal cavity before closure and administration of one or two doses of dexamethasone after surgery.

Microsurgical tenets were proven to decrease adhesion formation and to increase pregnancy rates in open and laparoscopic surgery [10, 11]. The relative importance of each of these factors that decrease acute inflammation and adhesion formation was investigated only recently in a laparoscopic mouse model with proof of concept trials in human [9]. However, the addition of low doses of N_2O which is the single most effective factor was investigated during laparoscopic surgery with an insufflation pressure only. Since there is no insufflation pressure in open surgery, we, therefore, decided to evaluate the effect of N_2O in a mouse model for open surgery before undertaking a trial in human.

Methods

Animals and the experimental set-up (anaesthesia, ventilation, laparoscopic surgery, adhesion induction and scoring) were as previously described [3, 12, 13].

Animals

Inbred 9 to 10-week-old female BALB/c OlaHsd mice of 18 to 20 g (Harlan Laboratories B.V., Venray, The Netherlands) mice were used to decrease experimental variability. They were kept under standard laboratory conditions and diet at the animal facilities of the Katholieke Universiteit Leuven (KUL). The study was approved by the Institutional Review Animal Care Committee (KUL: P040/2010).

The laparoscopic mouse model

Following anaesthesia and pneumoperitoneum induction (Thermoflator, Karl Storz, Tüttlingen, Germany) with humidified gas (Humidifier, 204,320 33, Karl Storz) and standardised 10 × 1.6 mm bipolar lesions (20 W, standard coagulation mode, Autocon 350, Karl Storz, Tüttlingen, Germany) were made on both right and left uterine horns and on abdominal walls using a 2 mm endoscope (Karl Storz, Tüttlingen Germany) and two 14-gauge catheters (Insyte-W, Vialon, Becton Dickinson, Madrid, Spain) as secondary ports. The insufflation pressure was 15 mmHg. Since adhesion formation increases with body temperature, the latter was strictly controlled [13]. Therefore, mice and equipment were placed in a closed chamber at 37 °C (heated air, WarmTouch, Patient Warming System, model 5700, Mallinckrodt Medical, Hazelwood, MO). Anaesthesia and ventilation [14] and the timing between anaesthesia (T_0), intubation (at 10 min, T_{10}) and the onset of the experiment (at 20 min, T_{20}) were standardised.

The only variable in this model of adhesion formation thus was the duration of the pneumoperitoneum and the type and humidification of the gas used.

A mouse model for open surgery

All factors validated for the laparoscopic model were kept identical, i.e. animals, anaesthesia, intubation, ventilation, temperature control, timing, type of lesions, the equipment used for gas insufflation and humidification and the scoring of adhesions. The only difference was that instead of a laparoscopy with a pneumoperitoneum, a laparotomy was performed and the mice were kept with the open abdomen in a box exposed to the specific gas environment.

Following some pilot experiments, the model was standardised as follows. Following anaesthesia (T_0), shaving and disinfection of the abdomen, the mouse was placed on a warm pillow in a transparent plexiglas box measuring 22 ×10 ×30 cm, closed with a sliding transparent cover that could be removed to perform at 20 min, T_2 surgery and lesions (Fig. 1). The box had one hole that accommodates the ventilation tube without gas leaks and two holes of 1 cm diameter each. The upper hole permitted escape of gas without pressure. The lower hole permitted insufflation of gas standardised in these experiments at 2 L/min. Since densities of CO_2 and N_2O are higher than air ($\delta CO_2 = 1.842$, $\delta N_2O = 1.872$, $\delta_{air} = 1.205$ at room temperature and atmospheric pressure), the box fills progressively until the gas escapes by overflow. In order to perform the surgical procedure, the box had to be opened; this causes the insufflated gas to partially mix with the ambient air. A midline xyphopubic incision was performed, and the abdomen kept open with two pins. Standard 10×2 mm bipolar lesions were created similar to the laparoscopic model. Following surgery, the cover was placed over the box and the mouse kept with the abdomen open exposed to the insufflated gas. This cover was necessary, since otherwise the insufflated gas would mix partially with the ambient air varying with the height of the box, the diameter of the opening and the flow rate of the gas insufflated. At the end of the experiment, the abdomen was closed with nylon 3-0 sutures.

Scoring of adhesions

Postoperative adhesions were scored blindly after 7 days as previously described during a second laparotomy using a stereomicroscope. The terminology of Pouly et al. [15] was used to describe de novo adhesion formation as adhesions formed at non-surgical sites.

Study design

Randomisation and factorial design

All experiments were block randomised by day as done in all previous experiments. Thus, one animal of each experimental group was operated at random on the same day in order to avoid eventual differences by day.

A factorial design [16] was used since a two by two factorial design results for each of the two variables in an almost similar statistical power as if two experiments had been performed with the same total number of animals in each experiment.

Mixture of N_2O and CO_2

In these experiments, we used either premixed gas with 90% CO_2 and 10% N_2O (Ijsfabriek, Strombeek, Belgium) or two Thermoflators one delivering CO_2 and the other N_2O, or the premixed gas. The gases from both insufflators were subsequently mixed in a mixing chamber, and the excess gas was permitted to escape from a water valve, the flow of both gases entering the box was limited to 2 L/min with a stopcock.

Pilot experiments

The first pilot experiment for open surgery consisted of mice ($n = 3$) with the abdomen open exposed to the ambient air at 37 °C (chamber at 37 °C) for 60 min. After 60 min, bowels were macroscopically dry and all mice died within 2 days. Mortality was thought to be caused by desiccation and maybe the damaging effect of 20% of O_2 in air. Therefore, the box was designed as described in order to control the gas environment, and CO_2 was

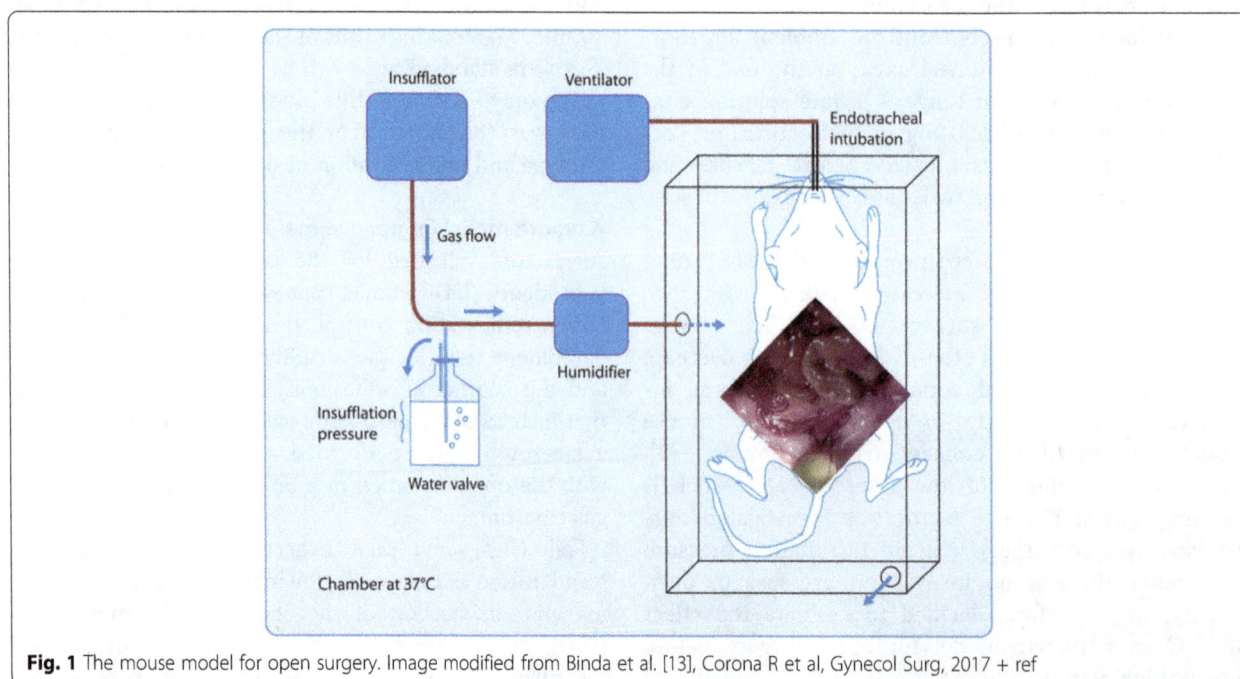

Fig. 1 The mouse model for open surgery. Image modified from Binda et al. [13], Corona R et al, Gynecol Surg, 2017 + ref

used as a carrier gas in order to be comparable with laparoscopy and because CO_2 is heavier than air and thus will fill the box progressively from the bottom.

A second pilot experiment was performed to evaluate in open surgery gas conditions known from the laparoscopy model. Humidified CO_2 for 60 min confirmed the absence of mortality with humidification; humidified 50% CO_2 + 50% N_2O and humidified 100% N_2O confirmed the strong adhesion preventing the effect of N_2O in concentrations over 5% (six mice, two mice per group).

Experiment I

The first experiment was designed to evaluate in open surgery the effect of humidification and of the duration of exposure to either 100% CO_2 or 100% N_2O or 96% CO_2 + 4%O_2 upon adhesion formation. A factorial design was used with non-humidified or humidified gas (two factors), during 30 or 60 min (two factors), and the three gas compositions (three factors). With three mice/ cell for two humidification factors and two duration factors and three gas factors (total mice = 3×2×2×3 = 36), an almost similar statistical power for each variable was obtained as if in three consecutive experiments with 36 mice each would have been done.

Experiment II

A dose response of the addition of various concentrations of N_2O to the CO_2 was evaluated in open surgery. Mice were exposed for 30 min to humidified CO_2 with concentrations of N_2O varying from 0 to 0.3, 1, 3, 10 and 100%. For 100% CO_2, 100% N_2O and 10% N_2O + 90% of CO_2, a Thermoflator was used with CO_2, N_2O or a premixed gas (10% N_2O + 90% CO_2), respectively. For the other concentrations two Thermoflators were used, one with CO_2 and the other with premixed gas (10% N_2O + 90% CO_2). The final concentrations of 3, 1, and 0.3% N_2O were obtained by combining various flow rates of 4 and 2 L/min, 9 and 1 L/min and 14.5 and 0.5 L/min of 100% CO_2 and premixed gas with 10% of N_2O (six mice/group, total mice = 36).

Experiment III

The third experiment was designed in order to compare adhesion formation following laparoscopic and open surgery and to evaluate whether the addition of 4% of O_2 had an additive effect when 10% of N_2O had been added to the CO_2. Using a factorial design, mice were exposed for 60 min to humidified 90% CO_2 + 10% N_2O or to 86% CO_2 + 10% N_2O + 4% O_2 either during laparoscopy or during open surgery. Since adhesions were known to be very low with 10% of N_2O, 10 mice per cell were used in order to have a power of almost 40 mice for each factor (total mice = 40).

Statistics

Differences were calculated with the SAS System (SAS Institute, Cary, NC) [17] using Wilcoxon/Kruskal Wallis unpaired test for comparison of individual data and a two-way analysis of variance (Proc GLM) for experiments with a factorial design. Results are expressed as a mean and standard deviations unless indicated otherwise.

Results

Experiment I

As observed in the pilot experiment for open surgery with non-humidified air for 60 minutes, open surgery with non-humidified CO_2 for 60 min resulted in 100% mortality (3/3). Even exposure to 30 min non-humidified CO_2 resulted in 33.3% mortality (1/3) (Fig. 2). As expected, there was no mortality when humidified gas was used. To our surprise, there was also no mortality when 10% of N_2O or 4% of O_2 were added to the non-humidified CO_2.

Adhesions at the surgical lesion site increased when the duration of exposure was longer ($p < 0.0001$) and when non-humidified gas was used ($p < 0.0001$) When 100% N_2O was used, adhesions were very scant in comparison with 100% CO_2 and 96% CO_2 + 4%O_2 with and without humidification (all comparisons $p < 0.0001$). When 96% CO_2 + 4% O_2 was used, adhesions were slightly less than with 100% CO_2 (non-humidified gas for 30 min $p < 0.0001$; humidified gas for 30 min $p = 0.0011$ and for 60 min $p = 0.003$).

Whereas in the laparoscopic mouse model, de novo adhesions in the upper abdomen have never been observed; in this experiment, de novo adhesions were seen in the upper abdomen between bowels, and between bowels and sidewalls when non-humidified CO_2 or non-humidified 96% CO_2 + 4%O_2 were used (Fig. 2).

Experiment II

The addition of increasing concentrations of N_2O to CO_2 decreases exponentially adhesion formation, with a

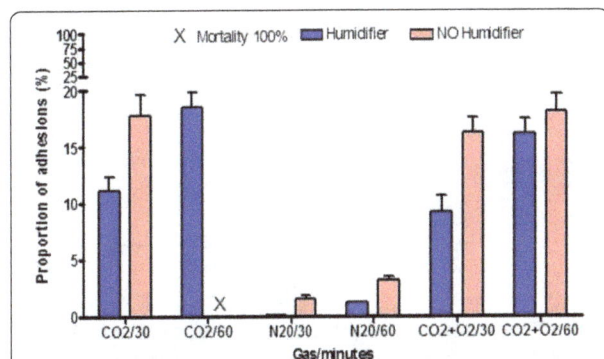

Fig. 2 Effect of duration, humidification and gas type upon mortality and adhesion formation during open surgery: 30 or 60 min of non-humidified or humidified CO_2, N_2O or 96% CO_2 + 4%O_2 Corona R et al, Gynecol Surg, 2017 + ref were used. Proportions of adhesions are given (mean and SD)

half maximum effect around 2.5% and a maximal effect from 5% onwards (Fig. 3). The difference between 10 and 100% N_2O was not significant ($p = 0.1551$). Differences between 0 and 3%, 0 and 10% and between 3 and 10% N_2O were $p = 0.0061$, $p = 0.0006$ and $p = 0.03$, respectively.

Experiment III

When humidified CO_2 with 10% of N_2O was used, adhesion formation was as expected very low in all groups (Fig. 4). The extent of adhesions was similar after both laparoscopic and open surgery with (NS) or without (NS) 4% of oxygen. The addition of 4% of oxygen to CO_2 with 10% of N_2O had a very small additive effect which however turned out to be significant ($p < 0.01$) caused by the high power of 20 mice in each group (factorial design, 10 mice/cell) and the low variability of inbred strains,

Discussion

These experiments confirm that the prevention of adhesion formation by conditioning is similar in both open and laparoscopic surgery. The main damaging effect of CO_2, thus, is caused by mesothelial cell hypoxia and retraction, and less by tissue and ischaemia-reperfusion. Adhesions indeed increase with the duration of exposure to CO_2 and with desiccation. N_2O in concentrations of more than 5% appears to be the single most effective factor with a marginal beneficial effect when 4% of oxygen is added to this gas mixture. Although not all observations made during laparoscopic surgery were repeated in open surgery, we conclude that the mechanisms involved are similar in both open and laparoscopic surgery. The key factors are mesothelial cell damage and acute inflammation in the

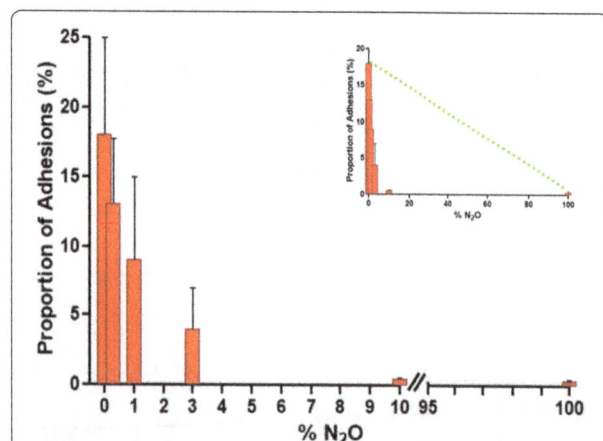

Fig. 4 The additional effect of 4% of O_2 on adhesion formation when 10% of N2O is used was investigated during laparoscopic and open surgery using humidified CO_2. Adhesion formation was comparable between laparoscopic and open surgery. The additive effect of 4% of O_2 was marginal ($p < 0.01$). Proportions of adhesions are given (mean and SD) Corona R et al, Gynecol Surg, 2017 + ref

entire peritoneal cavity, as a reaction to trauma, hypoxia, ROS, oxidative stress and desiccation.

The exact mechanisms involved in the peritoneal cavity that enhance or prevent adhesion formation are not fully understood. The half maximal effect around 2.5% of N_2O indicates that N_2O has a drug-like effect, the mechanism of which is unknown. It is also not understood why mortality is 100% after exposure for 60 min to non-humidified CO_2 and no mortality when non-humidified N_2O is used, although the desiccated aspect of the bowels is the same. We only can speculate that mortality is not only caused by the desiccation but mainly by the severity of the inflammatory process since N_2O strongly and O_2 slightly decrease the inflammatory reaction [18].

The observed effects of 5 to 10% of N_2O in open surgery at atmospheric pressure shed new light on the pathophysiology of adhesion formation. CO_2 pneumoperitoneum at an insufflation pressure of 15 mmHg decreases peritoneal oxygenation, triggers hypoxemia inducible factor (HIF) and decreases tissue plasminogen activator and upregulates PAI for several days. These effects of CO_2 pneumoperitoneum are less and/or of shorter duration at lower insufflation pressures and disappear at insufflation pressures below 8 mmHg in human and 2 mmHg in mice [3, 6–8]. Taking into account the differences in size between man and mice and Pascal's law, these pressures are considered the pressures at which vascular compression of the peritoneum, hypoxia and oxidative stress start. Since at atmospheric pressure N_2O still decreases adhesion formation caused by the CO_2 environment, we must conclude that key mechanism driving the subsequent events is mesothelial hypoxia

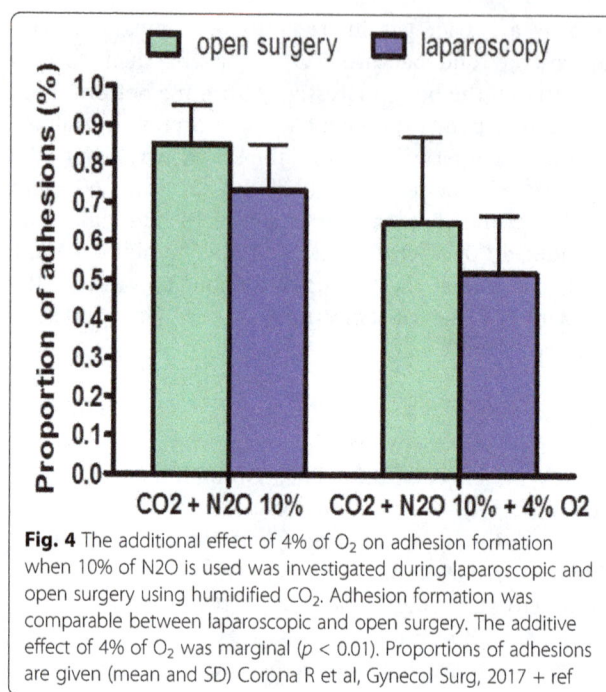

Fig. 3 Dose-response curve of the addition of 0.3 to 100% N_2O to humidified CO_2 upon adhesion formation during open surgery demonstrating the drug-like effect. In inset, the dotted yellow line indicates adhesion formation if the effect of N_2O would have been by replacing CO_2 irritation. Proportions of adhesions are given (mean and SD) Corona R et al, Gynecol Surg, 2017 + ref

and retraction. In addition, the observations that with laparoscopic surgery in the presence of a 10% N_2O environment at 15 mmHg pressure, the extent of adhesion formation is similar to open surgery at atmospheric pressure strongly suggests that 10% of N_2O prevents mesothelial cell oxidative stress hypoxia and its consequences including mesothelial cell retraction and decreased fibrinolysis enhanced adhesion formation and postoperative pain. However, whether N_2O also has a protective effect on oxidative stress caused by partial oxygen pressures higher than 75 mmHg (or more than 10% O_2 at atmospheric pressure) as in air remains to be investigated.

Despite the differences that exist between oxidative stress caused by 20% CO_2 in ambient air in open surgery and the detrimental effect of the CO_2 pneumoperitoneum and insufflation pressure, the prevention of adhesion formation and postoperative pain are similar in both open and laparoscopic surgery. Beside the use of a proper atraumatic surgical technique and precise haemostasis, the important adhesion preventive factors in open surgery are to avoid ROS formation, caused by the 20% oxygen concentration in ambient air; the use of N_2O in concentrations of 5% or more; cooling the peritoneal cavity; avoiding desiccation; the use of Ringer's lactate solution instead of saline; being toxic for mesothelial cells [19–25] for intraoperative irrigation and terminal thorough lavage and administration of one or two doses of dexamethasone after surgery. Although, it has not been investigated as yet whether N_2O can prevent the damaging effects of exposure to 20% of oxygen concentration, the flooding of the surgical site in open surgery with 5 to 10% of N_2O will require a carrier gas for which both CO_2 and nitrogen (N_2) seem suitable. The importance of cooling in open surgery has indirectly been confirmed in rats using cold saline infusions [26, 27]. Adhesions were also less when the abdominal cavity was exposed to the atmosphere of the operating theatre (21% O_2, 21 °C, 40–47% relative humidity) than to CO_2 + 4% of oxygen and 95–100% relative humidity at 37 °C [28]. Prevention of desiccation is much more important in open surgery than in laparoscopic surgery considering the 100% mortality of mice when exposed to dry CO_2 for 60 min. The toxicity of saline for the peritoneum was known since the early 1970s [19, 20] and has recently been confirmed [21–25]. The use of dexamethasone and another tenet of microsurgery was only proven to be effective after conditioning in laparoscopic surgery in an animal model. In any case, adhesion formation following open and laparoscopic surgery appears to be remarkably similar in an atmosphere of 10% N_2O in CO_2 without desiccation.

The implementation of these principles to open surgery should be carried out judiciously. That saline should be abandoned, and a richer solution should be used for irrigation is obvious. Prevention of desiccation can be achieved by continuous irrigation as done in microsurgery, by covering bowels with moistened inert towels and/or by flooding the operative field with humidified CO_2 [29, 30]. The latter indeed decreased adhesion formation in open cardiac surgery. The instillation of humidified CO_2 deep into the surgical field also decreased oxidative stress since the organs were no longer exposed to the 20% of O_2 in ambient air. A similar effect was achieved by shielding the organs in microsurgery. The exposure of the surgical field to the temperature of the operating theatre has never been an issue in open surgery. We can be happy today that cooling unexpectedly has a beneficial effect. The administration of dexamethasone after surgery, eventually at the end of surgery, may be beneficial to reduce inflammation and adhesion formation and accelerate recovery, while its use might aggravate an eventual infection. The proven very strong beneficial effect of 5 to 10% of N_2O with no explosion risk demands a trial in open surgery. As described for humidified CO_2 in cardiac surgery, [29, 30] the deep instillation of gases heavier than air will fill and flood progressively the operation field. CO_2 seems obvious as a carrier gas since it is heavier than air with minimal irritative effect at atmospheric pressure. N_2O, which fortunately also is heavier than air, should be used in concentrations of 5 to 10% of N_2O. For this reason, we used the same combination for these experiments, the efficacy of which had furthermore already been proven in animal models. It will obviously be necessary to prevent or reduce contamination of the operating theatre with N_2O. The suggested upper threshold for N_2O is 25 ppm [31]. We speculate that this can be achieved with aquarium-like drapings extending above the operating field with aspiration at the borders to prevent overflow; the opening of the draping would be a compromise between being sufficiently large to permit surgery but small enough to prevent mixture with the ambient air. Indeed even without aspiration contamination with 2 L/min with 10% of N_2O would result in only 15 ppm N_2O in a normal sized (e.g. 40 m^3) and ventilated (e.g. refresh rate of 20 cycles/h) operating room.

Conclusions

In conclusion, the mechanisms of mesothelial cell damage and their prevention are the same with open and with laparoscopic surgery. The application of microsurgical tenets, which enabled to decrease inflammation in the peritoneal cavity, reduce adhesion formation and improve fertility outcomes, can benefit further from flooding the operative field with 5 to 10% of N_2O, which has proven to be a most effective factor. Prevention of mesothelial cell damage and the subsequent acute inflammation may even be more important in open surgery than in laparoscopic surgery, especially when bowels are exteriorised and subjected to desiccation and exposed to ambient air that creates oxidative stress. Since both CO_2 and N_2O are heavier than air, it is also possible to instil humidified CO_2 with 5 to 10% of N_2O deep into the abdominal cavity during the procedure. Given the absence of side effects, as demonstrated in laparoscopic surgery, a study in open surgery may well demonstrate a virtually adhesion free surgery, a reduction of postoperative pain and a shortened recovery period, as has been observed in laparoscopic surgery.

Acknowledgements
We thank Anastasia Ussia (Rome, Italy), Karina Mailova (Moscow, Russia), Jasper Verguts (Hasselt, Belgium) and Michel Camus and Herman Tournaye (Brussels, Belgium) for the review and discussions. eSaturnus NV (Sony), Fisher and Paykel and Storz AG are acknowledged for supplying the equipment for these experiments. This research did not receive any specific grant from funding agencies in the public, commercial or not-for-profit sectors, except royalties from patents hold at the university.

Condensation
Peritoneal conditioning is equally important for open surgery as for laparoscopic surgery to prevent postoperative adhesions and pain.

Authors' contributions
RC and MMB carried out the experiments (study design, data collections) coordinated by PK. RC, MMB and PK have performed the data analysis and writing. LA made the basic observations on N_2O, and all were closely involved with the design and finalisation of the study. VG actively contributed to the understanding of these observations as an update of microsurgical tenets. All authors read and approved the final manuscript.

Competing interests
Roberta Corona, Maria Mercedes Binda, Leila Adamyan and Victor Gomel have nothing to declare. Philippe R Koninckx is a stockholder of EndoSAT NV.

Author details
[1]Department of Obstetrics and Gynaecology, KU Leuven – Catholic University of Leuven, 3000 Leuven, Belgium. [2]Barbados Fertility Centre, Seaston House, Hastings, Barbados. [3]Department of Reproductive Medicine and Surgery, Moscow State University of Medicine and Dentistry, Moscow, Russia. [4]Department of Obstetrics and Gynaecology, University of British Columbia, Women's Hospital, Vancouver, British Columbia, Canada. [5]KU Leuven, Vuilenbosstraat 2, 3360 Bierbeek, Belgium.

References
1. Mutsaers SE, Prele CM, Pengelly S, Herrick SE (2016) Mesothelial cells and peritoneal homeostasis. Fertil Steril 106:1018–1024
2. Koninckx PR, Gomel V, Ussia A, Adamyan L (2016) Role of the peritoneal cavity in the prevention of postoperative adhesions, pain, and fatigue. Fertil Steril 106:998–1010
3. Corona R, Verguts J, Schonman R, Binda MM, Mailova K, Koninckx PR (2011) Postoperative inflammation in the abdominal cavity increases adhesion formation in a laparoscopic mouse model. Fertil Steril 95:1224–1228
4. Matsuzaki S, Jardon K, Maleysson E, D'Arpiany F, Canis M, Bazin JE, Mage G (2010) Carbon dioxide pneumoperitoneum, intraperitoneal pressure, and peritoneal tissue hypoxia: a mouse study with controlled respiratory support. Surg Endosc. 2010;24:2871–80
5. Donnez J, Binda MM, Donnez O, Dolmans MM (2016) Oxidative stress in the pelvic cavity and its role in the pathogenesis of endometriosis. Fertil Steril 106:1011–1017
6. Shimomura M, Hinoi T, Ikeda S, Adachi T, Kawaguchi Y, Tokunaga M, Sasada T, Egi H, Tanabe K, Okajima M, Ohdan H (2013) Preservation of peritoneal fibrinolysis owing to decreased transcription of plasminogen activator inhibitor-1 in peritoneal mesothelial cells suppresses postoperative adhesion formation in laparoscopic surgery. Surgery 153:344–356
7. Matsuzaki S, Botchorishvili R, Jardon K, Maleysson E, Canis M, Mage G (2011) Impact of intraperitoneal pressure and duration of surgery on levels of tissue plasminogen activator and plasminogen activator inhibitor-1 mRNA in peritoneal tissues during laparoscopic surgery. Hum Reprod 26:1073–1081
8. Diamond MP (2016) Reduction of postoperative adhesion development. Fertil Steril 106:994–997
9. Koninckx PR, Corona R, Timmerman D, Verguts J, Adamyan L (2013) Peritoneal full-conditioning reduces postoperative adhesions and pain: a randomised controlled trial in deep endometriosis surgery. J Ovarian Res 6:90
10. Gomel V, Koninckx PR (2016) Microsurgical principles and postoperative adhesions: lessons from the past. Fertil Steril 106:1025–1031
11. Gomel V (2016) Reconstructive tubal microsurgery and assisted reproductive technology. Fertil Steril 105:887–890
12. Corona R, Verguts J, Koninckx R, Mailova K, Binda MM, Koninckx PR (2011) Intraperitoneal temperature and desiccation during endoscopic surgery. Intraoperative humidification and cooling of the peritoneal cavity can reduce adhesions. Am J Obstet Gynecol 205:392–397
13. Binda MM, Molinas CR, Hansen P, Koninckx PR (2006) Effect of desiccation and temperature during laparoscopy on adhesion formation in mice. Fertil Steril 86:166–175
14. Molinas CR, Tjwa M, Vanacker B, Binda MM, Elkelani O, Koninckx PR (2004) Role of CO_2 pneumoperitoneum-induced acidosis in CO_2 pneumoperitoneum-enhanced adhesion formation in mice. Fertil Steril 81:708–711
15. Pouly JL, Seak-San S (2000) Adhesions: laparoscopy versus laparotomy. Peritoneal surgery. Springer-Verlag, New York
16. Armitage P, Berry G (1987) Factorial designs. Statistical methods in medical research, 2nd edn, Oxford: Blackwell Scientific Publications; 227–39
17. Inc SI (1988). In: Inc SI (ed) Sas/stat users guide. Cary NC : SAS Institute Inc,
18. Corona R, Binda MM, Mailova K, Verguts J, Koninckx PR (2013) Addition of nitrous oxide to the carbon dioxide pneumoperitoneum strongly decreases adhesion formation and the dose-dependent adhesiogenic effect of blood in a laparoscopic mouse model. Fertil Steril 100:1777–1783
19. Ryan GB, Grobety J, Majno G (1971) Postoperative peritoneal adhesions. A study of the mechanisms. Am J Pathol 65:117–148
20. Ryan GB, Grobety J, Majno G (1973) Mesothelial injury and recovery. Am J Pathol 71:93–112
21. Cwalinski J, Breborowicz A, Polubinska A (2016) The impact of 0.9% NaCl on mesothelial cells after intraperitoneal lavage during surgical procedures. Adv Clin Exp Med 25:1193–1198
22. Cwalinski J, Staniszewski R, Baum E, Jasinski T, Mackowiak B, Breborowicz A (2015) Normal saline may promote formation of peritoneal adhesions. Int J Clin Exp Med 8:8828–8834
23. Polubinska A, Breborowicz A, Staniszewski R, Oreopoulos DG (2008) Normal saline induces oxidative stress in peritoneal mesothelial cells. J Pediatr Surg 43:1821–1826
24. Breborowicz A, Polubinska A, Breborowicz M, Simon M, Wanic-Kossowska M, Oreopoulos DG (2007) Peritoneal effects of intravenous iron sucrose administration in rats. Transl Res 149:304–309
25. Breborowicz A, Oreopoulos DG (2005) Is normal saline harmful to the peritoneum? Perit Dial Int 25(Suppl 4):S67–S70
26. Lin HF, Wu CY, Wu MC, Chou TH, Lin GS, Yen ZS, Chen SC (2014) Hypothermia decreases postoperative intra-abdominal adhesion formation. Am J Surg. 2014;208:419–24
27. Fang CC, Chou TH, Lin GS, Yen ZS, Lee CC, Chen SC (2010) Peritoneal infusion with cold saline decreased postoperative intra-abdominal adhesion formation. World J Surg 34:721–727
28. de Vries A, Marvik R, Kuhry E (2013) To perform operative procedures in an optimized local atmosphere: can it reduce post-operative adhesion formation? Int J Surg 11:1118–1122
29. Frey JM, Janson M, Svanfeldt M, Svenarud PK, van der Linden JA (2012) Local insufflation of warm humidified CO_2 increases open wound and core temperature during open colon surgery: a randomized clinical trial. Anesth Analg 115:1204–1211
30. van der Linden J, Persson M (2009) CO_2 field flooding may also reduce oxidative stress in open surgery. Anesth Analg 109:683–684

18

Fetoscopic endoluminal tracheal occlusion and reestablishment of fetal airways for congenital diaphragmatic hernia

Lennart Van der Veeken[1], Francesca Maria Russo[1], Luc De Catte[1], Eduard Gratacos[2,3], Alexandra Benachi[2,4,14], Yves Ville[2,5], Kypros Nicolaides[2,6], Christoph Berg[2,7,8], Glenn Gardener[2,9], Nicola Persico[2,10], Pietro Bagolan[2,11,14], Greg Ryan[2,12], Michael A. Belfort[2,13] and Jan Deprest[1,2,14*] (iD)

Abstract

Background: Congenital diaphragmatic hernia (CDH) is a congenital anomaly with high mortality and morbidity mainly due to pulmonary hypoplasia and hypertension. Temporary fetal tracheal occlusion to promote prenatal lung growth may improve survival. Entrapment of lung fluid stretches the airways, leading to lung growth.

Methods: Fetal endoluminal tracheal occlusion (FETO) is performed by percutaneous sono-endoscopic insertion of a balloon developed for interventional radiology. Reversal of the occlusion to induce lung maturation can be performed by fetoscopy, transabdominal puncture, tracheoscopy, or by postnatal removal if all else fails.

Results: FETO and balloon removal have been shown safe in experienced hands. This paper deals with the technical aspects of balloon insertion and removal. While FETO is invasive, it has minimal maternal risks yet can cause preterm birth potentially offsetting its beneficial effects.

Conclusion: For left-sided severe and moderate CDH, the procedure is considered investigational and is currently being evaluated in a global randomized clinical trial (https://www.totaltrial.eu/). The procedure can be clinically offered to fetuses with severe right-sided CDH.

Keywords: FETO, Fetal endoluminal tracheal occlusion, CDH, Congenital diaphragmatic hernia, Fetal surgery, Fetoscopy

Background

Congenital diaphragmatic hernia (CDH) is a life-threatening condition affecting up to 3 in 10,000 live born babies [1]. The diaphragmatic defect allows abdominal organs to herniate into the thorax which prevents normal lung development. Depending on the side and size of the defect, this may be the liver, bowel, spleen, and/or stomach. The majority of defects are left sided (LCDH 85%). Thirteen percent are right sided (RCDH), and bilateral defects or other forms occur very rarely.

Associated anomalies are frequent and should be ruled out by imaging and genetic testing as they independently influence survival and morbidity. In most registries currently, survival is approximately 70% depending on the case mix and location of treatment [2]. Surviving patients may suffer from not only medium and long-term morbidity predominantly respiratory in nature, but also gastro-esophageal reflux, failure to thrive, and less common orthopedic or other problems.

Individualized prognosis of isolated CDH can be made prenatally by using the lung size, the presence of the liver in the thorax, and the side of the defect [3]. Patients with predicted poor prognosis can be offered experimental fetal therapy. To improve survival, the intervention should reverse pulmonary hypoplasia (i.e., stimulate lung growth) before birth. Historically, this

* Correspondence: jan.deprest@uzleuven.be
[1]Academic Department of Development and Regeneration, Woman and Child, Biomedical Sciences, and Clinical Department of Obstetrics and Gynaecology, KU Leuven, Herestraat 49, 3000, Leuven, Belgium
[2]TOTAL (Tracheal Occlusion To Accelerate Lung Growth Trial) Consortium, Leuven, Belgium
Full list of author information is available at the end of the article

was attempted by anatomical repair of the defect in utero. The results of this approach were suboptimal [4]. Also, the anatomic defect itself can be relatively easily managed after birth hence it is not the problem. An alternative strategy, based on the clinical observation that fetuses with laryngeal atresia have larger lungs, led to animal experiments that demonstrated that fetal tracheal occlusion reverses experimental pulmonary hypoplasia [5]. Tracheal occlusion leads to accumulation of lung fluid which in turn causes lung stretch. This activates a pathway that leads to proliferation and increased growth of the airways and pulmonary vessels, nicely summarized in the acronym PLUG: "Plug the Lung Until it Grows" (PLUG) [6]. However, when the occlusion is maintained until birth, the number of type II pneumocytes is abnormally low, leading to a relative surfactant deficiency [7]. By reversing the tracheal occlusion before birth, the balance between type I and type II pneumocytes at birth is more optimal. This is captured in the concept "plug-unplug sequence," and reversal of occlusion is an important component in the fetal treatment strategy [7]. Nowadays, tracheal occlusion is uniquely performed by minimally invasive fetal endoluminal tracheal occlusion (FETO) and performed under sono-endoscopic guidance. This is a percutaneous procedure in which a latex balloon is endoscopically positioned

above the carina and inflated to occlude the trachea [8] (Fig. 1). The present paper describes the instrumentation and the technical aspects of the FETO procedure as currently performed by the above clinical research consortium within their clinical trial.

Methods
Selection of fetuses
CDH is typically diagnosed during mid-gestation on screening ultrasound. Following the diagnosis (or suspicion thereof), patients are best referred to a tertiary center where this condition is routinely managed after birth. Patients will be reassessed with targeted ultrasound and magnetic resonance imaging (MRI) and will be offered genetic testing (today this is by micro-array analysis) [9]. This has two purposes, (1) to rule out associated structural or genetic anomalies, which themselves may worsen the prognosis dramatically and (2) to assess the severity of the pulmonary hypoplasia. This information is used to make a personalized prognosis and lead multidisciplinary counseling. Additional evaluation frequently reveals some elements of discordance with the initial assessment at the referring site and may well result in a changed perspective and different parental decisions [10]. Therefore, it is considered prudent to limit prognostic advice at first diagnosis.

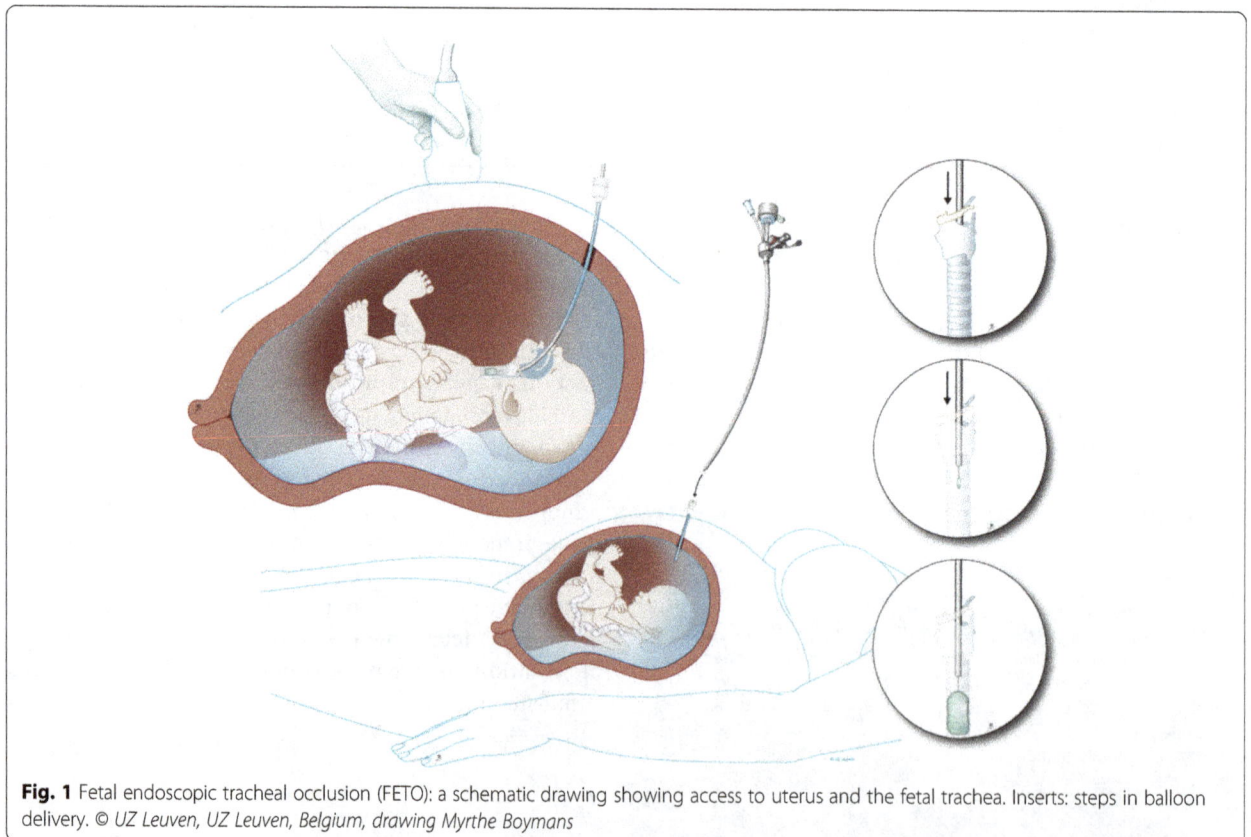

Fig. 1 Fetal endoscopic tracheal occlusion (FETO): a schematic drawing showing access to uterus and the fetal trachea. Inserts: steps in balloon delivery. © UZ Leuven, UZ Leuven, Belgium, drawing Myrthe Boymans

In isolated cases, personalized prediction of outcome is based on measurements of lung size, liver position, and the side of the defect [11]. Although other characteristics are being investigated among which stomach position, pulmonary circulatory parameters, and cardiac ventricular size as additional prognostic indicators, the lung-to-head-ratio (LHR) remains the best studied parameter for prediction. The lung contralateral to the lesion is measured in the standard plane for a four-chamber view of the heart, and the head circumference is measured in a standard biparietal view (Fig. 2a, b) [12]. The most accurate way of measuring the lung is by tracing its outline [13]. The LHR measured in the index case (observed) is expressed as a percentage (o/e LHR; %) of what one would expect in a normal fetus at a similar gestational age (expected). MRI is now almost ubiquitously used in tertiary centers for evaluation of congenital anomalies. In CDH cases, MRI allows for volumetric measurement of both lungs, the ability to quantitate the degree of liver herniation, and a detailed assessment of stomach position. So far, fetal MRI lung volumetry in CDH does not provide improved outcome prediction over ultrasound; hence, we do not use it for

decisions regarding FETO. The predictive value of imaging methods in terms of pulmonary hypertension or extra-corporeal membrane oxygenation needs is currently under review [14].

Fetuses from singleton pregnancies with a predicted poor postnatal outcome are the target group for fetal intervention. The o/e LHR, presence of the liver in the thorax, and the side of the defect are used so stratify these fetuses [15] (Fig. 2c, d). Babies born beyond 30 weeks with a left-sided CDH, a herniated liver, and an o/e LHR < 25% who are managed with standard postnatal therapy have a survival rate that is < 20% [11]. These parameters were therefore used to define that group of fetuses with severe pulmonary hypoplasia, and they formed the initial study population for prenatal therapy. Despite encouraging early experience with FETO [16], fetal surgery for isolated CDH is still considered experimental. Patients with a fetus who has an isolated LCDH and *severe* lung hypoplasia are currently being offered participation in a global randomized clinical trial (https://www.totaltrial.eu/) comparing outcomes of FETO to expectant management during pregnancy, followed by standardized postnatal therapy

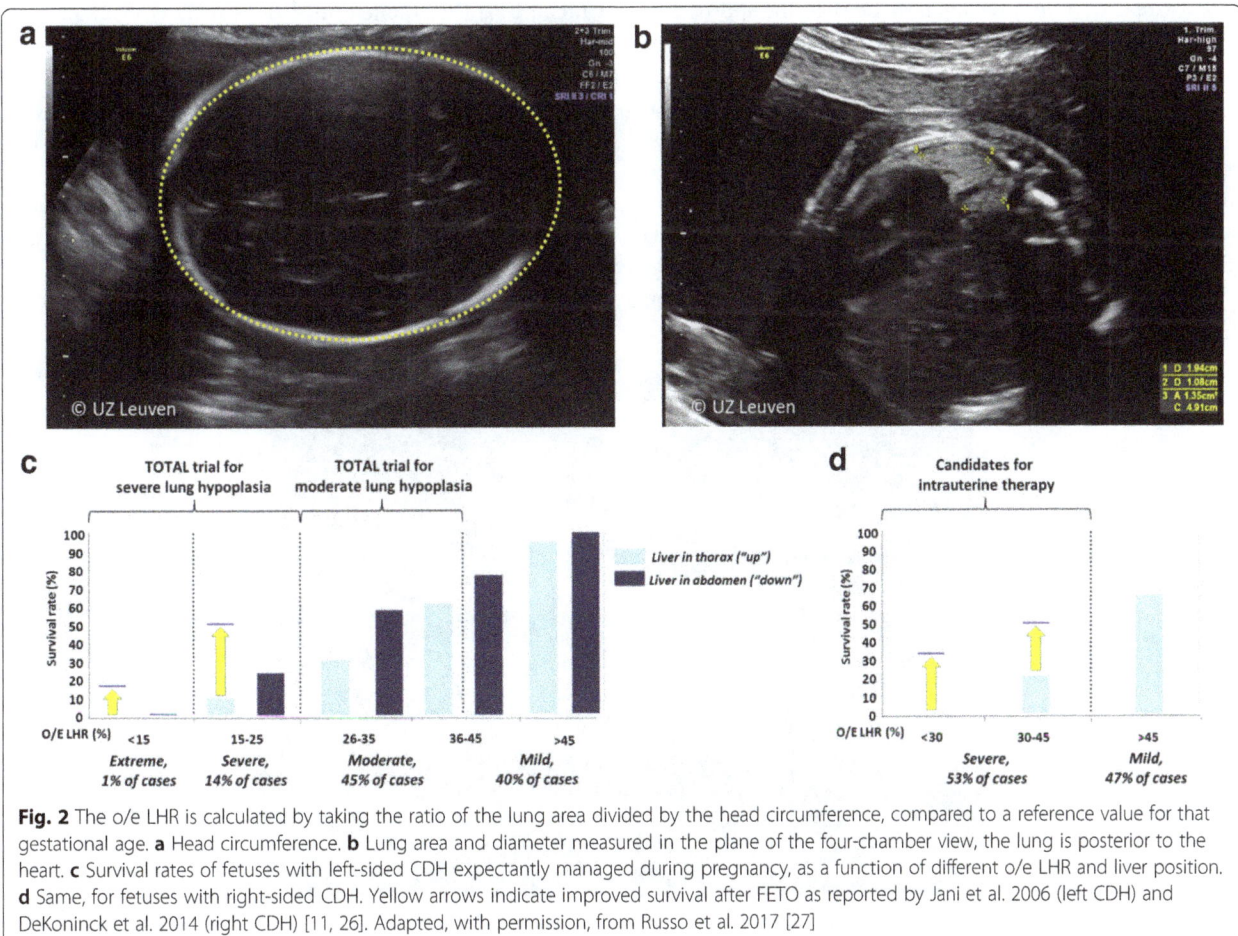

Fig. 2 The o/e LHR is calculated by taking the ratio of the lung area divided by the head circumference, compared to a reference value for that gestational age. a Head circumference. b Lung area and diameter measured in the plane of the four-chamber view, the lung is posterior to the heart. c Survival rates of fetuses with left-sided CDH expectantly managed during pregnancy, as a function of different o/e LHR and liver position. d Same, for fetuses with right-sided CDH. Yellow arrows indicate improved survival after FETO as reported by Jani et al. 2006 (left CDH) and DeKoninck et al. 2014 (right CDH) [11, 26]. Adapted, with permission, from Russo et al. 2017 [27]

[17]. In a second experimental arm to this trial, patients with a CDH fetus with *moderate* pulmonary hypoplasia (which has a 50% or greater survival rate) are randomized to FETO or expectant management, in an effort to reduce oxygen dependency at 6 months of age. For RCDH, fetal therapy is offered in case of severe hypoplasia (o/e LHR < 45%) because they have a predicted survival rate of 17%. For patients who have a more complex presentation with additional findings, a more individualized approach can be taken, yet in the absence of proof of benefit, this is debatable[18, 19].

FETO or PLUG procedure

FETO was initially performed at 24–28 weeks only in cases of severe CDH and under epidural anesthesia. Today, the procedure is typically performed under local anesthesia at 27–29 weeks with conscious sedation optional, yet locoregional can be done when clinically required. In moderate cases, FETO is done at 30–32 weeks. We use prophylactic tocolysis (atosiban or alternatively indomethacin or nifedipine) and antibiotics (cefazolin 2 g i.v. 8 hourly) until 24 h after the procedure. The patient is positioned in a dorsal supine position (with lateral tilt to prevent caval compression) such that there is direct access to the fetal mouth. External fetal manipulation may be required. Once in the appropriate position, we administer pancuronium (0.2 mg/kg) or equivalent, atropine (20 μg/kg), and fentanyl (15 μg/kg) intra-muscularly through a 22 G needle to the fetus to provide analgesia, immobilization, and prophylaxis against bradycardia. After sterile draping, the insertion trajectory is infiltrated with local anesthesia (lidocaine 1% 10–20 mL). A skin-incision is made and a disposable flexible 10 Fr cannula (3.3 mm; RCF 10.0 Check-Flo Performer, Cook, Bloomington, IN) loaded with a pyramidal trocar (11650TG, Karl

Storz, Tutlingen, Germany) is inserted into the amniotic cavity under ultrasound guidance, in an area devoid of placenta and as perpendicular as possible to the nose tip (Additional file 1: Video S1; Fig. 3). Some introduce the cannula using the Seldinger technique [20].

The fetoscope is a 1.3-mm fiber optic endoscope (11540AA, Karl Storz) housed within a curved 3.3-mm sheath (11540KE; Karl Storz) with a delivery catheter (Baltacci-BDPE-100 0.9 mm; Balt, Montmorency, France) that is loaded with a detachable inflatable latex balloon with integrated one-way valve (Goldbal2). These are used "off-label" as they were originally designed for endovascular occlusion. The inflated balloon accommodates for an increasing tracheal diameter during pregnancy. A stylet (11506P; Karl Storz) and grasping forceps (11510C, Karl Storz) are available to puncture and remove the balloon should it be incorrectly positioned (Fig. 4). We flush warmed crystalloid (Hartmann's solution or Ringer's Lactate) through the fetoscope sheath in order to distend the larynx, clear the debris, and improve vision.

Landmarks for balloon insertion are progressively the tip of the nose, philtrum, tongue, the raphe of the palate, uvula, epiglottis, and ultimately the vocal cords (Additional file 2: Video S2; Fig. 5). The fetoscope is advanced into the trachea until the carina is visualized, or if that is not possible, at least to a point where the tracheal rings and pars membranacea can be positively identified. The balloon is then advanced out of the fetoscope, positioned between the cords and the carina, and inflated with 0.6 mL of isotonic saline. Once inflated, the balloon is detached (Additional file 3: Video S3; Fig. 6a). Finally, excessive amniotic or irrigation fluid is drained until a normal volume is achieved. In our initial experience, the median duration of FETO

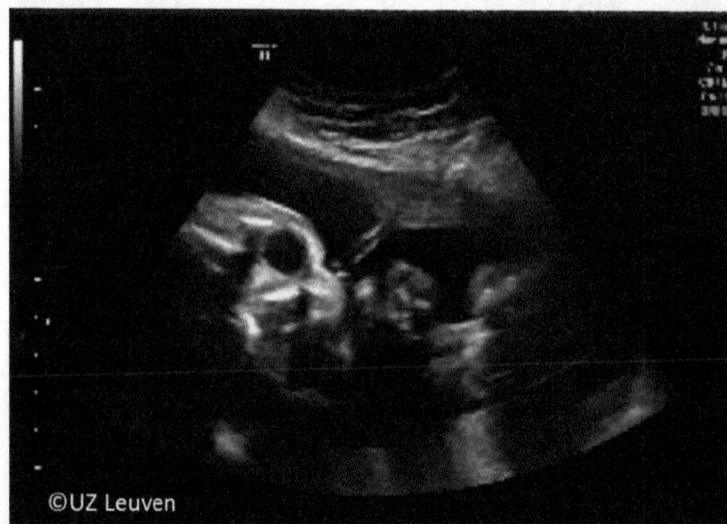

Fig. 3 Transabdominal trocar entry in the direction of the tip of the nose. © *UZ Leuven, UZ Leuven, Belgium*

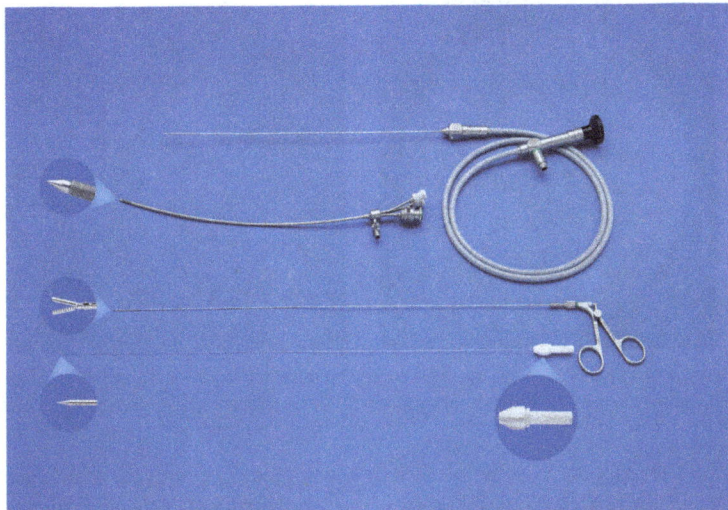

Fig. 4 Fetoscope, fetoscopic forceps, and stylet, courtesy of *KARL STORZ Endoskope, Tuttlingen, Germany*

was 10 min (range 3–93 min). Operating time depends mainly on operator experience and on the position of the fetus and is directly related to the risk of chorionic membrane separation and amniorrhexis.

Follow-up

Patients are followed with ultrasound every 1 to 2 weeks until the preset time for reversal of the occlusion. The fetus is evaluated for growth, movement, general wellbeing and routine antenatal care, and the cervical length is measured to estimate the risk for preterm birth. Amniotic fluid volume is measured to exclude polyhydramnios as this is common in CDH and can increase the risk of amniorrhexis and/or preterm labor. Amniodrainage is performed when the deepest vertical pool exceeds 12 cm. The membranes are inspected for amnion-chorion membrane separation. At each visit, the balloon is visualized since spontaneous deflation has been described [21]. The tracheal balloon appears on ultrasound as a hypoechoic fluid-filled structure without color Doppler flow and positioned just beneath the vocal cords between the common carotid arteries (Fig. 6b). Within a week following FETO, the fetal lung in responders becomes hyperechogenic. The parenchymal dimensional changes are quantified via the o/e LHR or MRI. Volume changes precede the vascular response. In case of amniorrhexis or preterm labor, the patients are admitted and management is individually planned for timely and safe balloon removal. Chorioamnionitis is the most common complication of membrane rupture and may mandate balloon removal and delivery. Antepartum hemorrhage has been described yet is in our experience uncommon [21].

UNPLUG or balloon removal

Our policy is to remove the balloon in utero even if delivery is imminent. It triggers lung maturation, increases survival chances, reduces morbidity [22, 23], and permits

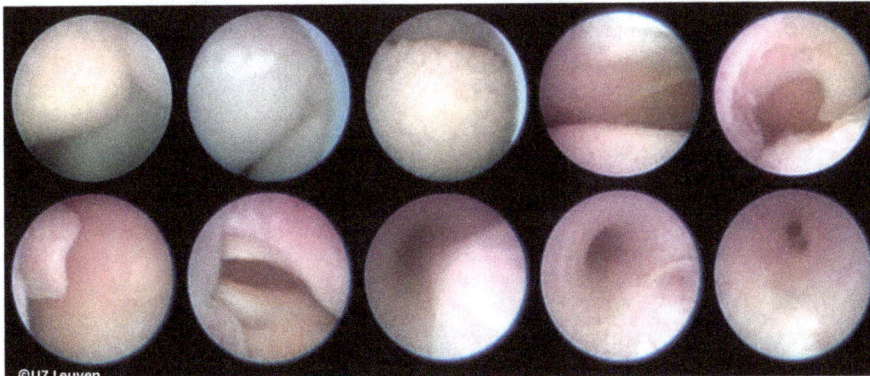

Fig. 5 Landmarks used for guidance from the tip of the nose to trachea. Up from left to right: tip of nose, upper lip, tongue, raphe palate, and uvula. Down from left to right: epiglottis, vocal cords, trachea with inwards bulging pars membranacea, trachea more expanded and also better visualization of the tracheal rings, and carina. © *UZ Leuven, UZ Leuven, Belgium*

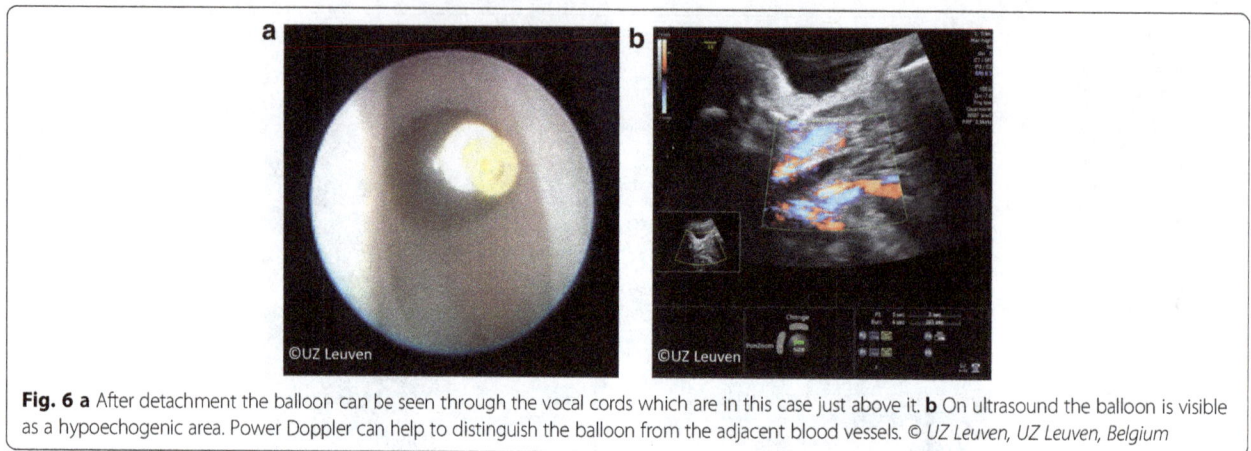

Fig. 6 a After detachment the balloon can be seen through the vocal cords which are in this case just above it. **b** On ultrasound the balloon is visible as a hypoechogenic area. Power Doppler can help to distinguish the balloon from the adjacent blood vessels. © *UZ Leuven, UZ Leuven, Belgium*

vaginal delivery. Removal of the balloon is scheduled at 34 weeks gestational age based on observations in sheep. In 28% of cases, balloon removal will be indicated earlier because of impending delivery [23]. Steroids are given to enhance lung maturation. The removal takes place in essentially the same preparation as described above for balloon placement, with the same fetal and maternal medications. The balloon can be punctured directly using a 20-22G needle under ultrasound guidance and in our experience is expulsed spontaneously. (Additional file 4: Video S4). In such cases, tracheal patency can be confirmed by demonstration of tracheal fluid movement with Doppler (Additional file 5: Video S5), change in tracheal diameter, or by MRI. The balloon can also be fetoscopically removed, which provides direct visualization of unobstructed airways (Additional file 6: Video S6). In the event that fetoscopic in utero removal is not possible, we resort to tracheoscopic removal (Table 1 for instruments) with the baby on placental circulation under loco-regional anesthesia (Fig. 7 and Additional file 7: Video S7). The fetal head and shoulders are delivered and direct laryngo-tracheoscopy is performed. In the worst (and not desirable) scenario, postnatal puncture from above the manubrium sterni is used, with or without ultrasound guidance, or by tracheoscopy. In a report on 302 cases, 67% of balloon removals were by fetoscopy, 21% by puncture, and 10% by tracheoscopy on placental circulation, and 1% ex utero [23]. In that study, the technique used

Table 1 Overview of the fetoscopic instruments used for FETO and UNPLUG

Fetal tracheoscopy	Description	ID
1.3 mm endoscope	Miniature telescope, with remote eyepiece 0° straight forward, 30.6 cm working length	11540AA
3.3 mm sheath	Blunt curved sheath, with sand-blasted echogenic tip with stop cock for irrigation and two side openings	11540KE
1.0 mm forceps	Retrieval forceps, double action jaws, 35 cm long	11510C
0.4 mm stylet	Single use puncture stylet with adjustable torque, 50 cm long	11506P
0.9 mm needle	Puncture needle to protect the catheter or for aspiration, length 35 cm, can house the stylet	11540KD
3.3 mm trocar	10 Fr pyramidal tipped trocar for use with flexible cannula RCF-10.0 (Cook, Check Flo Performer)	11650TG
0.6 mL balloon	Goldbal 2 detachable latex balloon with radio-opaque inclusion, outer diameter 1.5 mm (inflated: 7.0 mm); length 5.0 mm (inflated 20.0 mm)	Goldbal 2 (Balt)
0.9 mm microcatheter	catheter loaded with mandrel, and Touhy Boost Y-connection, max outer diameter 0.9 mm, tapered to 0.4 mm, 100 cm in length	"Baltacci" e BDPE 100 (Balt)
Direct bronchoscopy 1.3 mm endoscope	Miniature telescope, with remote eyepiece 0° straight forward, 18.8 cm working length	10040AA
Straight bronchoscopic sheath	4.2 mm outer, 3.5 mm inner diameter 18.5 cm length (size 2.5), is conventional neonatal "Doesel-Huzly" bronchoscope, with blanking and suction plug	10339F 10924SP 10315RV
Telescope bridge	Houses telescope and has side opening for irrigation 1.5 mm outer diameter	10338LCl
1.0 mm forceps	19 cm semi-flexible forceps for balloon retrieval	10338H
0.4 mm stylet	Single use puncture stylet with adjustable torque, 50 cm long	11506P

Endoscopic instruments were developed by Karl Storz Endoskope, supported by the European Commission in the 6th framework program. The balloon system is an adapted version of a commercially available vascular occlusion device. Most instruments and devices are used off label

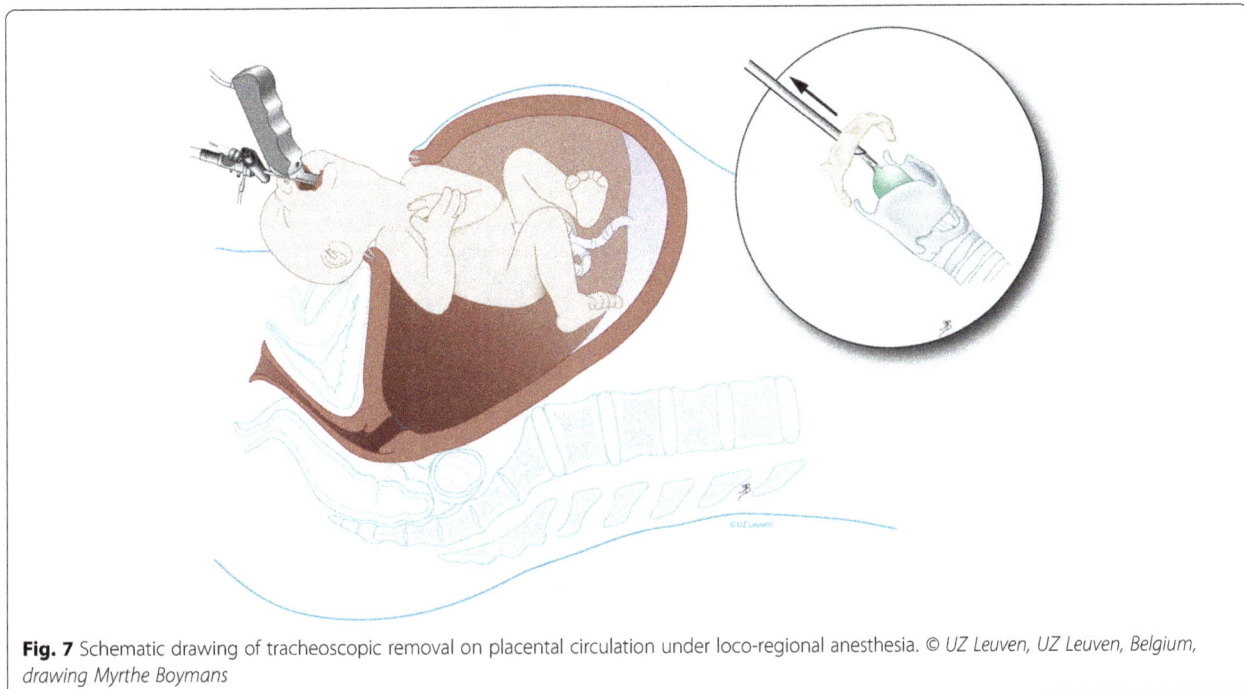

Fig. 7 Schematic drawing of tracheoscopic removal on placental circulation under loco-regional anesthesia. © UZ Leuven, UZ Leuven, Belgium, drawing Myrthe Boymans

appeared to be dictated mainly by operator preference. There was no difference in gestational age at delivery whether the balloon was punctured or removed by fetoscopy. The importance of immediate availability of trained and experienced operators who can remove a FETO balloon rapidly and safely cannot, and must not, be underestimated. To our knowledge, the only neonatal deaths directly due to balloon removal difficulties that have occurred happened when delivery took place in an unprepared and/or inexperienced environment [23].

Reported adverse events and side effects with FETO are rare. Fetal tracheomegaly is a recognized entity that usually presents as a barking cough on effort and then resolves over time with minimal long-term implications. There are a few neonates who have had significant long-term tracheal issues, and these appear to have been related to traumatic balloon removal or early insertion < 26 weeks [24]. This is however an aspect that requires more detailed and long-term follow-up. The main maternal-fetal complication is that of chorionic membrane separation and PPROM with resultant preterm birth. Although the median gestational age at birth is 35 weeks, up to one in three patients deliver prior to 34 weeks, potentially offsetting the effect of the fetal intervention.

Results

To date, the published data are predominantly based on observational trials and small case series [8]. There is one randomized controlled trial [25, 26] that showed benefit of FETO; however, in that study all deliveries were by EXIT procedure, there was a case mix of right and left CDH, and

the methodology was substantially different to what is currently being practiced in Europe and the USA.

Compared to historical controls of similar severity, FETO increases survival rate from 24 to 49% in LCDH with o/eLHR < 25% and from 17 to 42% in RCDH with o/eLHR < 45% [21, 26] (Fig. 2c, d). FETO also seems to reduce early neonatal respiratory morbidity.

Discussion

This potential benefit is now being investigated in two parallel randomized clinical trials (RCT) "Tracheal Occlusion To Accelerate Lung growth" (https://www.totaltrial.eu/), in fetuses with LCDH and either severe or moderate lung hypoplasia (NCT01240057 and NCT00763737). Current fetal treatment centers are in Leuven, Belgium; Paris, France; London, UK; Barcelona, Spain; Milan and Rome, Italy; Bonn, Germany; Toronto, Canada; Brisbane, Australia; and Houston, Texas, USA. These centers have a high volume fetoscopy program, completed a minimum learning curve of 15 FETO procedures, and committed to strict adherence to a prenatal and postnatal management protocol. The trial has recruited at the time of writing over 165 (moderate) and over 50 (severe) patients. Results are expected within the next 2 years at the current recruitment rate (moderate). We anticipate that more centers in the USA and in Japan will be joining the task force which may accelerate recruitment.

Conclusions

FETO may alter the natural history of congenital diaphragmatic hernia, and early clinical results look promising. It is hoped that the ongoing TOTAL trial will result in proof of benefit. FETO is an invasive technique associated with a significantly increased risk for preterm birth which potentially tempers its benefits. The procedure requires specific skills and instrumentation and permanent services and is at present limited to a select group of centers. If proven effective, this procedure is likely to be implemented more widely and appropriate dissemination will require an extensive training program and careful oversight in order to ensure safe implementation.

Additional files

Additional file 1: Video S1. The trocar is inserted into the amniotic cavity under ultrasound guidance, in an area devoid of placenta and as perpendicular as possible to the nose tip.

Additional file 2: Video S2. The subsequent landmarks are seen as the fetoscope is advanced to the fetal trachea. Chronologically: lower lip, tongue, uvula, soft palate, epiglottis, vocal cords, and tracheal pars membranacea.

Additional file 3: Video S3. The balloon is inflated with 0.6 mL of isotonic saline solution and fills the trachea just distal to the cords, following which it is detached.

Additional file 4: Video S4. The balloon is punctured under ultrasound guidance using a 20–22 G needle. The needle is inserted as close as possible to the anterior shoulder, which enables to pass the umbilical cord which is lying on the neck. As the balloon is punctured, the trachea can be seen collapsing.

Additional file 5: Video S5. After puncturing, the balloon tracheal patency can be confirmed by demonstration free tracheal fluid movement with Doppler.

Additional file 6: Video S6. Fetoscopic unplugging provides direct documentation of free airways. As the lung fluid egresses, the pressure drops and the trachea will slightly collapse.

Additional file 7: Video S7. If not possible to puncture the balloon ultrasound guided or fetoscopic guided, we can resort to tracheoscopic removal on placental circulation under loco-regional anesthesia.

Abbreviations

CDH : Congenital diaphragmatic hernia; EXIT: Ex utero intrapartum treatment; FETO : Fetal endoluminal tracheal occlusion; LCDH: Left-sided congenital diaphragmatic hernia; LHR: Lung-to-head-ratio; MRI : Magnetic resonance imaging; o/e LHR: Observed to expected lung-to-head-ratio; PLUG: Plug the Lung Until it Grows; PPROM: Preterm and Prelabor Rupture Of Membranes; RCDH: Right-sided congenital diaphragmatic hernia; RCT : Randomized clinical trial; TOTAL: Tracheal Occlusion To Accelerate Lung growth

Funding

JD is partly funded by the Great Ormond Street Hospital Charity Fund. LVDV is supported by the Erasmus+ Programme of the European Commission (2013-0040). FMR is supported by the KU Leuven (C32/17/054). Our research is in part supported by an Innovative Engineering for Health award by the Wellcome Trust (WT101957), the Engineering and Physical Sciences Research Council (NS/A000027/1), and the Fetal Health Foundation (USA).

Authors' contributions

LVDV, FMR, and JDP wrote the initial manuscript. EG, AB, YV, KN, CB, GG, NP, PB, GR, MAB, JDP are members of the FETO task force and were involved in development of the technique, collection of data, and editing of the manuscript. LDC and JDP acquired the images and clips. All authors read and approved the final version of the manuscript.

Authors' information

LVDV, FMR, LDC, and JD are in the Academic Department of Development and Regeneration, Woman and Child, Biomedical Sciences, and Clinical Department of Obstetrics and Gynaecology, KU Leuven, Leuven, Belgium. EG, AB, YV, KN, CB, GG, NP, PB, GR, MAB, and JD are members of the TOTAL (Tracheal Occlusion To Accelerate Lung Growth Trial) Consortium. EG is head of the Barcelona Center for Maternale Fetal and Neonatal Medicine (Hospital Clínic and Hospital Sant Joan de Déu), IDIBAPS, University of Barcelona, and Centre for Biomedical Research on Rare Diseases (CIBER-ER), Barcelona, Spain. AB is head of the Department of Obstetrics, Gynaecology and Reproductive Medicine, Hôpital Antoine-Béclère, University Paris Sud, Clamart, France. YV is head of the Fetal Medicine Unit, Obstetrics and Fetal Medicine Department, Necker-Enfants Malades Hospital, Université Paris Descartes, Sorbonne Paris Cité, Paris, France. KN is head of the Fetal Medicine Center, Harris Birthright Centre, King's College Hospital, London, UK. CB is head of the Division of Fetal Surgery, Department of Obstetrics and Prenatal Medicine, University of Bonn, and Department of Obstetrics and Gynecology, University of Cologne, Germany. GG is head of the Mater Health Services, Mater Research UQ, Brisbane, Australia. NP is in the Department of Obstetrics and Gynecology "L. Mangiagalli," Fondazione IRCCS "Ca' Granda" - Ospedale Maggiore Policlinico, Milan, Italy. PB is head of Neonatal Surgery Unit, Department of Medical and Surgical Neonatology, Bambino Gesù Children's Hospital, IRCCS, Piazza S. Onofrio, 4, 00165 Rome, Italy. GR is head of the Fetal Medicine Unit, Mt. Sinai Hospital, and University of Toronto, Toronto, Canada. MAB is head of the Department of Obstetrics and Gynecology, Baylor College of Medicine and Texas Children's Fetal Center, Houston, Texas, USA. AB, PB, and JD are members of the European Reference Network on Rare and Inherited Congenital Anomalies "ERNICA."

Competing interests

The authors declare that they have no competing interests.

Author details

[1]Academic Department of Development and Regeneration, Woman and Child, Biomedical Sciences, and Clinical Department of Obstetrics and Gynaecology, KU Leuven, Herestraat 49, 3000, Leuven, Belgium. [2]TOTAL (Tracheal Occlusion To Accelerate Lung Growth Trial) Consortium, Leuven, Belgium. [3]BCNatal – Barcelona Center for MaternaleFetal and Neonatal Medicine (Hospital Clínic and Hospital Sant Joan de Déu), IDIBAPS, University of Barcelona, and Centre for Biomedical Research on Rare Diseases (CIBER-ER), Barcelona, Spain. [4]Department of Obstetrics, Gynaecology and Reproductive Medicine, Hôpital Antoine-Béclère, University Paris Sud, Clamart, France. [5]Fetal Medicine Unit, Obstetrics and Fetal Medicine Department, Necker-Enfants Malades Hospital, Université Paris Descartes, Sorbonne Paris Cité, Paris, France. [6]Harris Birthright Centre, King's College Hospital, London, UK. [7]Division of Fetal Surgery, Department of Obstetrics and Prenatal Medicine, University of Bonn, Bonn, Germany. [8]Department of Obstetrics and Gynecology, University of Cologne, Cologne, Germany. [9]Mater Health Services, Mater Research UQ, Brisbane, Australia. [10]Department of Obstetrics and Gynecology, "L. Mangiagalli," Fondazione IRCCS "Ca' Granda" - Ospedale Maggiore Policlinico, Milan, Italy. [11]Neonatal Surgery Unit, Department of Medical and Surgical Neonatology, Bambino Gesù Children's Hospital, IRCCS, Piazza S. Onofrio, 4, 00165 Rome, Italy. [12]Fetal

Medicine Unit, Mt Sinai Hospital, University of Toronto, Toronto, Canada. [13]Department of Obstetrics and Gynecology, Baylor College of Medicine and Texas Children's Fetal Center, Houston, Texas, USA. [14]European Reference Network on Rare and Inherited Congenital Anomalies "ERNICA", Rotterdam, The Netherlands.

References

1. EUROCAT. EUROCAT statistical monitoring report – 2012
2. Harting MT, Lally KP (2014) The congenital diaphragmatic hernia study group registry update. Semin Fetal Neonatal Med 19:370–375
3. Claus F, Sandaite I, Dekoninck P, Moreno O, Cruz Martinez R, Van Mieghem T, Gucciardo L, Richter J, Michielsen K, Decraene J, Devlieger R, Gratacos E, Deprest JA (2011) Prenatal anatomical imaging in fetuses with congenital diaphragmatic hernia. Fetal Diagn Ther 29:88–100
4. Harrison MR, Langer JC, Adzick NS, Golbus MS, Filly RA, Anderson RL, Rosen MA, Callen PW, Goldstein RB, de Lorimier AA (1990) Correction of congenital diaphragmatic hernia in utero, V. Initial clinical experience. J Pediatr Surg 25: 47–55 discussion 56-7
5. Wilson JM, DiFiore JW, Peters CA (1993) Experimental fetal tracheal ligation prevents the pulmonary hypoplasia associated with fetal nephrectomy: possible application for congenital diaphragmatic hernia. J Pediatr Surg 28: 1433–1439 discussion 1439-40
6. Hedrick MH, Estes JM, Sullivan KM, Bealer JF, Kitterman JA, Flake AW, Adzick NS, Harrison MR (1994) Plug the lung until it grows (PLUG): a new method to treat congenital diaphragmatic hernia in utero. J Pediatr Surg 29:612–617
7. Flageole H, Evrard VA, Piedboeuf B, Laberge JM, Lerut TE, Deprest JA (1998) The plug-unplug sequence: an important step to achieve type II pneumocyte maturation in the fetal lamb model. J Pediatr Surg 33:299–303
8. Deprest J, Gratacos E, Nicolaides KH, Group FT (2004) Fetoscopic tracheal occlusion (FETO) for severe congenital diaphragmatic hernia: evolution of a technique and preliminary results. Ultrasound Obstet Gynecol 24:121–126
9. Brady PD, Delle Chiaie B, Christenhusz G, Dierickx K, Van Den Bogaert K, Menten B, Janssens S, Defoort P, Roets E, Sleurs E, Keymolen K, De Catte L, Deprest J, de Ravel T, Van Esch H, Fryns JP, Devriendt K, Vermeesch JR (2014) A prospective study of the clinical utility of prenatal chromosomal microarray analysis in fetuses with ultrasound abnormalities and an exploration of a framework for reporting unclassified variants and risk factors. Genet Med 16:469–476
10. Done E, Gucciardo L, Van Mieghem T, Devriendt K, Allegaert K, Brady P, Devlieger R, De Catte L, Lewi L, Deprest J (2017) Clinically relevant discordances identified after tertiary reassessment of fetuses with isolated congenital diaphragmatic hernia. Prenat Diagn 37:883–888
11. Jani J, Nicolaides KH, Keller RL, Benachi A, Peralta CF, Favre R, Moreno O, Tibboel D, Lipitz S, Eggink A, Vaast P, Allegaert K, Harrison M, Deprest J, Antenatal CDHRG (2007) Observed to expected lung area to head circumference ratio in the prediction of survival in fetuses with isolated diaphragmatic hernia. Ultrasound Obstet Gynecol 30:67–71
12. Deprest JA, Flemmer AW, Gratacos E, Nicolaides K (2009) Antenatal prediction of lung volume and in-utero treatment by fetal endoscopic tracheal occlusion in severe isolated congenital diaphragmatic hernia. Semin Fetal Neonatal Med 14:8–13
13. Jani J, Peralta CF, Benachi A, Deprest J, Nicolaides KH (2007) Assessment of lung area in fetuses with congenital diaphragmatic hernia. Ultrasound Obstet Gynecol 30:72–76
14. Russo FM, Eastwood MP, Keijzer R, Al-Maary J, Toelen J, Mieghem TV, Deprest JA (2016) Lung size and liver herniation predict the need for extra corporeal membrane oxygenation but not pulmonary hypertension in isolated congenital diaphragmatic hernia: a systematic review and meta-analysis. Ultrasound Obstet Gynecol, 2017. 49(6):704–13.
15. Metkus AP, Filly RA, Stringer MD, Harrison MR, Adzick NS (1996) Sonographic predictors of survival in fetal diaphragmatic hernia. J Pediatr Surg 31:148–151 discussion 151-2
16. Al-Maary J, Eastwood MP, Russo FM, Deprest JA, Keijzer R (2016) Fetal tracheal occlusion for severe pulmonary hypoplasia in isolated congenital diaphragmatic hernia: a systematic review and meta-analysis of survival. Ann Surg 264:929–933
17. Deprest J, Brady P, Nicolaides K, Benachi A, Berg C, Vermeesch J, Gardener G, Gratacos E (2014) Prenatal management of the fetus with isolated congenital diaphragmatic hernia in the era of the TOTAL trial. Semin Fetal Neonatal Med 19:338–348
18. Seravalli V, Jelin EB, Miller JL, Tekes A, Vricella L, Baschat AA (2017) Fetoscopic tracheal occlusion for treatment of non-isolated congenital diaphragmatic hernia. Prenat Diagn 37:1046–1049
19. Van Mieghem T, Cruz-Martinez R, Allegaert K, Dekoninck P, Castanon M, Sandaite I, Claus F, Devlieger R, Gratacos E, Deprest J (2012) Outcome of fetuses with congenital diaphragmatic hernia and associated intrafetal fluid effusions managed in the era of fetal surgery. Ultrasound Obstet Gynecol 39:50–55
20. Deprest JA, Van Schoubroeck D, Van Ballaer PP, Flageole H, Van Assche FA, Vandenberghe K (1998) Alternative technique for Nd: YAG laser coagulation in twin-to-twin transfusion syndrome with anterior placenta. Ultrasound Obstet Gynecol 11:347–352
21. Jani JC, Nicolaides KH, Gratacos E, Valencia CM, Done E, Martinez JM, Gucciardo L, Cruz R, Deprest JA (2009) Severe diaphragmatic hernia treated by fetal endoscopic tracheal occlusion. Ultrasound Obstet Gynecol 34:304–310
22. Done E, Gratacos E, Nicolaides KH, Allegaert K, Valencia C, Castanon M, Martinez JM, Jani J, Van Mieghem T, Greenough A, Gomez O, Lewi P, Deprest J (2013) Predictors of neonatal morbidity in fetuses with severe isolated congenital diaphragmatic hernia undergoing fetoscopic tracheal occlusion. Ultrasound Obstet Gynecol 42:77–83
23. Jimenez JA, Eixarch E, DeKoninck P, Bennini JR, Devlieger R, Peralta CF, Gratacos E, Deprest J (2017) Balloon removal after fetoscopic endoluminal tracheal occlusion for congenital diaphragmatic hernia. Am J Obstet Gynecol 217:78 e1-78 e11
24. Deprest J, Breysem L, Gratacos E, Nicolaides K, Claus F, Debeer A, Smet MH, Proesmans M, Fayoux P, Storme L (2010) Tracheal side effects following fetal endoscopic tracheal occlusion for severe congenital diaphragmatic hernia. Pediatr Radiol 40:670–673
25. Ruano R, Yoshisaki CT, da Silva MM, Ceccon ME, Grasi MS, Tannuri U, Zugaib M (2012) A randomized controlled trial of fetal endoscopic tracheal occlusion versus postnatal management of severe isolated congenital diaphragmatic hernia. Ultrasound Obstet Gynecol 39:20–27
26. DeKoninck P, Gomez O, Sandaite I, Richter J, Nawapun K, Eerdekens A, Ramirez JC, Claus F, Gratacos E, Deprest J (2015) Right-sided congenital diaphragmatic hernia in a decade of fetal surgery. BJOG 122:940–946
27. Russo FM, De Coppi P, Allegaert K, Toelen J, van der Veeken L, Attilakos G, Eastwood MP, David AL, Deprest J (2017) Current and future antenatal management of isolated congenital diaphragmatic hernia. Semin Fetal Neonatal Med 22:383–390

19

Clinical characteristic and intraoperative findings of uterine perforation patients in using of intrauterine devices (IUDs)

Xin Sun, Min Xue*, Xinliang Deng, Yun Lin, Ying Tan and Xueli Wei

Abstract

Background: Intrauterine devices (IUDs) are the most popular form of contraception used worldwide; however, IUD is not risk-free. IUD migrations, especially uterine perforations, were frequently occurred in patients. The aim of this study was to investigate the clinical characteristics and intraoperative findings in patients with migrated IUDs.

Results: 29 cases of uterine perforation associated with migrated IUDs and 69 control patients were followed between January 2008 to March 2015. Patients who used IUDs within first 6 months from the last delivery experienced a characteristically high rate of the perforation of the uterine wall. A significantly larger number of IUD insertion associated with uterine perforation were performed in rural hospitals or operated at a lower level health care system. There was no clear difference in the age and presented symptoms in patients between two groups. Majority of contraceptive intrauterine devices was the copper-releasing IUDs. Furthermore, patients who used V-shaped IUD showed significantly higher incidence of pelvic adhesions when compared with the users of O-shaped IUDs.

Conclusions: Unique clinical characteristics of IUD migration were identified in patients with uterine perforation. Hysteroscopy and/or laparoscopy were the effective approaches to remove the migrated IUDs. Improving operating skills is required at the lower level of health care system.

Keywords: IUD, Uterine perforation, Hysteroscopy, Laparoscopy

Background

Intrauterine devices (IUDs) are the most popular form of contraception used by millions of women worldwide, particularly in developing countries [1]. Currently, two major types of IUDs are used, the copper-releasing intrauterine device (IUD) and the levonorgestrel-releasing intrauterine system (LNG-IUS) [2, 3]. However, IUDs are not risk-free, and lots of complications have been reported, including expulsion, malpositioning, and uterine perforation [4]. Among them, the majority were missing the IUDs, and most of the missing IUDs were found in the uterus [2]; however, the device would also pass through the uterine serosa causing uterine perforation. Uterine perforation is rare, but it may cause serious problems, including pain, abnormal bleeding, bowel or bladder perforation, and fistula formation, when IUDs migrate into the pelvic peritoneal space invading the adjacent organs. Thus far, the invasion of omentum, pouch of Douglas, the serosa of the ileum, the bladder, and the rectum has been reported in patients with uterine perforation [3, 5–8]. The rate of uterine perforation was 0.3–2.6 in every 1000 users of copper IUD insertion, and the respective rate for LNG-IUS insertion was 0.3–2.2 [9–15]. Uterine perforation can be primary (at the time of insertion) or secondary (4 weeks or more after the insertion took place). Lots of risk factors were proposed for uterine perforation, including immediate postpartum period [10, 16], breastfeeding [14, 17], extremes of uterine posture [18], intrauterine device shape not fitting well with uterine cavity [19], inexperience of the

* Correspondence: xuemin5908@sina.com
Department of Obstetrics and Gynecology, The 3rd Xiangya Hospital of Central South University, 138 Tongzipo Rd, Changsha, Hunan 410013, China

inserter, and inappropriate technique during the IUD insertion [15, 16, 20].

Specifically, the use of intrauterine devices has been changing in parallel with social-economic development of China. In the 1980s, 90% of all IUDs were stainless steel rings; they were cheaper than copper T-shaped IUDs but were also less effective and had a greater rate of expulsion [1]. In the 1990s, the use switched to T-shaped copper IUDs, although a large population of women was still using the steel rings [21]. Today, there are dozens of different types of IUDs available on the market that clearly mirror their clinical application [22–24]. Most of the IUDs used in China are manufactured in China, and the majority is the copper-releasing IUDs, including all types of T-shaped and V-shaped copper-releasing IUDs. Recently, some overseas products, as LNG-IUS [25] and GyneFix [26], have also been introduced to China.

Although lots of factors have been proposed, the precise cause of uterine perforation is not well understood [27]. The risk factors associated with use of IUDs by Chinese women were not reported. In this retrospective study, we attempted to evaluate all potential risk factors for uterine perforation associated with the use of IUDs by Chinese women and provide suggestions possibly useful for the management of IUD migrations.

Methods
Patients enrolled and surgery management
Patients admitted to the 3rd Xiangya Hospital of Central South University (CSU) at Hunan, China, from January 2008 to March 2015 were reviewed for uterine perforation. Uterine abnormalities were evaluated by by B-scan ultrasonography (B-scan), X-rays, or computed tomography (CT). Two groups of patients with (1) uterine perforation and (2) non-uterine perforation were enrolled into the study. In the event of uterine perforation, the IUD devices passed through the uterus and caused uterine injury; 29 cases were included in this study. In the patients without uterine perforation ("non-uterine perforation"), there was a displacement of IUD, but the device was still located in the uterus; 69 cases were included in the study. Patients who had preexisting IUDs but could not find the missing IUDs, which might be due to expulsion, were excluded from the study. This study was approved by the Review Board and Ethics Committee of the 3rd Xiangya Hospital of Central South University (# 2008-S010). All patients signed a statement of consent to participate under the "ethics, consent, and permissions" heading and another informed consent to the publication of collected data.

In patients with non-uterine perforation, the IUDs were malpositioned in the uterine or embedded in the uterine myometrium but did not cause perforation of the organ. All these patients underwent hysteroscopy as initial step in removing the dislocated IUDs. Patients with uterine perforation had partially or completely perforated organ throughout the uterine serosa. In these patients, laparoscopy and/or hysteroscopy or cystoscopy were applied to remove the migrated IUDs. Since one patient showed perforated ileum; laparotomy was performed to repair the intestine after the removal of the IUD.

Patient information and intraoperative findings
Patient information, including age, medical history, history of previous pregnancy outcome, symptoms encountered by the patient, the time of IUD insertion after the last delivery, the time from the IUD insertion to diagnosis, and health facility where IUD insertion was conducted, was collected when the patients came to the hospital.

The intraoperative findings were recorded during the surgical operations, which include type and location of IUD, site of uterine perforation, surgical management, and pelvic adhesion. These and other associated complications were also recorded during hysteroscopy and/or laparoscopy, cystoscopy, and laparotomy.

Statistical analysis
Data analysis was performed using GraphPad Prism ver. 6 (GraphPad Software, La Jolla, CA). A nonparametric, the Mann-Whitney U test was used to assess the differences in parameters between the uterine perforation and non-uterine perforation groups, while Fisher's exact test was applied in the evaluation of the incidence of these two groups.

Results
Multiple factors contributed to uterine perforation occurrence
The patients' characteristics were summarized in Table 1. The average age of all patients was 37, and there was no significant difference between the groups of patients (Mann-Whitney test, $p > 0.05$). The median age was 35 (range 22–60) for uterine perforation and 38 (range 20 to 71) for non-uterine perforation groups (Table 1).

In this study, we found 10 patients (34.5%) with the uterine perforation showing no signs or symptoms of a disease at hospital arrival screens. Thirty-two patients (46.4%) in the non-uterine perforation group did not have symptoms, either. While a large number of patients were encountered with different symptoms, most of them were presented as pelvic and/or abdominal pain. Ten patients (34.5%) in the uterine perforation group had pain, and 15 (21.7%) of those with pain were observed in the non-uterine perforation group. Pain prevalence was followed by menstrual disorders affecting 10.3% of patients in the uterine perforation and 17.4% of them in the group of non-uterine perforation.

Pregnancy occurred in 17.2% in the uterine perforation group and 5.8% of cases in the non-uterine perforation.

114

Gynecological Surgery: New Frontiers

Table 1 Characterization of 98 patients with uterine perforation and without uterine perforation in Chinese women of IUD insertion

Characteristic	Uterine perforation (n = 29)	Non-uterine perforation (n = 69)
Age (years)		
Median (range)	35 (22–60)	38 (20–71)
Symptoms		
Asymptomatic	10 (34.5)	32 (46.4)
Pain (pelvic and/or abdominal)	10 (34.5)	15 (21.7)
Menstrual disorders	3 (10.3)	12 (17.4)
Unintended pregnancy	5 (17.2)	4 (5.8)
Missing strings	4 (13.8)	4 (5.8)
Vaginal bleeding	0 (0)	3 (4.3)
History of previously pregnancy outcome		
Cesarean section	7 (24.1)	27 (39.1)
Vaginal birth	22 (75.9)	42 (60.9)
Diagnosis of IUD migration		
B-scan ultrasonography (B-scan) only	13 (44.8)	52 (75.4)
X-radiation (X-rays) only	3 (10.3)	1 (1.4)
B-scan + X-rays	6 (20.7)*	3 (4.3)
Others	7 (24.1)	13 (18.8)
IUD insertion after last delivery (months)		
Median (range)	16 (3–60)	24 (3–120)
≤ 6	15 (51.7)*	17 (24.6)
> 6 to ≤ 12	4 (13.8)	15 (21.7)
≥ 12	8 (27.6)	20 (29.0)
Not postpartum	2 (6.9)	17 (24.6)
Time from insertion to diagnosis (months)		
Median (range)	114 (1–408)	93 (1–480)
≤ 12	8 (27.6)	13 (18.8)
> 12 to ≤ 60	6 (20.7)	27 (39.1)
> 60 to ≤ 120	6 (20.6)	15 (21.7)
≥ 120	9 (31.0)	14 (20.3)
Institution for operation of IUD inserting		
Rural hospital or lower level	26 (89.7)*	48 (69.6)
Urban hospital	3 (10.3)	21 (30.4)
Type of IUD		
T-shaped copper, made in China	10 (34.5)	20 (29.0)
V-shaped copper, made in China	13 (44.8)	31 (44.9)
O-shaped, made in China	4 (13.8)	10 (14.5)
GyneFix, made in Belgium	1 (3.4)	3 (4.3)
Others	1 (3.4)	5 (7.2)

Non-uterine perforation was subjected to IUD malposition without uterine perforation. The data are presented as n (%) unless stated otherwise
*p < 0.05, analyzed by Fisher's exact test

About 13.8% of patients with uterine perforation were associated with IUD missing strings and 5.8% of those with non-uterine perforation. Three cases of vaginal bleeding were observed, all of them in the group of non-uterine perforation (Table 1).

The time interval between IUD insertion and the time of last delivery was shorter in the uterine perforation group when compared with the group of non-uterine perforation. A half of the patients (n = 15, 51.7%) with the uterine perforation inserted the device within

6 months after delivery, which is significantly higher than in the patients of the no uterine perforation group ($n = 17$, 24.6%;Table 1, Fisher's exact test, * = $p < 0.05$). The time passed from the insertion of IUD to diagnosis of uterine perforation (duration of IUD placement) tended to be longer (14 months in average) when compared with 93 months for the conditions of non-uterine perforation (Table 1).

There are three major types of IUDs that were typically used: T- and V-shaped copper-releasing IUDs and O-shaped IUDs (O-shaped IUDs referred to as stainless steel single or double rings). Our findings showed that uterine perforation cannot be associated with a particular type of IUD (Table 1). However, 89.7% ($n = 26$) of patients with uterine perforations inserted IUDs in rural hospitals or at lower level health care systems, in comparison with 69.6% ($n = 48$) of those with no uterine perforation treated in the same setting Table 1).

Intraoperative findings were associated with uterine perforation

If the IUDs were going through the uterine serosa, or entirely outside the uterus, invading the organs in the pelvic abdominal cavity would make it difficult to remove devices. This invokes an increased risk for severe complications.

There was not a clear pattern of the organs affected by displaced and protruding IUDs through the uterine. Myometrium appeared on the top of the scattered pattern of organ injury ($n = 6$, 20.7%) and greater omentum ($n = 6$, 20.7%), followed by the sigmoid colon ($n = 5$, 17.2%) (Fig. 2), left sacrouterine ligament ($n = 3$, 10.3%), bladder ($n = 3$, 10.3%), pouch of Douglas ($n = 2$, 6.9%), and rectal serosa ($n = 2$, 6.9%). One patient (3.4%) had injured uterus isthmus and affected ileum was observed in the other one (3.4%; Table 2).

We identified five types of IUDs that were implanted (Fig. 1A (a–e). Most of them are T-shaped copper-

containing device ($n = 10$, 34.5%) and V-shaped copper-containing device ($n = 13$, 44.8%), which showed a random invasion of the pelvic peritoneum. The O-shaped IUDs predominantly invaded the left sacrouterine ligament (3/4, 75%; Table 2).

Uterine perforation frequently causes pelvic adhesion as reported before [6], but it is still unknown whether any typical type of IUD that is made in China is associated with pelvic adhesion. In our study, we found that V-shaped copper-releasing IUDs (12/13, 92.3%) induced significantly higher rate of pelvic adhesion when compared with the O-shaped IUDs (1/4, 25%) (Fig. 1B (a), Fisher's exact test, * = $p < 0.05$). The pain induction could not be related to any particular device evaluated in this study (Fig. 1B (b)).

Laparoscopy and/or hysteroscopy were applied to remove the migrated IUDs

Once the patients were diagnosed with uterine perforation and the device's location was identified, they underwent surgical removal of migrated IUDs. Five patients (17.2%) out of 29 underwent laparoscopy for removal of the IUDs, while 22 patients (75.9%) underwent hysteroscopy along with laparoscopy (Table 3 and Fig. 2). Since one patient experienced ileum injury, it underwent laparotomy for exploration, IUD removal, and the wound repair. In the other patient, the IUD migrated into the bladder, and the device was removed by cystoscopy (Table 3). All the patients showed signs of healthy recovery during hospitalization and were discharged within 1 week.

Discussion
Uterine perforation is a serious complication associated with IUD use. The precise mechanism of induction of uterine perforation is not well understood. A lot of risk factors were proposed for the induction of uterine perforation [10, 14, 15, 19]. In this study, we found that the

Table 2 Location and type of IUDs identified in uterine perforation

Location	Occurrence of patients	Type of IUDs				
		T-shaped copper	V-shaped copper	O-shaped	GyneFix	Others
Myometrium	6/29 (20.7)	1/10 (10.0)	4/13 (30.8)	1/4 (25.0)	0/1 (–)	0/1 (–)
Greater omentum	6/29 (20.7)	1/10 (10.0)	4/13 (30.8)	0/4 (–)	1/1 (100)	0/1 (–)
Sigmoid colon	5/29 (17.2)	2/10 (20.0)	3/13 (23.1)	0/4 (–)	0/1 (–)	0/1 (–)
Left sacrouterine ligament	3/29 (10.3)	0/10 (–)	0/13 (–)	3/4 (75.0)	0/1 (–)	0/1 (–)
Bladder	3/29 (10.3)	2/10 (20.0)	1/13 (7.7)	0/4 (–)	0/1 (–)	0/1 (–)
Pouch of Douglas	2/29 (6.9)	2/10 (20.0)	0/13 (–)	0/4 (–)	0/1 (–)	0/1 (–)
Serosa of rectum	2/29 (6.9)	1/10 (10.0)	1/13 (7.7)	0/4 (–)	0/1 (–)	0/1 (–)
Isthmus	1/29 (3.4)	1/10 (10.0)	0/13 (–)	0/4 (–)	0/1 (–)	0/1 (–)
Ileum	1/29 (3.4)	0/10 (–)	0/13 (–)	0/4 (–)	0/1 (–)	1/1 (100)

The data are presented as n (%) unless stated otherwise

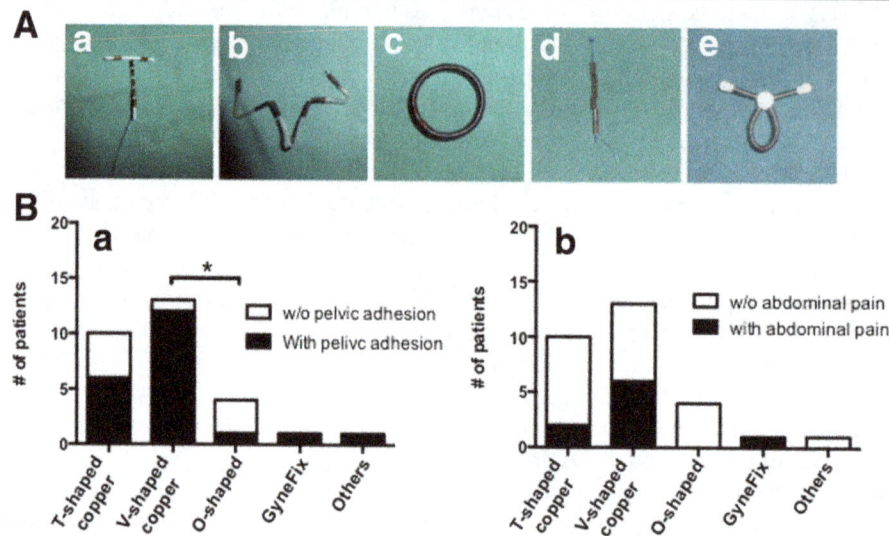

Fig. 1 IUDs and complications were associated with uterine perforation. **A** Different types of IUDs were identified in the patients with uterine perforation, including T-shaped copper (**a**), V-shaped copper (**b**), O-shaped (**c**), GyneFix (**d**), and other type (**e**) of IUDs. **B** Pelvic adhesion and abdominal pain were associated with uterine perforation. Five major types of IUDs were correlated with the intraoperative finding of pelvic adhesion (**a**) and clinical symptom of abdominal pain (**b**). Please note that significantly higher ratio of pelvic adhesions were observed in V-shaped copper IUD patients of 12/13 (92.3%) compared with O-shaped IUD patients of 3/4 (75%) with uterine perforation (Fisher's exact test, *p < 0.05), while the abdominal pains were no different among all the types of IUDs used with uterine perforation. Note, w/o means without

time of IUD insertion after the last delivery is shorter in the uterine perforation group when compared with the subjects without uterine perforation. A sharp increase of the uterine perforation rate occurred in the subjects with IUD inserted up to 6 months after delivery. The incidence of uterine perforation within the first 6 months was significantly higher when compared with the subjects treated under the same conditions but without uterine perforation (Table 1, 51.7 vs. 24.6%, p < 0.05). At this stage, most patients were still in the breastfeeding period, and all 15 subjects in the lactation period were diagnosed with uterine perforation. This finding is consistent with previous reports that women in the lactation period are at a high risk of uterine perforation [14, 17]. In addition, most of the patients with the uterine perforation had received an IUD at rural hospitals or a lower level of health care systems. Typically, the experience and technique of an obstetrician-gynecologist in rural hospitals or lower level health care systems are poorer when compared to those in urban hospitals in China. Many obstetrician-gynecologists in rural hospital or a lower level of health care systems are lacking an efficient

Table 3 Surgical approaches for uterine perforation cases

Approaches	Treatment of patients, n (%)
Laparoscopy	22/29 (75.9)
Hysteroscopy + laparoscopy	5/29 (17.2)
Laparotomy	1/29 (3.4)
Cystoscopy	1/29 (3.4)

training on handling of IUD insertion, which may directly cause perforation at the insertion time. As it was reported before, IUD migrations at the time of insertion may directly contribute to uterine perforation [14, 17, 28].

The IUD use in China has a long history, and it can be found as earlier as 1979 [1]; however, the IUD devices were still not well managed. In the early years, most IUDs were steel rings (designated as O-shaped in this study) due to its low cost, and the devices were provided free of charge in some hospitals [1, 22]. Later, the copper-releasing IUDs replaced the steel rings as many problems were encountered by using the rings [29].Nowadays, copper-releasing IUDs have become the prevailing devices in clinical application in China [22, 24]. Recently, the levonorgestrel intrauterine system (LNG-IUS) along with other optimized IUDs were also provided to Chinese women [25]. In this study, the majority of devices that induced uterine perforation were copper-releasing IUDs with T-shaped copper (n = 10) followed by V-shaped copper IUDs (n = 13) and four of those with O-shaped IUDs (Table 1). A larger number of patients is required to assess the risk factors associated with different types of IUDs, including the LNG-IUS that are used in China.

Pelvic adhesions as a consequence of uterine perforation also frequently occurred in the patients, but the mechanism is still unknown; it may due to different actions of the devices [3]. In our study, we found that 12 out of the 13 patients with V-shaped contraceptive

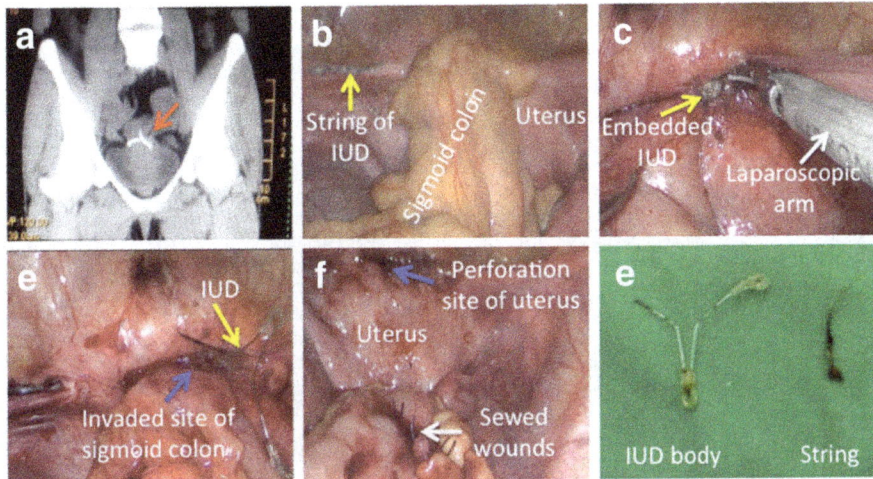

Fig. 2 Migrated IUD was removed by laparoscopy in a typical case of uterine perforation. **a** A 36-year-old patient was visiting the 3rd Xiangya Hospital for checking of hysteromyoma in January 2015, and this patient was experienced with two types of IUD insertions, and because of that, she assumed that the first IUD was expelled. However, after she took out the second IUD, another IUD was monitored unexpectedly by computed tomography (CT), indicating that the first IUD had undergone uterine perforation. Note that the red arrow showed the IUD. **b–f** The laparoscopy was applied for the removal of the migrated IUD. It was shown that the IUD completely perforated through the uterine serosa and invaded into the sigmoid colon and, finally, the IUD was removed and the wounds were sewn under laparoscopy. Note that the migrated IUD was shown in yellow arrows, and the perforation site at the uterus and the invaded site of the sigmoid colon were shown in blue arrows. **e** The IUD was identified as a V-shaped copper IUD, and the string was already separated from the IUD body

intrauterine devices had pelvic adhesions (Fig. 1B). This is significantly higher when compared with the patients that used O-shaped IUDs. The reason(s) for the higher rate of pelvic adhesions in patients who used V-shaped IUD is unknown at present. This issue requires a thorough investigation.

If the IUDs were missing, a method of searching for the strings or IUDs in the uterine cavity is sweeping by using uterine forceps. However, there are many IUDs used by Chinese women that do not have any string [23] (Fig. 1). The exploration success rate highly varies and is dependent on the experience and applied technique by the obstetrician-gynecologist who removes the IUDs using forceps or hooked instruments [30]. Under these aggravating circumstances, hysteroscopy and/or laparoscopy are suggested procedures, which secure a very high success rate [6–8, 31]. If the IUDs migrated into the pelvic peritoneal cavity, the procedures become dubious. Currently, the WHO recommends that all misplaced IUDs should be surgically removed once they are identified [32]. Some researches, however, suggest that if the migrated IUDs do not cause serious complications or significant symptoms, their removal is not necessary [33, 34]. In our study, all displaced IUDs associated with uterine perforation were successfully removed using laparoscopy and/or hysteroscopy that was accompanied with significant complications. Laparoscopy and/or hysteroscopy provide a high success rate in the removal of migrated IUDs in the patients with uterine perforation.

Conclusions

Potential risk factors associated with IUD use for the uterine perforation in Chinese population of patients are identified in a retrospective observational study. Hysteroscopy and/or laparoscopy are effective approaches in removing of displaced IUDs. A tailored training program planned to meet patients' needs in rural areas and at a lower level of health care system may be justified.

Acknowledgements
The authors thank all the members in the Department of Obstetrics and Gynecology, the 3rd Xiangya Hospital of Central South University, for their helpful assistance during the data collection.

Funding
None

Authors' contributions
XS and MX designed the studies, performed the surgical operations, and analyzed the data; XD performed the surgical operations and analyzed the data; YL, YT and XW collected the data and images; and XS wrote the manuscript. All authors read and approved the final manuscript.

Competing interests
The authors declare that they have no competing interests.

References

1. d'Arcangues C (2007) Worldwide use of intrauterine devices for contraception. Contraception 75(6 Suppl):S2–S7
2. Marchi NM, Castro S, Hidalgo MM, Hidalgo C, Monteiro-Dantas C, Villarroel M et al (2012) Management of missing strings in users of intrauterine contraceptives. Contraception 86(4):354–358
3. Kaislasuo J, Suhonen S, Gissler M, Lahteenmaki P, Heikinheimo O (2013) Uterine perforation caused by intrauterine devices: clinical course and treatment. Hum Reprod 28(6):1546–1551
4. Boortz HE, Margolis DJ, Ragavendra N, Patel MK, Kadell BM (2012) Migration of intrauterine devices: radiologic findings and implications for patient care. Radiographics 32(2):335–352
5. Rahnemai-Azar AA, Apfel T, Naghshizadian R, Cosgrove JM, Farkas DT (2014) Laparoscopic removal of migrated intrauterine device embedded in intestine. JSLS 18(3):e2014.00122.1-5
6. Kho KA, Chamsy DJ (2014) Perforated intraperitoneal intrauterine contraceptive devices: diagnosis, management, and clinical outcomes. J Minim Invasive Gynecol 21(4):596–601
7. Agacayak E, Tunc SY, Icen MS, Oguz A, Ozler A, Turgut A et al (2015) Evaluation of predisposing factors, diagnostic and treatment methods in patients with translocation of intrauterine devices. J Obstet Gynaecol Res 41(5):735–741
8. Mosley FR, Shahi N, Kurer MA (2012) Elective surgical removal of migrated intrauterine contraceptive devices from within the peritoneal cavity: a comparison between open and laparoscopic removal. JSLS 16(2):236–241
9. Heinemann K, Reed S, Moehner S, Minh TD (2015) Risk of uterine perforation with levonorgestrel-releasing and copper intrauterine devices in the European Active Surveillance Study on intrauterine devices. Contraception 91(4):274–279
10. Caliskan E, Ozturk N, Dilbaz BO, Dilbaz S (2003) Analysis of risk factors associated with uterine perforation by intrauterine devices. Eur J Contracept Reprod Health Care 8(3):150–155
11. Harrison-Woolrych M, Ashton J, Coulter D (2003) Uterine perforation on intrauterine device insertion: is the incidence higher than previously reported? Contraception 67(1):53–56
12. Harrison-Woolrych M, Zhou L, Coulter D (2003) Insertion of intrauterine devices: a comparison of experience with Mirena and Multiload Cu 375 during post-marketing monitoring in New Zealand. N Z Med J 116(1179):U538
13. Kaislasuo J, Suhonen S, Gissler M, Lahteenmaki P, Heikinheimo O (2012) Intrauterine contraception: incidence and factors associated with uterine perforation—a population-based study. Hum Reprod 27(9):2658–2663
14. Van Houdenhoven K, van Kaam KJ, van Grootheest AC, Salemans TH, Dunselman GA (2006) Uterine perforation in women using a levonorgestrel-releasing intrauterine system. Contraception 73(3):257–260
15. Zhou L, Harrison-Woolrych M, Coulter DM (2003) Use of the New Zealand Intensive Medicines Monitoring Programme to study the levonorgestrel-releasing intrauterine device (Mirena). Pharmacoepidemiol Drug Saf 12(5):371–377
16. Andersson K, Ryde-Blomqvist E, Lindell K, Odlind V, Milsom I (1998) Perforations with intrauterine devices. Report from a Swedish survey. Contraception 57(4):251–255
17. Heartwell SF, Schlesselman S (1983) Risk of uterine perforation among users of intrauterine devices. Obstet Gynecol 61(1):31–36
18. Zakin D, Stern WZ, Rosenblatt R (1981) Complete and partial uterine perforation and embedding following insertion of intrauterine devices. I. Classification, complications, mechanism, incidence, and missing string. Obstet Gynecol Surv 36(7):335–353
19. Wildemeersch D, Hasskamp T, Goldstuck N (2015) Intrauterine devices that do not fit well cause side effects, become embedded, or are expelled and can even perforate the uterine wall. J Minim Invasive Gynecol 22(2):309–310
20. Harrison-Woolrych M, Ashton J, Coulter D (2002) Insertion of the Multiload Cu375 intrauterine device; experience in over 16,000 New Zealand women. Contraception 66(6):387–391
21. Li Yong Ping KLB, Rowe PJ, De Wei Z, Xian WS, Yin ZH, Wu Z (1994) The demographic impact of conversion from steel to copper IUDs in China. Int Fam Plan Perspect 20(4):124–130
22. Cheung VY (2010) Sonographic appearances of Chinese intrauterine devices. J Ultrasound Med 29(7):1093–1101
23. Cheung VY (2010) A 10-year experience in removing Chinese intrauterine devices. Int J Gynaecol Obstet 109(3):219–222
24. Zhang S, Li Y, Yu P, Chen T, Zhou W, Zhang W et al (2015) In vitro release of cupric ion from intrauterine devices: influence of frame, shape, copper surface area and indomethacin. Biomed Microdevices 17(1):19
25. Zhao S, Deng J, Wang Y, Bi S, Wang X, Qin W et al (2014) Experience and levels of satisfaction with the levonorgestrel-releasing intrauterine system in China: a prospective multicenter survey. Patient Prefer Adherence 8:1449–1455
26. Cao X, Zhang W, Gao G, Van Kets H, Wildemeersch D (2000) Randomized comparative trial in parous women of the frameless GyneFix and the TCu380A intrauterine devices: long-term experience in a Chinese family planning clinic. Eur J Contracept Reprod Health Care 5(2):135–140
27. Goldstuck ND, Wildemeersch D (2014) Role of uterine forces in intrauterine device embedment, perforation, and expulsion. Int J Womens Health 6:735–744
28. Goldstuck ND, Holloway G (1988) IUD insertion forces: effects of recent childbirth and lactation. Adv Contracept 4(2):159–164
29. Bilian X (2007) Chinese experience with intrauterine devices. Contraception 75(6 Suppl):S31–S34
30. Su S, Zhao Z, Feng S, Dong B (2012) A novel medical device for removal of intrauterine devices under direct vision. Contraception 86(5):583–586
31. Balci O, Mahmoud AS, Capar M, Colakoglu MC (2010) Diagnosis and management of intra-abdominal, mislocated intrauterine devices. Arch Gynecol Obstet 281(6):1019–1022
32. World Health Organization (1987) Mechanism of action, safety and efficacy of intrauterine devices. Report of a WHO Scientific Group. World Health Organ Tech Rep Ser 753:1-91
33. Markovitch O, Klein Z, Gidoni Y, Holzinger M, Beyth Y (2002) Extrauterine mislocated IUD: is surgical removal mandatory? Contraception 66(2):105–108
34. Adoni A, Ben CA (1991 Jan) The management of intrauterine devices following uterine perforation. Contraception 43(1):77–81

20

Safety aspects of hysteroscopy, specifically in relation to entry and specimen retrieval: a UK survey of practice

S. H. Walker[*] and L. Gokhale

Abstract

Background: The purpose of this study is to evaluate current practice amongst gynaecologists across the UK, regarding safety aspects of inpatient hysteroscopy under anaesthesia, specifically in relation to entry and specimen retrieval.

A survey was created using survey monkey. The first round was circulated to all registrar trainees and consultant gynaecologists across Wales. Following a good response, the survey was then circulated to all members of the British Society of Gynaecological Endoscopy (BSGE).

Results: There were 212 responses including, 140 consultants, 36 senior registrars, 17 junior registrars and 18 clinical nurse specialists. In total, 136 out of 212 (64.7%) always perform a vaginal examination prior to hysteroscopy. 10.4% always sound the uterus, and 5.2% always dilate the uterus prior to insertion of the hysteroscope. Twenty-three consultants, six senior registrars, three junior registrars and one clinical nurse specialist knew how to position the internal cervical os as visualised through the scope when using a 30° hysteroscope. 35.8% of candidates always perform a post-procedure cavity check, and 9% use suction to flush the cavity to aid vision during the post-procedure cavity check. The majority (76%) predicted dilatation as the stage most likely to cause uterine perforation and predicted the most likely site for perforation as the posterior uterine wall in the anteverted uterus and the anterior uterine wall in the retroverted uterus.

Conclusion: This study highlights varied practice across the UK regarding safety aspects of hysteroscopy, in relation to entry and specimen retrieval. There is a need for increased awareness of the risks of hysteroscopy and paramount precautions that should be performed routinely as part of their practice. Standardised guidelines may be a beneficial tool to help bring about this change in practice, leading to a reduction in uterine perforation rates.

Keywords: Hysteroscopy, Uterine perforation, Specimen retrieval

Background

The hysteroscope has become a standard part of a gynaecologists' armamentarium, with operative hysteroscopy increasing as a surgical alternative for various gynaecological problems [1]. Uterine perforation is an uncommon but potentially serious complication of hysteroscopy. Guidance from the Royal College of Obstetricians and Gynaecologists (RCOG) on best practice in outpatient hysteroscopy estimates a perforation rate of 0.007–1.7% [2]. With higher rates of

* Correspondence: sarah.walker30@nhs.net
Department of Obstetrics and Gynaecology, Royal Gwent Hospital, Aneurin Bevan University Health Board, Newport, UK

1.6% reported for operative hysteroscopy [3, 4]. Risk factors include cervical stenosis, tortuous cervical canal and deviated uterine cavity as a result of fibroids [2, 5].

Outpatient hysteroscopy with or without the use of local anaesthesia is now an established technique [1]. It is associated with a lower incidence of uterine trauma due to being performed with smaller-diameter hysteroscopes and under direct vision [2]. The main reasons for failure to successfully perform outpatient hysteroscopy includes cervical stenosis, severe pain, vasovagal reaction and high body mass index (BMI) making access difficult [2, 6]. Consequently, there will always be a necessity for inpatient hysteroscopy under general anaesthetic, and this cohort of women are at higher risk of complications due to increasing operative complexity, higher incidence of cervical stenosis, postmenopausal cervical atrophy and co-morbidities [7].

It has been estimated that 55% of uterine perforations are entry related (i.e. secondary to sounding, dilatation and insertion of hysteroscope) and 45% are related to technique used and improper use of the probe [1, 8].

Hysteroscopy carries small risks that cannot be eliminated completely, but preventing hysteroscopy complications starts by raising awareness of risks and precautions [1]. Currently there are no clear guidelines regarding safety aspects of inpatient diagnostic and operative hysteroscopy under general anaesthetic.

The aim of this study is to evaluate current practice amongst gynaecologists across the UK regarding safety aspects of inpatient hysteroscopy under general anaesthetic, specifically in relation to entry and specimen retrieval. Results from the survey may help determine if practice needs to change and whether there is a need for standardised guidelines on inpatient hysteroscopy under general anaesthetic.

Method

A survey was created using survey monkey. The first round was circulated to all gynaecological speciality-training registrar doctors in their third to seventh year of training (ST3-7 trainees) and consultant gynaecologists across Wales in December 2016. Following a good response to this, the survey was then circulated to all members of the British Society of Gynaecological Endoscopy (BSGE) in June 2017. No ethical approval was required as the survey was optional and anonymous and study aims explained to all candidates prior to performing the survey.

Questions were based on safety aspects of all the stages of hysteroscopy, which can lead to uterine perforation. The survey specified for inpatient hysteroscopy under general anaesthetic. Question 1 was whether they routinely perform a vaginal examination prior to hysteroscopy. The next four questions were entry-related; whether they routinely sound and dilate the uterus prior to entry of the hysteroscope, the type of hysteroscope used and technique used when inserting the hysteroscope. Question 6 related to specimen retrieval. Questions 7 and 8 were whether they perform a post-procedure cavity check and whether they use suction to flush the cavity to aid this step.

An additional three questions were included in the survey when it was circulated to members of the BSGE. These included; the anatomical location the candidate thought you are most likely to perforate during hysteroscopy, during which stage of hysteroscopy they are most likely to perforate, and finally whether they use a standard proforma for documentation of their findings in their department.

Results were collated on an excel spreadsheet and analysed. For analysis the grades were split up into consultants, senior registrars (ST5-7), junior registrars (ST3-4) and clinical nurse specialists.

Results

In total, 212 responses were included in analysis, 83 out of 170 responses (48.8%) from the first round to gynaecologists across Wales (13 junior registrars, 15 senior registrars, 55 consultants) and 129 out of 983 responses (13.1%) from the second round to members of the BSGE covering all regions of the UK (18 clinical nurse specialists, 5 junior registrars, 21 senior registrars, 85 consultants).

Hysteroscopic approach and entry-related safety precautions

As shown in Table 1, in total, 64.2% (136/212) always carry out a vaginal examination prior to hysteroscopy, with a higher proportion of junior registrars (88.9%) compared to consultants (59.3%) always carrying out vaginal examination prior to hysteroscopy. In total, 10.4% (22/212) always sound the uterus before inserting the hysteroscope (15 consultants, 2 senior registrars, 4 junior registrars and 1 clinical nurse specialist). In total, 5.2% (11/212) always dilate, 22.6% (48/212) never dilate and 72.2% (153/212) sometimes dilate before inserting the hysteroscope (Table 1).

When asking which type of hysteroscope candidate's use, the majority of registrars never use a 0° hysteroscope, with 13.6% of consultants and 33.3% of clinical nurse specialists only using a 0° hysteroscope. Table 2 summarises the responses given when candidates were asked how they position the internal cervical os as visualised through the scope when using a 30° scope. Only 16.7% (34/204) knew the correct position being, 'the 6 o'clock position for anteverted uterus and 12 o'clock position for retroverted uterus.' The commonest answer given by 34.8% (71/204) was 'always the 6 o'clock position,' which is the correct answer for an anteverted uterus, followed by 'the way the hysteroscope naturally goes,' for which 32.4% gave as their answer (66/204).

Hysteroscopic technique

Table 3 demonstrates the instruments used by candidates for specimen retrieval. The majority of candidates use a range of instruments depending on availability. Overall, more candidates used polyp forceps (71%) and curette (58%), both being blind procedures compared to specimen retrieval under direct vision including myosure (24%) and resectoscope (10%).

Table 1 Summary of response to questions related to safety aspects of hysteroscopy

Questions	Response	Number (percentage)				
		Consultants	Senior registrar	Junior registrar	Clinical nurse specialist	Total
Do you carry out a vaginal examination before hysteroscopy?	Always	83 (59.3)	31 (86.1)	16 (88.9)	6 (33.3)	136 (64.2)
	Never	7 (5)	1 (2.8)	0	2 (11.1)	10 (4.7)
	Sometimes	50 (35.7)	4 (11.1)	2 (11.1)	10 (55.6)	66 (31.1)
Do you Sound the uterus before inserting the hysteroscope?	Always	15 (10.7)	2 (5.6)	4 (22.2)	1 (5.6)	22 (10.4)
	Never	77 (55)	20 (55.6)	8 (44.4)	13 (72.2)	118 (55.7)
	Sometimes	48 (34.3)	14 (38.9)	6 (33.3)	4 (22.2)	72 (34)
Do you dilate before inserting the hysteroscope?	Always	7 (5)	3 (8.3)	1 (5.6)	0	11 (5.2)
	Never	36 (25.7)	8 (22.2)	1 (5.6)	3 (16.7)	48 (22.6)
	Sometimes	97 (69.3)	25 (69.4)	16 (88.9)	15 (83.3)	153 (72.2)
Following collection of specimen, do you carry out post-procedure cavity check?	Always	63 (45)	7 (19.4)	4 (22.2)	2 (11.1)	76 (35.8)
	Never	12 (8.6)	4 (11.1)	2 (11.1)	9 (50)	27 (12.7)
	Sometimes	65 (46.4)	25 (69.4)	12 (66.7)	7 (38.9)	109 (51.4)
When carrying out post-procedure cavity check, do you use suction to flush the cavity?	Always	16 (11.4)	2 (5.6)	1 (5.6)	0	19 (9)
	Never	84 (60)	22 (61.1)	13 (72.2)	17 (94.4)	136 (64.2)
	Sometimes	40 (28.6)	12 (33.3)	4 (22.2)	1 (5.)	57 (26.9)

$N = 212$, with percentages in brackets. Grades of candidates are divided up in the columns

As shown at the bottom of Table 1, in total, 35.8% candidates (76/112) always carry out post-procedure cavity checks. A higher proportion of consultants (45%) carry out post-procedure cavity checks compared to junior registrars (22.2%) and clinical nurse specialists (11.1%). Only 9% of candidates (19/212) use suction to flush the cavity to aid vision during the post-procedure cavity checks (16 consultants, 2 senior registrars and 1 junior registrar).

For the additional three questions asked to the 129 candidates from the BSGE, the biggest response given by 41.9%; when asked what anatomical location they felt you are most likely to perforate during hysteroscopy, was the 'posterior uterine wall in the anteverted uterus and the anterior uterine wall in the retroverted uterus' (Fig. 1). The majority (76%) predicted dilatation as the

stage of hysteroscopy most likely to cause uterine perforation (Fig. 2). Lastly, 41.1% (53/129) use a standard proforma for documentation of their findings following hysteroscopy.

Discussion

Main findings

The results from this survey show varied practice amongst gynaecologists across the UK. This is reflected through limited information being available in the literature regarding safety aspects of hysteroscopy, specifically in relation to entry and specimen retrieval. There are guidelines available from the RCOG on best practice in outpatient hysteroscopy [2], but no guidelines available on inpatient diagnostic and operative hysteroscopy under general anaesthetic.

Table 2 Summary of response by candidates to the question of how they position the internal cervical os as visualised through the scope during insertion of a 30° hyster scope

How do you position the internal cervical os as visualised through the 30° hysteroscope?	Number (percentage)				
	Consultants	Senior registrar	Junior registrar	Clinical nurse Specialist	Total
Always 6 o'clock position	42 (30.2)	15 (44.1)	8 (44.4)	6 (46.2)	71 (34.8)
Always 12 o'clock position	12 (8.6)	4 (11.8)	0	1 (7.7)	17 (8.3)
The way the hysteroscope naturally goes	52 (37.4)	6 (17.6)	3 (16.7)	5 (38.5)	66 (32.4)
6 o'clock position for anteverted uterus, 12 o'clock position for retroverted uterus	23 (16.5)	6 (17.6)	4 (22.2)	1 (7.7)	34 (16.7)
12 o'clock position for anteverted uterus, 6 o'clock position for retroverted uterus	10 (7.2)	3 (8.8)	3 (16.7)	0	16 (7.8)

$N = 204$, with the percentages in brackets. Grades of candidates are divided up in the columns

Table 3 Summary of instruments used for specimen retrieval during hysteroscopy

Instrument used for specimen retrieval	Consultant	Senior registrar	Junior registrar	Clinical nurse specialist	Total
Polyp forceps	49	9	6	7	71
Currette	38	9	6	5	58
Versapoint	15	1	0	0	16
Myosure	19	1	0	4	24
Pipelle	8	0	0	5	13
All of above 5 options depending on availability	61	25	9	3	98
Resectoscope	7	2	0	1	10
Truclear	4	0	0	0	4

Candidates were able to give one or more responses and the columns separate out the different grades of gynaecologists

When asked if candidates perform a vaginal examination prior to hysteroscopy, 64.2% stated that they always do, 31.1% sometimes and 4.7% never. Literature highlights bimanual assessment being a vital step to perform to correctly identify the size, position and attitude of the uterus, helping to determine the direction to insert the hysteroscope, and reducing the risk of uterine perforation [9–11]. However, if the patient has had an ultrasound scan indicating the uterine position then this step may be omitted, provided the surgeon is aware of the ultrasound report.

Whether or not to sound the uterus prior to hysteroscopy is debatable, with limited evidence for its use in literature. In the survey, of concern, 10.4% of candidates stated that they always sound the uterus prior to insertion of the hysteroscope. Some articles report it as a useful step to help determine the length and direction of the internal os and uterine cavity, thereby reducing your chance of perforation and suspecting perforation when the sound goes beyond the expected size of the uterus [10–12]. However, it is another instrument introduced into the uterus, increasing the risk of perforation and should only be used on occasion with proper technique of a gentle approach holding the sound like a pen, not a skewer to avoid perforation [10].

Dilatation is reported to be when most cervical trauma and uterine perforations occur [5]. One study reported 50% of their perforations occurred during dilatation of the cervix [8]. Dilatation is not recommended for diagnostic procedures [1]. However,

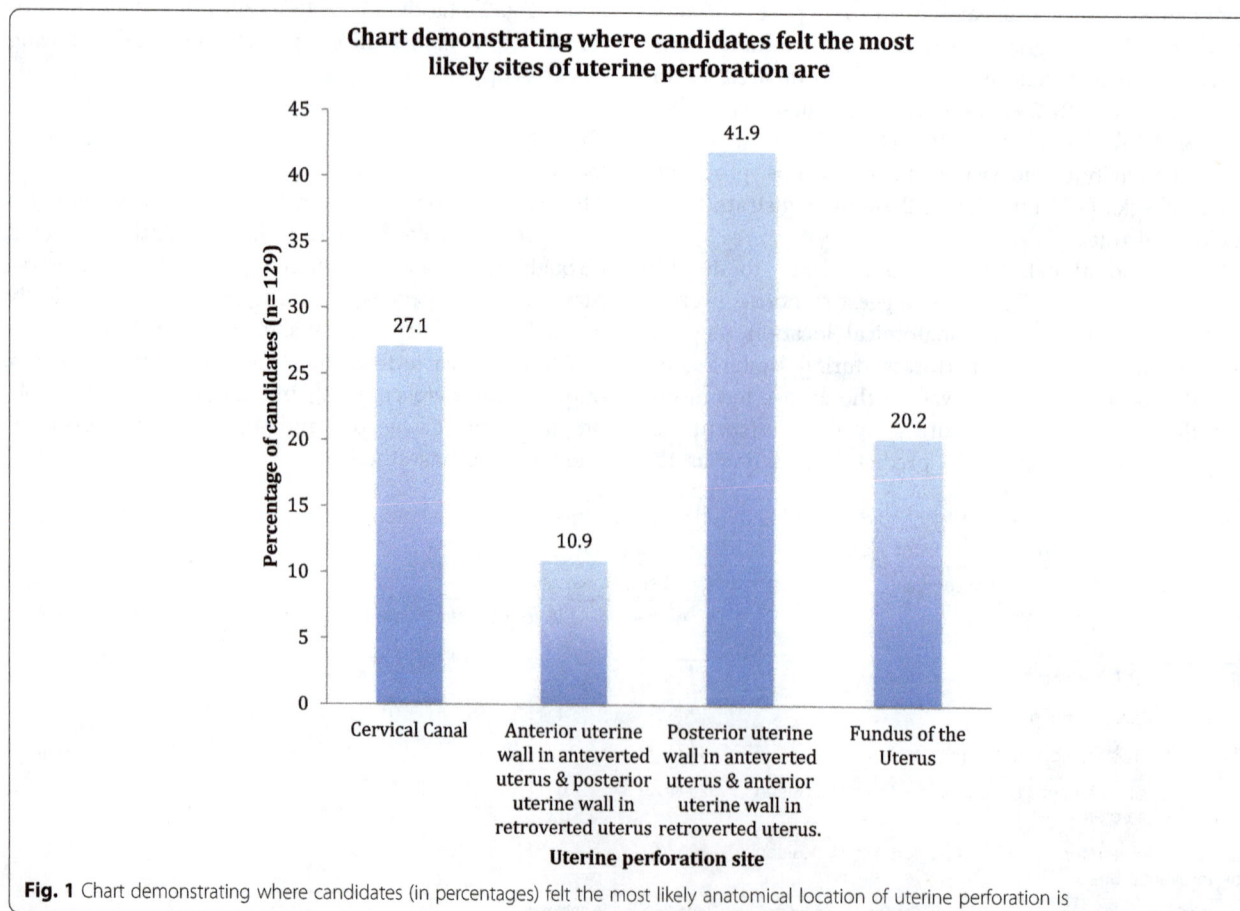

Fig. 1 Chart demonstrating where candidates (in percentages) felt the most likely anatomical location of uterine perforation is

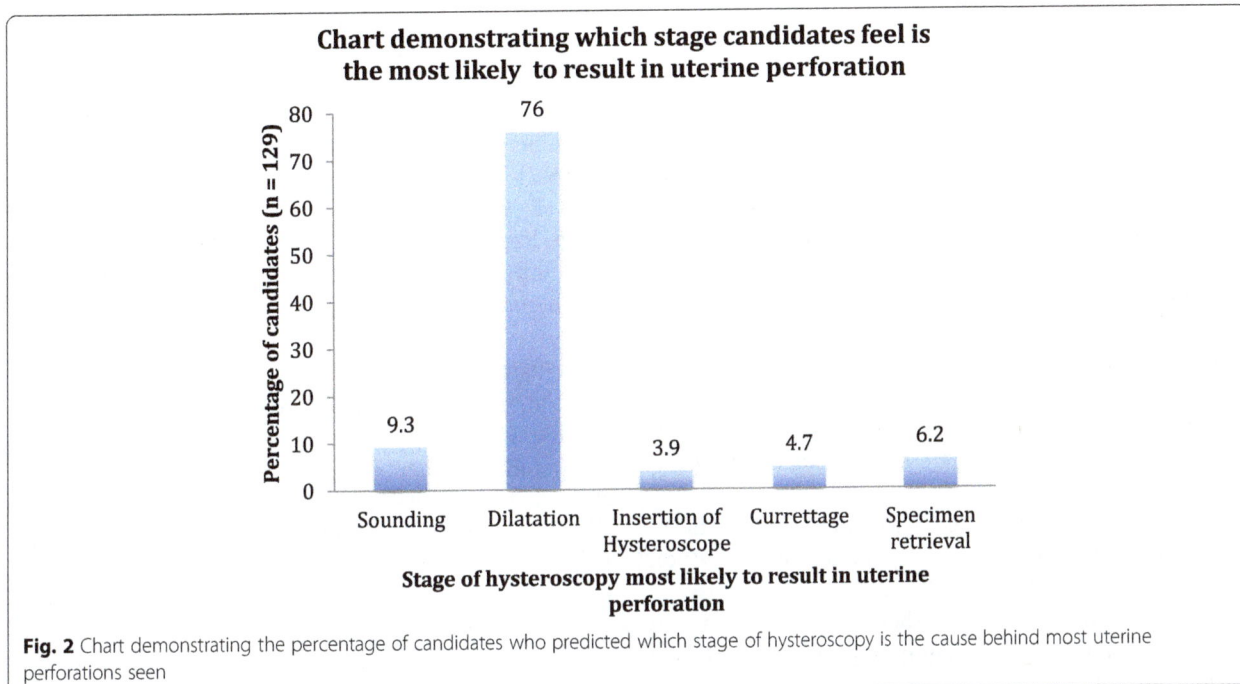

Chart demonstrating which stage candidates feel is the most likely to result in uterine perforation

Percentage of candidates (n = 129)

Stage of hysteroscopy most likely to result in uterine perforation

Fig. 2 Chart demonstrating the percentage of candidates who predicted which stage of hysteroscopy is the cause behind most uterine perforations seen

gradual cervical dilatation is sometimes required in cervical stenosis. Articles report the importance of avoiding excessive force and the use of half-size dilators to reduce the risk of perforation [9]. In the present study, candidates were aware of the risk of dilatation with 76% determining dilatation to be the commonest step to result in uterine perforation; however, 5.2% stated they always perform dilatation prior to insertion of the hysteroscope (Fig. 2).

There is limited information available on how to position the internal cervical os as visualised through the scope when inserting a 30° hysteroscope. This was reflected in the study with only 16.7% knowing the

correct technique. The correct technique to avoid perforation, for an anteverted uterus, is to guide the hysteroscope along the posterior cervical wall keeping the internal os at the 6 o'clock position and in a retroverted uterus to guide the hysteroscope along the anterior cervical wall keeping the internal os at the 12 o'clock position (see Fig. 3). The correct technique not only allows for a smooth procedure but also prevents perforation and creation of a false passage [13]. A review article titled, 'the perforated uterus' published in 2013 highlights the commonest site of uterine perforation being the anterior uterine wall, which was also the commonest response given by candidates in this study [9]. This

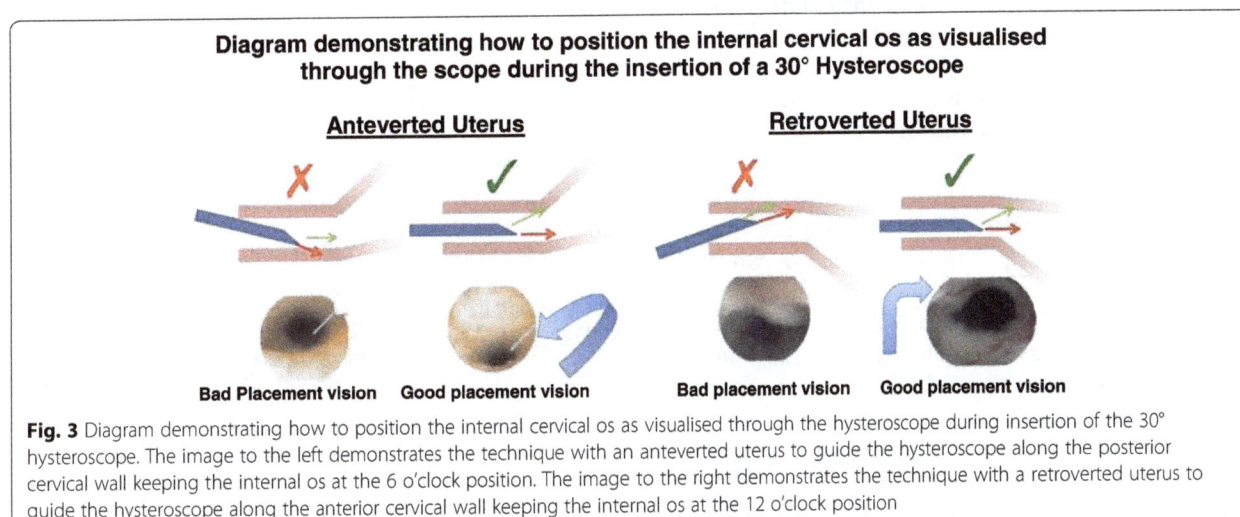

Diagram demonstrating how to position the internal cervical os as visualised through the scope during the insertion of a 30° Hysteroscope

Anteverted Uterus   **Retroverted Uterus**

Bad Placement vision   Good placement vision   Bad placement vision   Good placement vision

Fig. 3 Diagram demonstrating how to position the internal cervical os as visualised through the hysteroscope during insertion of the 30° hysteroscope. The image to the left demonstrates the technique with an anteverted uterus to guide the hysteroscope along the posterior cervical wall keeping the internal os at the 6 o'clock position. The image to the right demonstrates the technique with a retroverted uterus to guide the hysteroscope along the anterior cervical wall keeping the internal os at the 12 o'clock position corresponds to the site of perforation in the retroverted uterus which being the less common uterine anatomy often catches the gynaecologist off guard, highlighting the importance of good technique in determining the attitude of the uterus to avoid this mistake.

Continual advancement in technology and improvement in surgical instruments has resulted in a range of instruments available for specimen retrieval. Some instruments including polyp forceps and curette have a higher chance of uterine perforation due to being a blind procedure compared to myosure and resectoscope, which are performed under direct vision. The survey demonstrates a range of instruments used resulting from different health board funds and training of the staff. It also reflects limited knowledge of the risks of using different instruments.

Post-procedure cavity checks aid identification of an unsuspected uterine perforation. Sudden loss of vision during hysteroscopic procedures due to collapse of the uterus and bleeding together with a large deficit of distension medium is highly suggestive of uterine perforation [9, 11]. In this survey, only 35.8% always perform a post-procedure cavity check and 9% always use suction to aid vision during a post-procedure cavity check.

The study shows a range in practice amongst the different groups of practitioners. In general, a higher proportion of junior and senior registrars (88.9 vs 86.1%) always perform a vaginal examination (VE) compared to the consultants (59.3%) and nurse specialists (33.3%). This is expected as consultants through years of experience, performing multiple hysteroscopies in their working day, do not necessarily perform a VE as they know what to expect. Double the proportion of junior registrars (22.2%) always sound the uterus compared to 10.7% consultants, which might reflect what is being taught to the juniors. A higher proportion of consultants compared to registrars and nurse specialists perform post-procedure cavity checks. This would be expected, as consultants are more likely to do complex operative hysteroscopy with higher risk of perforation.

Strengths and limitations

This study provides a good overview about a national group of physicians and their methods of work. We were looking very specifically at entry techniques and specimen retrieval and hence the questionnaire focussed on this aspect. We did not include questions regarding other complications such as fluid absorption and its implications.

Limitations include a bias towards the practice in Wales as 39% of the responses were from Wales. Even though the study focused on inpatient

hysteroscopy under general anaesthetic, it would have been good to expand on the differences in practice between outpatient hysteroscopy under local anaesthetic and inpatient hysteroscopy under general anaesthetic. Outpatient hysteroscopy uses a vaginoscopic approach; therefore, they are less likely to perform vaginal examination, sounding and dilatation and more likely to use ultrasound. This would help to also differentiate the difference between diagnostic and operative hysteroscopies.

Conclusion

The study highlights varied practice across the UK regarding safety aspects of hysteroscopy, in relation to entry and specimen retrieval. Some gynaecologists are still using questionable techniques. The high percentage of gynaecologists who sound and/or dilate the cervix before hysteroscopy, and the low rate of specialists who correctly know how to position the internal cervical os on the hysteroscope was surprising and raises the question of whether the juniors are being taught the correct techniques. There is a need for increased awareness of the risks of hysteroscopy and paramount precautions that should be performed routinely as part of their practice. Standardised guidelines regarding safety aspects of inpatient diagnostic and operative hysteroscopy, taking into account patient caveats, may be a beneficial tool to help bring about this change in practice, leading to a reduction in uterine perforation rates.

Abbreviations
BMI: Body mass index; BSGE: British Society of Gynaecological Endoscopy; RCOG: Royal College of Obstetricians and Gynaecologists; ST3-7: Speciality-training registrar doctors in their 3rd to 7th year of training; UK: United Kingdom

Acknowledgements
None.

Funding
None required.

Declarations
None declared.

Authors' contributions
LG conceived and designed the study and revised the article for intellectual content. SHW helped design the study, collected the data, completed the statistical analysis and drafted the article. All authors approved the version for publication.

Competing interests
The authors declare that they have no competing interests.

References

1. Jansen FW et al (2000) Complications of hysteroscopy: a prospective, multicenter study. Obstet Gynaecol J 96(2):266–270
2. Best Practice in Outpatient Hysteroscopy (2011) Green-top Guideline No. 59. RCOG/BSGE Joint Guideline
3. Agostini A, Cravello L, Bretelle F, Shohai R, Roger V, Blanc B (2002) Risk of uterine perforation during hysteroscopic surgery. J Am Assoc Gynaecol Laparosc 9(3):264–267
4. Passini A, Belloni C (2001) Intraoperative complications of 697 consecutive operative hysteroscopies. Minerva Gynaecol J 53(1):13–20
5. Petrozza JC (2015) Hysteroscopy Treatment & Management. In: Rivlin ME (ed) eMedicine.com Found at: http://emedicine.medscape.com/article/267021-treatment#d13. Accessed 13 Oct 2017
6. Munro MG, Christianson LA (2015) Complications of hysteroscopic and uterine resectoscopic surgery. Clin Obstet Gynaecol 58(4):765–797
7. Cutner A, Erian J (1996) Who should have outpatient hysteroscopy? Gynaecol Endosc J 5:231–234
8. Paschopoulos M et al (2006) Safety issues of hysteroscopic surgery. N Y Acad Sci 1092:229–234
9. Shakir F, Diab Y (2013) The perforated uterus. Obstet Gynaecol 15:256–261
10. Hulka JF (2008) Surgical techniques: dilatation and curettage. Glob Libr Women's Med. https://doi.org/10.3843/GLOWM.10037
11. Bradley LD, Dayaratna SD (2008) Hysteroscopy. Gynaecol Board Rev Manual 11(4):2–11
12. Crane JMG (2007) How to overcome a resistant cervix for hysteroscopy and endometrial biopsy. Obstet Gynaecol Manag 19(11):37–46
13. Medhekar M Complications in hysteroscopy. Mumbai Obstet Gynaecol Soc Found at: http://www.mogsonline.org/complications_in_enewsletter_article.html. Accessed 13 Oct 2017

21

Surgical outcomes of laparoscopic hysterectomy with concomitant endometriosis without bowel or bladder dissection: a cohort analysis to define a case-mix variable

Evelien M. Sandberg[1], Sara R. C. Driessen[1], Evelien A. T. Bak[1], Nan van Geloven[2], Judith P. Berger[1,3], Mathilde J. G. H. Smeets[3], Johann P. T. Rhemrev[3] and Frank Willem Jansen[1,4,5*]

Abstract

Background: Pelvic endometriosis is often mentioned as one of the variables influencing surgical outcomes of laparoscopic hysterectomy (LH). However, its additional surgical risks have not been well established. The aim of this study was to analyze to what extent concomitant endometriosis influences surgical outcomes of LH and to determine if it should be considered as case-mix variable.

Results: A total of 2655 LH's were analyzed, of which 397 (15.0%) with concomitant endometriosis. For blood loss and operative time, no measurable association was found for stages I ($n = 106$) and II ($n = 103$) endometriosis compared to LH without endometriosis. LH with stages III ($n = 93$) and IV ($n = 95$) endometriosis were associated with more intra-operative blood loss ($p = < .001$) and a prolonged operative time ($p = < .001$) compared to LH without endometriosis. No significant association was found between endometriosis (all stages) and complications ($p = .62$).

Conclusions: The findings of our study have provided numeric support for the influence of concomitant endometriosis on surgical outcomes of LH, without bowel or bladder dissection. Only stages III and IV were associated with a longer operative time and more blood loss and should thus be considered as case-mix variables in future quality measurement tools.

Keywords: Concomitant endometriosis, Laparoscopic hysterectomy, Case-mix correction, Surgical outcome measures

Background

Measuring surgical outcomes to improve quality of health care has received increasing attention over the past decades. Consequently, many national registration systems have been developed to collect hospital data and compare surgical outcomes between hospitals or even surgeons. An important limitation of most of these registrations is the lack of correction of case-mix variables [1]. Case-mix variables are defined as specific patient characteristics that are known to independently influence surgical outcome measures and that are potentially explaining the differences in outcomes between hospitals and/or surgeons [1, 2]. Thus, for an appropriate and reliable interpretation of the surgical outcomes, a case-mix correction is absolutely mandatory.

Specific for the laparoscopic hysterectomy (LH), studies have demonstrated that BMI, uterine weight, and previous procedures influence surgical outcome measures [1, 2]. As a result, a case-mix correction for these variables has been recommended when comparing outcomes of LH [1, 2]. In a recent systematic review on this topic, pelvic endometriosis

* Correspondence: f.w.jansen@lumc.nl
[1]Department of Gynecology, Leiden University Medical Centre, Leiden, the Netherlands
[4]Department BioMechanical Engineering, Delft University of Technology, Delft, the Netherlands
Full list of author information is available at the end of the article

was also found to be a potential factor influencing surgical outcomes of LH [2]. However, no further conclusions on concomitant endometriosis could be drawn in this review as available evidence was limited. Indeed, only three retrospective studies were found that demonstrated an association between endometriosis and prolonged operative time and increased complication risk of LH [3–5]. Furthermore, none of these studies applied a correction for the known case-mix variables, which may have potentially resulted in an over- or underestimation of the impact of endometriosis.

The objective of this study was firstly to analyze to what extent concomitant endometriosis influences surgical outcomes of LH and secondly, to determine if concomitant endometriosis should be considered as case-mix variables in future quality tools.

Methods

In this study, all hysterectomies registered, between April 2014 and September 2016, in the web-based application of QUSUM (https://www.qusum.org) were included [1]. Detailed information on this database has been described elsewhere [1], but briefly, data were obtained by asking gynecologists performing laparoscopic surgery to register anonymously their consecutive LH's for benign indication and low-grade malignancy (e.g., cervical and endometrial dysplasia). All Dutch gynecologists performing LH's were recruited via a personal e-mail invitation, and gynecologists from abroad were asked to participate in the study at international meetings and conferences. The Institutional Review Board (IRB) of Leiden University Medical Centre, Leiden, the Netherlands reviewed the study and exempted it from IRB approval.

To evaluate the association between endometriosis and surgical outcomes, we retrospectively compared surgical outcomes of patients undergoing LH with and without concomitant endometriosis. Only procedures with hysterectomies as only surgery were considered, including LH's with concomitant adnexal surgery. Hysterectomies including bowel or bladder dissection of endometriosis were excluded. Indeed, it did not seem fair to compare these operations to 'simple' LH's for benign indication or low-grade malignancy.

We considered as primary outcomes the following three surgical outcome measures: intra-operative blood loss (ml), operative time (listed as time from incision to closure), and complications (up to 6 weeks postoperatively). Complications were defined according to the internationally accepted classification of the Dutch Society of Obstetrics and Gynecology

(Appendix 1) [6]. The severity of the complications was graded according to the following classification: level A, recovery without reoperation; level B, reoperation indicated; level C, permanent injury and loss of function; level D, death [6]. Only reactive conversions to laparotomy, as defined by Blikkendaal et al., were included [7]. To adequately compare LH's with and without endometriosis, a correction of the three known case-mix variables BMI (kg/m^2), uterine weight (grams), and previous abdominal procedures (previous laparotomy and therapeutic laparoscopy) was applied [2].

For each LH registered in the QUSUM database, we abstracted the data of the three primary outcomes, the three case-mix variables, and the following baseline characteristics: the presence and stage of concomitant endometriosis, the age of the patients at procedure (years), the type of hysterectomy (total laparoscopic hysterectomy (TLH)), supracervical laparoscopic hysterectomy (SLH), laparoscopic-assisted vaginal hysterectomy (LAVH) and robotic hysterectomy (RH)), and the experience of the surgeons (years of experience, number of LH's per year, and total number of LH's performed). Gynecologists were asked to enter the information on experience at initial registration in the web application [1].

Endometriosis was classified into four stages, according to the revised definition of the American Society for Reproductive Medicine [8]. Stage I was defined as minimal endometriosis with only superficial lesions and a few filmy adhesions; stage II, the mild variant, included additional deep lesions in the Douglas cavity; stage III was a moderate stage where, in addition to the previous stages, endometriomas on the ovary are observed together with more dense adhesions. Finally, stage IV, the severe endometriosis, included large endometriomas and extensive adhesions.

Statistics

For the statistical analysis, SPSS version 23.0 (SPSS Inc., Chicago, IL, USA) and R statistical software version 3.3.1 were used [9]. Categorical data were presented as frequency with percentages (%) and continuous data were presented as mean with standard deviation (SD) or as geometric mean with geometric standard deviation (GSD), if data were skewed. To assess significant differences between the baseline characteristics of the group with endometriosis and the one without, independent sample t tests, Fisher's tests, and chi-square with trends were used as appropriate. Statistical significance was defined as a p value $< .05$. A (generalized) linear mixed model regression (univariable and multivariable analysis) was

Table 1 Baseline patient characteristics and surgical outcomes of LH with and without endometriosis

	LH with endometriosis n = 397	LH without endometriosis n = 2258	p value
Patient characteristics			
Age, years, mean ± SD	43.5 ± 7.7	49.8 ± 11.9	< .001
BMI, kg/m², mean ± SD	27.9 ± 5.5	28.6 ± 6.4	.04
Uterine weight, gram, geometric mean; GSD*	149.31 ± 1.8	162.5 ± 2.1	< .001
Previous abdominal procedures, n (%)			< .001
None	152 (38.3)	1290 (57.1)	
One	124 (31.2)	592 (26.2)	
Two	64 (16.1)	234 (10.4)	
> Two	57 (14.4)	142 (6.3)	
Stage of endometriosis, n (%)			
Stage I	106 (26.7)	–	
Stage II	103 (25.9)		
Stage III	93 (23.4)		
Stage IV	95 (23.9)		
Procedure type, n (%)			.03
TLH	376 (94.7)	2036 (90.2)	
SLH	13 (3.3)	109 (4.8)	
LAVH	6 (1.5)	88 (3.9)	
Robotic	2 (0.5)	25 (1.1)	
Surgical outcomes			
Blood loss (ml), geometric mean; GSD*	80 ± 3.1	67 ± 3.4	ϕ
Operative time (min), geometric mean; GSD*	94 ± 1.5	91 ± 1.5	ϕ
Complications, n (%)	24 in 22 patients (5.5%)	175 in 153 patients (6.8%)	ϕ
Lesion			
Bladder	3 (0.8)	27 (1.2)	
Ureter	1 (0.3)	9 (0.4)	
Vessel	–	1 (< 0.1)	
Bowel	2 (0.5)	7 (0.3)	
Hemorrhage	5 (1.3)	41 (1.8)	
> 1000 mL intra-operative	5 (1.3)	13 (0.6)	
Wound dehiscence	–	6 (0.3)	
Thrombosis	–	3 (0.1)	
Dysfunction ileus	–	2 (0.1)	
Infections	1 (0.3)	50 (2.2)	
Dysfunction incontinence	–	10 (0.4)	
Other	2 (0.5)	11 (0.5)	
Conversion	10 (2.5)	8 (0.4)	.16

Table 1 Baseline patient characteristics and surgical outcomes of LH with and without endometriosis (Continued)

	LH with endometriosis n = 397	LH without endometriosis n = 2258	p value
Severity of complications, n (%)			
Level A–recovery	18 (4.5)	113 (5.0)	
Level B–reoperation	3 (0.8)	39 (1.7)	
Level C–permanent injury	1 (0.3)	0	
Level D–death	0	1 (< 0.1)	

Data are presented as number (percentage) or as mean ± standard deviation or as geometric mean (GM) with geometric standard deviation (GSD)
Interpretation of the GSD: 95% of the data are expected to lie in the range of GM/(GSD)² to GM(GSD)²
Statistics: independent t test for continuous data; Fisher's test for categorical data; chi-square with trend for number of previous procedures
ϕThis means that for every tenfold increase in uterine weight, blood loss and operative time increased by the stated percentages and odds of complication increased by the stated OR
SD standard deviation, GSD geometric standard deviation, LH laparoscopic hysterectomy, TLH total laparoscopic hysterectomy, SLH supracervical laparoscopic hysterectomy, LAVH laparoscopic-assisted vaginal hysterectomy

performed to define the association between endometriosis and surgical outcomes. The case-mix variables BMI, uterine weight, and previous procedures were included as co-variables [1, 10]. The characteristic "previous procedures" was dichotomized into no previous procedures or at least one. Data with a skewed distribution were transformed for analysis into log values. We found that blood loss, operative time, and uterine weight needed a log transformation, which resulted in normalization of the distribution. In 55 cases (including five patients with endometriosis) surgeons reported no blood loss after procedure (0 ml). Blood loss was therefore transformed into $\log(x + 1)$.

To correct for the fact that surgeons entered various procedures, analyses were performed with a random intercept for the performing surgeon. For blood loss and operative time, findings of the regression analyses were presented as percentage increase or decrease with 95% confidence interval (95% CI). The results for complication risk were reported as odds ratio with 95% CI. To make data easier to interpret, an index patient was used to demonstrate the additional effect of the different stages of endometriosis on surgical outcomes. The other case-mix characteristics of this index patient were fixed and based on the mean values of the entire cohort.

Results

During the study period, a total of 2655 LH's were analyzed of which 397 cases (15.0%) with concomitant endometriosis. Table 1 gives an overview of the baseline patient characteristics and surgical outcomes. Patients in the endometriosis group were younger (43.5

(7.7) versus 49.5 (11.9), $p < .001$), had lower uterine weight (149.3 (1.8) gram versus 162.5 (2.1), $p < .001$), lower BMI (27.9 (5.5) versus 28.6 (6.4), $p = .04$), and had had more previous abdominal surgeries (61.6 versus 42.9%, $p < .001$).

Most of the hysterectomies performed were TLH (94.7% in the endometriosis group versus 90.2%). The four stages of endometriosis were almost equally divided in the group with endometriosis (stage I: $n = 106$ (26.7%); stage II: $n = 103$ (25.9%); stage III: $n = 93$ (23.4%); stage IV: $n = 95$ (23.9%)). A total of 199 complications occurred in 175 patients (6.6%), including 22 patients with endometriosis. Regarding the severity of the complications, no difference between the group with and without endometriosis was observed ($p = .16$). Specifically, no increased risk was observed in the endometriosis group for the different organ injuries (bladder, ureter, and bowel). No p values were calculated for the three primary surgical outcomes, as these data were used in the regression analysis (Table 3).

As demonstrated in Table 2, a total of 93 surgeons registered on average 33 (30.6) procedures during the study period, performed yearly 31 (17.5) LH's and had on average 6 years (4.5) of experience. As the data were entered anonymously, it is unknown how many hospitals were involved. A significant difference was observed for the overall surgical experience and LH's performed with and without endometriosis ($p < .001$). In 50.1% of the cases with endometriosis, procedures were performed by surgeons with an experience of at least 200 LH's, compared to 34.8% in the group without endometriosis. Of note, no significant correlation was observed between the number of LH's registered in the application and the overall experience of the surgeons (Spearman's rho = 0.145, $p = .169$, Appendix 2).

Table 3 summarizes the association between the different case-mix variables, the stages of endometriosis, and surgical outcomes, using the mixed model regression analysis (univariate and multivariate analysis). For BMI, uterine weight and previous abdominal procedures, significant associations were observed with blood loss and operative time. Regarding endometriosis, we demonstrated that for blood loss and operative time, no measurable association was found for stages I and II endometriosis compared to LH's without endometriosis (geometric mean blood loss: no endometriosis: 67 (3.4) mL; stage I: 71.4 (3.2), $p = .48$; stage II: 79.0 (2.8), $p = .10$; operative time: no endometriosis 90.6 (1.5) min; stage I: 88.1 (1.5), $p = .23$; stage II: 81.9 (1.5), $p = .68$). Compared to LH's without endometriosis, LH's with stage III and IV endometriosis were associated with more intra-operative blood loss (stage III: 70 (3.6), $p = .01$) and stage IV: 106.4 (2.9), $p = <.001$) and a prolonged operative time (stage III: 95.1 (1.5), $p = <.001$ and stage IV: 117.6 (1.6), $p = <.001$). No significant association was found between endometriosis (all stages) and complication rates ($p = .62$).

For an index patient with stage IV endometriosis, a mean intra-operative blood loss of 140.8 ml (109.4–180.9) was expected compared to a mean of 65.7 ml (57.2–75.6) for a patient with the same characteristics but without endometriosis. Also, an additional mean operative time of 47 min was demonstrated for an

Table 2 Surgeon's characteristics

Surgeon characteristics*	Total $n = 93$ surgeons$^\phi$			
Number of procedures registered in QUSUM	33 (30.6), (1–130)			
Number of procedures per year	31 (17.5), (10–140)			
Years of experience	6 (4.5), (0–21)			
Overall experience	160 (158.9), (0–800)			
Total surgical experience for the LH's with and without endometriosis**	Total $n = 93$ surgeons$^\phi$	LH's with endometriosis $n = 397$	LH's without endometriosis $n = 2258$ LH	p value
Overall experience				< .001
0–99	42 (45.2)	125 (31.5)	954 (43.4)	
100–199	21 (22.6)	73 (18.4)	518 (21.8)	
200–299	10 (10.8)	99 (24.9)	347 (15.4)	
≥ 300	19 (20.4)	100 (25.2)	437 (19.4)	

*Data are presented as mean (SD), (minimum-maximum)
**Data are presented as number (percentage)
$^\phi$For one surgeon no information on experience was available
Statistics: chi-square test for trend
LH laparoscopic hysterectomy
Number of procedures per year is the number of LH they perform an average on a yearly basis
Years of experience is defined as the number of years of experience since they have finished residency
Overall experience is defined as the total number of LH's performed by a gynecologist during his or her career as attending, including the teaching cases

Table 3 Influence of each covariate on blood loss, operative time and complications

Blood loss	(Geometric) mean + (G)SD[§] or number (%)	Crude analysis		Adjusted analysis		
		Percentage increase (95% CI)	p value of univariate analysis	Percentage increase (95% CI)	Index patient* Data expressed in ml (95% CI)	p value of multivariate analysis
Patient characteristics		–				
[10]LOG uterine weight[φ]	153.6; 2.0			84.8 (74.5–95.4)		< .001
BMI (increase/1 kg/m²)	28.5 ± 6.2			2.4 (1.8–3.0)		< .001
Previous procedures		–				
Yes (versus no)	1213 (45.7)			13.1 (4.3–22.6)		< .001
Stage of endometriosis			< .001			< .001
No endometriosis	67.3; 3.4	Reference		Reference	65.7 (57.2–75.6)	
Stage I	71.4; 3.2	4.9 (−16.1–31.2)	.68	7.6 (− 12.3–31.9)	70.7 (55.7–89.7)	.48
Stage II	79.0; 2.8	16.0 (− 7.3–44.9)	.20	18.8 (− 3.2–45.6)	78.0 (61.4–99.2)	.10
Stage III	70.0; 3.6	27.9 (1–62.1)	.04	34.0 (8.0–66.4)	88.1 (68.7–113.0)	.01
Stage IV	106.4; 2.9	98.8 (56.7–152.4)	< .001	114.3 (72.1–166.7)	140.8 (109.4–180.9)	< .001
Operative time	Number (%)	Percentage increase (95% CI)	P-value of univariate analysis	Percentage increase (95% CI)	Index patient* Data expressed in min (95% CI)	p value of multivariate analysis
Patient characteristics		–				
[10]LOG uterine weight[φ]				20.0 (18.1–21.8)		< .001
BMI (increase/1 kg/m²)				1.0 (0.8–1.2)		< .001
Previous procedures		–				
Yes (versus no)				3.8 (1.5–6.1)		<.001
Stage of endometriosis			< 0.001			< .001
No endometriosis	90.6; 1.5	Reference		Reference	92.0 (87.4–96.9)	
Stage I	88.1; 1.5	− 4.4 (− 10.1–1.7)	.16	− 3.3 (− 8.6–2.1)	88.9 (82.7–95.7)	.23
Stage II	81.9; 1.5	0.3 (− 5.7–6.7)	.93	1.2 (− 4.3–6.9)	93.1 (86.5–100.3)	.68
Stage III	95.1; 1.5	15.3 (8.0–23.1)	< .001	17.0 (10.3–24.0)	107.7 (99.8–116.2)	< .001
Stage IV	117.6; 1.6	47.6 (38.0–57.6)	< .001	51.0 (42.3–60.3)	139.1 (128.8–150.1)	< .001
Complications	Number (%)	Odds ratio (95% CI)	p value of univariate analysis	Odds ratio (95% CI)	–	p value of multivariate analysis
Patient characteristics		–				
[10]LOG uterine weight[φ]				0.69 (0.56–0.82)		< .001
BMI (increase/1 kg/m²)				1.00 (0.98–1.03)		.935
Previous procedures		–				
Yes (versus no)				1.17 (0.87–1.58)		.305
Stage of endometriosis			.72			.62
No endometriosis	153 (6.8)	Reference		Reference		
Stage I (versus no)	5 (2.9)	1.27 (0.55–2.95)	.57	1.27 (0.54–2.98)		.59
Stage II	7 (4.0)	0.69 (0.33–1.43)	.32	0.67 (0.32–1.36)		.26

Table 3 Influence of each covariate on blood loss, operative time and complications *(Continued)*

		Crude analysis		Adjusted analysis	
Stage III	4 (2.3)	1.23 (0.48–3.10)0.76	.67	1.16 (0.45–2.96)	.76
Stage IV	6 (3.4)	(0.34–1.65)	.48	0.67 (0.30–1.50)	.34

§Interpretation of the geometric standard deviation (GSD): 95% of the data are expected to lie in the range of GM/(GSD)^2 to GM*(GSD)^2
*Index patient with BMI of 28.5, uterine weight of 161.3 g, and 50% previous procedures
ⱷThis means that for every tenfold increase in uterine weight, blood loss, and operative time increased by the stated percentages and odds of complication increased by the stated OR
Statistics: linear mixed model (for outcome blood loss and operative time) and generalized linear mixed model (with logistic link function) (for outcome complications)
95% CI 95% confidence interval
BMI body mass index, *GM* geometric mean, *GSD* geometric standard deviation

index patient with stage IV endometriosis compared to a patient with the same characteristics but without endometriosis (139.1 min (128.8–150.1) versus 92 min (87.4–96.9)).

Discussion
Main findings
In this present study, we demonstrated that LH with concomitant stages I or II endometriosis had no measurable and clinical relevant associations with surgical outcome measures compared to LH without endometriosis. Stages III and IV endometriosis, however, appeared to be of influence for the outcomes blood loss and operative time.

Strengths and limitations
A limitation of our study was that gynecologists registered themselves the procedures and that these data could not be verified as entered anonymously. As a result, we cannot guarantee that the surgeons included all their consecutive cases. Yet, this is similar to daily clinical practice where data are also entered by the surgeons. Moreover, previous studies have shown that these self-reported data are often accurate and reliable [10, 11].

Another limitation is the fact that information regarding the setting, the indication of surgery, or the participation of a fellow or resident during the procedure was missing. This might have biased the outcomes. Although these data would have been interesting, the baseline characteristics (BMI, uterine weight, and previous procedures), known to influence outcomes were analyzed and therefore we believe our comparison is reliable. Regarding the participation of a trainee we believe that it is the responsibility of the principle surgeon to judge if his or her involvement remains acceptable and therefore, no correction for this factor was applied. Additionally, it would have been interesting to know if surgeons knew pre-operatively of the presence of endometriosis as this

might be relevant for the choice of the surgeon and the surgical planning.

Although the outcome "previous surgeries" has been demonstrated to be associated with worse surgical outcome [2, 10], collecting data on adhesions would have been interesting as well. The advantage of the registration we used was that the number of previous procedures was an objective measure, whereas adhesions and their grading would have been more at risk for intra-observer variations [12]. Finally, in our study, surgery with bowel and bladder dissection of endometriosis was excluded. This might have resulted in an underestimation of the impact of endometriosis on surgery in general. Our data should thus not be generalized to all endometriosis cases but are limited to LH with concomitant endometriosis. Because the aim of our study was to determine the influence of concomitant endometriosis during LH, we believe that it would not be correct to compare these advanced cases to hysterectomies for benign indication or low-grade malignancy. Similar studies should be performed analyzing specifically surgical outcomes of procedures with bladder and/or bowel dissections. Strengths of this study included the relatively large database and number of cases with endometriosis. Also, the high number of surgeons with varying experience adds to the generalizability of the data.

Interpretation
Although endometriosis is often mentioned as complicating factor during LH, the additional surgical risks associated with LH's with concomitant endometriosis have not been well established. Yet, for a reliable interpretation and comparison of surgical outcome measures between surgeons and/or hospitals, numeric support of the impact of concomitant endometriosis during LH is necessary. This is also relevant for determining if concomitant endometriosis should be considered a case-mix variable. In this study, we firstly demonstrated that stages III and IV

endometriosis were associated with more intra-operative blood loss compared to the group without endometriosis. This finding has, to our knowledge, not been observed in previous studies [3–5, 10]. Although the amount of blood loss was twice as much in the group with stage IV endometriosis compared to the group without, the mean blood loss was still low (141 mL for stage IV). The clinical relevancy for patients is therefore questionable, yet, for the surgeons, it is important to be aware of this potentially increased amount of blood loss. Furthermore, our finding demonstrated that concomitant endometriosis independently influence surgical outcome and therefore should be taken into consideration when applying a case-mix correction.

In agreement with previous studies [4, 13], stages III and IV endometriosis was associated with a prolonged operative time, up to 47 min for stage IV endometriosis. This finding is important to consider for pre-operatively scheduling but also as prolonged operative time has been associated with increased morbidity [14, 15]. One study even demonstrated that every additional hour of surgery during LH increases the risk of postoperative complications by 22% [15].

Regarding complications, previous studies have demonstrated an increased risk for LH's with endometriosis compared to LH's without endometriosis. [3–5, 13] Specifically for LH's with moderate-severe endometriosis (stages III and IV), one of the studies showed an almost fourfold increase in the risk of complications compared to controls [13]. Interestingly, in our study, no significant difference in complication risk was observed (5.5% for the endometriosis group versus 6.8% for the non-endometriosis group). This could be explained by the fact that in previous studies, patients undergoing bowel and bladder resection were included. Other explanations could be related to the overall low number of complications in our study and hence the lack of power to demonstrate a significant difference and/or the high surgical experience for LH with endometriosis [16]. Indeed, LH's with stages III and IV endometriosis were significantly more often performed by surgeons with more experience, and this might have affected the outcomes. However, we explicitly did not correct for surgical experience in our model as we aimed to demonstrate how patient's characteristics independently influence surgical outcomes. In daily clinical practice, surgical experience cannot be used either to justify worse surgical outcomes. We want to underline that it is the responsibility of the surgeon to know his individual limitations when counseling a patient. This pre-operative awareness was reflected in our study as most severe endometriosis cases were performed by the more experienced surgeons, and this selection most probably has improved overall surgical outcomes. However, it is important to keep in mind that a high surgical volume does not necessarily directly stand for better surgical outcomes [1]. Although high surgical experience is often associated with positive outcomes, it is not a guarantee. As such, we would recommend surgeons to monitor their individual surgical performances over time rather than to focus on the number of surgeries Table 4 [1].

Conclusions

For a reliable comparison of surgical outcomes between hospitals and/or surgeons, it is necessary to correct for the patient characteristics that are independently influencing these outcomes. For LH, previous studies have already demonstrated that a case-mix correction for BMI, uterine weight, and previous procedures is required [1, 2]. The findings of our study have provided numeric support for the influence of concomitant endometriosis on the surgical outcomes of LH. We demonstrated that stages III and IV endometriosis were associated with a longer operative time and more blood loss. These specific stages should thus be considered as case-mix variable for these outcomes in future quality measurement tools.

Appendix 1

Table 4 Complication classification according to the NVOG

Main category	Complication
Infection	- Local - Organ - Systemic
Injury	- Vascular - Bowel - Bladder - Ureter - Other
Wound dehiscence	–
Hemorrhage	- > 1000 mL - Post-operative bleeding
Thrombo-embolism	–
Dysfunction	- Urinary retention - Incontinence - Ileus - Liver - Kidney
Systemic	- Medication error - Adverse drug event - Other
Technical	- Failed procedure - Retained foreign body
Reactive conversion	–
Other	–

Appendix 2

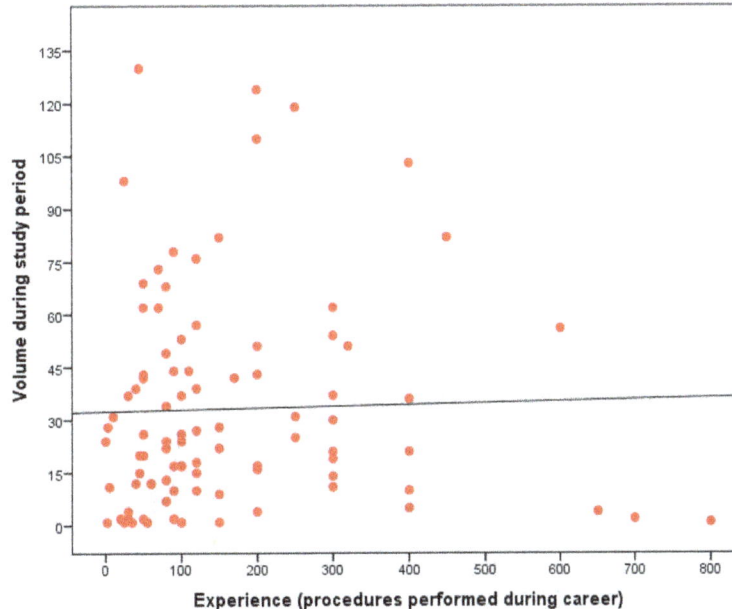

Fig. 1 Scatter plot presenting surgeon's experience versus the number of procedures registered during the study

Acknowledgements
None

Funding
Evelien M. Sandberg has received a research grant from the Bronovo
Research Fund (Bronovo Hospital, the Hague, the Netherlands). The funding
source had no involvement in the conduct of the study.

Authors' contributions
All authors contributed to the work presented in this paper. EMS was
responsible for the project development, the acquisition, analysis and
interpretation of data, as well as the drafting and finalization of the
manuscript. EATB and SRCD were also responsible for the acquisition of data
and contributed to the analysis and interpretation of the data as well as the
finalization of the manuscript. NvG contributed to the analysis and
interpretation of data as well as the finalization of the manuscript. JPB,
MJGHS, and JPTR contributed to the acquisition, the analysis and
interpretation of data as well as the finalization of the manuscript. FWJ was
responsible for the conception of the study and contributed to the
acquisition and interpretation of data and the finalization of the manuscript.
All authors take responsibility for this study and its findings. All authors read
and approved the final manuscript.

Competing interests
The authors declare that they have no competing interests.

Author details
[1]Department of Gynecology, Leiden University Medical Centre, Leiden, the
Netherlands. [2]Department of Medical Statistics, Leiden University Medical
Centre, Leiden, the Netherlands. [3]Department of Gynecology, Haaglanden
Medical Centre, the Hague, the Netherlands. [4]Department BioMechanical
Engineering, Delft University of Technology, Delft, the Netherlands.
[5]Department of Gynecology, Minimally Invasive Surgery, Leiden University
Medical Centre, PO Box 9600, 2300, RC, Leiden, the Netherlands.

References
1. Driessen SR, van Zwet EW, Haazebroek P et al (2016) A dynamic quality
    assessment tool for laparoscopic hysterectomy to measure surgical
    outcomes. Am J Obstet Gynecol 2016;215(6):754.e1-754.e8
2. Driessen SR, Sandberg EM, la Chapelle CF, Twijnstra AR, Rhemrev JP,
    Jansen FW (2016) Case-mix variables and predictors for outcomes of
    laparoscopic hysterectomy: a systematic review. J Minim Invasive
    Gynecol 23:317-330
3. Brummer TH, Jalkanen J, Fraser J et al (2011) FINHYST, a prospective study
    of 5279 hysterectomies: complications and their risk factors. Hum Reprod
    26:1741-1751
4. Song T, Kim TJ, Kang H et al (2012) Factors associated with
    complications and conversion to laparotomy in women undergoing
    laparoscopically assisted vaginal hysterectomy. Acta Obstet Gynecol
    Scand 91:620-624
5. Patzkowsky KE, As-Sanie S, Smorgick N, Song AH, Advincula AP (2013)
    Perioperative outcomes of robotic versus laparoscopic hysterectomy for
    benign disease. JSLS 17:100-106
6. Twijnstra AR, Zeeman GG, Jansen FW (2010) A novel approach to
    registration of adverse outcomes in obstetrics and gynaecology: a feasibility
    study. Qual Saf Health Care 19:132-137
7. Blikkendaal MD, Twijnstra AR, Stiggelbout AM, Beerlage HP, Bemelman WA,
    Jansen FW (2013) Achieving consensus on the definition of conversion to
    laparotomy: a Delphi study among general surgeons, gynecologists, and
    urologists. Surg Endosc 27:4631-4639
8. American Society for Reproductive Medicine (1997) Revised American
    Society for Reproductive Medicine classification of endometriosis: 1996.
    Fertil Steril 67:817-821
9. R Development Core Team (2008). R: A language and environment for
    statistical computing. R Foundation for Statistical Computing, Vienna,
    Austria. http://www.R-project.org
10. Twijnstra AR, Blikkendaal MD, van Zwet EW, van Kesteren PJ, de Kroon CD,
    Jansen FW (2012) Predictors of successful surgical outcome in laparoscopic
    hysterectomy. Obstet Gynecol 119:700-708
11. Van Leersum NJ, Snijders HS, Henneman D et al (2013) The Dutch surgical
    colorectal audit. Eur J Surg Oncol 39:1063-1070

12. Corson SL, Batzer FR, Gocial B, Kelly M, Gutmann JN, Maislin G (1995) Intra-observer and inter-observer variability in scoring laparoscopic diagnosis of pelvic adhesions. Hum Reprod 10:161–164

13. Uccella S, Marconi N, Casarin J et al (2016) Impact of endometriosis on surgical outcomes and complications of total laparoscopic hysterectomy. Arch Gynecol Obstet 294:771–778

14. Catanzarite T, Saha S, Pilecki MA, Kim JY, Milad MP (2015) Longer operative time during benign laparoscopic and robotic hysterectomy is associated with increased 30-day perioperative complications. J Minim Invasive Gynecol 22:1049–1058

15. Hanwright PJ, Mioton LM, Thomassee MS et al (2013) Risk profiles and outcomes of total laparoscopic hysterectomy compared with laparoscopically assisted vaginal hysterectomy. Obstet Gynecol 121:781–787

16. Maruthappu M, Gilbert BJ, El-Harasis MA et al (2015) The influence of volume and experience on individual surgical performance: a systematic review. Ann Surg 261:642–647

22

Survey among ESGE members on leiomyosarcoma morcellation incidence

Vasilios Tanos[1,2]* ⓘ, Hans Brölmann[3†], Rudi Leon DeWilde[4†], Peter O'Donovan[5†], Elina Symeonidou[6†] and Rudi Campo[7†]

Abstract

Background: Increased awareness of leiomyosarcoma (LMS) risk during myomectomy or hysterectomy is essential. Objective and correct reasoning should prevail on any decision regarding the extent and type of surgery to employ. The anticipated risk of a sarcoma after myoma or uterus morcellation is low, and the frequency of leiomyosarcoma especially in women below the age of 40 is very rare. The prevalence data has a wide range and is therefore not reliable. The European Society of Gynaecological Endoscopy (ESGE) initiated a survey among its members looking into the frequency of morcellated leiomyosarcoma after endoscopic surgery.

The ESGE Central office sent 3422 members a structured electronic questionnaire with multiple answer choices for each question. After 3 months, the answers were classified with a unique number in the EXCEL spread sheet. Statistical analysis was done using the SPSS v.18.

Results: Out of 3422 members, 294 (8.6%) gynaecologists replied to the questionnaire; however, only 240 perform myomectomies by laparoscopy and hysteroscopy and hysterectomies by laparoscopy. The reported experience in performing laparoscopic myomectomy, hysteroscopic myomectomy, laparoscopic hysterectomy (LH), and laparoscopic subtotal hysterectomy (LSH) on an average was 10.8 (1–32) years. The vast majority of 67.1% had over 5 years of practice in laparoscopic surgery. The total number of 221 leiomyosarcoma was reported among 429,777 minimally invasive surgeries (laparoscopic and hysteroscopic myomectomies and LH and LSH), performed by all doctors in their lifetime. The overall reported sarcoma risk of all types of endoscopic myoma surgeries has been estimated to be 1.5% of operations which is very rare. Categorizing by type, 57 (0.06%) LMS were operated by laparoscopic myomectomy and 54 (0.07%) by hysteroscopic myomectomy, while 38 (0.13%) leiomyosarcoma operated by laparoscopic subtotal hysterectomy and 72 (0.31%) by laparoscopic hysterectomy. The probability of a sarcoma after morcellation to be falsely diagnosed by histopathology as a benign tumour and later identified as a sarcoma in a later examination has been reported and calculated to be 0.2%. The low risk of a sarcoma is also reflected by the small number of surgeries, where only 32 doctors reported that they operated once, 29 twice, and 18 operated on 3–10 sarcomas by laparoscopy during their lifetime.

Conclusion: The survey demonstrated that myomectomy by hysteroscopy or laparoscopy has similar risks of sarcoma with an estimated incidence of 0.07%, much lower than that by laparoscopic hysterectomy and subtotal hysterectomy. Hence, for young patients with myoma infertility problem and low risk for LMS, myomectomy by MIS can be the first option of treatment. The fact that only 12.5% (216/1728) of uterine sarcoma cases are operated laparoscopically demonstrates the surgeons' awareness and alertness about LMS and the potential of spreading sarcomatous cells after myoma/uterus power morcellation.

Keywords: Leiomyoma uteri, Leiomyosarcoma, Leiomyosarcoma incidence, Laparoscopy, Morcellation, Power morcellation complication

* Correspondence: v.tanos@aretaeio.com
†Equal contributors
[1]St. Georges Medical School, Nicosia University, Nicosia, Cyprus
[2]Department of Obstetrics and Gynaecology, Aretaeio Hospital, Nicosia, Cyprus
Full list of author information is available at the end of the article

Background

Morcellation has been used for a long time during minimally invasive surgery (MIS) to extract pathological tissue from the abdominal cavity through a trocar or via the vagina. The FDA did a meta-analysis of the data from 18 studies and reported a risk of a uterine sarcoma in patients with presumed fibroids to be 0.28% [1]. It was then advised to avoid morcellation of uterine myomas suspicious for sarcoma in order to prevent the spread of sarcomatous cells and upstaging of the cancer status of the patient. The professional community and representatives of many scientific societies published their opinions on the matter [2–7], however, were unable to unanimously recommend for or against laparoscopic myomectomy or hysterectomy due to lack of solid scientific data. The dilemma of whether to counsel patients with fibroids to choose laparoscopic surgery with its established benefits or laparotomy to escape the small risks related to fibroid morcellation is still an open discussion [8].

Uterine fibroids are a common disorder with an estimated incidence of 20–40% in women during their reproductive years [9, 10]. In contrast, leiomyosarcoma (LMS) of the uterus is a rare entity with an annual incidence quoted between 0.014–0.28% [1, 11, 12]. Excluding the carcinosarcoma or Mixed Müllerian Tumour (MMT), LMS accounts for 70% and stromal sarcoma for 30% of all uterine sarcomas [13]. The true prevalence of uterine sarcoma in presumed fibroids is not known, and meta-analyses based on retrospective trials have shown a wide range of prevalence (0.014–0.45%). Age and certain imaging characteristics such as 'lacunes' suggesting necrosis and increased central vascularisation of the tumour are associated with a relatively higher risk of uterine sarcoma, although the overall risk remains low. There is not enough evidence to estimate this risk in individual patients [8]. Uterine sarcomas represent 2–7% of all uterine malignancies. Reliable figures for the incidence of smooth muscle tumours of unknown malignant potential (STUMP) and cellular fibroids are poorly documented. A LMS may spread locally, regionally, or by haematogenous dissemination. Local and regional spread may result in an abdominal or pelvic tumour causing gastrointestinal and/or urinary tract symptoms. Haematogenous dissemination most often spreads to the lungs. LMS typically appears around a median age of 50–55 years and is highly malignant, and in most cases, recurrences are detected within 2 years. A major prognostic factor is the extent of tumour spread [13]. Five-year survival ranges from 17 to 55%. Survival of patients with a LMS is strongly associated with the number of mitoses per 10 high power fields (× 100 magnification): 1–4, 98%; 5–9, 42%; ≥10; 15%. A LMS embedded and confined to the uterus that is removed 'end bloc' is associated with a better survival rate of up to 83% [14, 15].

Increased awareness of sarcoma risk is essential, but objective and correct reasoning should predominate any decision regarding the extent and type of surgery selected. The currently available data on prevalence of a LMS when operating on a presumed leiomyoma is imprecise and unreliable. Recently, Pritts et al. analysed 67 prospective studies in which 5951 women underwent surgery for fibroids and only two were found to have LMS (1 in 2975 or 0.03%). When they analysed an additional 66 retrospective studies, out of 23,926 women having surgery for fibroids, 22 were found to have LMS (1 in 1087 or 0.09%) [15].

The European Society of Gynaecological Endoscopy (ESGE), in an effort to be as objective as possible, initiated a survey among its members to collect data from each centre and surgeon individually. The survey results have assisted in the evaluation of sarcoma frequency after myoma morcellation in absolute numbers, reflecting European surgeons' current endoscopic surgery practices.

Methods

The ESGE central office sent its 3422 members a structured electronic questionnaire with multiple answer choices in July, 2014. Free text options and comments were also available for some of the questions. A letter accompanied the questionnaire (see Table 1) explaining the reason for the survey and read as follows: "Recently case reports on fibroid morcellation disseminating unexpected malignancy attracted the attention of gynaecologists but also public attention mainly through various websites. ESGE, in an effort to gain more information on that very rare neoplasia but also critical issue, would like to run a survey among its members in order to be able to give more information and advice to gynaecologists performing laparoscopic surgery. The doctors were asked to answer the questions, taking into consideration their management on symptomatic fibroids and/or enlarged uterus before the press release from the FDA."

Using the ESGE server and website, in conjunction with the "Survey Monkey" programme, the central office sent the questionnaire out electronically. By mid-September 2014, the survey was closed and the doctors who responded were automatically identified in an EXCEL spread sheet. E-mail addresses were used for the identification of each individual, while a serial number was also used to separate and establish the study group, thereby avoiding mistakes and enabling anonymous statistical analysis.

The probability of LMS was based on the average of individual results from each gynaecologist. The probability of a surgeon identifying a sarcoma while performing MIS (any type of surgery) has been estimated individually based on the total number of sarcomas divided by the total number of surgeries performed in a lifetime (number of surgeries performed annually multiplied by

Table 1 Descriptive statistics according to survey questions

Questions	Number of answers	Mean	Mode	Standard deviation	Sum	Pearson's correlation coefficient	
Q1: How many years have you been practicing laparoscopic myomectomy and hysterectomy?	240	10.78	5	7.265	2587		
Q2: How many uterine sarcomas have received a laparoscopic surgical approach?	280	.77	0	2.023	216	Q3	.427
						Q5	.451
						Q9	.461
Q3: How many uterine sarcomas have you seen in your lifetime practice?	280	6.17	2	9.008	1728	Q2	.427
Q4: How many laparoscopic myomectomies do you perform annually?	238	29.08	0	47.632	6920	Q5	.412
Q5: How many sarcomas did you encounter until today after laparoscopic myomectomies?	236	.24	0	.916	57	Q2	.451
						Q4	.412
						Q9	.492
Q6: How many laparoscopic subtotal hysterectomies you do per year?	237	28.81	0	52.492	6828	Q7	.484
Q7: How many sarcomas did you have until today after laparoscopic subtotal hysterectomies?	236	.16	0	.470	38	Q6	.484
Q8: How many laparoscopic hysterectomies you do per year?	237	43.90	30	49.018	10.404		
Q9: How many sarcomas did you have until today after laparoscopic hysterectomies?	235	.31	0	1.191	72	Q2	.461
						Q5	.492
Q10: How many hysteroscopic myomectomies do you perform annually?	233	31.10	20	29.233	7246		
Q11: How many sarcomas did you encounter until today after hysteroscopic myomectomies?	234	.23	0	1.087	54		
Q12: Myomectomy cases reported as leiomyoma and review of the slides revealed a sarcoma	233	.19	0	.556	44		

the years of practice). The overall probability is the average of each individual probability of sarcoma, presenting the mean of the means of each individual.

Statistical analysis

The statistical analysis was performed by using SPSS v.18 (Statistical Package for Social Sciences). The first part of the questionnaire consisted of 12 open-ended questions. Descriptive statistics (mean, mode, standard deviation, and sum) and frequency charts (bar charts) are used in order to give a screenshot of the sampled data. In order to present the data in bar charts, the quantitative data have been categorized in an ordinal form. Correlations, calculated with Pearson's correlation coefficient, are used as raw data (not categorized) in order to find the interaction between the answers. Pearson's correlation coefficient takes values between -1 and 1, where -1 proves strong negative correlation between the answers, zero value (0) shows no correlation and 1 proves strong positive correlation (Table 1). Where correlation coefficient exceeds or is close to $|1|$, the correlation is considered to be strong, and where the significance value (p value) is less than 0.01 is considered

to be statistically significant. Correlations are also visualized through clustered bar charts. Based on the sampled data, the probability of fact occurrence is also calculated.

Results

Out of 3422 ESGE members who received the questionnaire, 294 responded (8.6%) to the survey call. A total of 280 (95.2%) members were included in the final statistical analysis. Forty doctors received a second invitation because of incomplete survey answer. At the end, 14 respondents could not be included. Among 280 responders, 240 reported experience performing laparoscopic hysterectomies, myomectomies, and hysteroscopic myoma resections. The reported average experience in MIS was 10.7 years while the vast majority 67.1% had over 5 years of practice in laparoscopic surgery.

Survey results show that out of 1728 lifetime LMS seen by surgeons participating in this survey, 216 cases (12.5%) received laparoscopic surgery. The sum of the diagnosed sarcomas after each individual type of surgery in a lifetime as shown in Table 1 (sum (Q5 + Q7 + Q9 + Q11) = 221) which is verified by the sum of the general questions of the total number of uterine sarcomas calculated and seen in a lifetime (Table 1: sum Q2 = 216) strengthens the reliability of the answers given by the participants. The overall probability of finding a sarcoma after endoscopic surgery (myomectomy or hysterectomy) is 1.5%. The lowest probability of sarcoma is after laparoscopic myomectomy 0.6% and after hysteroscopic myomectomy 0.7% while the greatest probability of sarcoma is after laparoscopic hysterectomy 3.1%. The probability of sarcoma after laparoscopic subtotal hysterectomy is close to the overall probability and is equal to 1.3%. The number of doctors who participated in this survey as well as the high number of operations reported demonstrates the group's large exposure to gynaecological endoscopic surgery and strongly supports the reliability of these results.

Experience in MIS

The vast majority of responders (67.1%) reported over 5 years of practice in laparoscopic surgery, performing between 29 and 44 operations of each type (LH, LSH, LM, HM) of MIS on an annual basis. The overall exposure of doctors to laparoscopic surgery is demonstrated in Fig. 1. The rate of gynaecologists practicing laparoscopic myomectomy and hysterectomy according to number of years' (time interval) shows that majority of these surgeons (54.1%) have 1 to 10 years of experience and 32.3% have 11 to 20 years of experience in MIS. Only 4.6% of the doctors participated in our survey reported less than a year of experience while 9.2% of the most experienced surgeons reported more than 20 years of laparoscopic surgery experience. The experience of the surgeons according to the type and number of operations performed annually is demonstrated in Fig. 2. The first set of bars presents an average of 17% of doctors that do not perform the described endoscopic surgeries;

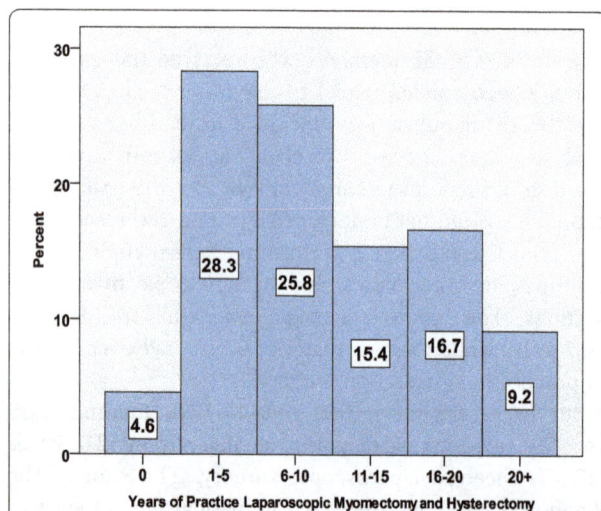

Fig. 1 The exposure of doctors to laparoscopic surgery. The percentage of gynae-surgeons practicing laparoscopic myomectomy and hysterectomy, according to years' interval

however, they still reported the number of sarcomas found during their lifetime. 49.3% reported that they perform 1–30 MIS and another 33.7% more than 30 MIS per year. The remaining 30% of the doctors reported that they do not perform LSH at all. Majority of doctors reported that they perform 30 laparoscopic hysterectomies and 20 hysteroscopic myomectomies on an annual basis. Statistical analysis revealed that the average number of annual LM is 29, LSH is 28, LH is 44, and HM is 31.

The most frequent type of endoscopic surgery performed is LH, and the least preferred surgical approach is LSH. Figure 2 demonstrates surgeons, with the least exposure to MIS (1–10 cases/annum), performed more myomectomies and subtotal hysterectomies than LH compared to more experienced surgeons with exposure to more than 11 endoscopic cases per year, on average. There was greater preference for LH than LSH by all experienced surgeons who performed more than 11 cases per year of MIS. The higher rate of hysteroscopic myomectomies, being 22.5 and 16.5%, were performed by surgeons reporting between 11–20 and 21–30 operations per year, respectively. Surgeons with exposure to MIS in more than 31 cases per year performed less hysteroscopic myomectomies, between 2.5 and 12%.

Incidence of uterine leiomyosarcomas

The total number of sarcomas encountered by all doctors after LM is 57, after LSH is 38, after LH is 72, and after HM is 54. The majority of doctors (71%), however, stated that they have never seen a sarcoma after any of these surgery approaches. The most frequent type of endoscopic surgery performed is the LH estimated to be 10,404 operations per year as calculated by all doctors together in this survey. The least frequent surgical approach is subtotal LM, for which 6828 cases are performed on an annual basis by all respondents.

All participants as a group have seen 1728 uterine sarcomas in their lifetime while the most common answer on an average is between two and six cases per lifetime, with a large standard deviation of 9008. Out of 1728 uterine sarcomas, only 216 cases have received a laparoscopic surgical approach. There is a positive and strong correlation between the number of uterine sarcomas encountered in a lifetime with the laparoscopic surgical approach (Pearson's $r = 0.427$), with the total number of sarcomas encountered after laparoscopic myomectomies (Pearson's $r = 0.451$), and with the total number of laparoscopic hysterectomies (Pearson's $r = 0.461$) which all reach statistically significant results (p value < 0.001) as shown in Table 1.

The total number of MIS surgeries described in Table 2 has been calculated by the years of endoscopic surgery experience multiplied by the number of doctors. The total number of LMS identified in a lifetime was based

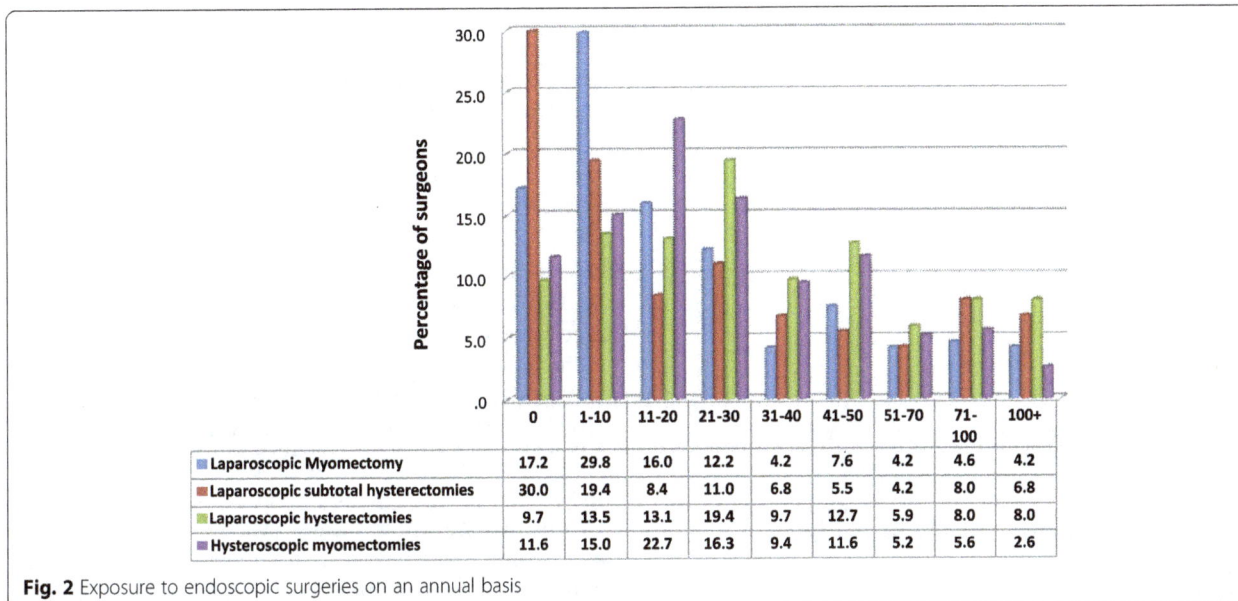

	0	1-10	11-20	21-30	31-40	41-50	51-70	71-100	100+
Laparoscopic Myomectomy	17.2	29.8	16.0	12.2	4.2	7.6	4.2	4.6	4.2
Laparoscopic subtotal hysterectomies	30.0	19.4	8.4	11.0	6.8	5.5	4.2	8.0	6.8
Laparoscopic hysterectomies	9.7	13.5	13.1	19.4	9.7	12.7	5.9	8.0	8.0
Hysteroscopic myomectomies	11.6	15.0	22.7	16.3	9.4	11.6	5.2	5.6	2.6

Fig. 2 Exposure to endoscopic surgeries on an annual basis

on the answer of the question 2 (sum = 216), which is validated by the sum of the questions 5, 7, 9, and 11 (sum = 221). The same exercise was calculated for each type of surgery as shown in Table 2. The overall sarcoma risk after endoscopic surgery including all types of surgeries in this group is 0.15% of operations. Analysis of Table 2 clearly demonstrates that the highest risk of sarcoma is after LH 3.1%, followed by LSH 1.3%, whereas the lowest risk appears after HM and LM being 0.7 and 0.6%, respectively.

The percentage of surgeons and the number of sarcomas operated by laparoscopy is demonstrated in Fig. 3. The vast majority of the gynaecological surgeons (71.1%) never had a LM or LH that histopathology later reported a sarcoma. Of the remaining 28.9% who did operate on sarcomas by laparoscopy during their lifetime, 11.4% experienced such an event only once, 0.4% twice, and 6.4% operated 3–10 times. The percentage of doctors and the number of uterine sarcomas seen in their lifetime is demonstrated in Fig. 4.

As demonstrated in Table 1, of those doctors who reported that they have seen sarcomas, most of them have

seen a maximum of two cases in their lifetime. Once the answers are categorized, the majority of the doctors (27.14%) are grouped in the 5–10 lifetime cases, and approximately half of the doctors (51.42%) have seen 1–4 sarcomas while the remaining 12.5% have seen more than 10 cases in their lifetime.

Figure 5 demonstrates that the majority, 62% (174/280), of endoscopic surgeons are aware of the sarcoma risk, and accordingly did not operate on sarcomas by laparoscopy during their lifetime. Among the 280 gynaecologists who operated by laparoscopy, 25 have never seen a uterine sarcoma during their lifetime practice. The 174 doctors that came across a sarcoma at least once during their lifetime practice did not perform laparoscopic surgery. However, 32 doctors reported that they operated once, 29 twice, and 18 doctors operated on 3–10 sarcomas by laparoscopy and only 2 operated more than 10 sarcomas by laparoscopy.

Only 0.2 per thousand of presumed and initially histologically diagnosed myomectomy cases turned out to be uterine sarcomas after the review of the slides. Among the 280 surgeons who participated in the survey, 30

Table 2 The frequency and probability of sarcoma in general and according to type of surgery as calculated by the number and types of operations performed in lifetime and the total number of sarcomas diagnosed in a lifetime by each surgeon

Type of surgery	Number of doctors	Total number surgeries by all doctors in their lifetime	Total number of sarcomas identified in their lifetime	Probability of sarcoma per 1000
All types of surgeries	218	429.777	221 ≈ 216[a]	1.5
Laparoscopic myomectomies	236	103.576	57	0.6
Laparoscopic subtotal hysterectomies	236	106.022	38	1.3
Laparoscopic hysterectomies	235	134.808	72	3.1
Hysteroscopic myomectomies	234	87.842	54	0.7

[a]The sum of the general question of the total number of uterine sarcomas calculated and seen in lifetime (Table 1: sum Q2 = 216). The sum of the diagnosed sarcomas after each individual type of surgery in lifetime as shown in Table 1: sum (Q5 + Q7 + Q9 + Q11) = 221)

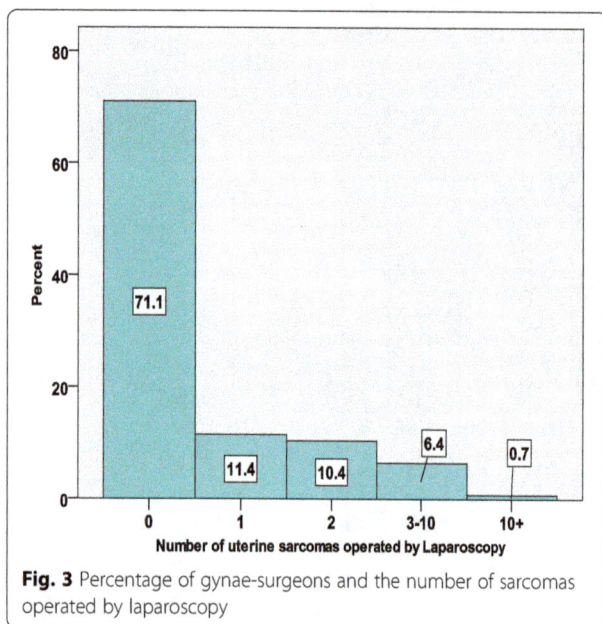

Fig. 3 Percentage of gynae-surgeons and the number of sarcomas operated by laparoscopy

surgeons reported 44 myomectomy cases that were initially reported as leiomyoma which after a histopathological review of the slides, due to clinical symptoms, revealed a sarcoma. Among these 30 surgeons, 19 reported that a false benign myoma histological answer happened to them once, 9 reported twice, 1 doctor reported 3 times, and one reported 4 times. The probability of a fibroid being falsely diagnosed by histopathology as a benign tumour and later revised as a sarcoma has been calculated to be 0.2 per 1000. This estimation has been calculated based on the total number of 429,777 endoscopic surgeries performed by all doctors in their lifetime, as reported in this review.

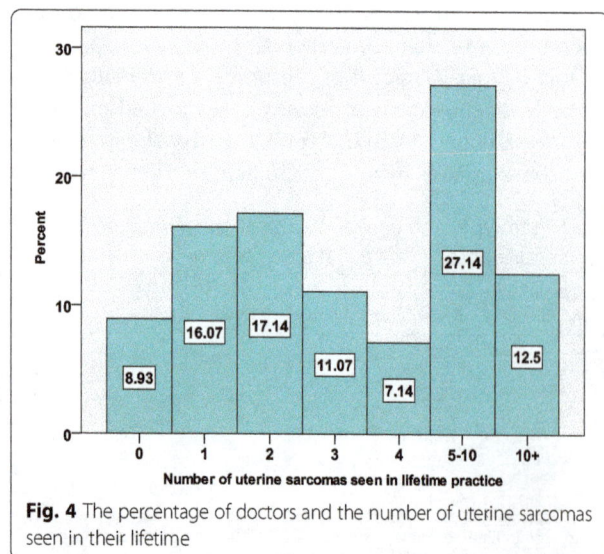

Fig. 4 The percentage of doctors and the number of uterine sarcomas seen in their lifetime

Discussion

The total number of 221 LMS was reported among 429,777 minimally invasive surgeries (laparoscopic and hysteroscopic myomectomies and LH and LSH), performed by all doctors in their lifetime. The overall reported sarcoma risk of all types of endoscopic myoma surgeries has been estimated to be 1.5% of operations. Categorizing by type, 57 (0.06%) LMS were operated by laparoscopic myomectomy and 54 (0.07%) by hysteroscopic myomectomy, while 38 (0.13%) LMS were operated by laparoscopic subtotal hysterectomy and 72 (0.31%) by laparoscopic hysterectomy.

The incidence of uterine sarcoma in presumed fibroids has been reported to be 0.14% (1:700) with a range from 0.014 to 0.49% (1:204), which is in agreement with our overall results after MIS 0.15% [2, 8, 9, 15]. The lower prevalence of sarcoma found in LSH 0.13% is also in agreement with other studies [12, 16–18]. Studies with laparoscopic supracervical hysterectomies, sometimes without the presumption of fibroids, will result in a lower reported prevalence. A difference in prevalence between studies where fibroids intended to be morcellated and the older (pathology) studies where all uteri and fibroids served as a denominator in the prevalence rate has also been demonstrated [17]. Table 3 presents several recent published studies with a large number of patients, where 7 studies including the present survey study, report the incidence of LMS after myomectomy to be between 0.03–0.09% and one study found 1.0%. A meta-analysis, based largely on peer-reviewed articles, demonstrated a prevalence of 0.14%, a similar result to literature reviews [1, 5]. However, a meta-analysis by Pritts et al., looking at prospective trials, detected 131 articles with 29,877 patients operated for fibroids and found a sarcoma prevalence of 1:7400 (0.014%) [12]. The large prevalence difference as compared to our results and the one reported in literature may be caused by a higher number of prospective trials (50%) of all languages and a statistical correction for low volume studies. A literature review addressing this apparent discrepancy concluded that the true prevalence of uterine sarcoma in presumed fibroids is not known. There is a wide range, from 0.014 to 0.45%, produced by meta-analyses mainly based on retrospective trials. The overall risk of not previously presumed sarcomatous change in the uterus from all papers was 0.14% (1 in 700). However, there were large differences between papers with figures varying from 0.49% (1 in 204) [19] to 0.056% (1 in 1788) [20] and that by Pritts et al. 2015 was even lower at 0.014% [12, 15].

The higher risk of sarcoma found after LH as compared to LM and HM in our series may be attributed to the older age of LH patients since myomectomy is reserved most often for younger women, who have not completed their families. An additional argument might

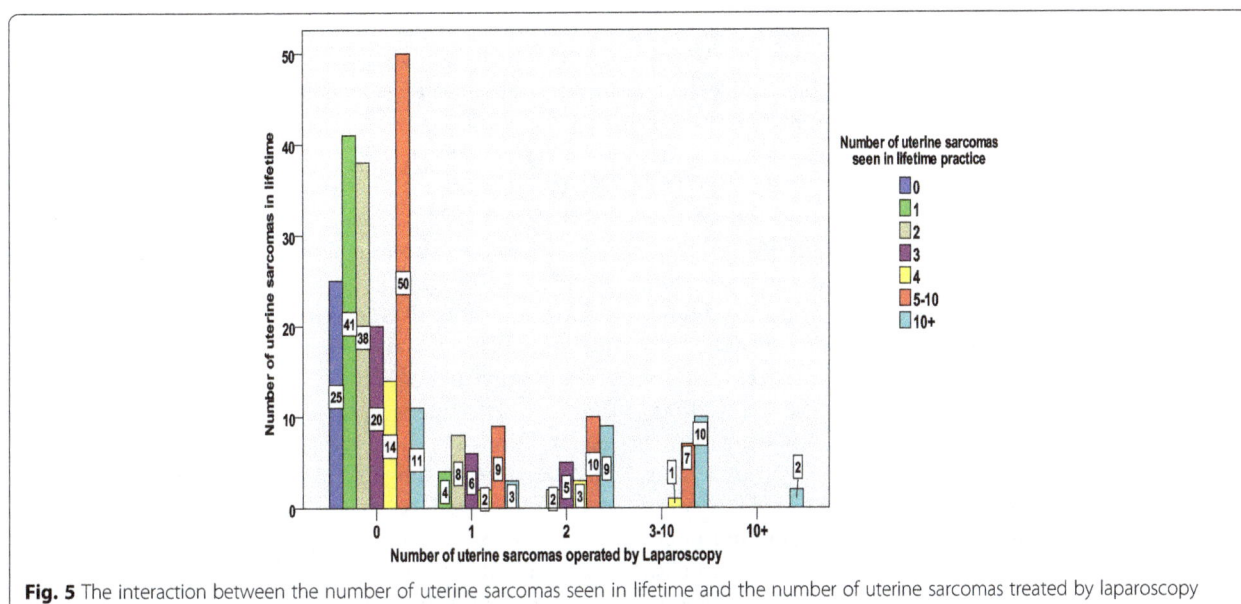

Fig. 5 The interaction between the number of uterine sarcomas seen in lifetime and the number of uterine sarcomas treated by laparoscopy

be that usually myomas treated by hysteroscopic myomectomy are significantly smaller in size compared to those found in enlarged uteri over 14 weeks. Usually, when fibroids are large in size, hysterectomy is the preferred surgery option, as in cases of peri- and postmenopausal women. According to literature the highest (absolute) number of sarcomas is found in the fourth decade, although the incidence is still extremely low [19]. The age over 40 remains the most reliable factor for triage between high and low risk for sarcoma fibroids [8]. Data on age and prevalence does not allow the estimation of an accurate risk of sarcoma in the individual patient scheduled for fibroid surgery but they may be taken into account to define a low and intermediate risk group of patients. The large variability of LMS prevalence reported reflects the rarity of the disease, the relatively small number of articles and series of patients published, and low quality of studies. In addition, the

vast majority of studies did not exclude STUMP's until recently, counting all types of sarcomatous changes hence falsely increasing the prevalence.

On average, each surgeon is expected to see two cases of LMS per lifetime while 71% of doctors stated that they have never seen a sarcoma after any of these surgery approaches, indicating the rarity of the disease. The fact that only 12.5% (216/1728) of uterine sarcomas cases are operated laparoscopically demonstrates the surgeons' awareness and alertness about LMS once they operate a myoma. The anticipation of a sarcoma when operating on a myoma is also reflected by the small number of doctors who reported that they have operated on a sarcoma by laparoscopy (Fig. 4).

LSH is the least performed operation, and 30% of the surgeons participated in this survey do not select this type of surgery as an option. In case of LMS after LSH, an additional operation is necessary. Since the risk of

Table 3 Myomectomy and LMS incidence publications compared to our survey results

Author and year	Journal	Study	No pts	LMS	LMS risk %
Tanos et al. present study [16]	Gyn Surg	Survey	103,576	57	0.06
Rodriguez et al. 2016 [33]	EJOG-RB	Database analysis	10,000	13	0.13
		< 49 years after myom/my			0.0012
Bojahr et al. 2015 [20]	Gyn Surg	Retrospective	8724	6	0.07
Pritts et al. 2015 [15]	Gyn Surg	Meta-analysis retrospective studies	23,926	22	0.09
Pritts et al. 2014 [12]	JMIS	Meta-analysis prospective studies	5951	2	0.03
Brohl A et al. 2015 (ref. [34])	The Oncologist	Retrospective 75–79 years	10,120		1.0
		< 30 years			< 0.002
Wright J et al. 2015 (ref. [35])	JAMA Oncol	Retrospective 496 hospitals	3220		0.09
Yuk J et al. 2015 (ref. [36])	Annals SurgOncol	National Korean population	32,085 Lpic		0.12–0.07
			69,955 Lmy		0.1–0.05

sarcoma is increased above the age of 40 probably, LSH should be reserved only for younger women [8]. When LH is performed, there is a high probability to extract the uterus vaginally without any need of power morcellation. It should be also noted that while vaginal hysterectomy allows extraction of the uterus via the vagina; however, it does not allow examination of the abdominal cavity like that in laparoscopic surgery. Hence, counselling patients with fibroids and especially young with small myoma size on the issue to choose laparoscopic surgery with its established benefits or laparotomy to escape the small LMS risks related to morcellation of the fibroid should be clear [8]. In a retrospective study by Bojahr et al. [20], reporting 10731 morcellated uteri after LSH, only 0.06% sarcoma and 0.07% endometrial carcinoma were detected. A very good prognosis in terms of survival was also found upon follow-up surgery according to the oncologic guidelines. In this ESGE survey, the overall sarcoma risk after endoscopic surgery including laparoscopic and hysteroscopic myomectomy and subtotal and total laparoscopic hysterectomy is estimated to be at 0.15% of operations as compared to 0.28% reported by FDA [1]. Our findings are in agreement with the majority of the published studies so far as demonstrated in Table 3.

The old common acceptance that rapid growth of a myoma (increasing uterine size by 6 weeks' size within 1 year) potentially indicates a uterine sarcoma is not valid since most women with a rapidly enlarging uterus do not have a sarcoma [21–25]. In addition, a sarcoma can remain indolent for a long period of time until suddenly it becomes more aggressive causing symptoms requiring further investigation. In a prospective MRI study, which evaluated 36 women with 101 fibroids at 3-month intervals for a year, rapid growth was noted mainly in myomas that were less than 5 cm in diameter while volume of more than 30% increase in 3 months was found in 37% of the myomas [21]. In a cohort study by Parker et al. among 1332 patients operated on for presumed leiomyoma, of 371 (28%) women operated for rapid growth of the uterus, only 1 patient found to have a sarcoma. None of 198 patients who met a published definition of rapid growth had a uterine sarcoma. Authors concluded the total incidence of uterine sarcoma among patients operated on for uterine leiomyoma was extremely low (0.23%) and among patients having surgery for 'rapidly growing' leiomyoma (0.27%) has results that do not support the concept of increased risk of sarcoma in these women [25].

There is no imaging modality that can reliably differentiate between benign leiomyomas and uterine sarcomas before deciding to morcellate or not. A retrospective nationwide cohort study during 2000–2012 from the Cancer Registry of Norway diagnosed 212 women with uterine LMS. In 54.2% (115/212) of women suffering from LMS, a malignant diagnosis was not suspected prior to surgery. The mean age at time of diagnosis was 58.1 years and the most frequent symptom was abnormal uterine bleeding in 51.9% (110/212) [26]. Parker et al. who reviewed 26 studies of uterine sarcoma published between 1962 and 1993 reported 580 patients, and the most common presenting symptom was abnormal bleeding, followed by pain and the presence of a pelvic mass [25].

LMS and fibroids are masses formed within the uterine musculature and both often have central necrosis. Trans vaginal sonography (TVS) is the first line examination to evaluate a potential uterine pathology and especially lesions concerning the myometrium. The usually described sonographic findings suggestive of sarcoma are mixed echogenic and poor echogenic parts, central necrosis, and findings of irregular vessel distribution, low impedance to flow and high peak systolic velocity as detected by colour Doppler. However, many of these characteristics may also be found in benign leiomyomas undergoing degeneration [14]. Computed tomography neither differentiates reliably between benign and malignant uterine tumours [27].

In magnetic resonance imaging (MRI), tumour irregular contour appearance and high signal intensity as well as absence of calcifications may be all suspicious but again not a reliable indicator of uterine sarcoma [24, 28]. Two small studies using different techniques of MRI with gadolinium contrast have reported specificities of 93 to 100% and positive predictive values of 53 to 100% [29, 30]. Baral et al. [30] reviewing MRI features of uterine sarcoma concluded that a combination of criteria including biological (elevated LDH and LDH isozyme), histological (transcervical-guided biopsies and expression of low-molecular mass polypeptide 2 and Ki-67), and imaging findings (solid mass with irregular margins, hyperintensity hemorrhagic changes T1-weighted fat suppressed images low value of apparent diffusion coefficient) may raise suspicion of the possibility of a malignant tumour. They also suggested that transcervical image-guided biopsy should be considered as a useful option in case of atypical imaging findings [31]. However, more prospective randomized controlled trials needed to extract firm conclusions. Positron emission tomography/CT with fluorodeoxyglucose (FDG) also failed to distinguish between leiomyomas and uterine sarcomas. Although the FDG uptake is high in LMS and low in leiomyomas, the high uptake variability among individual tumours, makes also this test unsuitable predicting the presumed myomas with sarcomatous changes [32].

Study limitations and potential biases
Although our survey results are consistent with other prospective and retrospective meta-analysis studies, this should be evaluated with caution. Several biases might

be involved and results should be elaborated with caution. The survey study has its limitations, however, which gives the opportunity to surgeons to disclose their complications without exposing directly their names. The strict data collection followed in a prospective or cohort studies is absent. The reliability of our results depends totally on the respondents, but probably balances with the method of survey since we are dealing with a rare disease and very low LMS incidence. A questionnaire has an important recall bias and uncertainty since the participants may forget the exact number of morcellated sarcomas once they are reporting their data just by memory. The fact is that most of the surgeons and especially high activity endoscopic surgery centres have been evaluating their results after the FDA announcement. In addition, the patients' electronic registrations and reports make easy the identification and recall of rare cases. However, the actual figures are also difficult to be collected in a prospective study of such rare cases like LMS.

Just over half of the respondents 54%, had 10 years or less experience with MIS. Given that uterine LMS is a rare finding, the estimation of the LMS incidence and the results accuracy found by our survey may carry a certain limitation since the respondents had relatively little experience. However, laparoscopic myomectomy demands high level suturing skills which is more prominent to younger laparoscopic surgeons. Also, proper teaching and guidance on laparoscopic teaching started only in the last decade. In order to bypass this potential bias, the frequency and probability of sarcoma was calculated by the number and types of operations performed in a lifetime and the total number of sarcomas diagnosed in a lifetime by each surgeon as shown in Table 2. The 8.6% response rate to ESGE survey call might also be considered another bias which, however, partially can be explained that a big group of ESGE members might not perform laparoscopic myomectomy and/or would not like to share their experience with LMS cases.

Conclusions

Taking into consideration the limitations of a survey study, our results show that laparoscopic hysterectomy and LSH carry higher risk of LMS than laparoscopic or hysteroscopic myomectomy cases, probably due to the older age of the patients and larger fibroids. Once LH is performed, the preferable way to remove the uterus is via the vagina when the size and circumstances are suitable. Probably, LSH should be discouraged in high-risk patients because the uterus should be morcellated to remove it from the pelvic cavity. According to our study, gynaecologists practicing MIS in Europe are aware of, and cautious about, LMS and the potential of spreading sarcomatous cells after power morcellation.

With reserve and including all biases mentioned above, it has also been demonstrated that myomectomy by hysteroscopy or laparoscopy may have similar risk of sarcoma about 0.07%. The survey results demonstrate the cautious surgery attitude of this specific group of gynae-endoscopist about morcellation of a LMS on a presumed myoma and a big uterus. Prospective, larger and multicentre data collection may clarify further the important issue of LMS prevalence.

Abbreviations
ESGE: European Society of Gynaecological Endoscopy; LH: Laparoscopic hysterectomy; LMS: Leiomyosarcoma; LSH: Laparoscopic subtotal hysterectomy

Acknowledgements
The authors thank Rhona O'Flaherty, Head ESGE Central Office, Diestsevest 43/0001, 3000 Leuven, Belgium, for her great assistance in the administration and data mining of the survey results.

Funding
Not applicable

Declaration
The authors declare that their relation with the companies mentioned above have no impact upon the scientific value and the content of the submitted article entitled "Survey among ESGE members on leiomyosarcoma morcellation incidence" assigned by manuscript number: GYNS-D-17-00043R1.

Authors' contributions
VT contributed in the design, data collection, analysis of the results, writing, and editing. HB took part in the design, analysis of the results, layout and composition, reviewing, and editing. RLDW is responsible for the analysis of the results and reviewing of the paper. POD took part in the analysis of the results, reviewing, and editing. ES did the review and analysis of data, statistical analysis of the data, and development of the figures. RC contributed in the design, analysis of the results, reviewing, and editing. All authors read and approved the final manuscript.

Competing interests
Dr. Rudi Campo: He is a consultant for Karl Storz endoscope.
Prof. Rudi Leon De Wilde: He receives reimbursement of travel expenses to the International congresses by the Karl Storz Company.
Prof. Hans Brölmann: He does research projects with Olympus, Gynesonics and Gedeon-Richter without any personal fees.
Prof. Peter O'Donovan: He has provided consultancy advice to both Karl Storz and Lina medical in the last year in the field of ambulatory gynaecology; nothing linked with morcellation.
Prof. Vasilios Tanos and Elina Symeonidou declare no conflict of interest.

Author details
[1]St. Georges Medical School, Nicosia University, Nicosia, Cyprus. [2]Department of Obstetrics and Gynaecology, Aretaeio Hospital, Nicosia, Cyprus. [3]Department

of Obstetrics and Gynaecology, VU University Medical Centre, De Boelelaan 1117, 1181HV Amsterdam, The Netherlands. [4]Clinic of Gynaecology, Obstetrics and Gynaecological Oncology, University Hospital for Gynaecology, Pius-Hospital Oldenburg, Medical Campus University of Oldenburg, Oldenburg, Germany. [5]Obstetrics and Gynaecological Oncology Yorkshire Clinic, Bradford Road, Bingley, West Yorkshire BD16 1TW, UK. [6]Nicosia, Cyprus. [7]European Society Gynaecological Endoscopy, European Academy for Gynaecological Surgery, LIFE, Tiensevest, 168, 3000 Leuven Leuven, Belgium.

References

1. FDA (2014) FDA discourages use of laparoscopic power morcellation for removal of uterus or uterine fibroids. Food Drug Adm 17:4 Ref Type: Internet Communication
2. Goff BA (2014) SGO not soft on morcellation: risks and benefits must be weighed. Lancet Oncol 15(4):e148–e2045
3. Patient safety must be a priority in all aspects of care (2014) Lancet Oncol. 15(2):123–2045
4. WGE (2014) Morcelleren: reactie vanWerkgroep Gynaecologische Endoscopie op FDA-advies; FDA ontraadt gebruik vanmorcellator. Ned Tijdschr Obstet Gynaecol 127:215
5. Knight J, Falcone T (2014) Tissue extraction by morcellation: a clinical dilemma. J Minim Invasive Gynecol 21(3):319–320
6. Kho KA, Nezhat CH (2014) Evaluating the risks of electric uterine morcellation. JAMA 311(19):905–906
7. Leung F, Terzibachian JJ (2012) Re: "The impact of tumor morcellation during surgery on the prognosis of patients with apparently early uterine leiomyosarcoma". Gynecol Oncol 124(1):172–173
8. Brölmann H, Tanos V, Grimbizis G, Ind T, Philips K, van den Bosch T, Sawalhe S, van den Haak L, Jansen FW, Pijnenborg J, Taran FA, Brucker S, Waiez A, Campo R, O'Donovan P, DeWilde RL (2015) Options on fibroid morcellation: a literature review. J Gynecol Surg 12:3–15
9. Ryan GL, Syrop CH, Van Voorhis BJ (2005) Role, epidemiology, and natural history of benign uterine mass lesions. Clin Obstet Gynecol 48(2):312–324
10. Wallach EE, Vlahos NF (2004) Uterine myomas: an overview of development, clinical features, and management. Obstet Gynecol 104(2):393–406
11. Felix AS, Cook LS, Gaudet MM, Rohan TE, Schouten LJ, Setiawan VW, Wise LA, Anderson KE, Bernstein L et al (2013) The etiology of uterine sarcomas: a pooled analysis of the epidemiology of endometrial cancer consortium. Br J Cancer 108(3):727–734
12. Pritts E, Parker WH, Brow J, Olive DL (2014) Outcome of occult uterine leiomyosarcoma after surgery for presumed uterine fibroids: a systematic review. J Min Invasive Gynecol 22(1):26–33
13. Tavassoli FA, Devilee P (eds) (2003) World Health Organization Classification of Tumours. Pathology and genetics of tumours of the breast and female genital organs, 3rd edn. IARC Press, Lyon
14. Amant F, Coosemans A, Debiec-Rychter M, Timmerman D, Vergote (2009) Clinical management of uterine sarcomas. Lancet Oncol 10:1188
15. Pritts EA, Vanness DJ, Berek JS, Parker W, Feinberg R, Feinberg J, Olive DL (2015) The prevalence of occult leiomyosarcoma at surgery for presumed uterine fibroids: a meta-analysis. Gyn Surg 12(3):165–77
16. Tanos V, Brölmann H, DeWilde RL, O'Donovan P, Campo R (2015) Myoma morcellation and leiomyosarcoma panic. Gynecol Surg 12:17–19
17. Brolmann H, Hehenkamp WJK, Huirne JAF (2014) Heeft het myoom zijn onschuld verloren? Ned Tijdschr Obstet Gynaecol 127:322–325
18. Oduyebo T, Rauh-Hain AJ, Meserve EE, Seidman MA, Hinchcliff E, George S et al (2014) The value of re-exploration in patients with inadvertently morcellated uterine sarcoma. Gynecol Oncol 132(2):360–365
19. Leibsohn S, D'Ablaing G, Mishell DR Jr, Schlaerth JB (1990) Leiomyosarcoma in a series of hysterectomies performed for presumed uterine leiomyomas. Am J Obstet Gynecol 162:968–974 discus: 968–974
20. Bojahr B, Leon De Wilde R, Tchartchian G (2015) Malignancy rate of 10731 uteri morcellated during laparoscopicsupracervical hysterectomy (LASH). Arch Gynecol Obstet 292:665–672
21. Baird DD, Garrett TA, Laughlin SK, Davis B, Semelka RC, Peddada SD (2011) Short-term change in growth of uterine leiomyoma: tumor growth spurts. Fertil Steril 95:242
22. DeWaay DJ, Syrop CH, Nygaard IE, Davis WA, Van Voorhis BJ (2002) Natural history of uterine polyps and leiomyomata. Obstet Gynecol 100:3

23. Peddada SD, Laughlin SK, Miner K, Guyon JP, Haneke K, Vahdat HL, Semelka RC, Kowalik A, Armao D, Davis B, Baird DD (2008) Growth of uterine leiomyomata among premenopausal black and white women. Proc Natl Acad Sci U S A 105:19887
24. Kawamura N, Ito F, Ichimura T, Shibata S, Tsujimura A, Minakuchi K, Ishiko O, Ogita S (1999) Transient rapid growth of uterine leiomyoma in a postmenopausal woman. Oncol Rep 6:1289
25. Parker WH, Fu YS, Berek JS (1994) Uterine sarcoma in patients operated on for presumed leiomyoma and rapidly growing leiomyoma. Obstet Gynecol 83(3):414–418
26. Skorstad M, Kent A, Lieng M (2016) Uterine leiomyosarcoma—incidence, treatment, and the impact of morcellation. A nationwide cohort study. Acta Obstet Gynecol Scand 95:984–990
27. Rha SE, Byun JY, Jung SE, Lee SL, Cho SM, Hwang SS, Lee HG, Namkoong SE, Lee JMSO (2003) CT and MRI of uterine sarcomas and their mimickers. AJR Am J Roentgenol 181:1369
28. Schwartz LB, Zawin M, Carcangiu ML, Lange R, McCarthy S (1998) Does pelvic magnetic resonance imaging differentiate among the histologic subtypes of uterine leiomyomata? Fertil Steril 70:580
29. Goto A, Takeuchi S, Sugimura K, Maruo T (2002) Usefulness of Gd-DTPA contrast-enhanced dynamic MRI and serum determination of LDH and its isozymes in the differential diagnosis of leiomyosarcoma from degenerated leiomyoma of the uterus. Int J Gynecol Cancer 12:354
30. Barral M, Place V, Dautry RI, Bendavid S, Cornelis F, Foucher R, Guerrache Y, Soyer P (2017) Magnetic resonance imaging features of uterine sarcoma and mimickers. Abdom Radiol 42:1762–1772
31. Tanaka YO, Nishida M, Tsunoda H, Okamoto Y, Yoshikawa H (2004) Smooth muscle tumors of uncertain malignant potential and leiomyosarcomas of the uterus: MR findings. J Magn Reson Imaging 20:998
32. Kitajima K, Murakami K, Kaji Y, Sugimura K (2010) Spectrum of FDG PET/CT findings of uterine tumors. AJR Am J Roentgenol 195:737
33. Rodriguez A, Zeybek B, Asoglu M, et al. (2016) Corrigendum to "Incidence of occult leiomyosarcoma in presumed morcellation cases: a database study" [Eur J Obstet Gynecol Reprod Biol 197(2016) 31–35]. 207:247. doi:10.1016/j.ejogrb.2016.10.007
34. Brohl A, Li L, Andikyan V, Običan S, Cioffi A, Hao K, Dudle J, Ascher-Walsh C, Kasarskis A, Maki R (2015) Age-stratified risk of unexpected uterine sarcoma following surgery for presumed benign leiomyoma. Oncologist 20(4):433–439
35. Wright J, Tergas A, Cui R, Burke W, Hou J, Ananth C, Chen L, Richards C, Neugut A, Hershman D (2015) Use of electric power morcellation and prevalence of underlying cancer in women who undergo myomectomy. JAMA Oncol 1(1):69–77
36. Yuk J, Ji H, Shin J, Kim L, Kim S, Lee J (2015) Comparison of survival outcomes in women with unsuspected uterine malignancy diagnosed after laparotomic versus laparoscopic myomectomy: a national, population-based study. Annals Surg Oncol 23(4):1287–1293

23

Laparoscopic sacrocolpopexy is as safe in septuagenarians or elder as in younger women

Karlien Vossaert[1], Susanne Housmans[1], Stefaan Pacquée[1], Geertje Callewaert[1], Laura Cattani[1], Frank Van der Aa[2], Albert Wolthuis[3], André D'hoore[3], Philip Roelandt[4,5] and Jan Deprest[1,6]* ⓘ

Abstract

Background: Data concerning laparoscopic sacrocolpopexy (LSCP) in elder women are scarce. We compared intra-operative and early-postoperative complications associated with laparoscopic colpo-, cervico-, or hysteropexy in women under and above 70 years.

Methods: Retrospective assessment by an independent investigator of a prospective cohort of 571 consecutive women undergoing LSCP in a tertiary unit over an 18-year period. Data included were patient demographics, operative variables, intra-operative, and early ($\leq$ 3 months) postoperative complications. Complications were graded according to the Clavien-Dindo classification and mesh complications categorized using the International Urogynaecological Association (IUGA)-classification.

Findings: Median age was 66 (IQR 15, range 27-91) and 204 (35.7%) patients were older than 70 years. There were no deaths. Strategic conversion rate was 2.3% (13/571), the majority because of extensive adhesions yet early in our experience. Reactive conversion rate was 0.7% (4/571). Among 554 patients who had a completed LSCP, there were 20 intra-operative complications (3.6%), mostly bladder (1.3%) and vaginal (1.1%) injuries. Eighty-four patients had a total of 95 early-postoperative Dindo $\geq$ II complications (15.1%). Most common complications were infectious and treated medically (Dindo II). Clinically major complications are rare (III = 3.1% and IV = 0.2%). Reoperation for suspected bleeding (IIIb = 0.7%) was the most common reintervention, typically without demonstrable cause. Most mesh complications were vaginal exposures. Septuagenarians were not more likely to have an intra-operative (4.0 vs 3.3% < 70 years, p = 0.686) or early-postoperative complication (13.6 vs 16.0% < 70 years, p = 0.455) than younger patients. Mesh complications were also equally uncommon.

Conclusions: LSCP is as well-tolerated by women above 70 years as by younger women.

Keywords: Laparoscopic sacropexy, Elder women, Elderly, Complication, Conversion, Laparoscopy

Background

Clinically visible pelvic organ prolapse (POP) occurs in up to 50% of parous women, half of them being symptomatic [1, 2]. When operated, most patients can be adequately managed by vaginal access. In case of apical descent or a multi-compartment prolapse yet with a so-called level-I defect, abdominal suspension is a better approach [3]. In sacrocolpopexy, the vaginal vault, cervix, or uterus is fixed by means of a graft to the anterior longitudinal ligament over the sacrum. This operation conserves vaginal length; hence, should not compromise its function. Historically, sacrocolpopexy was performed by laparotomy, competing with vaginal sacrospinous fixation, which has a shorter operation time, lower morbidity, and hospital cost, and which can be offered under loco-regional anesthesia. In the 90s, we moved towards laparoscopic sacrocolpopexy (LSCP) and earlier reported on the medium term outcomes [4, 5]. Since 2012, there is level-I evidence that LSCP yields as good anatomical and subjective outcomes as the same

* Correspondence: Jan.Deprest@uzleuven.be
[1]Pelvic Floor Unit Department of Gynaecology, University Hospitals Leuven, Leuven Herestraat 49, 3000 Leuven, Belgium
[6]Institute for Women's Health, University College London, London, UK
Full list of author information is available at the end of the article

operation by laparotomy [6]. Moreover, it is associated with less blood loss, less pain, and a shorter hospital stay. Conversely, operation time, return to normal activities, or functional effects were comparable for both modalities. More recently, this operation is also performed robotically, yet without any proven benefit [7].

Given that the population is aging and that symptomatic POP is more common among the elderly, the number of elder patients eligible for sacropexy will also increase. In 2016, 19.2% of the EU-28-popluation was over 65 years (5.4% > 80 years), and by 2030 that will be 23.9% (7.2% > 80 years) [8]. With increased activity and a healthier population, POP surgery in the elderly will therefore increase accordingly. In one study [9], the annual risk for POP surgery was 4.3/1000 women aged 71–73 years and in another one it was 5.0/1000 women aged 65–69 years [10]. With age, the prevalence of chronic illnesses and comorbidities increases, including poor cardiopulmonary reserve, not to forget, the prevalence of prior surgery [11]. Considering that POP is not a life-threatening condition, surgeons and anesthetists may be reluctant to perform complex and potentially risky operations in the elderly. However, we speculated that, particularly in this population, the choice of minimally invasive surgery is beneficial, because of reduced morbidity, lower transfusion rate, decreased postoperative pain, shorter hospital stay, and faster recovery hence quicker return to normal activity [12].

The relationship between age and complication risk is however controversial. At present, little is known on outcome of LSCP in the elderly. Currently available case series or cohort studies are small to medium sized (≤ 302 patients) with only one controlled study [2] [13] [14]. Most studies show similar complication rates in younger and elder patients, yet occasionally higher complication rates are observed, including for sacrocolpopexy [2]. In the latter study, age ≥ 65 years remained a significant predictor of complications after correction for BMI, estimated blood loss, and operating time (adjusted OR 2.28, 95% CI 1.21–4.29, $p = 0.01$). Herein, we aimed to determine whether in our setting there was an increased risk for intra- or postoperative complications when LSCP is offered to the elder patient. In our unit, sacrocolpopexy is the first choice for the surgical management of level I defects [5], also for elder patients who are judged to be fit for general anesthesia.

Methods

This is a retrospective analysis of a prospective cohort of consecutive patients scheduled for LSCP at the University Hospitals Leuven. Laparoscopy was the preferred route from September 1997 onwards, and all consecutive cases till December 2015 were included. Preoperatively patients were clinically assessed using the pelvic organ prolapse

quantification system (POP-Q) [15]. Sacropexy procedures were either vault suspension ($n = 419$), cervicopexy ($n = 136$), or hysteropexy ($n = 16$), according to the presence or absence of the uterus and the patient's desire to conserve it. The nature of concomitant pelvic floor or other surgery was also noted. LSCP was performed or supervised by an experienced surgeon with a standardized technique and structured training program [16, 17]. Over the years, the only change was the replacement of non-resorbable multifilament polyester by monofilamentary polydioxanone sutures, the abandoning of acellular collagen matrices, and increasingly lighter meshes [17, 18]. These changes were implemented irrespective of the age of the patient. All patients received prophylactic antibiotics (cefazolin and metronidazole unless known allergies). Low molecular weight heparin injections were given until discharge, or longer in case of a history of venous thromboembolism. Midstream urine culture was taken after removal of the catheter. Patients were typically reassessed within 3 months after the operation.

For this study, the electronic medical records were screened by a physician not involved in the surgery or management of the patient. She identified any planned and unplanned hospital visits or any evidence of management for adverse events within 12 weeks after surgery. This includes visits elsewhere at a hospital using our network's electronic medical record system. In the absence of data, the general practitioner was contacted for a follow-up. Post hoc, postoperative complications were categorized using the modified Clavien-Dindo surgical complication classification system [19] and mesh complications by the terminology of the International Urogynecological Association (IUGA) [20]. Previous studies on rectal sacropexy considered Dindo grade III complications as clinically being relevant, hence severe [21]. Other data retrieved included pre-operative characteristics (age, body mass index, menopausal status, diabetes, smoking habits, previous surgery), operative details (operation time, estimated blood loss), and the occurrence and nature of any intra-operative and early postoperative (≤ 12 weeks) complications. Conversions were categorized into either a *strategic* conversion, i.e., instances where the surgeon as a precaution decided to open up the abdomen or to proceed vaginally, or *reactive*, i.e., as a result of an intra-operative complication which the surgeon felt was better managed through open abdomen [22, 23].

Data were entered into a purpose designed database, and statistical analysis was performed using SPSS software (version 24.0, IBM, Armonk, New York, USA). Normality testing was done using the Kolgomorov-Smirnov test. Continuous data were compared using the unpaired Student's t test and categorical data using the χ^2 Fisher exact two-tailed test. Our ongoing prospective follow-up study as well as this audit was approved by the ethical committee on clinical studies (MP10810).

Findings

Patient data

During this 18-year period, 571 consecutive patients had a LSCP (Table 1). Their median age was 66.3 years (range 27-91; IQR 14.5). Two hundred four (35.7%) patients were above 70. Of these, 101 (17.7%) patients were above 75, including 26 (4.6%) above 80 and two (0.4%) above 90 years. 73.4% underwent a LSCP after previous hysterectomy, 24.2% had a cervicopexy with concomitant laparoscopic-assisted subtotal hysterectomy (LASH) and 2.8% had a hysteropexy. Twenty-six were redo-sacropexies (4.6%). Concomitant rectopexy, incontinence surgery, or vaginal prolapse surgery was performed in 5.3, 3.7, and 3.0%, respectively.

Conversions

The overall conversion rate was 3.0% or 17 patients with a median age of 68 (range 44-81; IQR 12). There were 13 strategic conversions. In 11 cases, conversion was because of adhesions (1.9%; median age = 67; range 56–76; IQR 11); 9 were completed as open sacropexies (median age 67; range 56–73, IQR 11), and 2 had a vaginal suspension (age 67 and 76) instead. There were two additional patients (age 68 and 72) where visualization of presacral vascular anatomy was judged problematic, and an uneventful open sacropexy was done.

There were four *reactive* conversions (0.7%). One patient (age 68) was converted because of hypercapnia after > 120 min of surgery. Her sacropexy was uneventfully completed via laparotomy. In one patient (aged 81), a large bowel perforation occurred at the time of open laparoscopy. Primary repair of the perforation was done and sacropexy was uneventfully completed by open access, using a non-cross linked 8-layered small intestinal submucosa graft (SIS, Cook, Bloomington, IN) [18]. The postoperative course was uneventful. There were two additional conversions for vascular injury early in the operation, one for epigastric artery injury (age 44) and one left iliac vein laceration (age 60). In both bleeding was controlled by open access and an uneventful open sacropexy was done. None of these patients required a blood transfusion. Overall conversion rate was similar in both age groups (11/367 = 3.0% < 70 vs 6/204 = 2.9%, p = 0.969). In retrospect, there was an early (< 60 cases) peak of strategic conversions, yet thereafter conversions were rare and equally distributed along the experience (Fig. 1). These 17 patients are not further included in statistical analysis as they did not undergo a complete LSCP.

Intra-operative complications without need for conversion

Twenty additional patients had an intra-operative complication, their nature displayed in Table 2 (20/554 = 3.6%). The majority were lesions to the bladder (n = 10),

Table 1 Patient characteristics of the cohort and operative variables for all patients broken down by age category (under and above 70 years)

	Median or %	≤ 70 years	> 70 years	
Number of patients	Total 571 (100%)	367 (64.3%)	204 (35.7%)	
Baseline patient characteristics				p
Age (years)	66 (IQR 15)	61 (IQR 11)	75 (IQR 6)	0.000
BMI (kg/m²)	25 (IQR 5)	25 (IQR 5)	25.5 (IQR 4)	0.917
Menopausal	90.7%	87.2%	100%	0.000
Diabetes mellitus (all types)	10.8%	9.5%	13.4%	0.344
Current smoker	12.2%	15.7%	3.9%	0.001
Prior hysterectomy	73.4%	70.3%	78.9%	0.025
Prior POP surgery	72.1%	68.9%	77.8%	0.022
Prior LSCP	4.6%	5.7%	2.5%	0.072
Nature of procedures (index operation)				
Sacrocolpopexy	73.4%	70.3%	78.9%	0.025
Concomitant LASH + cervicopexy	24.2%	27.0%	19.1%	0.036
Hysteropexy	2.8%	3.0%	2.5%	0.705
Concomitant rectopexy	5.3%	5.5%	4.9%	0.783
Concomitant incontinence surgery	3.7%	3.6%	3.9%	0.814
Concomitant vaginal surgery	3.0%	3.3%	2.5%	0.584

Abbreviations: BMI = body mass index, *LASH* = laparoscopic subtotal hysterectomy, *LSCP* = laparoscopic sacrocolpopexy. Absolute values not displayed; missing values range from prior surgery 0% to certitude on menopausal status 26.4%

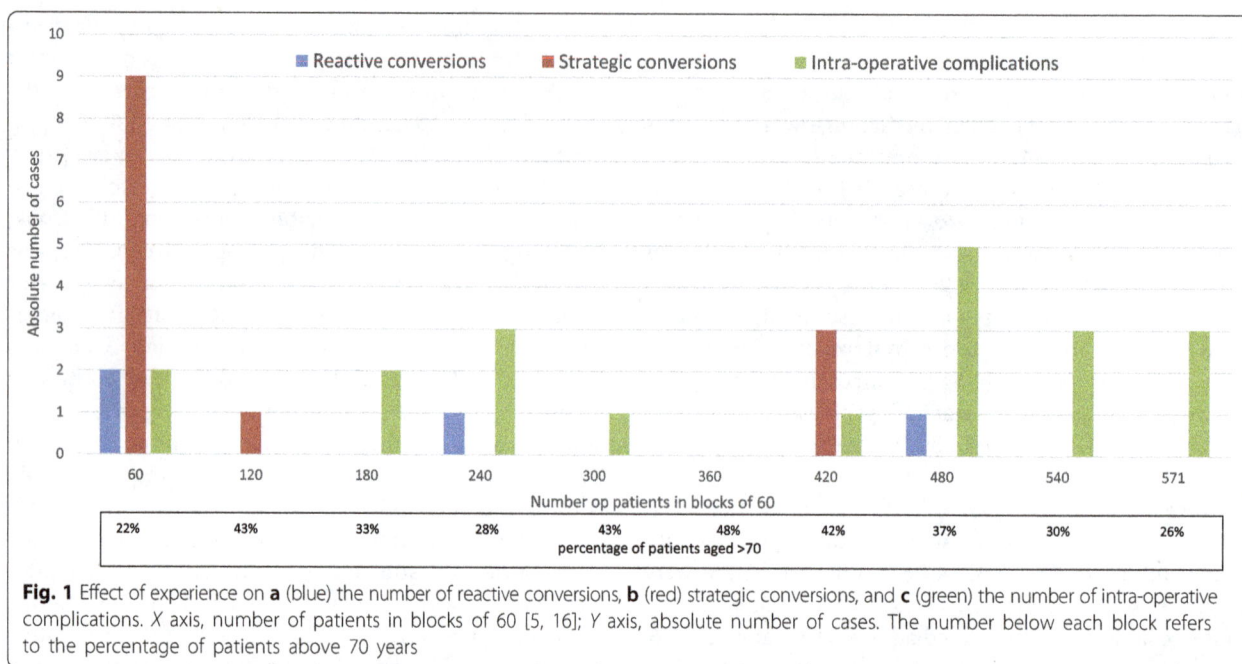

Fig. 1 Effect of experience on **a** (blue) the number of reactive conversions, **b** (red) strategic conversions, and **c** (green) the number of intra-operative complications. *X* axis, number of patients in blocks of 60 [5, 16]; *Y* axis, absolute number of cases. The number below each block refers to the percentage of patients above 70 years

vagina ($n = 6$), or epigastric arteries ($n = 2$), which were managed laparoscopically. In one patient with hypercapnia, the operation was temporarily suspended for hyperventilation, yet could eventually be completed by laparoscopy. She was afterwards briefly observed in the intensive care unit (ICU), which is a deviation from the normal protocol. In one patient, a suturing needle got

detached, fell in the abdomen, and could only be laparoscopically retrieved under fluoroscopy.

Postoperative complications according to the Clavien-Dindo classification

The follow up rate was 100%. Eighty-four women ($84/554 = 15.2\%$) had in total 95 postoperative complications within 3 months (Dindo grade $\geq$ II; Table 3). Dindo II complications are those events that cause a deviation from the normal postoperative course and that prompt the use of drugs other than analgesics, antipyretics, antiemetics, diuretics, electrolytes, and physiotherapy. Among these, urinary tract infection was the most common (5.9%), the majority identified on urine culture and asymptomatic. Other common Dindo II complications were the need for blood transfusion (1.9%) and the occurrence of postoperative fever/asymptomatic CRP rise treated with antibiotics (1.9%). Dindo III and higher were categorized as major, as earlier described for rectopexy [21]. Interventions without the need for general anesthesia (Dindo IIIa) were for patients with urinary retention and in one patient in office mesh removal and administration of intravenous antibiotics, because of frank mesh extrusion and obvious local infection. She recovered completely and remained without any reintervention without recurrence beyond the observation period.

Reintervention under general anesthesia (Dindo IIIb), and ICU admission (Dindo IV) are clinically very relevant complications. These were rare ($n = 13$, 2.3%). There were four early second look laparoscopies for suspected hemorrhage. Despite a hemoperitoneum, in none of them a true source could be identified.

Table 2 Rate and nature of complications in 554 consecutive patients who had their sacrocolpopexy completely by laparoscopy

Per-operative complications	n (%)	≤ 70 years	> 70 years	p value
Number of patients	554	356 (64.3%)	198 (36.7%)	
Visceral injuries	16 (2.9%)	10 (2.8%)	6 (3.0%)	0.882
Bladder	7 (1.3%)	5 (1.4%)	2 (1.0%)	–
Ureter	3 (0.5%)	3 (0.8%)	0 (0.0%)	–
Vaginal	6 (1.1%)	2 (0.6%)	4 (2.0%)	–
Vascular injury	2 (0.4%)	0 (0.0%)	2 (1.0%)	0.127
Epigastric artery bleeding	2 (0.4%)	0 (0.3%)	2 (1.0%)	–
Anesthetic problems	1 (0.2%)	1 (0.3%)	0 (0.0%)	1.000
Hypercapnia	1 (0.2%)	1 (0.3%)	0 (0.0%)	–
Other	1 (0.2%)	1 (0.3%)	0 (0.0%)	1.000
Needle detachment	1 (0.2%)	1 (0.3%)	0 (0.0%)	–
Total number	20 (3.6%)	12 (3.3%)	8 (4.0%)	0.686

Abbreviations: –, not calculated because of low number per individual cell.
p values are based on χ^2 testing (Fisher exact)

Table 3 Nature and number of 95 early postoperative complications in 83 patients broken down according to the Dindo classification and categorized by age groups. When several complications occurred, the patient was counted in the highest category applicable

Early postoperative complications	n	≤70 years	> 70 years	p value
Number of patients	554	356	198	
Number of patients with complications (% of the population)	84 (15.2%)	57 (16.0%)	27 (13.6%)	0.455
Number of complications	95	61	34	
Dindo II—any deviation from the normal postoperative course requiring pharmacological treatment with drugs other than such allowed for grade I complications	77	53 (14.9%)	24 (12.1%)	0.372
Antibiotics for asymptomatic or symptomatic urinary tract infection	33	24	9	
Antibiotics for postoperative fever and/or CRP rise	11	9	2	
Treatment of vaginal infection	4	3	1	
Antibiotics for umbilical/trocar wound infection	4	4	0	
Antibiotics for chronic obstructive pulmonary disease exacerbation/pneumonia	2	2	0	
Antibiotic prophylaxis after vomiting during extubation	1	1	0	
Blood transfusion	11	6	5	
Administration of (additional) drugs (amlodipine, perindopril, digoxin, bisoprolol, haloperidol)	7	1	6	
Low molecular weight heparin for treatment of deep venous thrombosis/pulmonary embolism	4	3	1	
Dindo IIIa—complication requiring surgical, endoscopic, or radiologic intervention not under general anesthesia	4	1 (0.3%)	3 (1.5%)	0.100
Infection with mesh extrusion, vaginally removed in the office	1	0	1	
Urinary retention, catheterization	3	1	2	
Dindo IIIb—complication requiring surgical, endoscopic, or radiologic intervention under general anesthesia	13	7 (2.0%)	6 (3.0%)	0.429
Reoperation for prolapse	1	0	1	
Reoperation for suspected hemorrhage	4	2	2	
Reoperation for ureter reimplantation	1	1	0	
Reoperation for mesh removal	2	1	1	
Reoperation for exposure sling	1	1	0	
Reoperation: cholecystectomy	2	2	0	
Reoperation for bowel obstruction	2	0	2	
Dindo IV—life-threatening complication	1	0 (0.0%)	1 (0.5%)	0.357
ICU admission for cardiac decompensation and pulmonary edema	1	0	1	

Abbreviations: CRP, C-reactive protein. Statistics were done on individual patient basis for each Dindo category

There were three directly prolapse surgery-related additional surgeries. One 63-year-old heavy-smoking chronic obstructive pulmonary disease (COPD) patient developed vault detachment when awakening with vomiting and coughing. She was reinduced to reattach the mesh to the vault. Because of bronchitis, she was heavily coughing in the postoperative period, leading again to recurrence. Once in remission, we performed a successful abdominal sacropexy 2 weeks later. She remained asymptomatic. There were two reinterventions for mesh-related complications. One 60-year-old patient developed spondylodiscitis (IUGA 6CT2S4), from which she recovered after 9 weeks of antibiotic therapy (including 3 weeks intravenously). She later had a mesh exposure fixed. One 74-year-old patient developed a severe pelvic infection for which the mesh was removed laparoscopically on day 6. She was postoperatively admitted to ICU (Dindo IV) because of severe dyspnea disappearing with diuretics. She remained under intravenous antibiotics for 14 days. She recovered and did not develop recurrence. In retrospect, this patient had multiple co-morbidities among which essential thrombocytosis, for which she was on the antitumoral agent hydroxycarbamide.

Two patients had a reintervention for bowel obstruction. One 80-year-old had bowel herniation in an abdominal wall hernia. Another 78-year-old had a laparotomy for adhesions 7 weeks postoperatively, requiring partial small bowel resection. Four patients experienced complications away from the operation field. One had a reintervention for a symptomatic sling exposure. Two patients suffered from cholecystitis for which they were operated. One patient who underwent simultaneous LASH was postoperatively diagnosed with a ureteric obstruction at the level of the uterine artery and underwent reimplantation.

Mesh-related complications

There were 15 (2.7%) mesh-related complications, including some already mentioned above (Table 4). Six patients had clinical signs of infection in the mesh area, yet four without loss of vaginal epithelial integrity (IUGA 1CT2 or T3). These were managed by intravenous administration of antibiotics (making them Dindo II complications). Further, there were two patients earlier mentioned. One was the patient with symptomatic exposed mesh removed in the office (3CT2), and the other one was the IUGA 6CT2S4 patients with spondylodiscitis. There were nine small (< 1 cm) suture exposures, eight asymptomatic, and one symptomatic. Most were successfully managed in the outpatient clinic by suture removal. There were no graft-related urinary tract (category 4) or bowel (category 5) complications.

Complications by age group and other patient characteristics

Outcomes in patients under and above 70 years of age are displayed in Tables 1–3. In terms of patient demographics, younger patients were four times more likely

Table 4 Mesh-related complications broken down according to the IUGA classification; with left and right column displaying numbers per age category (under (left) or above (right) 70). Statistics were done by age group for each IUGA CTS-category

General description↓/category→	A		B		C		D		All categories per age group		p value
	≤70 years	> 70 years	≤70 years	> 70 years	≤70 years	> 70 years	≤70 years	> 70 years	≤70 years	> 70 years	
Vaginal complications	Asymptomatic		Symptomatic		Infection		Abscess				
1 No epithelial separation	0	0	0	0	3	1	0	0	3/356 (0.8%)	1/198 (0.5%)	1.000
2 Smaller ≤ 1 cm exposure	7	1	1	0	0	0	0	0	8/356 (2.2%)	1/198 (0.5%)	0.168
3 Larger > 1 cm exposure	0	0	0	0	0	1	0	0	0/356 (0.0%)	1/198 (0.5%)	0.357
4 Urinary tract	Small intraoperative defect		Other lower urinary tract complication or urinary retention		Ureteric or upper urinary tract complication						
	0	0	0	0	0	0			0/356 (0.0%)	0/198 (0.0%)	–
5 Rectal or bowel	Small intraoperative defect		Rectal injury or compromise		Small or large bowel injury or compromise		Abscess				
	0	0	0	0	0	0	0	0	0/356 (0.0%)	0/198 (0.0%)	–
6 Skin and/or musculoskeletal	Asymptomatic, abnormal finding		Symptomatic		Infection		Abscess				
	0	0	0	0	1	0	0	0	1/356 (0.3%)	0/198 (0.0%)	1.000
7 Patient	Bleeding complication		Major degree of resuscitation or intensive care		Mortality						
	0	0	0	0	0	0			0/356 (0.0%)	0/198 (0.0%)	–
Graft-related Complications									12/356 (3.3%)	3/198 (1.5%)	0.277

to smoke. Elder patients were more likely to have undergone previous pelvic floor surgery and/or hysterectomy. Conversely, younger patients were more likely to undergo cervico- or hysteropexy. Operating time was comparable between both age groups as well as length of hospital stay.

When considering by age category, there were no differences in occurrence of *intra-operative* complications (Table 2). Early *postoperative* Dindo categories II, III, or IV complications were not tied to age either. Because of the low numbers in the subcategories of complications, no detailed statistics for those were attempted. Short-term mesh problems were also comparable in both age groups (Table 4).

When analyzing the entire data set, the only correlation with occurrence of complications was having a prior hysterectomy. These patients were less likely to have a complication (RR 0.539 [0.33-0.88]). Actually, this applied in particular to patients under 70, not above. The other factors such as diabetes, menopausal status, prior POP surgery, or prior sacropexy were not associated with an increased likelihood for complications in this data set.

Conclusions

In when reviewing this prospective cohort, an independent researcher meticulously scrutinized the records for any adverse event during their hospital stay and during the first three postoperative months after LSCP. The occurrence of post-discharge complications was based on findings on the routine postoperative visit with us (95.1%), elsewhere with a specialist or in its absence by contact with the general practitioner (4.9%). This resulted in a 100% short-term follow-up rate, which is possible in a small country like Belgium. In addition, our complication and conversion rate is comparable to what was observed in other large series [2, 24]. Therefore, we think the results of our study are representative.

Though the use of terms as "severe," "major," or "minor" for complications is discouraged [19], the clinical relevance of the occurrence of what we categorized as "severe" cannot be debated, because of their potential life-threatening impact. There were a few severe intra-operative complications, some of them leading to reactive conversions. The most relevant ones were hemorrhagic in nature. Three were epigastric bleedings, which early on in our experience still prompted a conversion in one, yet later such complication was easily managed laparoscopically. Epigastric artery bleeding is also reported by others, yet is to some extent avoidable [2, 24]. We report one laceration at the inferior border of the iliac vein, a well-known and feared complication of sacropexy. That is probably the reason why we were ready to compress the vein immediately with a swab.

Despite adequate control of the situation, the vascular surgeon preferred to perform an open repair. Others have reported laparoscopic management of such event [25]. There was one bowel perforation diagnosed during entry by open laparoscopy, hence without clinical consequences. In case of potential bacterial contamination, we do not use durable mesh as it may get permanently colonized, yet use in that case resorbable biografts despite poorer outcomes [18, 26]. The other intra-operative complications, such as bladder or vaginal perforations, can easily be managed laparoscopically with no clinical consequences. These were also frequently reported by others [2, 14, 24]. Also, hypercapnia can be managed, either by conversion or by pausing the intervention. None of the above intra-operative complications seem to us directly age-related neither are they are avoidable by cautious patient selection.

There were also a number of severe *postoperative* complications. There was the patient with discitis, which required prolonged use of antibiotics, yet no mesh removal. Discitis is a debilitating complication, which may require multiple reinterventions. It has been tied to the use of staples or tackers, yet it has also been reported when sutures are used and after open repair [27, 28]. Discitis is uncommon so typically individual cases are reported or will only surface in large series. We do not see any reason why it would be age-related. We had another severe local infectious complication. This woman presented with clinical signs of pelvic infection so we thought the mesh was infected. She was so sick she was admitted to ICU and underwent mesh removal, after which she fully recovered. In retrospect, we probably underestimated her co-morbidities and could have offered her an alternative surgical technique. A third complication, which was also in part infectious, was the COPD patient with chronic cough and respiratory infection, in whom coughing caused early release of the vault. She was successfully reoperated (Dindo IIIb) when her respiratory problems were solved. We preoperatively felt she should have sacrocolpopexy after two earlier failed vaginal repairs. There were also two obstructions, one because of adhesions. Though we always peritonealize, adhesions are unavoidable, except when choosing a vaginal extraperitoneal alternative, like sacrospinous fixation. Another striking complication is postoperative bleeding. Though clinically there was intra-abdominally convincing evidence of previous bleeding, we could never identify an active source. Postoperative hemorrhage is not the privilege of abdominal procedures, neither is it more likely in the elderly.

This study was essentially undertaken to investigate whether LSCP is justifiable in the elder population. In our series, we did not find a higher risk in patients above 70 years of age. This was neither the case when we took a lower (65 years) or higher age cut off (data not shown). The same observation was made by others, though all studies with another age cut off (range 65–80 years) [2, 13, 14]. This is also in line with observations following abdominal sacrocolpopexy [29]. Conversely, Turner et al. observed a higher major complication rate following laparoscopic or robotic sacrocolpopexy in women ≥ 65 years, both unadjusted (OR 1.84, 95% CI 1.02–3.35, p = 0.04), yet also after adjustment for BMI, estimated blood loss (EBL) and operating room time (OR 2.28, 95% CI 1.21–4.29, p = 0.01). The authors were unable "to reliably attribute the increased risk in the elderly" to the particularities of minimal invasive surgery in this population [2]. We did not correct for EBL or operating time, as they are dependent on concomitant surgery and because EBL cannot be accurately measured. Also, BMI was comparable in our patients with and without severe complications. Also in other surgical disciplines, laparoscopy is the preferred access route in the elderly, such as for cholecystectomy [30] or colonic surgery, including for cancer [31, 32]. Also rectopexy, which technically is very comparable to LSCP, can be safely offered to the elderly [33]. In brief, elder patients are in fact the ones who benefit the most of avoiding a laparotomy.

Our study definitely has its weaknesses. One limitation is generic in nature as it is due to the inherent limitations of the used classifications systems. The Clavien-Dindo grading system does not necessarily refer to the clinically most relevant complications. On the one hand, it identifies asymptomatic urinary tract infections (UTI) treated by a single course of oral antibiotics (or any other one time used drug such as an antihypertensive) as a Dindo II complication. Short lasting per-oral drug administration is barely considered as a complication by patients and physicians. Moreover, some of these complications, like UTI, are only picked up because one screens for it, hence may never be symptomatic. Along the same lines, also the IUGA mesh complication system identifies asymptomatic exposures as a grade 2A complication, including a suture exposure. Such complications are obviously clinically irrelevant, whatever the age of the patient. Conversely, the Dindo classification system underestimates relevant incidents like transient neurological symptoms, such as sensory or motoric dysfunction in the lower limbs, which we tied to wrong positioning of the patient [5]. Though they only required prolonged physiotherapy and other conservative measures, and eventually fully recovered, this is a tangible complication for the patient and the healthcare system. It however qualifies as a Dindo I complication, hence was not included here. Moreover, in the elderly any limitation in mobility is adversely influencing outcome. Briefly, the limitation of the Dindo classification is that it is based on the nature of the intervention prompted by the complication. In that respect, the IUGA/ICS mesh-complication classification is more patient-centered.

We acknowledge a number of other limitations. Though based on a large prospective cohort, it remains a retrospective audit on what eventually stays a selected population of women judged to be fit for general anesthesia (hence, not the others). Retrospective studies have the potential of underreporting. We have tried to tackle this limitation, by [1] including all consecutive cases; [2] having the data audited by a third person not involved in the management of the patient [3]; in the absence of physical postoperative visit of the patient, we used the electronic medical record system used in a network of hospitals and [4] contacted where necessary the general practitioner of the patient. The latter two increased the follow-up rate from 95 to 100%, yet it is possible that a number of events may have been missed. Another potential confounder is that quite some patients had concomitant procedures, which on themselves may have caused complications. We decided to assume they were tied to the LSCP, which might be an overestimation. Conversely, we reported reactive conversions separately, hence did not include them in the statistics of procedures done completely by laparoscopy, as did Vandendriessche et al. [34]. In order to disclose them, we reported them separately in detail.

Another problem is that, despite the large cohort, the ultimate incidence of rare events limits statistical comparison between age groups. We therefore aggregated categories of complications to reach reasonable numbers. Obviously, these small numbers also limit the justified use of multivariate analysis for other factors than age. Further, we do not report outcomes on alternative procedures, such as sacrospinous fixation or colpocleisis, performed during the same period. This would be neither correct, as the selection criteria for these procedures were not exactly the same. To finish, we realize this is only a report on short-term outcomes, yet the functional and long-term outcome of this cohort is the subject of another study.

This study has however its strengths. To our knowledge, this is the largest cohort study looking into complications with a 100% short-term follow-up rate. It is a consecutive series of standardized operations at a single center, yet with both experienced operators and subspecialists in training. Finally, the assessment was done by a clinician not involved in the surgical management of the patients. Given that our overall outcomes fall in the range of what is expected, we believe the conclusion of this study stands.

In conclusion, in this large prospective cohort intraoperative and severe (Dindo III and IV), early postoperative complications occurred in 3.6 and 2.3%, respectively. Older age at the time of intervention was not associated with additional morbidity. Therefore, we conclude that LSCP appears to be well-tolerated and safe in elderly women with level I defects and without contra-indication for general anesthesia.

Abbreviations
BMI: Body mass index; CI: Confidence interval; COPD: Chronic obstructive pulmonary disease; EBL: Estimated blood loss; EU-28-population: European Union of the 28 countries-population; ICU: Intensive care unit; IQR: Interquartile range; IUGA: International Urogynaecological Association; LASH: Laparoscopic-assisted subtotal hysterectomy; LSCP: Laparoscopic sacrocolpopexy; OR: Odds ratio; POP: Pelvic organ prolapse; POP-Q: Pelvic organ prolapse quantification; RR: Relative risk; SPSS: Statistical Package for the Social Sciences; UTI: Urinary tract infection

Disclosures
Our research program has previously received support from Bard, Covedien, FEG Textiltechnik, Ethicon, Blasingame and Garrard Law. All provided unconditional grants managed by the transfer office Leuven Research and Development of the KU Leuven. The investigators design the protocols, are owners of the results, and publish these independently of the above. JDP is a proctor for Ethicon Endosurgery in their side-by-side teaching program.

Authors' contributions
KV, SH, SP, GC, FVDA, AW, ADH, PR, and JDP did the clinical management of the patients involved, both at the pre- and postoperative outpatient setting and perioperative follow-up. KV, SP, GC, and LC did the data collection. KV and JDP did the data analysis. All authors contributed to manuscript writing, read, and approved the manuscript.

Competing interest
We received an investigator-initiated research grant from Johnson & Johnson for an initial audit of sacropexy patients. Both the study protocol, data analysis, interpretation and reporting, as well as the manuscript were made without interference of the company.

Authors' information
JD was a fundamental clinical researcher for the Fonds Wetenschappelijk Onderzoek Vlaanderen (1801207) till 2015. He now is funded by the Great Ormond Street Hospital Charity Fund.

Author details
[1]Pelvic Floor Unit Department of Gynaecology, University Hospitals Leuven, Leuven Herestraat 49, 3000 Leuven, Belgium. [2]Department of Urology, University Hospitals Leuven, Leuven, Belgium. [3]Department of Abdominal Surgery, University Hospitals Leuven, Leuven, Belgium. [4]Departments of Gastroenterology, University Hospitals Leuven, Leuven, Belgium. [5]Academic Department of Development and Regeneration, Group Biomedical Sciences, Katholieke Universiteit Leuven, Leuven, Belgium. [6]Institute for Women's Health, University College London, London, UK.

References
1. Glazener C, Elders A, MacArthur C, Lancashire RJ, Herbison P, Hagen S et al (2013) Childbirth and prolapse: long-term associations with the symptoms and objective measurement of pelvic organ prolapse. BJOG Int J Obstet Gynaecol 120(2):161–168
2. Turner LC, Kantartzis K, Lowder JL, Shepherd JP (2014) The effect of age on complications in women undergoing minimally invasive sacral colpopexy. Int Urogynecol J 25(9):1251–1256
3. Maher C, Feiner B, Baessler K, Christmann-Schmid C, Haya N, Brown J (2016) Surgery for women with apical vaginal prolapse. Cochrane Database Syst Rev 10:CD012376
4. Claerhout F, De Ridder D, Roovers JP, Rommens H, Spelzini F, Vandenbroucke V et al (2009) Medium-term anatomic and functional results of laparoscopic sacrocolpopexy beyond the learning curve. Eur Urol 55(6):1459–1467
5. Claerhout F, Roovers JP, Lewi P, Verguts J, De Ridder D, Deprest J (2009) Implementation of laparoscopic sacrocolpopexy–a single centre's experience. Int Urogynecol J Pelvic Floor Dysfunct 20(9):1119–1125
6. Freeman RM, Pantazis K, Thomson A, Frappell J, Bombieri L, Moran P et al (2013) A randomised controlled trial of abdominal versus laparoscopic sacrocolpopexy for the treatment of post-hysterectomy vaginal vault prolapse: LAS study. Int Urogynecol J 24(3):377–384
7. Callewaert G, Bosteels J, Housmans S, Verguts J, Van Cleynenbreugel B, Van der Aa F et al (2016) Laparoscopic versus robotic-assisted sacrocolpopexy for pelvic organ prolapse: a systematic review. Gynecol Surg 13:115–123
8. http://ec.europa.eu/eurostat/statistics-explained/index.php/Population_structure_and_ageing. Accessed 21 July 2017
9. Wu JM, Matthews CA, Conover MM, Pate V, Jonsson FM (2014) Lifetime risk of stress urinary incontinence or pelvic organ prolapse surgery. Obstet Gynecol 123(6):1201–1206
10. Smith FJ, Holman CD, Moorin RE, Tsokos N (2010) Lifetime risk of undergoing surgery for pelvic organ prolapse. Obstet Gynecol 116(5):1096–1100
11. Richardson JD, Cocanour CS, Kern JA, Garrison RN, Kirton OC, Cofer JB et al (2004) Perioperative risk assessment in elderly and high-risk patients. J Am Coll Surg 199(1):133–146
12. Bates AT, Divino C (2015) Laparoscopic surgery in the elderly: a review of the literature. Aging Dis 6(2):149–155
13. King SW, Jefferis H, Jackson S, Marfin AG, Price N (2017) Laparoscopic uterovaginal prolapse surgery in the elderly: feasibility and outcomes. Gynecol Surg 14(1):2
14. Boudy AS, Thubert T, Vinchant M, Hermieu JF, Villefranque V, Deffieux X (2016) Outcomes of laparoscopic sacropexy in women over 70: a comparative study. Eur J Obstet Gynecol Reprod Biol 207:178–183
15. Bump RC, Mattiasson A, Bo K, Brubaker LP, DeLancey JO, Klarskov P et al (1996) The standardization of terminology of female pelvic organ prolapse and pelvic floor dysfunction. Am J Obstet Gynecol 175(1):10–17
16. Claerhout F, Verguts J, Werbrouck E, Veldman J, Lewi P, Deprest J (2014) Analysis of the learning process for laparoscopic sacrocolpopexy: identification of challenging steps. Int Urogynecol J 25(9):1185–1191
17. Manodoro S, Werbrouck E, Veldman J, Haest K, Corona R, Claerhout F et al (2011) Laparoscopic sacrocolpopexy. Facts, views & vision in ObGyn 3(3):151–158
18. Deprest J, De Ridder D, Roovers JP, Werbrouck E, Coremans G, Claerhout F (2009) Medium term outcome of laparoscopic sacrocolpopexy with xenografts compared to synthetic grafts. J Urol 182(5):2362–2368
19. Dindo D, Demartines N, Clavien PA (2004) Classification of surgical complications: a new proposal with evaluation in a cohort of 6336 patients and results of a survey. Ann Surg 240(2):205–213
20. Haylen BT, Freeman RM, Swift SE, Cosson M, Davila GW, Deprest J et al (2011) An international Urogynecological association (IUGA) / international continence society (ICS) joint terminology and classification of the complications related directly to the insertion of prostheses (meshes, implants, tapes) and grafts in female pelvic floor surgery. Int Urogynecol J Pelvic Floor Dysfunct 22(1):3–15
21. Consten EC, van Iersel JJ, Verheijen PM, Broeders IA, Wolthuis AM, D'Hoore A. Long-term outcome after laparoscopic ventral mesh rectopexy: an observational study of 919 consecutive patients. Ann Surg 2015;262(5):742-747; discussion 7-8
22. Blikkendaal MD, Twijnstra AR, Stiggelbout AM, Beerlage HP, Bemelman WA, Jansen FW (2013) Achieving consensus on the definition of conversion to laparotomy: a Delphi study among general surgeons, gynecologists, and urologists. Surg Endosc 27(12):4631–4639
23. Twijnstra AR, Blikkendaal MD, van Zwet EW, Jansen FW (2013) Clinical relevance of conversion rate and its evaluation in laparoscopic hysterectomy. J Minim Invasive Gynecol 20(1):64–72
24. Vandendriessche D, Giraudet G, Lucot JP, Behal H, Cosson M (2015) Impact of laparoscopic sacrocolpopexy learning curve on operative time, perioperative complications and short term results. Eur J Obstet Gynecol Reprod Biol 191:84–89

25. Jafari MD, Pigazzi A (2013) Techniques for laparoscopic repair of major intraoperative vascular injury: case reports and review of literature. Surg Endosc 27(8):3021–3027

26. Claerhout F, De Ridder D, Van Beckevoort D, Coremans G, Veldman J, Lewi P et al (2010) Sacrocolpopexy using xenogenic acellular collagen in patients at increased risk for graft-related complications. Neurourol Urodyn 29(4):563–567

27. Rajamaheswari N, Agarwal S, Seethalakshmi K (2012) Lumbosacral spondylodiscitis: an unusual complication of abdominal sacrocolpopexy. Int Urogynecol J 23(3):375–377

28. Brito LG, Giraudet G, Lucot JP, Cosson M (2015) Spondylodiscitis after sacrocolpopexy. Eur J Obstet Gynecol Reprod Biol 187:72

29. Richter HE, Goode PS, Kenton K, Brown MB, Burgio KL, Kreder K et al (2007) The effect of age on short-term outcomes after abdominal surgery for pelvic organ prolapse. J Am Geriatr Soc 55(6):857–863

30. Lill S, Rantala A, Vahlberg T, Gronroos JM (2011) Elective laparoscopic cholecystectomy: the effect of age on conversions, complications and long-term results. Dig Surg 28(3):205–209

31. Denet C, Fuks D, Cocco F, Chopinet S, Abbas M, Costea C et al (2017) Effects of age after laparoscopic right colectomy for cancer: are there any specific outcomes? Dig Liver Dis 49(5):562–567

32. Sklow B, Read T, Birnbaum E, Fry R, Age FJ (2003) Type of procedure influence the choice of patients for laparoscopic colectomy. Surg Endosc 17(6):923–929

33. Gultekin FA, Wong MT, Podevin J, Barussaud ML, Boutami M, Lehur PA et al (2015) Safety of laparoscopic ventral rectopexy in the elderly: results from a nationwide database. Dis Colon Rectum 58(3):339–343

34. Vandendriessche D, Sussfeld J, Giraudet G, Lucot JP, Behal H, Cosson M (2017) Complications and reoperations after laparoscopic sacrocolpopexy with a mean follow-up of 4 years. Int Urogynecol J 28(2):231–239

24

Feasibility and safety of total laparoscopic hysterectomy for huge uteri without the use of uterine manipulator: description of emblematic cases

Antonio Macciò[1*], Clelia Madeddu[2], Paraskevas Kotsonis[1], Giacomo Chiappe[1], Fabrizio Lavra[1], Ivan Collu[1] and Roberto Demontis[3]

Abstract

Background: Uterine manipulator is a very useful tool in performing total laparoscopic hysterectomy (TLH) for large uteri; however, in some cases, it cannot be used due to unfavorable anatomical conditions. The feasibility and safety of TLH for very large uteri without the use of uterine manipulator has not yet been established.

Results: We describe two emblematic cases of TLH for huge fibromatous uteri: the first one for a uterus weighing 5700 g, which is the largest uterus laparoscopically removed to date reported in literature, and the second one for a uterus of 3670 g associated with a severe lymph node neoplastic disease.

In both cases, TLH was successfully and safely performed even without the use of uterine manipulator, thus allowing a rapid recovery, especially in the second case, which was essential for a fast start of the most appropriate oncological treatment, the best quality of life and undoubtedly cosmetic advantages.

Conclusions: Although we believe in the great usefulness of the uterine manipulator in performing TLH for huge uteri, in the present paper, we demonstrate the feasibility and safety of such complex surgery also when the use of this tool is not possible due to unfavorable anatomical condition.

Keywords: Uterine fibromatosis, Total laparoscopic hysterectomy, Huge uteri, Uterine manipulator

Background

Hysterectomy is one of the most commonly performed gynecological procedures. Since the first total laparoscopic hysterectomy (TLH) has been published in 1993 [1], surgeons have tried to identify tools and techniques that could make surgery simpler and safer. Uterine manipulators were among the first instruments introduced to improve laparoscopic performance [2]. Indeed, to date, most publications state that manipulators provide multifunctional assistance in gynecologic surgery, particularly during TLH [3]. Recently, we emphasized the usefulness of the uterine manipulator for laparoscopic removal of large fibromatous uteri ranging from 300 to 5320 g [4, 5]. We clarified that the manipulator aids in mobilizing the uterus to better define surrounding organs to display the vaginal fornices for easier culdotomy and to move the ureter from the uterine cervix to avoid damage. However, there are situations where, for anatomical reasons, the uterine manipulator cannot be used; for example, in the case of vaginal stenosis or other anatomic situations in which it is difficult to identify the uterine cervix. We believe that such situations should not prevent the use of laparoscopic surgery, even in the case of very large fibromatous uteri, and that these issues should be adequately explored and discussed. For this reason, we describe two emblematic cases of laparoscopic removal of a huge fibromatous uterus weighing 5700 and 3670 g, respectively, without the use of a uterine manipulator.

* Correspondence: a.maccio@tin.it
[1]Department of Gynecologic Oncology, Azienda Ospedaliera Brotzu, via Jenner, 09100 Cagliari, Italy
Full list of author information is available at the end of the article

Methods

The TLH was performed according to the procedure we previously reported [4, 5]. However, in this case, we omitted the use of the uterine manipulator due to unfavorable anatomical findings. A 12-mm trocar was positioned via an open entry technique nearly the xiphoid process, and a 10–14-mmHg pneumoperitoneum was obtained. Four 5-mm trocars were positioned laterally to the rectus abdominis; the lowest of these was used, in the absence of the uterine manipulator, to push cephalad the markedly enlarged uterus to reproduce the "traction-counter traction" effect and obtain both the displacement of the lower uterine segment aside from ureters and elevation of uterine arteries alongside the cervix. A 12-mm trocar was placed at the umbilicus, and another 5-mm trocar was inserted in the suprapubic position. The surgery table was positioned in the Trendelenburg orientation, and the stages of surgery were as previously described by the authors [5] for the removal of uterus of similar weight combined with bilateral adnexectomy, using Ligasure (Tyco Healthcare, Norwalk, CT, USA). The uterine arteries were skeletonized, coagulated with the BiClamp LAP forceps (ERBE GmbH, Tubingen, Germany), and then resected with Ligasure. After the introduction of a small surgical swab in the vagina, the cervicovaginal edge was laparoscopically identified and catted with monopolar scissor, and the colpotomy was completed using Ligasure. As is our routine practice, after the cervix dissection, a Foley catheter was inserted into the vagina to prevent losing of the pneumoperitoneum. The laparoscopic suture of the vaginal cuff was performed with a continuous closure using the V-Loc device (Covidien-Medtronic, Minneapolis, MN, USA). The uterus was then extracted from the abdomen via a very low transverse laparotomy cut of approximately 5 cm, to reduce operative time, utilizing a wound protector/retractor (Wound Edge Protector - 3MTM Steri-DrapeTM 1073, Diegem, Belgium), and morcellated outside the abdomen with a cold blade scalpel to avoid spillage. Finally, after suture of the low minilaparotomy, we laparoscopically cautiously evaluated the abdominal cavity and repeatedly washed it.

Results

Case 1

A 52-year-old, Caucasian, 1 para, obese (body mass index (BMI) 32.46) female presented to our department for progressive increase in abdominal circumference in the previous year associated with constipation and dyspnea. A fibromatous uterus had been diagnosed previously by pelvic magnetic resonance. Her surgical history included a previous cesarean section. No relevant disturbances of the menstrual cycle were referred by the patient. Physical exam showed an abdomen entirely occupied by a pelvic mass reaching the xiphoid process, which was especially evident when the patient laid supine (Fig. 1). On bimanual pelvic examination, the superior third of the vagina was making it impossible to visualize the cervix. Abdominal and vaginal ultrasound performed on hospital admission confirmed a huge fibromatous uterus. Cervicovaginal smear and endometrial sampling, to exclude potential endometrial cancer, could not be performed for the above reported anatomical reasons. The patient had normal hematological, the liver and renal function parameters. Tumor markers were within the normal range. The patient was counseled on the various surgical options and the associated risks, and she opted for a minimally invasive approach, if feasible. Then, detailed written informed consent, prepared by a forensic expert physician, was obtained for the procedure as well as for the publication of a case report and the accompanying images. The TLH was performed as described above. No intraoperative complications occurred; the operative time was approximately 200 min. Intraoperative blood loss was 300 ml due to bleeding at the time of skeletonization of the left uterine vein, which was particularly large and frail. The removed uterus weighed 5700 g. The histological examination revealed a benign fibroid uterus. The patient left the hospital on postoperative day 3 in a very good state. Seven days after discharge she was readmitted to our department because of fever with elevated C-reactive protein (CRP) level and white cell count associated with left basal thoracic pain; then, she underwent total body computed tomography (CT) that showed basal bronchopneumonitis, which resolved with antibiotics. The patient was discharged after 2 days and continued antibiotic therapy at home. One month after discharge, the patient was in excellent condition.

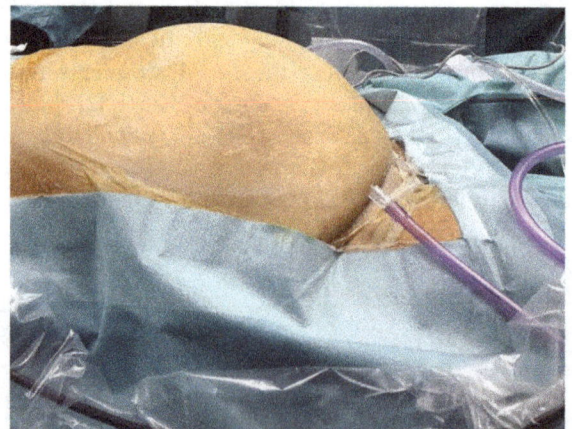

Fig. 1 Case 1: enlarged abdomen with the patient lying supine before surgery

Case 2

A 50-year-old obese (BMI 34.25) woman was referred to our department from another hospital because we are the Regional Referral Center for cancer disease, with the diagnosis of a huge abdominal mass and a large right pelvic lymph node mass associated with severe edematous enlargement of the ipsilateral lower limb, suspicious for thrombophlebitis. On bimanual pelvic examination, the vagina was occupied by a voluminous spherical mass, the size of a tennis ball. The mass originated from the right vaginal fornix, making it impossible to reach and evaluate the cervix. A large fibromatous mass, reaching the third space above the transverse umbilical line, filled entirely the abdomen. Total body CT showed a huge inhomogeneous uterus measuring more than 20 cm, occupying entirely the right pelvis (Fig. 2). This lesion appeared in continuity with another inhomogeneous mass, considered likely to be lymphatic in origin, measuring approximately 14×15 cm, extending to the proximal extremity of the right thigh (Fig. 3), and incorporating the vascular structures from the aortic bifurcation to the iliac-femoral venous axis. The large abdominal mass at the right iliac fossa constricted the vena cava, the bladder, and the right ureter with initial pyeloureteral dilatation. No pelvic effusion nor pathological findings outside the abdomen and pelvis were noted. On admission, laboratory analyses showed high levels of CA-125 (2195 U/ml, normal level < 35), C-reactive protein (0.3 mg/dL, normal range 0–0.10), fibrinogen (448 mg/dL, normal range 200–400), LDH (1976 U/L, normal range 0–248), and low hemoglobin

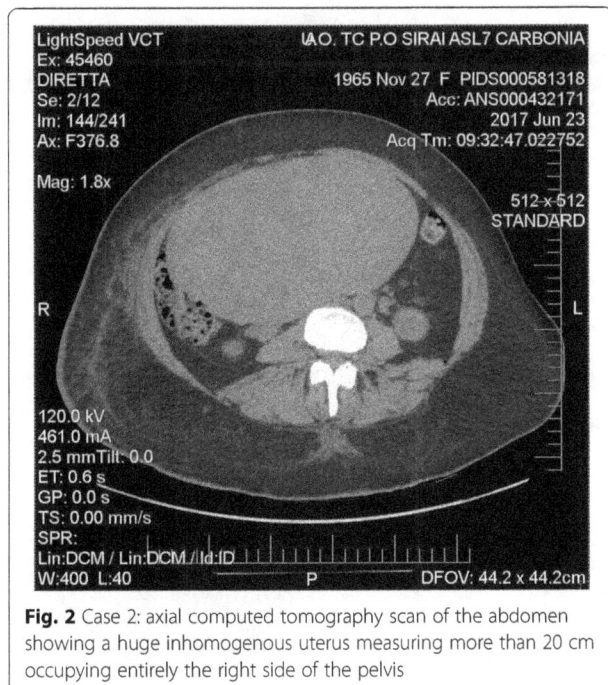

Fig. 3 Case 2: axial computed tomography scan showing the lymph node mass (14×15 cm) extending to the origin of the right thigh

(10.5 g/dl, range 12–15), iron (32 mg/dL, normal range 60–180), and ferritin (34 ng/mL, normal range 10–291). Assuming the presence of two pathologies, i.e., a massive fibromatous uterus and a myeloproliferative disease associated with thrombophlebitis of the right leg due to compression, we proposed that the patient underwent a mini-invasive exploratory laparoscopy with possible hysterectomy plus bilateral adnexectomy and lymph node biopsy. This approach was chosen based on the urgent need to decompress the pelvis from the massive uterine mass and to reduce the patient's delay in receiving the appropriate chemotherapy. The patient signed an informed consent and agreed to our surgical plan. The surgical technique was as described in the previous section, without the use of the uterine manipulator due to the unfavorable findings of the vagina occupied by the massive lymph node masses. In particular, the ureter isolation was required throughout its course, freeing it from the adhesions with the massive lymph nodes extending from the origin of the common iliac artery to the inguinal canal, including the hypogastric artery. Both uterine arteries were coagulated at the origin of the hypogastric artery. The surgery was subsequently carried out as reported above, with the support of a laparotomy incision of approximately 5 cm. Prior to the removal of the uterus, an extensive excision of the lymph node mass was performed at the level of the common right iliac artery, and the specimen was sent for intraoperative histological examination, with a diagnosis of lymphoproliferative disease. The definitive histology diagnosed a large B cell lymphoma, present in 20 out of 24 removed lymph nodes, with an ovarian secondary involvement.

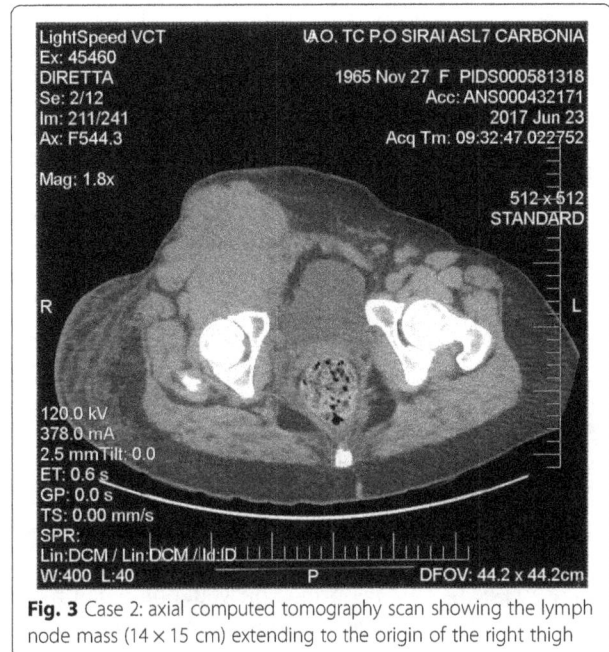

Fig. 2 Case 2: axial computed tomography scan of the abdomen showing a huge inhomogenous uterus measuring more than 20 cm occupying entirely the right side of the pelvis

The postoperative course was optimal and the patient was quickly transferred to the Department of Oncology/ Hematology at our Institute, where she is currently receiving the appropriate chemotherapy treatment.

Discussion

The central role that laparoscopy now plays in gynecological surgery is indisputable, especially in the case of TLH. A recent Cochrane analysis has reported that vaginal hysterectomy (VH) seems to be a superior minimal access method for benign gynecological disease in comparison to TLH, although the authors emphasized in their conclusions that the surgical approach to hysterectomy should be decided with the patient on the basis of the relative benefit and risks, which are dependent on the surgical expertise [6]. In fact, it must be clarified that, despite the widespread use of laparoscopic hysterectomy, this approach should be applied in those cases where VH cannot be performed or would be much more complex, or in case of adnexal disease or where laparoscopy avoids open surgery while offering certain advantages in efficacy, safety, time of hospitalization, and recovery. It should be added that, among the different procedures, TLH has higher costs in comparison to the vaginal and abdominal surgery [7]. Then, the comparison between various surgical procedures can be effectively performed only when the indications for surgery are similar, clear, and appropriate. The choice of surgical approach in the case of a large uterus presents an entirely different discussion. The precise surgical conditions that make the TLH technique for large uteri feasible, repeatable, and safe have been codified so that skilled and well-coordinated teams choose it as the first choice approach rather than laparotomy, even in the case of huge uteri. The publications of these working groups, including the current authors, have highlighted some central points regarding the performance of TLH for very large uteri, including pneumoperitoneum created in the neutral position, trocar number and location dependent upon the uterine size, modifying the trocar positions during the surgery for a better view, and the uterine vessel coagulation using the BiClamp to provide very good hemostasis [4, 8, 9]. With these two clinical cases, we describe the feasibility of performing TLH without the use of the uterine manipulator, even in the case of very large uteri. Such technical possibility has been already described [10], but for uteri of a size not comparable to the cases herein reported. Far from affirming the usefulness of the uterine manipulator, however, we demonstrated the feasibility and safety of such complex interventions even in its absence. We emphasize that only unfavorable conditions should lead to perform this surgery without this valuable tool. Moreover, we believe that the description of these interventions and their technical modalities should be a matter of discussion and may aid those

surgeons who choose this mini-invasive approach. The unique clinical features of our two cases should also be highlighted. In the first case, the uterus was extremely great, weighing 5700 g, similar to a case we previously reported of 5320 g [5]; this, therefore, constitutes the description of the largest uterus removed laparoscopically in the published literature to date. The second case is notable for the association of a massive fibromatous uterus with severe lymph node neoplastic disease, which created difficulty in providing an exact diagnosis and also in choosing the most appropriate surgical techniques for a successful outcome. In this second case, our approach allowed the patient's rapid healing and fast initiation of oncologic treatment.

Conclusions

These peculiar clinical cases reaffirm the efficacy and safety of TLH, even in the case of very large uteri, also without using an important instrument such as the uterine manipulator. The presence of other associated pathologies (i.e., the pelvic lymph node disease), while making the intervention more complex and lengthy, underlines that, also in such truly complex cases, TLH is a valid alternative to open surgery, provided that highly experienced and well-coordinated surgical teams perform it. The immediate recovery after TLH is also a major aspect in the patient comprehensive clinical management, as in the second case herein described where the patient was able to access the most appropriate antiblastic therapy as soon as possible in excellent postoperative conditions and, thus, with great therapeutic benefits.

Abbreviations
BMI: Body mass index; CT: Computed tomography; TLH: Total laparoscopic hysterectomy

Acknowledgements
The authors would like to thank Andreea Voicu, Claudia Vacca, Federica Concas, and Martina Trudu for their technical assistance.

Funding
This work supported by the "Associazione Sarda per la Ricerca in Ginecologia Oncologica - ONLUS".

Authors' contributions
AM participated in the study design and protocol development, data collection and management, data analysis, and manuscript writing. CM contributed to the data collection and management, data analysis, and manuscript writing. PKK contributed to the data collection, manuscript editing, and final approval of the manuscript. GC contributed to the data collection, manuscript editing, and final approval of the manuscript. FL contributed to the data collection, manuscript editing, and final approval of the manuscript. IC contributed to the data collection, manuscript editing, and final approval of the manuscript. RD contributed to the protocol development, preparation and acquisition of informed consent, data analysis, and manuscript writing. All authors read and approved the final manuscript.

Feasibility and safety of total laparoscopic hysterectomy for huge uteri without the use of uterine...

159

Competing interests

The authors declare that they have no competing interests.

Author details

[1]Department of Gynecologic Oncology, Azienda Ospedaliera Brotzu, via Jenner, 09100 Cagliari, Italy. [2]Department of Medical Sciences and Public Health, University of Cagliari, Cagliari, Italy. [3]Department of Medical Sciences and Public Health, Section of Forensic Medicine, University of Cagliari, Cagliari, Italy.

References

1. Reich H, McGlynn F, Sekel L (1993) Total laparoscopic hysterectomy. Gynaecol Endosc 2:59–63
2. Nassif J, Wattiez A (2010) Clermont Ferrand uterine manipulator. Surg Technol Int 20:225–231
3. Van den Haak L, Alleblas C, Nieboer TE, Rhemrev JP, Jansen FW (2015) Efficacy and safety of uterine manipulators in laparoscopic surgery: a review. Arch Gynecol Obstet 292:1003–1011
4. Macciò A, Chiappe G, Kotsonis P, Nieddu R, Lavra F, Serra M, Onnis P, Sollai G, Zamboni F, Madeddu C (2016) Surgical outcome and complications of total laparoscopic hysterectomy for very large myomatous uteri in relation to uterine weight: a prospective study in a continuous series of 461 procedures. Arch Gynecol Obstet 294:525–531
5. Macciò A, Kotsonis P, Lavra F, Chiappe G, Sanna D, Zamboni F, Madeddu C (2017) Laparoscopic removal of a very large uterus weighting 5320 g is feasible and safe: a case report. BMC Surg 17(1):50
6. Aarts JW, Nieboer TE, Johnson N, Tavender E, Garry R, Mol BW, Kluivers KB (2015) Surgical approach to hysterectomy for benign gynaecological disease. Cochrane Database Syst Rev 8:CD003677
7. Sandberg EM, Twijnstra AR, Driessen SR, Jansen FW (2017) Total laparoscopic hysterectomy versus vaginal hysterectomy: a systematic review and meta-analysis. J Minim Invasive Gynecol 24:206–217 e22
8. Yavuzcan A, Caglar M, Ustun Y, Dilbaz S, Kumru S (2014) Evaluation of the outcomes of laparoscopic hysterectomy for normal and enlarged uterus (> 280 g). Arch Gynecol Obstet 289:831–837
9. Wu KY, Lertvikool S, Huang KG, Su H, Yen CF, Lee CL (2011) Laparoscopic hysterectomies for large uteri. Taiwan J Obstet Gynecol 50:411–414
10. Mebes I, Diedrich K, Banz-Jansen C (2012) Total laparoscopic hysterectomy without uterine manipulator at big uterus weight (> 280 g). Arch Gynecol Obstet 286:131–134

25

Fertility outcome after treatment of retained products of conception

Tjalina W. O. Hamerlynck[1*], Dora Meyers[2], Hannelore Van der Veken[1], Jan Bosteels[1,3] and Steven Weyers[1]

Abstract

Background: Treatment of retained products of conception (RPOC) can be expectant, medical or operative. Surgical removal of RPOC may lead to intrauterine adhesions (IUA) and Asherman's syndrome.

Objective: To evaluate how treatment options for RPOC affect future fertility by means of a systematic review.

Search strategy: MEDLINE, EMBASE, The Cochrane Library, and clinical trial registers were searched, and reference lists were scanned.

Selection criteria: Randomised controlled trials (RCT) comparing different treatment options for RPOC (conservative, medical or surgical treatment, including curettage and/or hysteroscopic techniques, with or without application of anti-adhesion therapy), in women of reproductive age, were eligible for inclusion.

Data collection and analysis: Reviewers independently performed data extraction and quality of evidence assessment. For dichotomous variables, results were presented as risk ratio (RR) with 95% CI.

Main results: Two studies were included. Nonsignificant differences were observed between the use of an anti-adhesion barrier gel versus no treatment after operative hysteroscopy in IUAs (RR 0.32, 95% CI 0.04 to 2.80, P value = 0.30) and clinical pregnancy (RR 2.22, 95% CI 0.67 to 7.42, P value = 0.19), and between hysteroscopic morcellation versus loop resection in IUAs (RR 0.86, 95% CI 0.06 to 13.12, P value = 0.91).

Conclusion: There is insufficient evidence on how different treatment options for RPOC affect future reproductive outcomes. Results from ongoing RCTs are needed to guide clinicians towards choosing the best treatment.

Keywords: Retained products of conception, Treatment, Fertility, Reproductive outcome, Systematic review

Introduction

Retained products of conception (RPOC) consist of intra-uterine tissue that develops after conception and persists after miscarriage, termination of pregnancy, delivery or caesarean section [1]. The occurrence of RPOC is not rare; however, the prevalence varies widely (from 0.5 to as much as 19%) depending on pregnancy duration, pregnancy outcome and the successive management [2]. There is no consensus in literature on the type of tissue RPOC comprise. Some authors describe RPOC as non-villous trophoblastic tissue, chorionic villi or foetal membranes, and they state that decidua alone does not fall within the

definition [3–5]. Others say that RPOC consist of the gestational sac, the decidua capsularis, chorionic villi or the embryo itself [6]. Still others argue that RPOC are from placental origin, and thus, that the presence of chorionic villi in RPOC is necessary [1, 7].

The diagnosis of RPOC remains a clinical challenge. The existence of RPOC may be suspected based on clinical history, with patients having symptoms of vaginal bleeding, abdominal or pelvic pain, and/or fever. However, RPOC may also be present in asymptomatic patients [8]. Ultrasound (US) findings such as a thickened endometrial echo complex or the presence of an endometrial mass with or without detectable vascularity at colour or power Doppler US are highly suggestive for RPOC [1]. Still, there is no consensus on the US criteria, and US alone may not be sensitive and/or specific

* Correspondence: tjalina.hamerlynck@ugent.be
[1]Women's Clinic, Ghent University Hospital, C. Heymanslaan 10, 9000 Ghent, Belgium
Full list of author information is available at the end of the article

enough to confirm the presence or absence of RPOC [1]. In order to avoid unnecessary procedures, diagnostic hysteroscopy may be of additional value to ultrasonography, although this needs further research [9, 10].

In case expectant management or medical treatment of RPOC fails, the surgical treatment traditionally consists of dilation and curettage, preferably under US guidance, using vacuum aspiration and/or a metal curette. Nevertheless, operative hysteroscopy is a suitable alternative to 'blind' curettage in the treatment of RPOC [5, 11–16]. These surgical procedures for RPOC, however, expose the uterus to additional trauma, which can cause intrauterine adhesions (IUAs) and Asherman's syndrome, clinically manifested by menstrual abnormalities, infertility and recurrent pregnancy loss [17].

The objective of the present study was to evaluate how the different treatment options for RPOC affect future fertility.

Methods

We specified the methods in advance and registered the protocol of the review on PROSPERO (CRD42016042444). We followed the PRISMA guidelines for writing a systematic review.

Criteria for selecting studies for this review
Types of studies

Published parallel-group randomised controlled trials (RCTs) were eligible for inclusion. Non-randomised studies (e.g. studies with evidence of inadequate sequence generation such as alternate days, participant numbers) were excluded, as they are associated with a high risk of bias.

Types of participants

Women of reproductive age with RPOC more than 24 h after end of pregnancy, without the presence of gestational trophoblastic disease or uterine malignancies. Trials that excluded women who wished to conceive were not eligible.

Types of interventions

We included the following randomly assigned comparisons:

- Expectant management versus medical treatment
- Expectant management versus surgical removal by curettage or hysteroscopy
- Medical treatment versus surgical removal by curettage or hysteroscopy
- Curettage versus hysteroscopy
- Technique A versus technique B for operative hysteroscopy
- Anti-adhesion therapy versus placebo or no treatment following surgical treatment

The last two comparisons were not pre-defined in our review protocol. We included these randomised comparisons because at present different hysteroscopic techniques are available for the treatment of RPOC and anti-adhesion therapy following surgical treatment of RPOC may affect subsequent reproductive outcome [18]. The findings of our review might be biased if these two comparisons were omitted.

Types of outcome measures
Primary outcomes:

- Live birth rate. Live birth was defined as the complete expulsion or extraction from its mother of a product of fertilisation, irrespective of the duration of the pregnancy, which, after such separation, breathes or shows any other evidence of life, such as heart beat, umbilical cord pulsation, or definite movement of voluntary muscles, irrespective of whether the umbilical cord has been cut or the placenta is attached. We count the delivery of singleton, twin or multiple pregnancies as one live birth.
- Presence of IUAs at second-look hysteroscopy.

Secondary outcomes:

- Time to conception, conception rate and clinical pregnancy rate. Clinical pregnancy was defined as a pregnancy diagnosed by ultrasonographic visualisation of one or more gestational sacs or definitive clinical signs of pregnancy. It includes ectopic pregnancy. Multiple gestational sacs are counted as one clinical pregnancy.
- Miscarriage rate. Miscarriage was defined as the spontaneous loss of a clinical pregnancy before 20 completed weeks of gestational age (18 weeks after fertilisation) or, if gestational age is unknown, the loss of an embryo/foetus of less than 400 g.

Eligible studies that could have measured the outcomes of interest were reviewed and any lack of data for the key outcomes was reported in the final review. We adhered as much as possible to terminology of the International Committee for Monitoring Assisted Reproductive Technology (ICMART) (http://www.icmartivf.org/) for key reproductive outcomes (live birth, pregnancy and miscarriage) [19]. We contacted primary study authors for clarification in cases of unclear definitions. We reported discrepancies or uncertainties in the final review.

Search methods for identification of studies

The following electronic bibliographic databases were searched: MEDLINE, EMBASE, and The Cochrane

Library (Cochrane Central Register of Controlled Trials (CENTRAL)). The search strategy included terms relating to or describing the disease (retained products of conception), management or intervention (expectant, medical or surgical) and outcome (fertility). The search terms were adapted for use to each bibliographic database, and a combination of both MeSH/Emtree and free-text terms was used (Additional file 1: Appendix S1). There were no language restrictions in the search, but we included only articles in English, French, German, Dutch, Italian and Portuguese, due to restraints in time and cost. In addition, the reference lists of eligible studies were scanned, and clinical trial registers were searched for ongoing and registered trials (World Health Organization (WHO) International Clinical Trials Registry Platform (ICTRP) search portal (http://apps.who.int/trialsearch/) and ClinicalTrials.gov (https://clinicaltrials.gov)).

Data collection and analysis
Selection of studies
Duplicates of the studies obtained by the search strategy were removed using specialised software (EndNote X7). The titles and abstracts of the remaining studies were screened independently and simultaneously by two review authors (D.M., H.V.d.V.). The full texts of the potentially eligible studies were retrieved and independently assessed by the same two review team members for compliance with the inclusion criteria, and studies eligible for inclusion in the review were selected. Any disagreement during the selection was resolved through discussion or, if required, by consulting a third and/or fourth review author (T.H., S.W.).

Data extraction and management
A pre-piloted form (Additional file 2: Appendix S2) was used by two review authors (T.H., H.V.d.V.) independently to extract data from the included studies for assessment of study quality and evidence synthesis. Discrepancies were identified and resolved through discussion, with a third and/or fourth author (J.B., S.W.) where necessary. When information regarding an essential topic was missing or unclear, contact with the authors was attempted.

Assessment of risk of bias in included studies
Risk of bias of the included studies was independently assessed by two authors (T.H., H.V.d.V.) according to the Cochrane risk of bias assessment (random sequence generation, allocation concealment, blinding of participants and personnel, blinding of outcome assessment, incomplete outcome data, selective outcome reporting and other potential sources of bias) [20]. Disagreements between the review authors over the risk of bias in particular studies

were resolved by discussion, with involvement of a third review author (J.B.) where necessary.

Measures of treatment effect
For dichotomous outcomes, we used risk ratios (RR) with 95% confidence intervals (CI).

Data synthesis
Statistical analysis was performed using the software REVIEW MANAGER 5.3 provided by the Cochrane Collaboration [21]. For dichotomous variables, results were presented as RR with 95% CI. We aimed to perform statistical pooling if enough studies were retrieved. However, in case of clinical diversity or evidence of substantial statistical heterogeneity, we provided a narrative synthesis of the findings rather than statistical pooling.

Results
Description of studies
A total of 777 citations were identified from searching electronic databases and trial registers, of which 185 duplicate citations were removed. The remaining 592 records were assessed for eligibility through checking the titles and/or abstracts. We excluded 567 records as being obviously irrelevant. The eligibility of the remaining 25 articles was assessed by reading the full text. We retrieved six potentially eligible studies, we included two randomised trials (Additional file 3: Table S1), one was excluded (Additional file 4: Table S2) and three studies are ongoing (NCT02201732, NTR4923, ChiCTR-INR-16009 074) (Additional file 5: Table S3). The PRISMA flow chart for study selection is shown in Fig. 1.

We included two parallel-design RCTs [10, 22]. The first trial was performed in a tertiary medical care centre in Israel [22]. Fifty-two women underwent hysteroscopic surgery because of suspected RPOC. The mean age was 29.5 years (standard deviation (SD) 5.1 years) in the intervention group and 31.4 years (SD 6.5 years) in the control group. The trial did not include women with primary subfertility. After hysteroscopic removal of RPOC, a viscoelastic gel, composed of polyethylene oxide and carboxymethylcellulose, was applied or not. All patients received postoperative sequential hormone treatment and antibiotics. The outcomes were clinical pregnancy and presence of IUAs. The second trial was a multicentre study from Belgium and the Netherlands [10]. Eighty-six women who underwent hysteroscopic surgery because of RPOC were included. The mean age was 32 years (SD 6 years) in the hysteroscopic morcellation group and 31 years (SD 4 years) in the loop resection group. RPOC were removed by hysteroscopic morcellation or loop resection. In the resection group, cold loop resection was attempted first, whereas the loop was electrically activated in case the RPOC were too adherent to

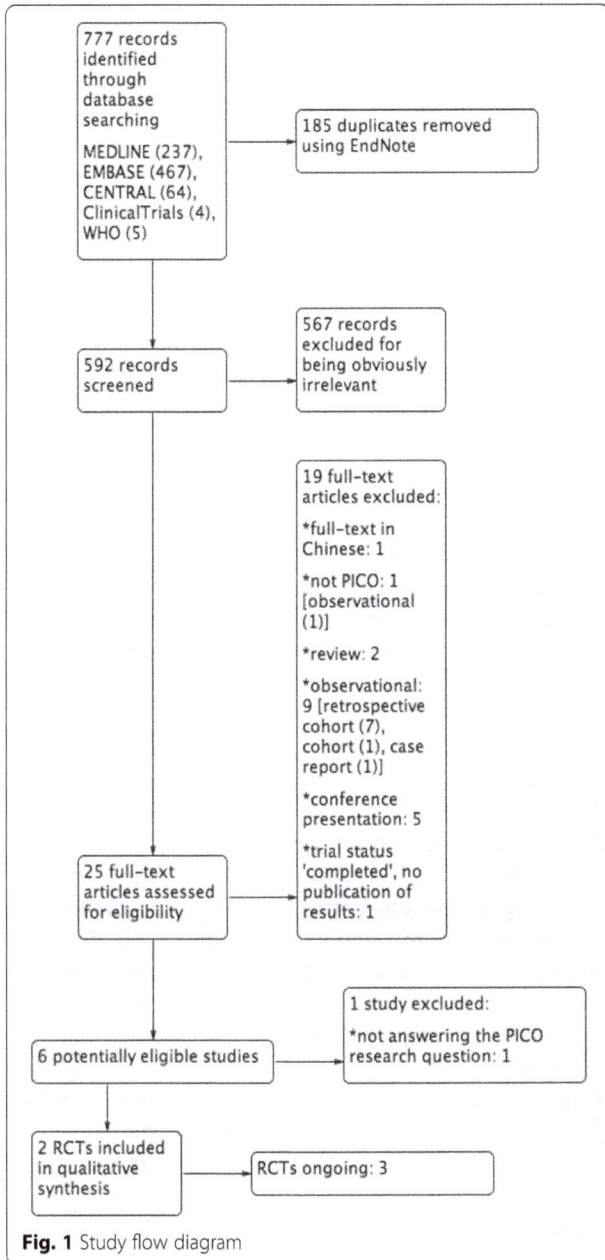

Fig. 1 Study flow diagram

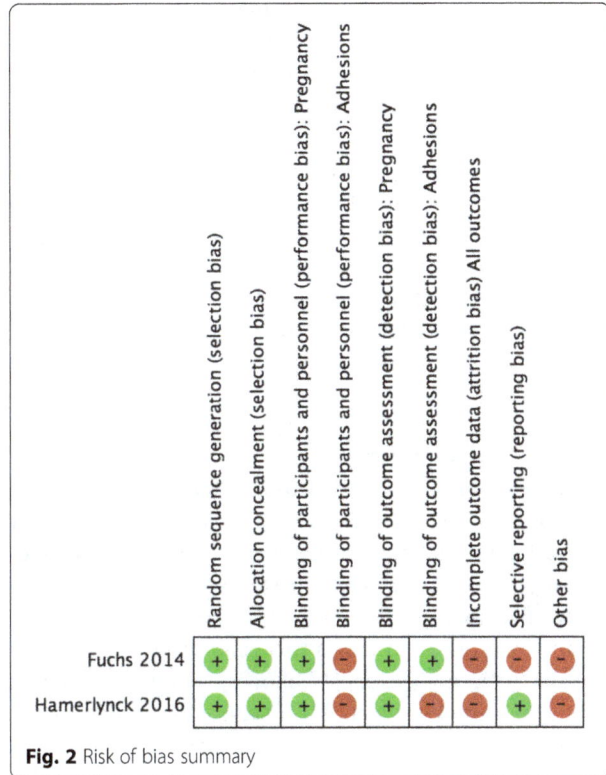

Fig. 2 Risk of bias summary

be removed by cold loop (4/39 cases, 10%). Patients did not receive any cervical ripening agents or standard antibiotic prophylaxis preoperatively. The outcome was the presence of IUAs.

Risk of bias in included studies

See: assessment of the risk of bias (Additional file 6: Table S4) and Fig. 2. We judged both trials to be at low risk for selection bias related to random sequence generation and allocation, because a computer-generated randomisation list and sequentially numbered opaque sealed envelopes were used. We judged both trials to be at low risk of performance and detection bias in relation

to blinding of participants, personnel and outcome assessors for the outcome of clinical pregnancy, because clinical pregnancy is an unequivocal outcome. For the outcome of presence of IUAs, we considered both trials to be at high risk of performance bias in relation to blinding of participants and personnel, because personnel were not blinded in the trial of Fuchs et al. and participants and personnel were not blinded in the trial of Hamerlynck et al. We found the trial of Fuchs et al. to be at low risk of detection bias for the key outcome of IUAs because outcome assessors were independent observers blinded to treatment allocation. However, we found the trial of Hamerlynck et al. to be at high risk of detection bias for the outcome of IUAs because outcome assessors were aware of the treatment allocation. We judged the trial of Fuchs et al. to be at high risk of attrition bias, because a high proportion of women were excluded after randomisation (11/52 or 21%) without clarification of the reasons. Similarly, in the trial of Hamerlynck et al., 9 of 44 participants and 6 of 39 participants undergoing hysteroscopic removal of placental remnants did not undergo second-look hysteroscopy (15/83 or 18%), leading to a high risk of attrition bias. We considered the trial of Fuchs et al. to be at high risk of selective reporting, because it failed to report data for the primary outcome of live birth despite a study duration of 27 months. The trial of Hamerlynck et al. was considered to be at low risk of selective reporting, because all pre-specified outcomes were reported. We found the trial of Fuchs et al. to be at high risk of other potential sources of bias, because at follow-up hysteroscopy co-treatment with hysteroscopic adhesiolysis was offered to women with AFS II or III IUAs. The differences in co-treatment between both comparison groups—three of 20 (14%) women in the control group and one of 21 (4%) women in the intervention group—may have affected the extent and course of the treatment effect. Similarly, in the trial of Hamerlynck et al., adhesiolysis was offered to women with IUAs, leading to a potential source of bias in relation to fertility outcome.

Effects of interventions

We retrieved no randomised studies for the comparisons of expectant management versus medical treatment or surgical removal, medical treatment versus surgical removal, or curettage versus hysteroscopy for the treatment of RPOC.

We found one randomised trial comparing anti-adhesion therapy with no treatment following surgical treatment [22]. There was no evidence of a statistically significant difference between both comparison groups for the outcome of IUAs at second-look hysteroscopy at 5 to 8 weeks (RR 0.32, 95% CI 0.04 to 2.80, P value = 0.30, one study, 41 women; Fig. 3). There were no statistically significant differences in clinical pregnancy rates between both comparison groups (RR 2.22, 95% CI 0.67 to 7.42, P value = 0.19, 1 study, 41 women; Fig. 3). We retrieved one randomised trial comparing hysteroscopic morcellation with loop resection for removal of RPOC [10]. There was no evidence of a statistically significant difference between both comparison groups for the outcome of de novo IUAs at second-look hysteroscopy at 6 to 8 weeks (RR 0.86, 95% CI 0.06 to 13.12, P value = 0.91, 1 study, 65 women; Fig. 4).

Discussion
Main findings
Our systematic review aimed at investigating the influence of the treatment of RPOC on reproductive outcome and the presence of IUAs. We searched for randomised trials comparing different treatment options (expectant management, medical and surgical treatment) for women of reproductive age with RPOC more than 24 h after end of pregnancy, in relation to fertility and/or the presence of IUAs.

We found only one randomised study containing 41 participants on the use of an anti-adhesion barrier gel versus no treatment after hysteroscopic treatment of RPOC and one randomised study containing 86 participants on hysteroscopic morcellation versus loop resection for removal of RPOC [10, 22]. Both studies had a high risk of bias on four out of seven items. According to the results of both studies, there is no evidence of statistically significant differences between both comparison groups for the outcomes of clinical pregnancy or the presence of IUAs at second-look hysteroscopy.

Strengths and limitations
We aimed to follow the guidelines recommended by the Cochrane Handbook as much as possible [20]. We excluded non-randomised studies to minimise bias. We aimed at investigating the influence of the treatment of RPOC on fertility. Selection of studies and extraction of data was performed by two review authors independently.

Only two relevant randomised studies were identified. The studies were at high risk of bias, so results should be interpreted with caution, and they did not report on the primary outcome of live birth. However, for the trial performed by our group, we are considering follow-up of reproductive outcome for the patients as randomised [10]. Moreover, in the trial that did report on pregnancy, relevant information was lacking regarding the histologic

1.1 Presence of intrauterine adhesions at second-look hysteroscopy

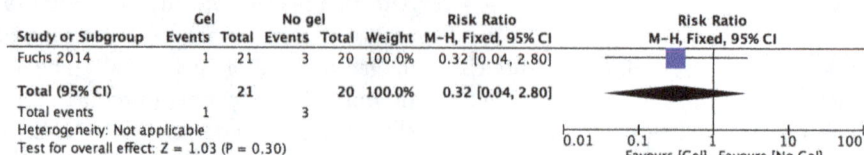

1.2 Clinical pregnancy

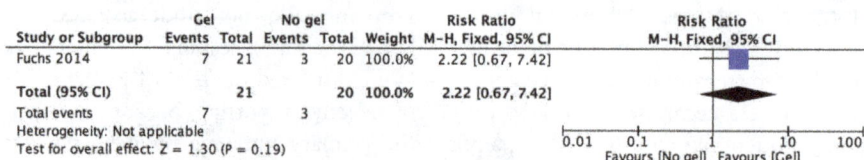

Fig. 3 Forest plot of comparison: 1 gel versus no treatment

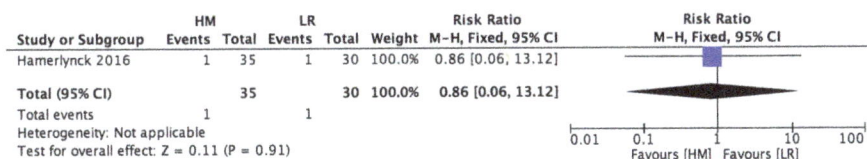

2.1 Presence of intrauterine adhesions at second-look hysteroscopy

HM = hysteroscopic morcellation; LR = loop resection

Fig. 4 Forest plot of comparison: 2 hysteroscopic morcellation versus loop resection

criteria for RPOC, absolute numbers of pathologic confirmation of RPOC per group, the relation between histologic confirmation of RPOC and/or IUAs and/or fertility, as well as the number of women actually trying to reconceive after treatment of RPOC [22]. Our query related to these topics remained unanswered by the authors.

Interpretation

Previous reviews have addressed the topic of reproductive outcome after treatment of RPOC [23, 24]. Both reviews identified only cohort studies and no randomised trials. The trials included in the reviews studied the treatment of RPOC by curettage, hysteroscopy or both. The results in relation to IUAs appear to be in favour of hysteroscopic treatment of RPOC; however, no significant differences in conception or ongoing pregnancy rates were demonstrated. Due to the low methodological quality and high risk of bias in the included cohort studies—although a formal assessment of the risk of bias was lacking in both reviews—, the results need to be interpreted with caution. Our review was limited to randomised trials in order to reduce the risk of bias. We could identify one randomised trial examining the use of an anti-adhesion barrier after operative hysteroscopy for RPOC [22]. The study did not show a significant difference in the presence of IUAs or clinical pregnancy rate between intervention and control group. This finding is in line with the results of the systematic review of Bosteels et al. stating that the effectiveness of anti-adhesion therapy in improving reproductive outcome or reducing IUAs following operative hysteroscopy in subfertile women is still unclear [18]. The second study identified was a randomised trial comparing two hysteroscopic techniques, namely, hysteroscopic morcellation with loop resection for removal of RPOC [10]. The trial did not show a significant difference in the presence of IUAs. However, both identified trials may have been too small to demonstrate a difference in the outcome measures, and other factors than the techniques under study may have contributed to the risk of IUA formation or influenced the reproductive outcome.

Conclusions

Implication for practice

For daily clinical practice, the effectiveness of anti-adhesion treatment in improving key reproductive outcomes or decreasing IUAs following operative hysteroscopy for RPOC in women wishing to conceive remains uncertain. Similarly, it is not clear whether hysteroscopic morcellation or loop resection of RPOC leads to better reproductive outcomes or a lower risk of IUAs.

Implication for research

Additional studies are needed to evaluate the influence of RPOC on fertility. Hypothetically, there may be causal mechanisms linking the risk for RPOC with adverse reproductive outcomes such as infertility and recurrent miscarriage. The diagnostic modalities for RPOC need to be evaluated, and histopathological definitions need to be reviewed, aiming at reaching a consensus and providing practical guidelines. Different treatment modalities including expectant management, medical and surgical treatment (curettage, different hysteroscopic techniques) need to be compared to study reproductive outcome and cost-effectiveness. The size of the study population needs to be sufficiently large, and follow-up should be long enough to study the outcomes of interest. Obstetric history and other factors related to the occurrence of RPOC as well as the development of IUAs need to be considered when performing research on the subject. Our RCT, included in this review, should be considered as a pilot trial for hypothesis testing. Our future research agenda includes a pragmatic multicentre trial studying IUAs and reproductive outcome after surgical treatment of RPOC (NTR4923). Hysteroscopic morcellation (TRUCLEAR) is compared with US guided electric vacuum aspiration, because the latter is still the most frequently applied treatment for RPOC in Belgium and the Netherlands. There are currently two other ongoing trials examining following comparisons for treatment of RPOC: operative hysteroscopy (resection) versus vacuum aspiration (NCT02201732; primary outcome: intrauterine pregnancy lasting up to at least 22 weeks of gestation), and hysteroscopic morcellation (MyoSure) versus hysteroscopic monopolar loop resection (ChiCTR-INR-16009074; secondary outcomes: IUAs and pregnancy rate).

Additional files

> **Additional file 1: Appendix S1.** Search strategy for systematic review on fertility outcome after treatment of retained products of conception.
>
> **Additional file 2: Appendix S2.** Items of the pilot-tested data extraction form.
>
> **Additional file 3: Table S1.** Characteristics of included studies.
>
> **Additional file 4: Table S2.** Characteristics of excluded studies.
>
> **Additional file 5: Table S3.** Characteristics of ongoing studies.
>
> **Additional file 6: Table S4.** Risk of bias table.

Abbreviations
ICTRP: International Clinical Trials Registry Platform; IUA: Intrauterine adhesion; RCT: Randomised controlled trial; RPOC: Retained products of conception; RR: Risk ratio; SD: Standard deviation; US: Ultrasound; WHO: World Health Organization

Acknowledgements
We thank Mrs. De Sutter, reference librarian KCGG of the Ghent University, for her assistance with the search strategy.

Capsule
There is insufficient evidence on how different treatments for retained products of conception affect future fertility.

Authors' contributions
TH took the lead in writing the manuscript. TH, DM, HVdV and SW contributed to the conception and design, as well as the acquisition of data. TH, DM, HVdV, JB and SW contributed to the analysis and interpretation of data, drafting, revising and final approval of the review.

Competing interests
T.H. received a Clinical PhD Fellowship grant from the Research Foundation–Flanders (FWO).

Author details
[1]Women's Clinic, Ghent University Hospital, C. Heymanslaan 10, 9000 Ghent, Belgium. [2]Faculty of Medicine and Health Sciences, Ghent University, C. Heymanslaan 10, 9000 Ghent, Belgium. [3]Department of Gynaecology, Imelda Hospital, Imeldalaan 9, 2820, Bonheiden, Belgium.

References
1. Sellmyer MA, Desser TS, Maturen KE et al (2013) Physiologic, histologic, and imaging features of retained products of conception. RadioGraphics 33:781–796
2. Hamerlynck TWO, Blikkendaal MD, Schoot BC et al (2013) An alternative approach for removal of placental remnants : hysteroscopic morcellation. J Minim Invasive Gynecol 20:796–802. https://doi.org/10.1016/j.jmig.2013.04.024
3. Sadan O, Golan A, Girtler O et al (2004) Role of sonography in the diagnosis of retained products of conception. J Ultrasound Med 23:371–374
4. Pather S, Ford M, Reid R, Sykes P (2005) Postpartum curettage: an audit of 200 cases. Aust New Zeal J Obstet Gynaecol 45:368–371. https://doi.org/10.1111/j.1479-828X.2005.00445.x
5. Dankert T, Vleugels M (2008) Hysteroscopic resection of retained placental tissue : a feasibility study. Gynecol Surg 5:121–124. https://doi.org/10.1007/s10397-007-0354-x
6. Inal MM, Yildirim Y, Ertopcu K, Ozelmas I (2006) The predictors of retained products of conception following first-trimester pregnancy termination with manual vacuum aspiration. Eur J Contracept Reprod Heal Care 11:98–103. https://doi.org/10.1080/13625180500456742
7. Kitahara T, Sato Y, Kakui K et al (2011) Management of retained products of conception with marked vascularity. J Obstet Gynaecol Res 37:458–464. https://doi.org/10.1111/j.1447-0756.2010.01363.x
8. van den Bosch T, Daemen A, Van Schoubroeck D et al (2008) Occurrence and outcome of residual trophoblastic tissue: a prospective study. J Ultrasound Med 27:357–361
9. Vitner D, Filmer S, Goldstein I et al (2013) A comparison between ultrasonography and hysteroscopy in the diagnosis of uterine pathology. Eur J Obstet Gynecol Reprod Biol 171:143–145. https://doi.org/10.1016/j.ejogrb.2013.08.024
10. Hamerlynck TWO, van Vliet HAAM, Beerens AS et al (2016) Hysteroscopic morcellation versus loop resection for removal of placental remnants: a randomized trial. J Minim Invasive Gynecol 23:1172–1180. https://doi.org/10.1016/j.jmig.2016.08.828
11. Goldenberg M, Schiff E, Achiron R, Lipitz S, Mashiach S (1997) Managing residual trophoblastic tissue: hysteroscopy for directing curettage. J Reprod Med 42:26–28
12. Cohen SB, Kalter-Ferber A, Weisz BS et al (2001) Hysteroscopy may be the method of choice for management of residual trophoblastic tissue. J Am Assoc Gynecol Laparosc 8:199–202
13. Faivre E, Deffieux X, Mrazguia C et al (2009) Hysteroscopic management of residual trophoblastic tissue and reproductive outcome: a pilot study. J Minim Invasive Gynecol 16:487–490. https://doi.org/10.1016/j.jmig.2009.04.011
14. Nicopoullos JDM, Treharne A, Raza A, Richardson R (2010) The use of a hysteroscopic resectoscope for repeat evacuation of retained products of conception procedures: a case series. Gynecol Surg 7:163–166
15. Golan A, Dishi M, Shalev A et al (2011) Operative hysteroscopy to remove retained products of conception: novel treatment of an old problem. J Minim Invasive Gynecol 18:100–103. https://doi.org/10.1016/j.jmig.2010.09.001
16. Rein DT, Schmidt T, Hess AP et al (2011) Hysteroscopic management of residual trophoblastic tissue is superior to ultrasound-guided curettage. J Minim Invasive Gynecol 18:774–778. https://doi.org/10.1016/j.jmig.2011.08.003
17. Yu D, Wong YM, Cheong Y et al (2008) Asherman syndrome-one century later. Fertil Steril 89:759–779. https://doi.org/10.1016/j.fertnstert.2008.02.096
18. Bosteels J, Weyers S, Kasius J et al (2015) Anti-adhesion therapy following operative hysteroscopy for treatment of female subfertility. Cochrane Database Syst Rev 11:CD011110. https://doi.org/10.1002/14651858.CD011110.pub2
19. Zegers-Hochschild F, Adamson GD, de Mouzon J et al (2009) International Committee for Monitoring Assisted Reproductive Technology (ICMART) and the World Health Organization (WHO) revised glossary of ART terminology, 2009*. Fertil Steril 92:1520–1524. https://doi.org/10.1016/j.fertnstert.2009.09.009
20. Higgins JPT, Green S (editors). Cochrane Handbook for Systematic Reviews of Interventions Version 5.1.0 [updated March 2011]. The Cochrane Collaboration, 2011. Available from www.handbook.cochrane.org
21. Review Manager 5 (RevMan 5) [Computer program]. Version 5.3. Copenhagen: Nordic Cochrane Centre, The Cochrane Collaboration, 2014.
22. Fuchs N, Smorgick N, Ben Ami I et al (2014) Intercoat (Oxiplex/AP gel) for preventing intrauterine adhesions after operative hysteroscopy for suspected retained products of conception: double-blind, prospective, randomized pilot study. J Minim Invasive Gynecol 21:126–130. https://doi.org/10.1016/j.jmig.2013.07.019
23. Smorgick N, Barel O, Fuchs N et al (2014) Hysteroscopic management of retained products of conception: meta-analysis and literature review. Eur J Obstet Gynecol Reprod Biol 173:19–22. https://doi.org/10.1016/j.ejogrb.2013.11.020
24. Hooker AB, Aydin H, Brölman HAM, Huirne JAF (2016) Long-term complications and reproductive outcome after the management of retained products of conception : a systematic review. Fertil Steril 105:156–164. https://doi.org/10.1016/j.fertnstert.2015.09.021

26

Cadaveric surgery in core gynaecology training

Chou Phay Lim[1]* (iD), Mark Roberts[2], Tony Chalhoub[2], Jason Waugh[3] and Laura Delgaty[4]

Abstract

Background: Fresh frozen cadaver training has been proposed as a better model than virtual reality simulators in laparoscopy training. We aimed to explore the relationship between cadaveric surgical training and increased surgical confidence.

To determine feasibility, we devised two 1-day cadaveric surgical training days targeted at trainees in obstetrics and gynaecology. Seven defined surgical skills were covered during the course of the day. The relationship between surgical training and surgical confidence was explored using both quantitative (confidence scores) and qualitative tools (questionnaires).

Results: Participants rated a consistent improvement in their level of confidence after the training. They universally found the experience positive and three overarching themes emerged from the qualitative analysis including self-concept, social persuasion and stability of task.

Conclusions: It is pragmatically feasible to provide procedure-specific cadaveric surgical training alongside supervised clinical training. This small, non-generalisable study suggests that cadaveric training may contribute to an increase in surgical self-confidence and efficacy. This will form the basis of a larger study and needs to be explored in more depth with a larger population.

Keywords: Cadaveric surgery, Laparoscopy training, Gynaecological surgery, Surgical confidence

Background

It is now an expectation that an integral part of surgical training should include meaningful simulation prior to live patient operating wherever possible. Training time in obstetrics and gynaecology has been reduced over the past 20 years following the introduction of shorter training programmes and work hour restrictions from bodies like the European Working Time Directive (EWTD) and the Accreditation Council for Graduate Medical Education (ACGME). As such there is an increasing opportunity for realistic surgical simulation to improve clinical training [1–9].

There are a number of simulation methods that suit acquisition of various skills. For example, neoprene surgical pads or animal tissue may be used to learn suturing and tissue handling, and laparoscopic 'boxes' or virtual simulation may improve hand-eye co-ordination [10].

There is difficulty, however, in simulating core procedures such as salpingectomy, which is one of the mandatory competencies in the curriculum for gynaecology trainees. Animal models lack anatomical accuracy and artificial models lack the realism of live tissue [11]. Fresh frozen cadaver training has been proposed as a better model than virtual reality simulators in laparoscopy training [12].

The use of cadaveric material was at one time a cornerstone of medical training, including undergraduate medical school anatomy teaching. More recently, students and trainees have little, if any, exposure to cadaveric material, those who do often only see prosected or preserved specimens. The concept of 'procedure-specific' cadaveric surgical training has been recently introduced in several specialities, including orthopaedics, trauma medicine and head and neck surgery [12–14]. This has become possible by advances in preserving human tissue for teaching purposes. Cadaveric simulation in gynaecology has been applied in some surgical settings such as gynaecological

* Correspondence: chouphay.lim@nhs.net
[1]Obstetrics and Gynaecology, Royal Victoria Infirmary, Newcastle upon Tyne Hospitals NHS Foundation Trust, Newcastle Upon Tyne NE1 4LP, UK
Full list of author information is available at the end of the article

oncology, targeted at advanced surgical trainees and established consultant specialists [7, 8] but not at junior trainees who are still at the stage of familiarising basic surgical skills and procedures.

The benefit of this training intervention is not easy to quantify, but it is postulated that improved self-belief in a task enhances self-confidence [15]. Self-confidence, for trainees, is the trust in one's abilities, qualities and judgement. Social cognitivist theory refers to this belief of self-ability as 'perceived self-efficacy', and this is one of the cognitive mechanisms underlying behavioural change [16]. Importantly, in this context, it is also one of the factors that predict performance success [17]. Literature suggests that those who expect to do well, demonstrating a high belief in their own self-efficacy, are more likely to do well than those who expect to do poorly [18]. Therefore, with the increasing constraints on surgical gynaecological training, educators must identify relevant factors that can increase skill acquisition and self-efficacy, or surgical confidence [16]. In the context of this study, it is anticipated that improved surgical confidence may be linked to surgical expertise and, therefore, competence. For educators, being aware of this relationship and, designing training programmes accordingly, is essential to surgical expertise and, ultimately, patient outcomes [19].

We aimed to explore the relationship between cadaveric surgical training and increased surgical confidence. We report the feasibility of introducing cadaveric surgical training into a basic training programme at year 3. To our knowledge, the use of cadaveric material in basic gynaecology training has never been reported.

Methods

Using a survey methodology, the relationship between cadaveric surgical training and improved confidence was explored. A mixed methods approach was used, which facilitated the collection of both quantitative and qualitative data.

Training resources

Postgraduate specialty training in obstetrics and gynaecology within England is run by 13 geographically separate Local Education Training Boards (LETB). Funding to introduce a cadaveric surgery programme for gynaecology trainees in Health Education England North East (HEE NE) was obtained from Health Education England. The programme was run at the Newcastle Surgical Training Centre (NSTC).

The Human Tissue Act 2004 established standards and guidance to institutions carrying out education and training using human cadaveric materials [20]. In collaboration with the department of Anatomy in Newcastle University, the Newcastle Surgical Training Centre

(NSTC) is licenced under the Human Tissue Authority (HTA). Details of the philosophy and ethical approval in the use of cadaveric material within this facility were described in another publication [14]. The cadaveric material is stored fresh frozen at -17 to -20 °C and defrosted before use.

Study design

Competency level of obstetrics and gynaecology trainees in the UK follows a standardised 7-year curriculum set out by the Royal College of Obstetricians and Gynaecologists (RCOG) [21, 22]. We devised two 1-day surgical training days targeted at trainees (year 3) to cover the surgical competencies in the training programme of the RCOG [21, 22]. The first day was set to be within the first 3 months of the training year and the second was set to be 8 months later. The content of the days were the same. We exclude any candidates who have taken a significant time away from the training programme within this timeframe for example for parental leave or long-term sick leave to maintain a homogenous level of training experience within the interval time period. Ethical consideration of the study was reviewed and approved from the Newcastle Clinical Research Facility. Informed consent was obtained from all participants included in the study.

The training days ran from 0900 to 1700 h. Each station was supplied with one female cadaver torso (assessed by CT scan to confirm that a uterus was present) allocated to two or three delegates and one trainer. The delegates were encouraged to perform the surgical procedures as the primary surgeon under the supervision and guidance of the trainer at their station. Seven defined surgical skills were covered during the course of the day including tubal clip sterilisation (laparoscopic), laparoscopic salpingectomy, laparoscopic oophorectomy, laparoscopic specimen retrieval, opening and closing the abdomen (suprapubic transverse incision), optimising the surgical field (open and laparoscopic), and abdominal hysterectomy.

The trainers were all consultant gynaecological surgeons from approved training units across the HEE NE region. All the members of faculty attended a pre-course briefing at the NSTC and were all asked to follow a set programme and standard technique for the purpose of this programme to keep training similar across cadaver groups. This is so that delegates are not confused by the variety of surgical techniques and preferences among different consultant trainers.

Outcome measures

We collected two types of data to investigate confidence. All data was anonymised:

1. Quantitative: self-assessed surgical confidence score (SCS)
2. Qualitative: Evaluation form

Analysis: surgical confidence score (SCS)

We designed a surgical confidence score (SCS) system to quantify the level of confidence the delegates had in approaching surgical cases (Fig. 1). The delegates score their level of confidence on a Likert scale from 0 to 10 (0 meaning 'no confidence' and 10 meaning 'full confidence') on the SCS. This was done at the beginning and the end of each day of the programme. For each of the surgical skills, we calculated the mean of the SCS and used two-tailed paired Student's t test to determine the change in the delegates' confidence.

Analysis: qualitative evaluation form

We invited the delegates to complete an evaluation at the end of each day. We asked the delegates whether they felt that the course delivered value for money, whether they felt the course should be funded from the trainee study leave budget in the future and general questions concerning individual experiences. The evaluation used a combination of simple rating scales for satisfaction and free text questions allowing for the collection of rich data. All free text data was analysed broadly following a method of qualitative content analysis described by Cohen et al. [23]. Codes were generated from the rough data and overarching themes or labels emerged. The themes were reviewed and refined.

Results

Data from the nine trainees at ST year 3 level within the HEE NE training programme who attended both days of the 2-day programme are reported. Figure 2 shows the linear changes in mean delegate SCS for the seven surgical competencies over the four time points. This is presented as a visual representation of all the results. A more detailed analysis is given in Tables 1, 2, 3 and 4 and in the text below.

n.s.t.c.

NHS
Health Education North East

Surgical Skills Training Programme
Pilot ST3 Obstetrics & Gynaecology SSTP

Course centre: NSTC, Freeman Hospital

TO BE COMPLETED BEFORE THE COURSE

Please rate your confidence in performing the following procedures unsupervised (assuming not complicated) in the clinical work place by circling 0 – 10 on the scales below

	No confidence Full confidence	RCOG level (1-3 RCOG)
a. Tubal clip sterilisation	0----1----2----3----4----5----6----7----8----9----10	________
b. Laparoscopic salpingectomy (ectopic pregnancy)	0----1----2----3----4----5----6----7----8----9----10	________
c. Laparoscopic oophorectomy	0----1----2----3----4----5----6----7----8----9----10	________
d. Laparoscopic specimen retrieval	0----1----2----3----4----5----6----7----8----9----10	________
e. Opening and closing the abdomen (SPT incision)	0----1----2----3----4----5----6----7----8----9----10	________
f. Optimising the surgical field (open/laparoscopic)	0----1----2----3----4----5----6----7----8----9----10	________
g. Abdominal hysterectomy	0----1----2----3----4----5----6----7----8----9----10	________

Fig. 1 Surgical confidence score (SCS)

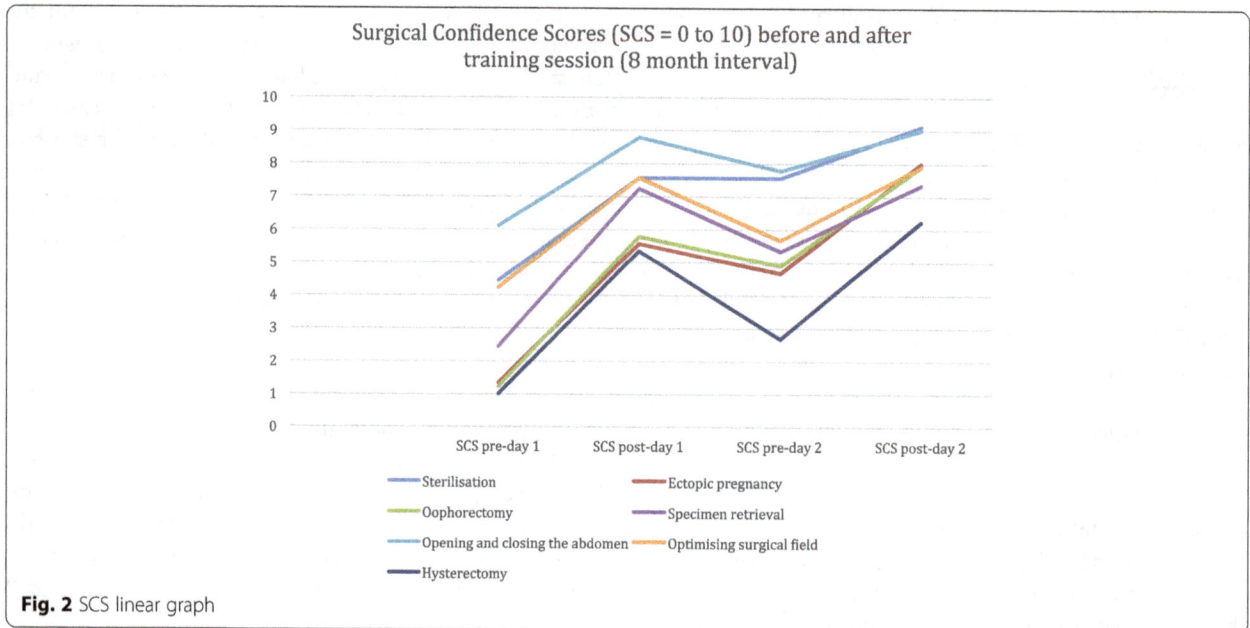

Fig. 2 SCS linear graph

Surgical confidence scores

There was a significant improvement in the mean SCS in all the seven surgical skills assessed. Table 1 shows the mean SCS for the nine delegates on each of the surgical skills across both training days and the respective improvement in the mean SCS. There was a mean increase in the SCS, ranging from 2.89 ($p < 0.05$) for opening and closing the abdomen to 6.67 ($p < 0.0001$) for ectopic pregnancy, with statistically significant improvements in SCS for all seven surgical skills assessed.

Sub-analysis of SCS (post-day 1 to pre-day 2)

Table 2 presents the data and statistical analysis that allows comparison of SCS at the end of day 1 to the start of day 2. This was designed to assess whether SCS was retained over the 8-month interval between training days.

Between the end of the first training day and the start of the second training day, there was a general trend of reduction in the SCS.

We were unable to report specific details on each delegates' case volume in the interim between the two training days because this information was not collected. However, all delegates remained in active training under the nationally approved specialty training programme during this time frame, with regular opportunity in assisting and performing live surgical cases under close supervision in each of their training hospital unit.

Sub-analysis of SCS (pre-day 1 and pre-day 2)

Table 3 presents the comparison of SCS before both training days. This was intended to assess whether the baseline SCS on day 2 was higher, given that trainees had already undergone day 1 followed by consolidation clinical training in the 8-month interval. There was a significant improvement for sterilisation, oophorectomy, salpingectomy, specimen retrieval, and abdominal hysterectomy. There was no difference in this comparison

Table 1 Analysis of Day 1 and Day 2 mean SCS

Procedures	Day 1 SCS			Day 2 SCS			Overall change
Trainees = 9	Pre day 1	Post day 1	Diff day 1	Pre day 2	Post day 2	Diff day 2	Pre-day 1 to post day 2
Sterilisation	4.44	7.56	3.12	7.56	9.11	1.55	4.67**
Ectopic	1.33	5.56	4.23	4.67	8.00	3.33	6.67****
Oophorectomy	1.22	5.78	4.56	4.89	7.89	3.00	6.67****
Specimen Retrieval	2.44	7.22	4.78	5.33	7.33	2.00	4.89***
Opening and Closing	6.11	8.78	2.67	7.78	9.00	1.22	2.89*
Optimising surgical field	4.22	7.56	3.34	5.67	7.89	2.22	3.67***
Hysterectomy	1.00	5.33	4.43	2.67	6.22	3.55	5.22***

($* = p < 0.05$, $** = p < 0.01$, $*** = p < 0.001$, $**** = p < 0.0001$)

Table 2 Sub analysis of SCS Post Day 1 to Pre Day 2

Procedures	Mean SCS after Day 1	Mean SCS before Day 2	Difference in Mean SCS	Student t-test p values
Sterilisation	7.56	7.56	0.00	1.000
Ectopic	5.56	4.67	−0.89	0.069
Oophorectomy	5.78	4.89	−0.89	0.138
Specimen Retrieval	7.22	5.33	−1.89	*0.033
Opening and Closing	8.78	7.78	−1.00	0.108
Optimising surgical field	7.56	5.67	−1.89	*0.023
Hysterectomy	5.33	2.67	−2.67	**0.007

(* = $p < 0.05$, ** = $p < 0.01$)

in opening and closing the abdomen ($p = 0.18$) and optimising the surgical field ($p = 0.09$).

Study day evaluation

The evaluation attracted universally positive feedback. None of the delegates found the experience unpleasant. All of the delegates responded to confirm that they would be willing to pay for the programme (cost £550) from their set annual training budget. We present the evaluation results from satisfaction scales in Table 4 with further analysis of the qualitative data below.

Analysis of qualitative data

i) Self-concept

The participants personalised their experiences suggesting that the opportunity presented allowed them to perform these procedures 'without fear' in comparison to a live patient and without 'feeling silly'. Furthermore, performing the procedures in 'real time' was clearly valuable and suggested transferability to actual surgical practice.

ii) Social persuasion

A perhaps unanticipated theme was one of social persuasion. The learners consistently suggested the value of the faculty and how it contributed to their overall gain in confidence. Having the support and guidance of these

individuals was essential. Also, the opportunity to 'discuss the techniques' both with faculty and their peers added to their experience and self-assurance.

iii) Stability of task

This final theme encompassed the very nature of the learning opportunity with cadaveric specimens. Participants overwhelmingly suggested the experience itself, the 'hands on' nature of it and the 'practical exposure' was valuable. There were specific codes making up this theme demonstrating the actual learning process in this stable environment. These included the specific procedures they were tasked to perform, the 'opportunity to identity anatomy' in cadaveric specimens and 'running through the actual steps'.

Discussion

This was intended as a feasibility study, and we have had an opportunity to demonstrate from here that cadaveric surgery improves surgical confidence.

Analysis of SCS at different stages of the study gives some insight into the value of cadaveric surgical simulation training. Firstly, it is noted that there was a universal improvement in confidence scores for all skills assessed (Table 1). The greatest improvement appeared to be for oophorectomy, salpingectomy and hysterectomy. These are procedures that year 3 trainees are often only just starting to undertake as supervised clinical cases, which may explain why the baseline SCS prior to

Table 3 Sub analysis of SCS Pre-Day 1 and Pre-Day 2

Procedures	Mean SCS before Day 1	Mean SCS before Day 2	Difference in Mean SCS	Student t-test p values
Sterilisation	4.44	7.56	3.11	*0.022
Ectopic	1.33	4.67	3.33	*0.022
Oophorectomy	1.22	4.89	3.67	**0.005
Specimen Retrieval	2.44	5.33	2.89	*0.022
Opening and Closing	6.11	7.78	1.67	0.179
Optimising surgical field	4.22	5.67	1.44	0.089
Hysterectomy	1.00	2.67	1.67	*0.028

(* = $p < 0.05$, ** = $p < 0.01$)

Table 4 Evaluation forms response

Satisfaction score overall rating	5	4	3	2	1
Cadaveric session 1	8	1	0	0	0
Cadaveric session 2	8	1	0	0	0
	YES		NO		
Do you feel the course should be funded from the study leave budget in the future?	9		0		
Did you find cadaveric surgery training unpleasant?	0		9		

day 1 were lower than for other procedures. Whereas for procedures that year 3 trainees were likely to be already experienced in, such as opening and closing the abdomen and optimising the surgical field (skills used in caesarean section), the baseline SCS prior to day 1 was higher and therefore the overall improvement was less as a result.

Table 2 demonstrates that SCS retention over 8 months was variable for different competencies. This retention of confidence is likely to be related to the trainees' actual surgical experiences over the 8-month interim. For example, trainees were almost as confident at the start of day 2 as the end of day 1 for procedures that were simple and likely to be a common part of supervised clinical training, such as sterilisation and opening and closing the abdomen. The greatest reduction in SCS between the two training days was for hysterectomy. This is likely to be because hysterectomy is more complex to undertake and trainees have less opportunities for supervised clinical training. Table 3 shows that despite some loss of confidence for some of the surgical competencies, trainees were universally more confident at the start of day 2 than day 1. This would suggest that the intervention of cadaveric simulation combined with supervised clinical training is an effective approach to teaching surgical procedures. Simulation training is an important adjunct rather than an alternative to clinical experience [24] but is likely to be of greatest value when simulation is timed to clinical exposure.

Three main themes emerged from the qualitative data: self-concept, social persuasion and stability of task. These are described in detail in the "Results" section. The responses were overwhelmingly positive, suggesting that trainees felt better equipped to engage with supervised clinical training. Not only did trainees highlight the value of real-time surgery and real anatomy but also the interaction with trainers and working in an environment where mistakes can be made before operating on live patients. This would suggest that it is not just the use of cadavers are important but also the structure of the training days.

Our study report results from the first nine participants to undertake both training days as a group. This was limited in part by the regional workforce for the population

and also our intention to study a homogenous group of trainees of similar level of experience. All delegates had more than 2 years but less than 3 years equivalent of full-time training within obstetrics and gynaecology. As this was a pilot intended as a feasibility study with a small sample size, we are cautious in claiming generalisability or drawing conclusions surrounding the benefit of cadaveric surgical training. As a feasibility study, the aim was to produce findings that help determine whether this intervention could be recommended for further studies.

This study suggests that more advanced surgical trainees can be trained with a similar model on more complex advance procedures. The process of training a surgeon to a level of higher confidence can also be supplemented with this model. Our group have begun work in implementing a more regular set of training days around similar models with cadaveric work throughout the training programme for the region.

In the absence of clinical training, confidence level varies greatly [25]. Clanton et al. reported in a study involving 150 medical students in basic surgical skills that there is a strong association between confidence and competence [19]. Hutton et al. reported a similar relationship between confidence and competence in chest tube insertion by junior doctors [26].

The values of surgical simulation training have been established in other medical disciplines [10, 11, 27, 28]. Palter et al. described 25 colorectal surgical residents who received ex vivo simulation training and demonstrated improved technical knowledge and performance in the operating room compared to conventional residency training [29]. Ahmed et al. described a series of 81 urology residents having undergone a cadaveric surgical programme. They reported that human cadaveric surgery was the best mode of simulation-based training with improvements in skills that were transferrable to the operating theatre based on evaluation surveys only [30]. This study may be criticised for its heterogeneity because of the varied levels of experience of the participating residents and that evaluation survey was the only tool they used to assess the success of the programme. However, it does demonstrate an appetite for realistic simulation training.

Our study demonstrates that it is feasible to integrate cadaveric surgery into core training curriculum. It is already accepted that trainees should have the opportunity to develop skills by simulation prior to operating on live patients. However, insufficient literature addresses the relationship between confidence and surgical skills [19]. The results presented here address this gap and demonstrate that cadaveric surgery may improve the confidence of trainees when introduced as an adjunct to conventional training. This is valuable as there is evidence that improved confidence in a task enhances self-efficacy [15]. Furthermore, an association between surgical skills and confidence has both educational and clinical implications [19]. We recognise that this is a study with a small sample size; however, using a mixed methods approach, we have assessed the complex construct of confidence and plan further studies with a larger cohort of trainees.

We acknowledge that surgical confidence depends on many factors within a training environment. We were not able to determine the relative merits of procedure-specific cadaver training versus dedicated skill training in the lab with a consultant surgeon in this study. Also, no comparison was made with other synthetic or virtual reality training tools. However, the results demonstrate that cadaveric surgical training is well received by trainees and appears to be an effective intervention.

In light of the findings of this study, we can conclude that it is feasible to integrate cadaveric surgical training into conventional gynaecology surgical training. Our next priority would be to reinforce the hypothesis of quantitative confidence improvements by incorporating a larger cohort of delegates.

This study gives some support to the notion that simulation training improves surgical technique; however, the concept of surgical competence is complex and whether simulation is an effective tool to teach or assess competence is beyond the scope of this study. It is therefore important to acknowledge that although cadaveric surgical training can serve as a valid adjunct to conventional training, it does not supersede live surgical training. This is expected to be addressed in the more senior years of training in the clinical environment.

Conclusions

It is pragmatically feasible to provide procedure-specific cadaveric surgical training alongside supervised clinical training. Assessment of this training can be achieved by a mixed quantitative and qualitative approach. This study will form the basis of a larger study. This work has implications surrounding the improvement of self-confidence and assisting educators in implementing interventions to optimise success and self-confidence during surgical skills acquisition.

Acknowledgements
The authors wish to acknowledge the support from the Newcastle Surgical Training Centre, including Sue Dent, Specialty surgical coordinator, Phil Jackson, Cadaveric Lab Practitioner, and Lorraine Waugh, Education Manager. The authors also wish to specially thank the consultant gynaecologists acting as faculty of the programme, including the following:
Karen Brown, Newcastle upon-Tyne Hospitals NHS Foundation Trust,
Michelle Russell, Newcastle upon-Tyne Hospitals NHS Foundation Trust,
Anthony Sproston, Northumbria Healthcare NHS Foundation Trust,
Ann Fisher, Northern Gynaecological Oncology Specialist Centre, Queen Elizabeth Hospital, Gateshead Health NHS Foundation Trust,
Jonathan Chamberlain, City Hospital Sunderland NHS Foundation Trust,
Partha Sengupta, County Durham and Darlington NHS Foundation Trust,
Remko Beukenholdt, County Durham and Darlington NHS Foundation Trust,
Mary George, North Tees and Hartlepool NHS Foundation Trust,
Paul Ballard, South Tees Hospitals NHS Foundation Trust,
Jeremy Twigg, South Tees Hospitals NHS Foundation Trust,
Pinky Khatri, South Tees Hospitals NHS Foundation Trust.
The authors also wish to specially dedicate this work to Mark Roberts, second author of this paper, who sadly passed away from pancreatic cancer just shortly before publication.

Funding
This initiative was funded entirely by NHS England via Health Education England North East.

Authors' contributions
JW secured the funding. CPL, MR, TC and JW conceived the project. CPL, MR and TC designed the programme. CPL and MR acquired the data. CPL, MR, JW and LD analysed and interpreted the data. CPL drafted the manuscript, and all authors critically revised the manuscript. All authors gave final approval of the submitted version of the manuscript.

Competing interests
The authors declare that they have no competing interests.

Author details
[1]Obstetrics and Gynaecology, Royal Victoria Infirmary, Newcastle upon Tyne Hospitals NHS Foundation Trust, Newcastle Upon Tyne NE1 4LP, UK. [2]Royal Victoria Infirmary, Newcastle Upon Tyne, UK. [3]Obstetrics and Gynaecology, Northern Deanery, HEE (NE), Newcastle Upon Tyne, UK. [4]Newcastle University, Newcastle Upon Tyne, UK.

References
1. British Medical Association. What is the European working time directive?. https://www.bma.org.uk/advice/employment/working-hours/ewtd (Accessed 18 Sept 2016)
2. The National Archives. General and specialist medical practice (education, training and qualifications) Order 2003. http://www.legislation.gov.uk/uksi/2003/1250/contents/made (Accessed 18 Sept 2016)
3. Tooke J, Ashtiany S, Carter D, Cole A, Michael J, Rashid A, Smith PC, Tomlinson S, Petty-Saphon K. Aspiring to excellence: final report of the independent enquiry into modernising medical careers. http://www.asit.org/assets/documents/MMC_FINAL_REPORT_REVD_4jan.pdf (Accessed 18 Sept 2016)
4. Wikipedia. Modernising medical careers. https://en.wikipedia.org/wiki/Modernising_Medical_Careers (Accessed 18 Sept 2016)
5. Garvin JT, McLaughlin R, Kerin MJ (2008) A pilot project of European working time directive compliant rosters in a university teaching hospital. Surgeon 6(2):88–93
6. Reid PC, Mukri S (2005) Trends in number of hysterectomies performed in England for menorrhagia: examination of health episode statistics, 1989 to 2002-3. BMJ 330(7497):938–939

7. English J. Launch of BSGE National Laparoscopic Hysterectomy Project. The Scope: Newsletter of the British Society of Gynaecological Endoscopy 2015; (2): 12. https://28x8koygrj92snigkorkjod2-wpengine.netdna-ssl.com/wp-content/uploads/2016/04/The-Scope-Issue-2.pdf (Accessed 18 Sept 2016)

8. BSGE. Launch of The National Laparoscopic Hysterectomy Training Programme (LAPHYST). The Scope: Newsletter of the British Society of Gynaecological Endoscopy 2016; Summer(4): 10. https://28x8koygrj92snigkorkjod2-wpengine.netdna-ssl.com/wp-content/uploads/2016/04/The-Scope-issue-4-WEB.pdf (Accessed 18 Sept 2016)

9. Accreditation Council for Graduate Medical Education, Common Program Requirements Section VI with Background and Intent:13-19. http://acgmecommon.org/2017_requirements (Accessed 14 Apr 2017)

10. Sutherland LM, Middleton PF, Anthony A, Hamdorf J, Cregan P, Scott D, Maddern GJ (2006) Surgical simulation: a systematic review. Ann Surg 243(3):291–300

11. Sarker SK, Patel BCK (2007) Simulation and surgical training. Int J Clin Pract 61(12):2120–2125

12. Sharma M, Horgan A (2012) Comparison of fresh-frozen cadaver and high-fidelity virtual reality simulator as methods of laparoscopic training. World J Surg 36(8):1732–1737

13. Gilbody J, Prasthofer AW, Ho K, Costa ML (2011) The use and effectiveness of cadaveric workshops in higher surgical training: a systematic review. Ann R Coll Surg Engl 93(5):347–352

14. Holland JP, Waugh L, Horgan A, Paleri V, Deehan DJ (2011) Cadaveric hands-on training for surgical specialties: is this back to the future for surgical skills development? J Surg Educ 68(2):110–116

15. Bandura A (1994) Self-efficacy. In: Ramachaudran VS (ed) Encyclopedia of human behaviour, vol 4. Academic, New York, pp 71–81

16. Geoffrion R, Lee T, Singer J (2013) Validatiing a self-confidence scale for surgical trainees. J Obstet Gynaecol 35:355–361

17. Cervone D (2000) Thinking about self-efficacy. Behav Modif 24:30–56

18. Bandura A (1989) Human agency in social cognitive theory. Am Psychol 44:1175

19. Clanton J, Gardner A, Cheung M, Mellert L, Evancho-Chapman M, George RL (2014) The relationship between confidence and competence in the development of surgical skills. J Surg Educ 71(3):405–412

20. Human Tissue Authority (HTA). Human Tissue Act 2004 (c30). https://www.hta.gov.uk/policies/human-tissue-act-2004 (Accessed 20 Nov 2016)

21. Royal College of Obstetricians and Gynaecologists. Core Module 5: Core surgical skills. https://www.rcog.org.uk/en/careers-training/specialty-training-curriculum/core-curriculum/core-module-5-core-surgical-skills/ (Accessed 7 Dec 2016)

22. Royal College of Obstetricians and Gynaecologists. Core Module 7: Surgical procedures. https://www.rcog.org.uk/en/careers-training/specialty-training-curriculum/core-curriculum/ core-module-7-surgical-procedures/ (Accessed 7 Dec 2016)

23. Cohen L, Manion L, Morrison K (2011) Research methods in education, seventh ed. Routledge, New York

24. Kneebone R, Aggarwal R (2009) Surgical training using simulation. BMJ 338:b1001

25. Suwanrath C, Samphao S, Prechawai C, Singha P (2016) Confidence in essential procedural skills of Thai medical graduates. Int J Clin Skills 10(1):6–10

26. Hutton IA, Kenealy H, Wong C (2008) Using simulation models to teach junior doctors how to insert chest tubes: a brief and effecting teaching module. Intern Med J 38:887–891

27. SSS T, Sarker SK (2011) Simulation in surgery: a review. Scott Med J 56(2):104–109

28. Nesbitt CI, Birdi N, Mafeld S, Stansby G (2016) The role of simulation in the development of endovascular surgical skills. Perspect Med Educ 5(1):8–14

29. Palter VN, Grantcharov TP (2012) Development and validation of a comprehensive curriculum to teach an advanced minimally invasive procedure: a randomized controlled trial. Ann Surg 256(1):25–32

30. Ahmed K, Aydin A, Dasgupta P, Khan MS, McCabe JE (2015) A novel cadaveric simulation in urology. J Surg Educ 72(4):556–565

27

Pushing the boundaries of laparoscopic myomectomy: a comparative analysis of peri-operative outcomes in 323 women undergoing laparoscopic myomectomy in a tertiary referral centre

Rebecca Mallick[*] [iD] and Funlayo Odejinmi

Abstract

Background: The aim of this study was to analyse the demographic data and peri-operative outcomes of women undergoing a laparoscopic myomectomy and assess what factors, if any, precluded using the laparoscopic approach.

Methods: A single surgeon observational study of 323 patients undergoing a laparoscopic myomectomy was undertaken. Data was collected prospectively over a 12-year period and analysed using SPSS. Surgical outcomes included operating time, estimated blood loss, conversion to laparotomy, intraoperative and postoperative complications and duration of inpatient stay.

Results: A total of 323 patients underwent a laparoscopic myomectomy over the 12-year period. The majority of fibroids removed were intramural (49%) and subserosal (33%). The mean size of fibroids removed was 7.66 ± 2.83 (7.34–7.99) cm, and the mean number was 4 ± 3.62 (3.6–4.39), with the greatest being 22 removed from a single patient. Average blood loss was 279.14 ± 221.10 (254.59–303.69) ml with mean duration of surgery and inpatient stay recorded as 112.92 ± 43.21 (107.94–117.91) min and 1.88 ± 0.95 (1.77–1.99) days, respectively. No major intraoperative complications were noted, and the conversion to laparotomy rate was 0.62%. All histology following morcellation was benign. Over the 12-year period despite increasingly large and more numerous fibroids being tackled, increasing experience resulted in a simultaneous reduction in overall blood loss, operating time and duration of inpatient stay.

Conclusions: Laparoscopic myomectomy is a safe and efficacious procedure that should be considered the gold standard surgical treatment option for fibroids. With experience, the procedure can be undertaken with minimal complications, a low risk of conversion to laparotomy and early discharge from hospital, even in cases of large and multiple fibroids that historically would have required the open approach. This allows even the most complex of cases to now benefit for the advantages of the minimal access approach.

Keywords: Laparoscopic myomectomy, Outcomes, Complications

* Correspondence: rmallick@doctors.org.uk
Department of Gynaecology, Barts Health NHS Trust, Whipps Cross University Hospital, London E11 1NR, UK

Background

Uterine fibroids remain the commonest benign tumour encountered in the female population. They affect around 20–25% of women with symptoms ranging from heavy menstrual bleeding and pressure to subfertility. The clinical features and treatment options offered are largely dependent on the type, number and position of the fibroids, and historically, the surgical treatment of choice was an open myomectomy or abdominal hysterectomy. However, many women, especially those of reproductive age, prefer more conservative uterine-preserving techniques, and the minimal access route offers significant benefits both in terms of recovery and future fertility [1–3]. These benefits are now well established in the wider literature, and the minimal access route should generally be considered the gold standard surgical treatment for such women. But is there a limit to what can be performed laparoscopically and what are the risks? Are there specific demographic features that can affect the surgical outcome and can help guide us when counselling patients and choosing the safest surgical procedure? Since the first laparoscopic myomectomy, described by Kurt Semm in 1979 [4], there have been significant technological advances and increasing expertise in minimal access surgery and the previously considered contra-indications to laparoscopic myomectomy [5, 6] may no longer exist in experienced hands. The aims of this study were to analyse the demographic data and perioperative outcomes of 323 women who underwent a laparoscopic myomectomy over a 12-year period in a tertiary referral centre in London and compare our findings to the published literature.

Methods

This is a prospective observational study of 323 patients who underwent a laparoscopic myomectomy from March 2004 to November 2016. All patients were operated on by a single surgeon at Whipps Cross University Hospital Trust. The only exclusion criteria was uterine size greater than 28 weeks size limiting access to the pelvis. A standardised technique was used; initial entry was through an intra-umbilical incision or palmer's point in cases where the uterine size was more than 14 weeks, with two 5 mm ancillary lateral ports and a suprapubic port. For haemostasis, 800 μg misoprostol was administered rectally and vasopressin injected intra-myometrially unless contraindicated. For uterine manipulation, a ClearView™ (Clinical Innovations) uterine manipulator was used to achieve the optimum uterine position. For most cases, the Harmonic™ (Ethicon) scalpel was used, but more recently, alternative ultrasonic energy devices such as Thunderbeat™ (Olympus) have been introduced. A 5 mm myoma screw and grasping forceps were used for traction and counter traction. Initially, the resulting defects were closed in two or three layers as required using polyglactin sutures

for the myometrium and monofilament sutures used for the serosa; however, more recently, self-retaining sutures such as V-loc™ (Covidien) and Stratafix™ (Ethicon) have been introduced. For adhesion prevention, due to the discontinuation of Sprayshield™ (Covidien), Interceed™ (Ethicon) has been used since 2014. Myomas were removed by electro-mechanical morcellation through the suprapubic port, currently without the use of containment/morcellation bags, and sent for histology. Initially, we used the Johnson and Johnson Ethicon morcellator; however, when it was withdrawn, we changed to the Roto-Cut morcellator (Stortz), and more recently, we have been using the LiNA morcellator.

All patients were assessed for suitability pre-operatively and had radiological fibroid mapping using either ultrasound or MRI. Patients were given written information regarding their procedure and counselled preoperatively about their recovery and anticipated discharged within 24 h. Also, following the concerns regarding the possibility of dissemination of malignant cells during the morcellation process [7], we considered the information provided by national and international societies [8, 9] and devised a leaflet explaining the risks of morcellation. This leaflet contained not only information about the potential risk of dissemination of malignancy and the risk of upstaging a leiomyosarcoma, but also the possible risks of visceral injury. All patients were also given antibiotics prophylaxis at induction of anaesthesia and appropriate thromboprophylaxis.

Patient demographics (age, BMI, parity), procedure details and patient outcomes were collected prospectively from 2004 onwards on an Excel spreadsheet and entered immediately following each procedure and on discharge from hospital. The data was analysed using SPSS (version 22). The t test was used for the comparison group analysis, but if the data failed the homogeneity assumption (Levene's test), a Mann–Whitney test was undertaken. A p value of 0.05 was considered significant. Formal ethical approval was not required as this was an evaluation of ongoing surgical practice.

Results

Three hundred twenty-three patients underwent a laparoscopic myomectomy over the 12-year period. There was almost a fivefold increase in the number of laparoscopic myomectomies performed in 2016 compared to 2004 (Fig. 1). Patient demographics are summarised in Table 1. 40.3% had undergone previous abdominal surgery with 27.6% undergoing a previous laparoscopic procedure and 12.7% undergoing a laparotomy.

A total of 1921 fibroids were removed with the size of the dominant fibroid ranging from 2 to 20 cm (mean 7.6 cm). The majority of fibroids removed were intramural (49%) and subserosal (33%) and less frequently submucosal (17%) and pedunclulated (1%). With regards

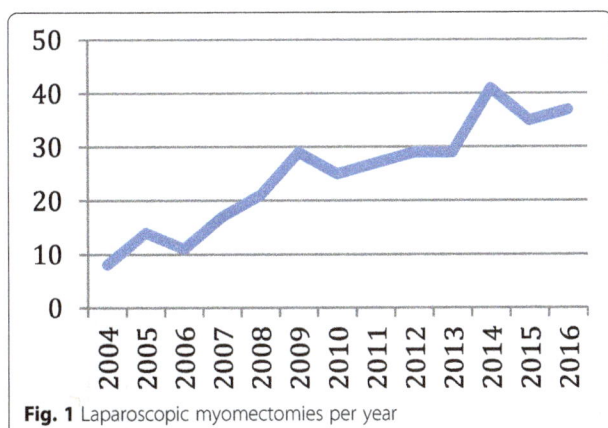

Fig. 1 Laparoscopic myomectomies per year

Table 2 Operative features

Variable	Value
Largest fibroid removed (cm)	7.66 ± 0.165 (7.34–7.99)
Number of fibroids removed	4 ± 0.202 (3.6–4.39)
Weight of fibroids removed (g)	216.28 ± 12.127 (192.42–240.14)
Blood loss (ml)	279.14 ± 12.477 (254.59–303.69)
Duration of surgery (min)	112.92 ± 2.533 (107.94–117.91)
Inpatient stay duration (days)	1.88 ± 0.055 (1.77–1.99)

Data presented as mean ± standard error of mean (95% CI)

to the position of the fibroids, the majority were posterior (40%), fundal (25%) and anterior (20%) with less common sites including broad ligament (9%), lateral (3%) and cervical (3%). Thirty-one percent of patients had a single fibroid removed, and the remaining 69% required multiple fibroid removal. The mean number of fibroids removed was 4, with the greatest being 22 removed from a single patient. Average blood loss was 279.14 ml with mean duration of surgery and inpatient stay recorded as 112.92 min and 1.88 days, respectively. Operative features are summarised in Table 2.

Twenty-three percent of patients had co-existing endometriosis, which was excised.

No major intraoperative complications were noted. Two procedures were converted to a mini laparotomy, one due to technical difficulties in closing the uterine incision and the other due to anaesthetic concerns with the patient's ventilation, giving a conversion rate of 0.62%. Nine patients required post-operative blood transfusions (2.79%). Seven patients had documented post-operative complications (2.17%); one patient returned to theatre on day 2 due to intra-abdominal bleeding, which was managed by a

Table 1 Patient demographics

Variable	Value
Age (years)	38 (24–56)
BMI	26.5 (16–46)
Parity	0 (0–6)
Ethnicity	
African/Afro-Caribbean	196 (60.7%)
Asian	43 (13.3%)
Caucasian	84 (26%)
Indications for surgery	
Bleeding	179 (55.2%)
Pain/pressure	77 (23.8%)
Infertility	68 (21%)

Data presented as median (range) or absolute number (%)

laparotomy and re-suturing. Two patients had postoperative urinary retention, and four patients developed port site hernias.

All specimens were removed using electo-mechanical morcellation, and in all cases, the histology was reported as benign. There were histological variants described and these included apoplectic myoma, adenomatoid tumour and symplastic tumour. These tumours are also benign and do not need any follow-up; however, one of the patients, who had an atypical myoma, opted for a laparoscopic hysterectomy and required no further treatment.

Between the onset of the study to January 2010, out of the 41% of patients who had surgery for infertility, 56% had conceived after surgery.

When comparing the number of fibroids removed and operative outcomes, there was a significantly greater blood loss and operating time in patients having multiple fibroids removed compared to those having a single myomectomy.

Fibroids over 9 cm also had a significantly greater blood loss and operating time when compared to those less than 8 cm. Both age and BMI did not appear to have any significant impact on operative outcomes (Table 3).

Learning curve of laparoscopic myomectomy

Over the time 12-year period, the cases have become increasingly complex with larger fibroids and more numerous fibroids being tackled in women who are increasingly more obese (Fig. 2). Despite this, the increasing experience and expertise has resulted in a simultaneous reduction in blood loss and operating time (Fig. 3). Inpatient stay has been also reduced by more than half from a mean of 3.5 days to 1.3 days.

Discussion

Since the first laparoscopic myomectomy in 1979, there has been a wealth of data published highlighting the benefits of the minimal access approach over the standard open approach. Benefits include reduced blood loss, shorter hospital stay, reduced post-operative pain and less adhesion formation, and many case series have been published worldwide [10–25] (Table 4). However, this series appears to one of the largest and the only prospective single surgeon series from the UK.

Table 3 Fibroid and patient factors impacting operative outcomes

	Single myomectomy	Multiple myomectomy	p value
Blood loss (ml)	218.5	308.45	0.001
Operating time (min)	85.6	125.43	< 0.001
Inpatient stay (days)	1.81	1.9	0.437
	Fibroid < 8 cm	Fibroid ≥ 9 cm	p value
Blood loss (ml)	121.34	192.03	< 0.001
Operating time (min)	105.30	130.12	< 0.001
Inpatient stay (days)	1.799	1.989	0.127
	BMI < 29.9	BMI > 30	p value
Blood loss (ml)	272	278	0.837
Operating time (min)	112	114	0.765
Inpatient stay (days)	1.85	1.64	0.062
	Age < 40	Age ≥ 40	p value
Blood loss (ml)	259	193	0.059
Operating time (min)	114	94	0.054
Inpatient stay (days)	1.9	1.7	0.408

Data presented as mean

Historically, the laparoscopic route had been reserved for smaller and less numerous fibroids due to the advanced technical skills required, and many recommendations have been made in the literature as to the "safe" limits of laparoscopic surgery. In 1996, Dubuisson et al. [10] advised that laparoscopic myomectomy should only be considered when the fibroids are less than 8 cm and in cases where there are less than two fibroids to be removed due to the high conversion to laparotomy rates. Other authors have suggested that the presence of more than four large fibroids greater than 4 cm in diameter or a solitary fibroid greater than 10 cm in diameter should be a contraindication to the laparoscopic approach [26, 27].

More recently, due to technological advances and increasing surgical expertise, these traditional boundaries are being pushed and larger. Sinha et al. [19] published a case series in 2008 assessing myomectomies for fibroids greater

than 10 cm in size and five in number. Our case series has an average fibroid size of 8 cm (range 2–20 cm), and the average number of fibroids removed was four (range 1–22), which is greater than the traditional limits and larger than the vast majority of published case series (Table 3). However, our complication rate remains low (2.17%) in keeping with other case series including those historical studies using more conservative limits [10, 17, 21]. To date, the largest laparoscopic myomectomy case series was described by Sizzi et al. [18] in 2007, which described a similarly low complication rate of 2.02% in 2050 cases, although in this case series, both the number (mean = 2.26) and size of fibroids (mean = 6.40) removed were significantly less than ours.

Historically, one of the most common complications encountered during a laparoscopic myomectomy was the need to convert to laparotomy. In one of the earliest case series, Dubusisson et al. [10] reported a conversion rate of 7.5% and attributed this to fibroid size, number and position. Furthermore in 2001, Dessolle et al. [11] reported a similarly high conversion rate of 14.8%. Over the last 10 years, with increasing experience and expertise, this has significantly dropped to reported rates in the literature of between 0 and 1.69% [15, 21, 22, 25]. We also report a low conversion to laparotomy rate of 0.62%. Reassuringly, however, our conversion rate remained low despite tackling larger and more numerous fibroids.

In our case series, the mean blood loss was 279 ml, which was comparable to the wider literature [17, 20, 21]. Nine patients required post-operative blood transfusions; however, in the majority of these cases (77%), the patients were anaemic pre-operatively and the need for transfusion was not directly related to operative blood loss. Maintaining haemostasis and bloodless enucleation are fundamental steps in a successful laparoscopic myomectomy, and a Cochrane review found a reduction in blood loss with the use of both misoprostol and vasopressin [28]. All the patients in our

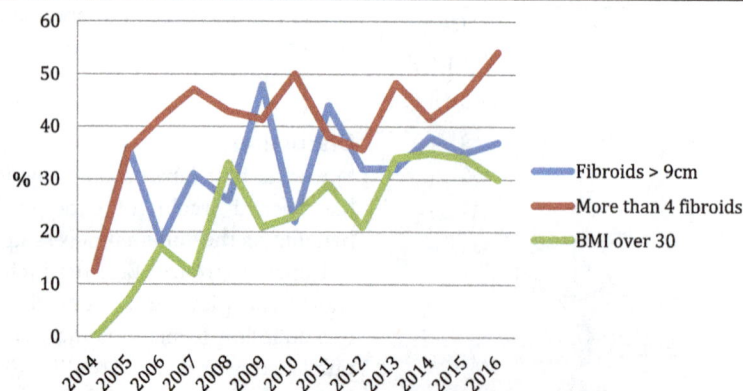

Fig. 2 Percentage of patients with fibroids size > 9cm, greater than four fibroids and a BMI over 30 over time

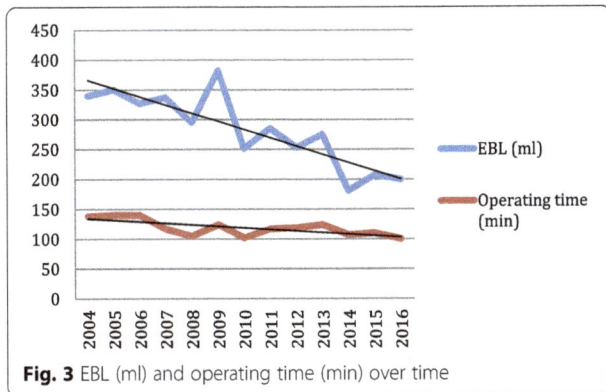

Fig. 3 EBL (ml) and operating time (min) over time

series were given both misoprostol 800 μg per rectum and intra-myometrial vasopressin, which helped reduce blood loss without any significant side effects.

The operating time in our case series was in keeping with the wider literature [17–19], and as one would expect, the greater the number and larger the size of fibroids, the longer the operating time, which is keeping with the findings of Sinha et al. [19]; however, this did not appear to have any significant effect on patient recovery/duration of inpatient stay. We have also found that using barbed sutures (V-loc™or Stratafix™) has helped reduce operating time, and in a recent multicenter study, the use of such barbed sutures has also been shown to significantly reduce operative blood loss [29].

The average duration of hospital stay (1.8 days) was comparable with other studies [18, 20, 21]. Sinha et al. [19] found that hospital stay increased with increasing number, size and weight of fibroids. However, our study reassuringly found no significant effect on the day of discharge in patients with large (> 9 cm) and numerous (> 4) fibroids. The reasons for this may be multifactorial, but a large factor is our extensive pre-operative counselling and well-established enhanced recovery practices.

One of the current controversies surrounding laparoscopic myomectomy is morcellation and the risk of undiagnosed sarcoma, and in April 2014, the FDA discouraged the use of electro-morcellation [7]. However, the most recent BSGE statement acknowledges the place of power

Table 4 A comparative analysis of case series of laparoscopic myomectomy from 1996 to 2017

	n=	Fibroids removed (n)	Largest fibroid removed (cm)	EBL (ml)	Operating time (min)	Inpatient stay (days)	Conversion rate (%)	Complication rate (%)
Dubisson 1996 [10]	213						7.5	3.8
Dessolle 2001 [11]	88	1.7 ± 0.6 (1–4)	6.2 ± 1.8 (3–11)		150 ± 60 (60–300)	3.0 ± 1 (1–10)	14.8	
Landi 2001 [12]	368				100.78 ± 43.83	2.89 ± 1.3		
Malzoni 2003 [13]	144		7.8 (5–18)		95 (58–180)	2.6 (2–5)	1.39	
Malzoni 2006 [16]	982	2.23 (1–8)	6.72 ± 2.71 (1–20)		104.5 (30–360)	2.02 ± 0.61	1.29	
Rosetti 2007 [24]	332	2.23 ± 1.7 (1–8)	6.2 ± 2.7 (1–20)		124.021 ± 52.2	2.0 ± 0.57	1.51	
Yoon 2007 [15]	51	2.2 ± 1.8	9.3 ± 1.8		85.6 ± 38.9	3.2 ± 0.9	0	
Sizzi 2007 [18]	2050	2.26 ± 1.8 (1–15)	6.40 ± 2.6 (1–20)		107.71 ± 43.42	1.99 ± 0.9		2.02
Sinha 2008 [19]	505	1.85 ± 5.706	5.86 ± 3.3	90 (40–2000)	60 (30–270)			
Paul 2010 [21]	1001	1.97 (1–17)	(1–20)	248 (20–1000)	93 (20–280)	1.5 (1–5)	0.1	2.62
Tinelli 2012 [25]	235		6.6 ± 3.5 (4–10)	118 ± 27.9	84 (25–126)		0	
Sankaran 2013 [22]	125	3.69 ± 2.96 (1–15)	7.68 ± 2.95 (2–15)	339.83 ± 254.15 (50–1500)	115.9 ± 42.09 (40–200)	2.38 ± 1.09 (1–7)	1.69	
Saccardi 2014 [23]	444		7.6 ± 2.7	184.1 ± 233.5	77.2 ± 33	2.54 ± 1.1		
Sandberg 2016 [20]	731	3.54 ± 4.10		181.54 ± 342.02		0.58 ± 1.00	1.09	
Bean 2017 [17]	514	1 (1–12)	7 (1–20)	73 (5–3000)		2 (0–24)	0.4	3.5

Data presented as mean ± SD (range) or %

morcellation and the benefits of laparoscopic myomectomy and highlights the importance of patient counselling regarding the potential risks although low [8]. Reassuringly, all the histology reported in our case series was benign. However, caution must be applied in the older age group, and to avoid the risk of undiagnosed malignancy patient selection and counselling is key. Red flag symptoms that should raise suspicion include new onset irregular or heavy vaginal bleeding, unexplained weight loss and systemic symptoms. None of the patients in this series were menopausal, and we would also not routinely offer laparoscopic myomectomy to peri-menopausal women; however, many prefer uterine conserving techniques and decline hysterectomy. In such women, detailed counselling is essential not only with regard to the potential up-staging of malignancy if they were found to have a sarcoma, but also with regard to the potential operative benefits of hysterectomy over myomectomy such as reduced blood loss, operating time and hospital stay as highlighted by Odejinmi et al. [30] when comparing myomectomy and hysterectomy in the older age group. An alternative approach is to use a morcellation bag, which contains the theoretical risk of spreading malignancy if present [31]. This practice is becoming increasingly popular, but national guidance is yet to recommend its general use. Consideration should also be given to the implementation of a national database to record outcomes following laparoscopic myomectomy and morcellation; this would also help with the counselling process and assessment of individual risk.

Conclusions

In conclusion, our study highlights that in experienced hands, laparoscopic myomectomy is a safe and efficacious procedure with low complication and conversion to laparotomy rates even when large (> 8 cm) and numerous (> 4) fibroids are tackled, unlike the earlier studies in the wider literature. As expected, blood loss and operating time are directly related to fibroid size and number; however, large, multiple fibroids can be tackled safely without any increase in patient morbidity and length of hospital stay. Experience, ongoing self-audit of outcomes and a dedicated enhanced recovery approach are essential to the improved outcomes demonstrated in this study.

Acknowledgements
Nothing to declare.

Funding
No specific funding was required.

Authors' contributions
FO devised the project and participated in data collection and manuscript writing. RM participated in the project development, data analysis and manuscript writing. Both authors approved the final manuscript.

Competing interests
The authors declare that they have no competing interests.

References
1. Peacock K, Hurst BS (2006) Laparoscopic myomectomy. Surg Technol Int. 15:141–145
2. Bhave Chittawar P, Franik S, Pouwer AW, Farquhar C (2014) Minimally invasive surgical techniques versus open myomectomy for uterine fibroids. Cochrane Database Syst Rev 21(10):CD004638
3. Takeuchi H, Kinoshita K (2002) Evaluation of adhesion formation after laparoscopic myomectomy by systematic second-look microlaparoscopy. J Am Assoc Gynecol Laparosc. 9(4):442–446
4. Semm K (1979) New methods of pelviscopy (gynecologic laparoscopy) for myomectomy, ovariectomy, tubectomy and adnectomy. Endoscopy 11(2): 85–93
5. Dubuisso JB, Fauconnier A, Babaki-Fard K, Chapron C (2000) Laparoscopic myomectomy: a current view. Hum Reprod Update 6(6):588–594
6. Glasser MH (2005) Minilaparotomy myomectomy: a minimally invasive alternative for the large fibroid uterus. J Minim Invasive Gynecol 12(3): 275–283
7. FDA. UPDATED Laparoscopic uterine power morcellation in hysterectomy and myomectomy: FDA safety communication (https://wayback.archive-it.org/7993/20161023125535/, http://www.fda.gov/NewsEvents/Newsroom/PressAnnouncements/ucm393689.htm). Accessed 1 Jan 2017
8. BSGE. BSGE STATEMENT ON POWER MORCELLATION https://bsge.org.uk/news/bsge-statement-power-morcellation/. Accessed 1 Jan 2017
9. Brölmann H, Tanos V, Grimbizis G, Ind T, Philips K, van den Bosch T et al (2015) Options on fibroid morcellation: a literature review. Gynecol Surg 12(1):3–15
10. Dubuisson J-B, Chapron C, Levy L (1996) Difficulties and complications of laparoscopic myomectomy. J Gynecol Surg 12(3):159–165
11. Dessolle L, Soriano D, Poncelet C, Benifla JL, Madelenat P, Darai E (2001) Determinants of pregnancy rate and obstetric outcome after laparoscopic myomectomy for infertility. Fertil Steril 76(2):370–374
12. Landi S, Zaccoletti R, Ferrari L, Minelli L (2001) Laparoscopic myomectomy: technique, complications, and ultrasound scan evaluations. J Am Assoc Gynecol Laparosc 8(2):231–240
13. Malzoni M, Rotond M, Perone C, Labriola D, Ammaturo F, Izzo A et al (2003) Fertility after laparoscopic myomectomy of large uterine myomas: operative technique and preliminary results. Eur J Gynaecol Oncol 24(1):79–82
14. Marret H, Chevillot M, Giraudeau B (2004) A retrospective multicentre study comparing myomectomy by laparoscopy and laparotomy in current surgical practice. What are the best patient selection criteria? Eur J Obstet Gynecol Reprod Biol 117(1):82–86
15. Yoon HJ, Kyung MS, Jung US, Choi JS (2007) Laparoscopic myomectomy for large myomas. J Korean Med Sci 22(4):706–712
16. Malzoni M, Sizzi O, Rossetti A, Imperato F (2006) Laparoscopic myomectomy: a report of 982 procedures. Surg Technol Int 15:123–129
17. Bean EMR, Cutner A, Holland T, Vashisht A, Jurkovic D, Saridogan E (2017) Laparoscopic myomectomy: a single-center retrospective review of 514 patients. J Minim Invasive Gynecol 24(3):485–493
18. Sizzi O, Rossetti A, Malzoni M, Minelli L, La Grotta F, Soranna L et al (2007) Italian multicenter study on complications of laparoscopic myomectomy. J Minim Invasive Gynecol 14(4):453–462
19. Sinha R, Hegde A, Mahajan C, Dubey N, Sundaram M (2008) Laparoscopic myomectomy: do size, number, and location of the myomas form limiting factors for laparoscopic myomectomy? J Minim Invasive Gynecol 15(3):292–300
20. Sandberg EM, Cohen SL, Jansen FW, Einarsson JI (2016) Analysis of risk factors for intraoperative conversion of laparoscopic myomectomy. J Minim Invasive Gynecol 23(3):352–357
21. Paul GP, Naik SA, Madhu KN, Thomas T (2010) Complications of laparoscopic myomectomy: a single surgeon's series of 1001 cases. Aust N Z J Obstet Gynaecol 50(4):385–390
22. Sankaran S, Odejinmi F (2013) Prospective evaluation of 125 consecutive laparoscopic myomectomies. J Obstet Gynaecol 33(6):609–612
23. Saccardi C, Gizzo S, Noventa M, Ancona E, Borghero A, Litta PS (2014) Limits and complications of laparoscopic myomectomy: which are the best predictors? A large cohort single-center experience. Arch Gynecol Obstet 290(5):951–956

Pushing the boundaries of laparoscopic myomectomy: a comparative analysis of peri-operative...

181

24. Rossetti A, Sizzi O, Chiarotti F, Florio G (2007) Developments in techniques for laparoscopic myomectomy. Jsls 11(1):34–40

25. Tinelli A, Hurst BS, Hudelist G, Tsin DA, Stark M, Mettler L et al (2012) Laparoscopic myomectomy focusing on the myoma pseudocapsule: technical and outcome reports. Hum Reprod 27(2):427–435

26. Ribeiro SC, Reich H, Rosenberg J, Guglielminetti E, Vidali A (1999) Laparoscopic myomectomy and pregnancy outcome in infertile patients. Fertil Steril 71(3):571–574

27. Marret H, Chevillot M, Giraudeau B (2006) Factors influencing laparoconversions during the learning curve of laparoscopic myomectomy. Acta Obstet Gynecol Scand 85(3):324–329

28. Kongnyuy EJ, Wiysonge CS (2014) Interventions to reduce haemorrhage during myomectomy for fibroids. Cochrane Database Syst Rev 15(8):CD005355

29. Tinelli R, Litta P, Angioni S, Bettocchi S, Fusco A, Leo L et al (2016) A multicenter study comparing surgical outcomes and ultrasonographic evaluation of scarring after laparoscopic myomectomy with conventional versus barbed sutures. Int J Gynaecol Obstet 134(1):18–21

30. Odejinmi F, Maclaran K, Agarwal N (2015) Laparoscopic treatment of uterine fibroids: a comparison of peri-operative outcomes in laparoscopic hysterectomy and myomectomy. Arch Gynecol Obstet 291(3):579–584

31. Cohen SL, Einarsson JI, Wang KC, Brown D, Boruta D, Scheib SA et al (2014) Contained power morcellation within an insufflated isolation bag. Obstet Gynecol 124(3):491–497

Chronic pelvic pain and the role of exploratory laparoscopy as diagnostic and therapeutic tool: a retrospective observational study

Géraldine Brichant[1], Marie Denef[1], Linda Tebache[1], Gaëlle Poismans[1], Serena Pinzauti[2], Valérie Dechenne[1] and Michelle Nisolle[1*]

Abstract

Background: Forty percent of exploratory laparoscopies are performed for chronic pelvic pain (CPP). However, a final diagnosis is still unreported in 35% of the patients. We decided to evaluate the identification of pathological lesions and the improvement of painful symptoms in patients with CPP and normal physical examination and imaging and who are scheduled for exploratory laparoscopy. The prospective study was designed in a tertiary referral center for endometriosis. Forty-eight patients complaining of CPP and scheduled for exploratory laparoscopy were included. Pelvic pain intensity was assessed using the visual analogue pain scale (VAS), and at inclusion, negative clinical and imaging assessments were required. During exploratory laparoscopy, the recognized lesions were reported and different surgical treatment options were performed depending on the location of the lesion.

Results: In 98% of the cases, exploratory laparoscopy demonstrated the presence of pelvic anomalies that had not been diagnosed at the time of clinical and imaging examination. After surgery, a significant improvement of CPP has been demonstrated in 24 (59%) patients with VAS < 5 postoperatively.

Conclusions: Exploratory laparoscopy is reasonable in patients complaining of CPP, allowing a final diagnosis in a high percentage of patients and a significant improvement in pain symptom in 59% of the cases. This study was retrospectively registered by our local Ethics Committee on February 7, 2018 (B412201835729).

Keywords: Chronic pelvic pain, Exploratory laparoscopy, Endometriosis, Excision of uterosacral ligaments

Background

Chronic pelvic pain (CPP) is defined as intermittent or constant pain lasting since at least 6 months in the lower abdomen or the pelvis. It can be localized in the pelvis, the anterior abdominal wall at the umbilicus or below, and the lumbosacral back or the buttocks and is sufficient to cause functional disability or lead to seek medical care [1]. Almost 15% of women between 18 and 49 years old complain of CPP, but less than a third seek medical advice [2]. CPP is responsible for about 10% of gynecological consultations and represents the surgical indication of 40% of exploratory laparoscopies [1]. CPP may be related to different causes, from gynecological diseases to gastro-intestinal and urological pathologies. Although less common in such patients, neurological, musculoskeletal, and psychological diseases should be considered [3]. In 25 to 50% of the cases, more than one anomaly can be found in a single patient, increasing the difficulties in diagnosing and alleviating the symptoms [4]. A full medical history, associated with a complete medical examination, is key in order to address patients' correct diagnosis and management. Nowadays, it becomes more and more obvious that a multidisciplinary approach is one of the best way to help the patient in an individualized manner [5].

* Correspondence: michelle.nisolle@chrcitadelle.be
[1]University Department of Obstetrics and Gynecology, CHR La Citadelle, Boulevard du Douzième de Ligne, 1, 4000 Liège, Belgium
Full list of author information is available at the end of the article

Considering our experience, we found that patients' history is often characterized by a long series of medical advices and wrong diagnoses before the final treatment.

The present study aims to establish if exploratory laparoscopy demonstrates the presence of pathological lesions in patients with normal physical and complementary examinations complaining of CPP and to evaluate the improvement of pain after the surgical procedures.

Methods

This study took place in a tertiary referral Center for endometriosis, in the University department of Obstetrics and Gynecology of Liège, Belgium, between October 2011 and April 2015. A total of 48 patients complaining of CPP and scheduled for a surgical treatment were included in the present study following guidelines of our Ethics Committee (B412201835729, retrospectively registered February 7, 2018).

In order to evaluate the role and the efficacy of exploratory laparoscopy in patients with CPP, women in reproductive age (range 18–45 years old) with CPP and negative clinical and imaging examination were considered as possible candidates in the study. CPP was assessed using a 10-point visual analogue pain scale (VAS), and only women with a VAS ≥ 8 were included in the study. Negative clinical examination or only a uterosacral ligament (USL) thickening or uterine retroversion were considered as inclusion criteria. All patients had had a negative ultrasound from their referent OB-GYN. Negative imaging assessments, such as barium enema, pelvic computerized tomography (CT), or pelvic magnetic resonance imaging (MRI), were also required at inclusion in the study. Exclusion criteria were an evidence of chronic disease at medical history or anatomic or endometriotic lesion on clinical examination and imaging assessments.

At inclusion, VAS score for chronic pelvic pain was noted for each patient. During exploratory laparoscopy, a complete examination of the abdominal and pelvic cavity was performed. The observed lesions were classified as endometriosis, thickening of USLs with suspicion of endometriosis, adhesions, uterine anomalies, adnexal anomalies, or any other anomalies. Patients had been counseled before surgery about the different treatment options offered: excision of endometriosis, excision of torus uterinum, adhesiolysis, total hysterectomy with or without bilateral salpingo-oophorectomy (SO), salpingectomy, oophorectomy, or any possible surgical treatment. More than one lesion could be observed in each patient, and subsequently more than one surgical procedure, performed. All specimens were sent for histological examination.

After surgery, VAS score for chronic pelvic pain was assessed at 3- and 24-month interval during consultations.

Depending on the VAS score, patients were divided into the following four groups: group A: VAS 0, no pain; group B: VAS 1–4, mild pain; group C: VAS 5–7, moderate pain; and group D: VAS 8–10, severe pain.

Statistical analysis

Data were collated in a secured data file and were analyzed thanks to the Excel software. Results were expressed as mean ± standard deviation for continuous variable or as percentages for discrete variables. A p value < 0.05 was considered as statistically significant.

Results

The characteristics of the patients are summarized in Table 1. Data were analyzed in 41 patients as 6 patients were lost to follow-up, and in one case, laparoscopy was unsuccessful due to severe adhesions secondary to bowel resection for necrotizing enterocolitis in infancy, leading to unacceptable surgical risks. At exploratory laparoscopy, the documented lesions were reported as follows: 19 (46%) endometriotic lesions such as deep infiltrating endometriosis nodule or peritoneal lesions; 19 (46%) endometriotic suspected lesion (USL thickening); 14 (31%) abdomino-peritoneal adhesions and adhesions between the adnexa and bowel or uterus and bladder; 5 (12%) uterine anomalies (increased uterine volume, abnormal vascularization, suspicion of adenomyosis); 7 (17%) adnexal anomalies (non-dilated hydrosalpinx, ovarian cyst of small size); and 1 (2%) normal pelvis (Fig. 1 and Table 2). In summary, exploratory laparoscopy demonstrated the presence of pelvic anomalies not previously detected in 98% of patients.

Considering surgical procedures, we performed excisions of visible endometriosis 17 patients (41%); excisions of USLs in 24 patients (59%); adhesiolysis in 10 patients (24%); total hysterectomies (1 with unilateral SO and 4 without) in 5 patients (12%); cystectomy, salpingectomies, SO, or other procedures on the adnexa in 7 patients (17%); excision of the post-hysterectomy vaginal scar in 2

Table 1 Characteristics of patients

Characteristics	Patients
Age	Range 18–45 years old; mean 32 years old
VAS score	Mean 8.8/10 (± 0.9)
Complementary examinations	
• Barium enema	27%
• Colonoscopy	5%
• Pelvic computerized tomography (CT)	17%
• Pelvic magnetic resonance imaging (MRI)	68%
Medical history of abdomino-pelvic surgery	
• Endometriosis	17%
• Other abdomino-pelvic surgery	56%
Parity	46% nulliparous

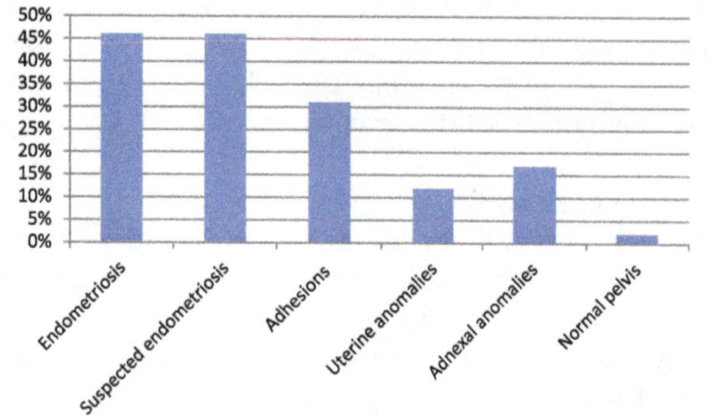

Fig. 1 Pathological lesions documented during laparoscopy

patients (5%); and treatment of uterine retroversion in 1 patient (2%). In one patient (2%), no surgical procedure was performed (Fig. 2 and Table 2). As previously mentioned, more than one lesion could have been described in a patient and subsequently more than one surgical procedure would then be performed. In all cases but one, adhesiolysis has been always associated with another surgical procedure. In two thirds of the patients undergoing excision of USLs, another procedure was performed. No intraoperative complications occurred during surgeries, and no abdominal conversion to laparotomy was needed.

The histological examination confirmed the presence of the corresponding pathological diseases in four cases (24%) of macroscopic endometriosis, in nine cases (38%) of suspected endometriosis (USL thickening), in five cases (100%) of uterine anomalies after hysterectomies (adenomyosis, salpingitis, leiomyomas, endometriosis), and in three cases (43%) of adnexal anomalies (Fig. 2).

Postoperative pain was assessed, and patients were divided into four groups as previously mentioned: 18

Table 2 Surgical procedures and number of patients improved depending on the procedure

Surgical procedures	Number of patients: n (%)	Number of patients improved (%)
Visible endometriosis	17 (41%)	9 (53%)
USLs excisions	24 (59%)	13 (54%)
Adhesiolysis	10 (24%)	6 (60%)
Total hysterectomies	5 (12%) (1 with unilateral SO)	5 (100%)
Other adnexal procedures: • Cystectomy • Salpingectomy • SO • others	7 (17%)	5 (71%)
Excision of post hysterectomy scar	2 (5%)	1 (50%)
Uterine retroversion treatment	1 (2%)	1 (100%)
Nothing	1 (2%)	0 (0%)

patients (44%) had no residual pain (VAS score 0), 6 patients (15%) had mild pain (VAS score between 1 and 4), 8 patients (19%) had moderate pain (VAS score between 5 and 7), and 9 patients (22%) had severe pain with no improvement of CPP and with VAS score ≥ 8 (Fig. 3).

Considering the single surgical procedures only, at the time of endometriotic lesion resection, 10 (53%) patients reported a significant improvement of pain (group A and group B), while excision of USLs, adhesiolysis, cystectomy or salpingectomies or SO, and hysterectomy led to a considerable improvement of pain in 13 (54%), 6 (60%), 5 (71%), and 5 (100%) of cases, respectively (Fig. 4 and Table 2).

Discussion

Chronic pelvic pain is a debilitating condition among women with a major impact on health-related quality of life, on work productivity, and on the health care system and concerns about 4% of women [1]. Identifying the origin of CPP is difficult as it may be caused by disorders of the reproductive tract, gastrointestinal system, urological organs, and musculoskeletal and psychoneurological systems [6]. Some conditions are often associated in the same patient, and many factors have to be evaluated and be taken care of. Pelvic lesions discovered during exploratory laparoscopy are not necessarily responsible for the pain described by the patient [2]. The medical history and physical examination of the patient are essential to allow an appropriate management of the disease.

Gynecologic conditions account for approximately 20% of cases of CPP [3, 7], and irritable bowel syndrome (IBS) and interstitial cystitis (IC) are the other most diagnosed pathology [8]. Considering the different specific gynecological pathologies, several studies describe endometriosis and adhesions as the most frequent causes of CPP (80 and 52%, respectively) [1, 2, 9]. In our series, the high incidence of endometriosis and adhesions in patients with CPP was confirmed, accordingly with previous results.

However, if the association between painful symptoms and endometriosis or adhesions is well accepted, the precise causal relationship is still poorly understood. Endometriosis is still found in 2–50% of asymptomatic women [4], confirming that the scientific research in this field remains a priority. The three most commonly suggested mechanisms for pain in endometriosis are the production of chemokines (growth factors and cytokines), the direct and indirect effects of active bleeding from endometriotic implants, and the irritation or direct invasion of pelvic floor nerves by infiltrating endometriotic lesions [10]. Central sensitization is also a mechanism involved in the pain process in patients with endometriosis. Becker et al. showed in their review that central changes might explain why pain could become more and more difficult to treat

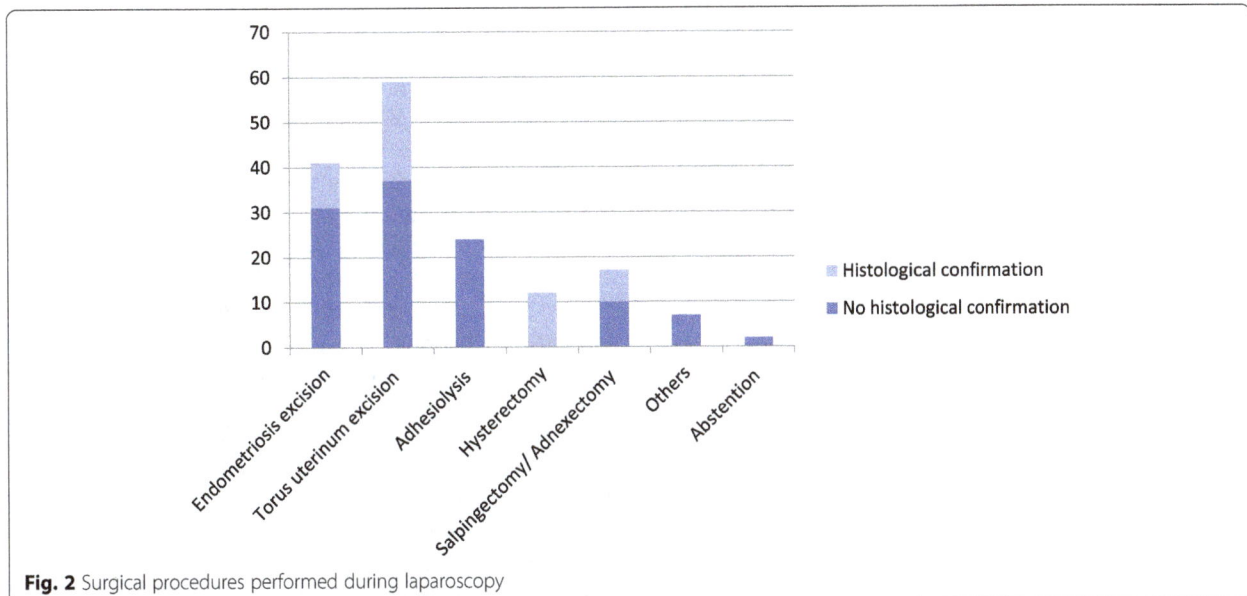

Fig. 2 Surgical procedures performed during laparoscopy

despite appropriate medication. This could also explain the gap sometimes existing between the extent of the disease and the importance of the pain and/or the persistence of the pain despite extensive surgery [11]. However, as the authors stated, further studies targeting central changes in women with proven endometriosis and their influence on pain symptoms and the response to treatment are needed.

Nowadays, the relationship between deep infiltrating endometriosis (DIE) and painful symptoms is well consolidated, even if the extent of lesions does not correlate with the severity of pain [12]. On the contrary, no strong evidence can be found for a relation between endometrioma and painful symptoms. Two reports suggested that painful endometriomas are frequently associated with pelvic adhesions, peritoneal implants, or deep infiltrating lesions, and the severity of pain is independent from the size of the endometrioma [13, 14].

Endometriotic lesions may have variable appearance. The histological distinction in peritoneal, ovarian, and deep-infiltrating endometriosis as three separate entities has been well established [15]. Endometriotic lesions

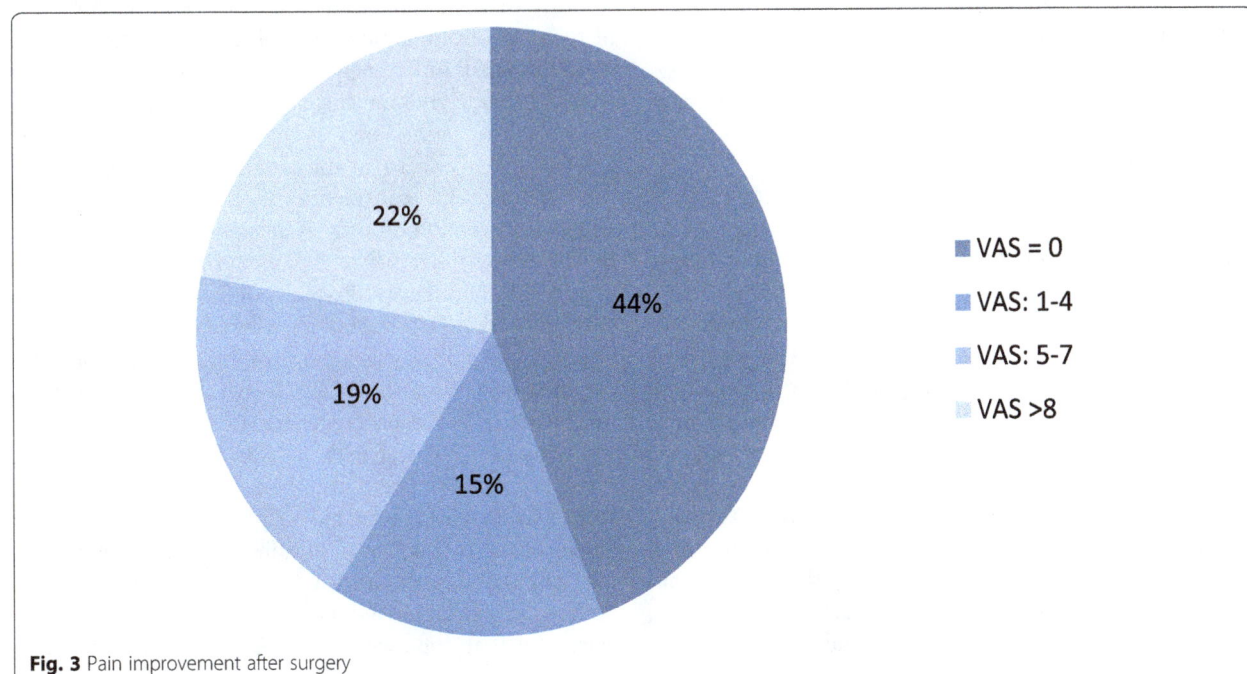

Fig. 3 Pain improvement after surgery

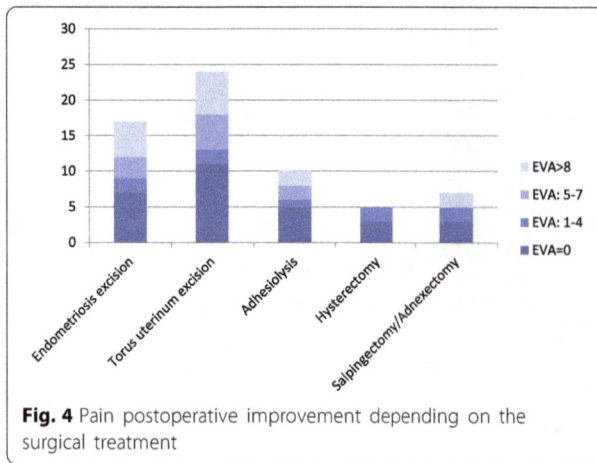

Fig. 4 Pain postoperative improvement depending on the surgical treatment

may have typical aspects, purple or blue nodules, or more atypical presentations in 15–30% of patients (peritoneum opacification or circular defects, glandular growths, inflammatory alterations, yellow spots, ovarian adhesions) that may be confused with other non-endometriotic lesions [16]. Even if the gold standard for endometriosis diagnosis remains the exploratory laparoscopy, this technique in unexperienced hands may still ignore some atypical or retroperitoneal endometriotic lesions. Nisolle et al. also showed that microscopic endometriosis, invisible at the laparoscopic assessment, can be diagnosed during anatomopathological analysis [17]. The old concept of microscopic endometriosis in visually normal peritoneum reported more than a decade ago and supported at that time by few series was recently confirmed by Khan et al. [18]. Clinical consequences of this endometriosis are unknown. However, some of the most recent papers studying microscopic intestinal endometriosis tend to be giving those tiny lesions some clinical relevance. Authors have proved the presence of microscopic endometriosis at a distance from macroscopic lesions that are resected. In those cases, radical segmental colectomy would not be more efficient than discoid resection as it would not remove the microscopic lesions [19, 20].

In summary, the increasing knowledge of the variability of endometriotic lesions appearance has led to a significant increase in endometriosis diagnosis. However, a high incidence of indefinite diagnosis is still reported in patients with CPP as no visible pathology can be found in 35% of cases [9]. This proportion of failure to diagnose an etiology for the CPP is high considering that exploratory laparoscopy remains an invasive surgical procedure with the inherent risks. In our series, the rate of negative exploratory laparoscopy is extremely low (2%) and this data may be explained by the fact that all patients had been carefully examined and investigated by a gynecologist specialized in CPP and endometriosis. The same experimented gynecologist performed all

surgical procedures. From data about the lesions' appearance, the development of other surgical procedures arises, such as the torus uterinum excision (or resection of uterosacral ligament(s)). Surgery is performed by removing all the USLs at the pararectal levels until their insertions on the cervix. This technique should be differentiated from the laparoscopic uterosacral nerve ablation (LUNA), consisting in a single uterosacral ligament section at 1–2 cm from their insertion on the cervix, and the pre-sacral neurectomy (PSN), consisting in the interruption of the sympathetic nervous fibers at the superior hypogastric plexus. Both LUNA and PSN are currently considered non-specific procedure for CPP and are no longer recommended of these patients [9]. In our experience, torus uterinum excision has been performed in patients whose USLs were tight and sore on clinical examination and/or if their thickened appearance was confirmed at the exploratory laparoscopy. More than half of our patients described less pain after the surgery even if their satisfaction was not always related to the histological confirmation of endometriosis. This procedure was efficient in 54% (group A and B) even if the presence of endometriosis was confirmed only for 5 patients on 13 (38%).

Our data on histological examination confirmed the presence of endometriosis in only 24% of treated patients for macroscopic endometriosis and in 38% of patients with USLs excision. Actually, negative histological examination cannot exclude endometriosis diagnosis because either all rigorous histological criteria might not be met or lesions might not visible because of hormonal suppression or histological exploration might be incomplete (i.e., small lesions surrounded by large sections of healthy tissue). There is no consensus about technics for histological examination. Histological examination is recommended but a negative histological examination cannot exclude endometriosis diagnosis [21, 22].

Considering adhesions, as previously reported, they are frequently related to the endometriotic process and may be actually considered as a possible cause of pain-related endometriosis. Adhesions may theoretically be caused by other pelvic inflammatory processes, such as pelvic inflammatory disease, inflammatory bowel disease, and previous abdominal-pelvic surgery but in 50% of cases the etiology is unknown [9]. The relationship between adhesions and CPP is controversial. Usually, studies show a similar frequency of adhesions between women with CPP and without CPP [9]. However, some series report some solid arguments in favor of a role of adhesions in CPP. Even as early as the 1980s, Kresch found a higher frequency of adhesions in women with CPP compared with women without CPP. In his study, he noted a characteristic aspect of adhesions in women with CPP that appeared to be restricting the motion or the expansibility of one or more organs [23]. More recently, the role of adhesions seemed to be confirmed by the laparoscopy conscious pain mapping where a laparoscopy is performed under local anesthesia. The study showed that under local anesthesia stimulation of adhesions elicited pain in patients [24]. In our series, adhesions were described in 31% of patients with CPP and we performed 10 (24%) of adhesiolysis with a significant improvement of pain symptomatology (groups A and B) in 60% of treated patients. Except in one case, this procedure has been always associated to another surgical procedure and it seems difficult to make a judgment on its benefit.

CPP represents 12% of all the indications for hysterectomy [25]. A recent review tells that in the absence of any obvious pathology, 60 to 79% of women report improvement in symptomatology after hysterectomy. In our series, we performed four (10%) total hysterectomies and one (2%) total hysterectomies with BSO when the uterus or adnexa had abnormal aspect, such as increased volume, and abnormal vascularisation or fibroid appearance. Histological examination confirmed pathologies such as adenomyosis, endosalpingiosis, salpingitis, endometritis, and leiomyoma in 100% of the specimen. All patients had significant improvement of pain after the procedure. Our data are similar to those of the literature, confirming that hysterectomy may be effective against pain, even in the absence of obvious anomalies of the uterus. However, it should be important to inform patients that in 21 to 40% of the cases the intervention will not help in improving CPP and rarely will it worsen the painful symptomatology. Hysterectomy should be categorized as a non-specific treatment. It should be kept in mind that 70% of CPP are non-gynecologic etiology such as irritable bowel syndrome, painful bladder syndrome, and pelvic floor myalgia. All women with CPP should undergo a multidisciplinary evaluation before surgery to exclude other causes of pain to maximize the chances of pain resolution [25].

We performed five (12%) interventions at adnexal level with one cystectomy and one salpingo-oophorectomy for cyst and three salpingectomies. Pelvic inflammatory disease is found in 5% of laparoscopy performed to CPP. One fourth of women who had acute salpingitis will develop CPP. The aftereffect of acute salpingitis can be variable and include adhesions, hydrosalpinx, and ovarian dystrophi [2]. Ovarian cysts are found in 3% of laparoscopy performed for CPP. Ovarian cysts are usually asymptomatic or cause acute pain. Recurrent functional ovarian cysts seem to be sometimes the cause of CPP. In our series, adnexal surgeries have been associated to another procedure except in one case of the adnexectomy for a cyst. In all those cases, the patient is pain free (group A).

Conclusion

In conclusion, our study demonstrated that exploratory laparoscopy provides a definitive diagnosis in 98% of women complaining of unexplained CPP. The surgical treatment of these lesions improves painful symptomatology in 59% of women with a total disappearance of pain in 44% of cases (VAS 0) and significant improvement in 15% of cases (VAS < 5). We believe that the exploratory laparoscopy is therefore justified in patients complaining of significant CPP. The candidates' selection should be meticulous, and patients should be investigated at urologic, gastroenterologic, and musculoskeletal level before surgery. We believe that women should be referred to experimented gynecologists in the field of CPP and endometriosis who can properly inspect the pelvic area and who are able to detect lesions potentially responsible of CPP. Despite that, 22% of women do not improve after surgery. This could either be because of the found anomaly wasn't the only one responsible for the painful symptoms and/or that normal anatomy couldn't be restored completely. We believe a better candidates' selection including the identification of poor prognostic factor such as psychosomatic syndrome could improve the results as well as a better identification of macroscopic and microscopic conditions. A better understanding of relationship between some type of lesions and CPP will help in alleviating the patients' symptoms.

Abbreviations

CPP: Chronic pelvic pain; CT: Computerized tomography; DIE: Deep infiltrating endometriosis; IBS: Irritable bowel syndrome; IC: Interstital cystitis; LUNA: Laparoscopic uterosacral nerve ablation; MRI: Magnetic resonance imaging; PSN: Pre-sacral neurectomy; SO: Salpingo-oophorectomy; USLs: Utero-sacral ligaments; VAS: Visual analogue pain scale

Acknowledgements

Special thanks to Marie Timmermans for her help in the data collection and analysis.

Authors' contributions

GB, MD, GP, and SP have collected the data. MN and VD performed the surgeries. GB, MD, and MN wrote the manuscript. All authors read and approved the final manuscript.

Competing interests

The authors declare that they have no competing interests.

Author details

[1]University Department of Obstetrics and Gynecology, CHR La Citadelle, Boulevard du Douzième de Ligne, 1, 4000 Liège, Belgium. [2]UO Ostetricia e Ginecologia, Ospedale Santa Maria alla Gruccia, Arezzo, Montevarchi, Italy.

References

1. Howard FM (2003) Chronic pelvic pain. Obstet Gynecol 101:594–611
2. Fauconnier A, Fritel X (2010) Algies pelviennes chroniques d'origine non endométriosique. J Gynecologie, Obstetrique et Biologie de la Reproduc 39: s1–S342
3. Steege JF, Siedhoff MT (2014) Chronic pelvic pain. Obstet Gynecol 124:616–629. https://doi.org/10.1097/AOG.0000000000000417
4. Moen MH, Stokstad T (2002) A long-term follow-up study of women with asymptomatic endometriosis diagnosed incidentally at sterilization. Fertil Steril 78:773–776
5. Morrissey D, Ginzburg N, Whitmore K (2014) Current advancements in the diagnosis and treatment of chronic pelvic pain. Curr Opin Urol 24:336–344. https://doi.org/10.1097/MOU.0000000000000062
6. Alcock A (1926) Chronic pelvic pain in women. Br Med J 1:609–612
7. Zondervan KT, Yudkin PL, Vessey MP, Dawes MG, Barlow DH, Kennedy SH (1999) Patterns of diagnosis and referral in women consulting for chronic pelvic pain in UK primary care. Br J Obstet Gynaecol 106:1156–1161
8. Vercellini P, Somigliana E, Vigano P, Abbiati A, Barbara G, Fedele L (2009) Chronic pelvic pain in women: etiology, pathogenesis and diagnostic approach. Gynecol Endocrinol 25:149–158. https://doi.org/10.1080/09513590802549858
9. Howard FM (2000) The role of laparoscopy as a diagnostic tool in chronic pelvic pain Bailliere's best practice & research. Clinical Obstetrics & Gynaecology 14:467–494
10. Berkley KJ, Rapkin AJ, Papka RE (2005) The pains of endometriosis. Science 308(5728):1587–1589. https://doi.org/10.1126/science.1111445
11. Morotti M, Vincent K, Becker CM (2017) Mechanisms of pain in endometriosis. Eur J Obstet Gynecol Reprod Biol. 209:8–13. https://doi.org/10.1016/j.ejogrb.2016.07.497
12. Fauconnier A, Chapron C, Dubuisson JB, Vieira M, Dousset B, Breart G (2002) Relation between pain symptoms and the anatomic location of deep infiltrating endometriosis. Fertil Steril 78:719–726
13. Fauconnier A, Chapron C (2005) Endometriosis and pelvic pain: epidemiological evidence of the relationship and implications. Hum Reprod Update 11(6):595–606. https://doi.org/10.1093/humupd/dmi029
14. Khan KN, Kitajima M, Fujishita A, Hiraki K, Matsumoto A, Nakashima M, Masuzaki H (2013) Pelvic pain in women with ovarian endometrioma is mostly associated with coexisting peritoneal lesions. Hum Reprod 28:109–118. https://doi.org/10.1093/humrep/des364
15. Nisolle M, Donnez J (1997) Peritoneal endometriosis, ovarian endometriosis, and adenomyotic nodules of the rectovaginal septum are three different entities. Fertil Steril 68:585–596. https://doi.org/10.1016/S0015-0282(97)00191-X
16. Lamvu G, Tu F, As-Sanie S, Zolnoun D, Steege JF (2004) The role of laparoscopy in the diagnosis and treatment of conditions associated with chronic pelvic pain. Obstet Gynecol Clin N Am 31:619–630. https://doi.org/10.1016/j.ogc.2004.05.003
17. Nisolle M, Paindaveine B, Bourdon A, Berliere M, Casanas-Roux F, Donnez J (1990) Histologic study of peritoneal endometriosis in infertile women. Fertil Steril 53:984–988
18. Khan KN, Fujishita A, Kitajima M, Hiraki K, Nakashima M, Masuzaki H (2014) Occult microscopic endometriosis: undetectable by laparoscopy in normal peritoneum. Hum Reprod 29:462–472. https://doi.org/10.1093/humrep/det438
19. Badescu A et al (2016) Mapping of bowel occult microscopic endometriosis implants surrounding deep endometriosis nodules infiltrating the bowel. Fertil Steril 105(2):430–434. https://doi.org/10.1016/j.fertnstert.2015.11.006
20. Darwish B, Roman H (2016) Surgical treatment of deep infiltrating rectal endometriosis: in favor of less aggressive surgery. Am J Obstet Gynecol 215(2):195–200. https://doi.org/10.1016/j.ajog.2016.01.189
21. Fritel X (2007) Endometriosis anatomoclinical entities. J Gynecologie, Obstetrique et Biologie de la Reproduc 36:113–118. https://doi.org/10.1016/j.jgyn.2006.12.003
22. Kennedy S et al (2005) ESHRE guideline for the diagnosis and treatment of endometriosis. Hum Reprod 20:2698–2704. https://doi.org/10.1093/humrep/dei135
23. Kresch AJ, Seifer DB, Sachs LB, Barrese I (1984) Laparoscopy in 100 women with chronic pelvic pain. Obstet Gynecol 64:672–674
24. Howard FM, El-Minawi AM, Sanchez RA (2000) Conscious pain mapping by laparoscopy in women with chronic pelvic pain. Obstet Gynecol 96:934–939
25. Lamvu G (2011) Role of hysterectomy in the treatment of chronic pelvic pain. Obstet Gynecol 117:1175–1178. https://doi.org/10.1097/AOG.0b013e31821646e1

29

A long-term cohort study of surgery for recurrent prolapse comparing mesh augmented anterior repairs to anterior colporrhaphy

Natasha Curtiss and Jonathan Duckett*⍟

Abstract

Background: There are safety concerns regarding the use of mesh in vaginal surgery with a call for long-term follow-up data. This study was designed to evaluate the long-term safety and efficacy of vaginal repairs performed for recurrent cystocele using Perigee (non-absorbable trans-obturator) mesh.

Methods: A retrospective consecutive cohort of 48 women who underwent surgery for recurrent prolapse between March 2007 and December 2011 in a single centre was reviewed. Satisfaction was assessed using the patient global impression of improvement (PGI-I). Symptoms were assessed with the pelvic floor distress inventory (PFDI). Women were questioned regarding pain, sexual activity and pelvic floor surgery performed since the original procedure and examined for erosion. Women were compared to 25 controls from a consecutive cohort of repeat anterior colporrhapies.

Results: The mean length of follow-up was 6.5 years (78 months; range 48–106). Significantly more women in the mesh group reported that they were "much better" or "very much better" (69 vs 40% $p = 0.02$). The rate of mesh erosion at follow-up was 11.6%. Two women in the mesh group required surgical excision of eroded mesh in the operating room (4%). The reoperation rate for a combination of de novo stress incontinence, recurrent prolapse and mesh exposure was similar in each group (33% mesh vs 32% native tissue).

Conclusions: A vaginal mesh repair using a non-absorbable trans-obturator mesh has improved satisfaction compared to an anterior colporrhaphy.

Keywords: Mesh, Perigee, Pelvic organ prolapse, Surgery, Colporrhaphy, Long term

Background

Pelvic organ prolapse (POP) is a common condition with considerable socio-economic, psychological and physical impact [1, 2]. Eleven percent of women will have undergone a surgical repair by the age of 80 [3]. The most common repair to be performed is an anterior vaginal wall repair [4].

There is a significant recurrent prolapse rate after primary native tissue repair [5]. Mesh repairs were introduced to reinforce the native tissues aiming to reduce recurrence rates. A Cochrane review suggested recurrence rates are lower using non absorbable mesh augmented repairs [6]. However, there are complications

unique to mesh repairs and 12% of patient will have a mesh complication and a proportion of these will require further surgical intervention to manage the complication [5, 6]. High rates of pain and dyspareunia have also been reported affecting patient satisfaction [7].

The reported complications of mesh-augmented repairs have resulted in interest from regulatory bodies including the FDA, the media and the patient support groups. The Scottish Government ordered an independent review of the use of transvaginal mesh in women and NHS England produced an interim report in October 2015 [8]. The long-term safety and prolapse recurrence is of concern to urogynecologists and their women, and there is currently a paucity of long-term evidence. This study aimed to look at the long-term

* Correspondence: jraduckett@hotmail.com
Department of Obstetrics and Gynaecology, Medway Maritime Hospital, Windmill Road, Gillingham, Kent ME7 5NY, UK

safety and efficacy of vaginal repairs performed using Perigee mesh for recurrent cystocele and compare them to native tissue repair/anterior colporrhaphy for recurrent cystocele. This was a single-center single-surgeon cohort study.

Methods

All women who had undergone a recurrent cystocele (symptomatic POP-Q stage 2) repair using either native tissue or a Perigee vaginal mesh repair at a single surgical centre were identified from a prospectively maintained database. This was cross-referenced with information from the British Society of Urogynaecology (BSUG) database. All procedures were performed by or under the supervision of a single surgeon. All procedures were carried out in an operating theatre under regional or general anaesthesia with administration of prophylactic antibiotics. Fascial plication was performed in the native tissue repairs using absorbable polyglactin sutures. A continuous locking polyglactin suture was used for vaginal skin closure. The same technique was used for mesh repairs other than the repair was augmented with placement of non-absorbable mesh under the fascial plication sutures. The mesh was placed in a tension-free fashion with the aim of supporting the whole of the anterior vaginal wall. The upper transobturator arm was placed 1/2 cm in front of the ischial spine. Women with vault prolapse (greater than or equal to stage 2) were treated with abdominal sacrocolpopexy and were excluded from this study.

A consecutive cohort of women receiving Perigee mesh vaginal repairs for recurrent cystoceles between March 2007 and December 2011 was contacted and asked to attend for clinical assessment. The time frame and number of women were purely dependent on the number of operations performed. A post hoc power calculation suggested that a study with 79 recruits had a 70% chance of demonstrating a difference in the patient global impression of improvement (PGI-I) with a p value of 0.05. Before 2007, mesh kits were not used. After 2011, very few meshes were inserted into the anterior vaginal wall due to concerns regarding safety and efficacy. No other anterior vaginal wall mesh kit was used before, during or after these dates. Meshes were not inserted for primary repairs. Demographic data and details regarding the surgery were gathered from the patient's clinical record. The primary outcome was based on the PGI-I (much better and very much better) with the presence of prolapse symptoms ascertained by the pelvic floor distress inventory (PFDI). Women were interviewed regarding their awareness of mesh complications reported in the media. Women were asked if they were sexually active before the surgery and whether they continued to be sexually active at follow-up. Women

were examined for mesh exposure. Women were assessed as having a mesh erosion if one was detected on examination or if the patient had undergone medical or surgical treatment for mesh erosion during the follow-up period. A single research fellow who was not previously known by the women undertook the clinical examinations. This person assessed the clinical notes and hence was not blinded to the previous surgery. Women who did not attend for clinical assessment were contacted by telephone, where possible, questionnaires and interviews were undertaken over the telephone.

Women who had undergone native tissue repairs at the same centre for recurrent cystocele during the same timespan completed the same questionnaires and were contacted and interviewed by telephone. Their notes were scrutinised, for demographic and operative details. There were limited cases in this cohort as women were primarily offered mesh repairs during this time. The same time frame was used so that women with a similar length of follow-up would be studied.

A symptomatic recurrence was assessed when either further surgery had been undertaken or if the woman had answered Somewhat, Moderately or Quite a Bit to the PFDI-6 question "usually have a bulge or something falling out that you can see or feel in your vaginal area". All definitions and terminology confirm to the joint International Urogynecology Association/International Continence Society terminology report [9]. T tests were used for continuous variables which were normally distributed, and proportions were compared using the Chi-squared test.

Ethical consent and permissions

Ethical approval for the study was given by the National Research Ethics Service (NRES) (Ref 15/LO/0158: 6th February 2015), and the study was registered with ClinicalTrials.gov (NCT02642835). Patients provided written informed consent. The research was performed in accordance with the Helsinki declaration.

Results

A total of 50 women were identified as having had a Perigee mesh vaginal repair for recurrent cystocele in the study period (see Fig. 1). Forty-eight women were assessed (five by telephone interview). Two women were lost to follow-up. One had died from unrelated causes. There were 38 women identified as having undergone a native tissue repair for recurrent cystocele in the same time period. Twenty-five were interviewed (66%) and one woman had died of unrelated causes. The mean length of follow-up was 6.5 years (78 months; range 48–106). There was no difference in the patient demographics (see Table 1). The population was predominantly white Caucasian (98%). There were no intra-operative

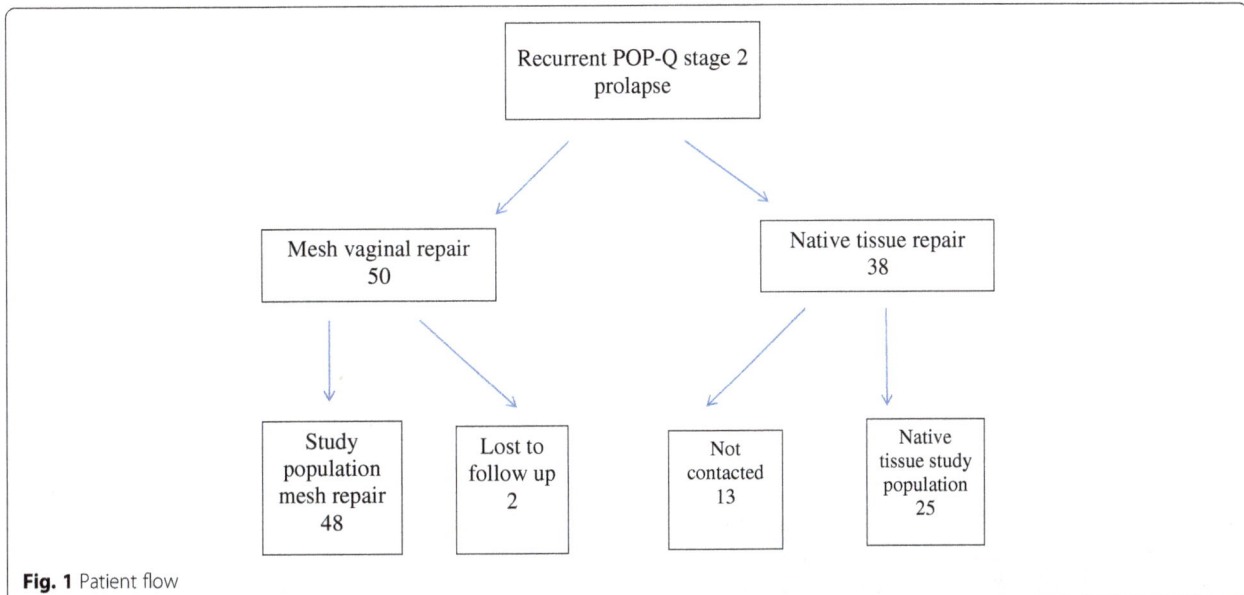

Fig. 1 Patient flow

complications in either group. No woman required a blood transfusion. The outcome data is presented in Table 2. Nine women (19%) interviewed in the Perigee group reported being aware of concerns regarding vaginal mesh in the media or from friends or family prior to receiving the invitation to be part of the study.

Significantly more women in the mesh group reported that they were "much better" or "very much better" (69 vs 40% $p = 0.02$). In the Perigee group, the rate of mesh erosion at follow-up was 11.6% (5/43). None of these occurred in either women with diabetes 3/48 or in smokers 7/48. Two erosions were treated with topical oestrogen alone, one was cut in clinic (IUGA graft complication code 2AT4S1) and the other two required surgical excision in the operating theatre (2/48; 4%) (3AT4S2). Three of the mesh erosions were identified for the first time during the study; two had symptoms of prolapse recurrence and the other overactive bladder symptoms but none had re-presented before invitation with these symptoms. These women were unaware of the mesh exposure and did not have exposure-specific symptoms. Mesh erosion is a complication that does not affect native tissue repairs. Table 3 describes the surgical

procedures that the women had undergone since the index procedure. When the need for repeat surgery for mesh exposure, surgery for de novo stress incontinence and repeat surgical treatment of prolapse are combined 33% (16/48) of the Perigee group and 32% (8/25) of the native tissue repairs needed further surgery ($p = 1$).

Discussion

More women in the anterior vaginal wall mesh group scored their prolapse as "very much better" or "much better" following surgery compared to those in the native tissue arm. The reoperation rate after the index procedure was similar in both groups with 33% in the mesh group and 32% in the native tissue group

Table 1 Demographic data

	Perigee ($n = 48$)	Native tissue ($N = 25$)	P value
Age (range)	66 (47–83)	62 (44–81)	0.10
BMI (mean)	27.4	30.0	0.12
Parity (median)	2	3	
Smoking (current)	7	4	1
Time to follow-up (months) (range)	82 (48–106)	69 (53–101)	0.01
Prior hysterectomy	98% (47/48)	88% (22/25)	0.11

Table 2 Post operative outcomes

	Perigee ($n = 48$)	Native tissue ($N = 25$)	P value
Much or very much better PGI-I	33 (68.8)	10 (40%)	0.02
Sexually active preoperatively	37 (75.5%)	15 (60%)	0.0002
Stopped sexually active after most recent repair	17/37 (46%)	6/15 (40%)	0.77
Operation for SUI during follow-up	5 (10.4%)	2 (8%)	1
Reoperation for POP: same compartment	1 (2.1%)	2 (8%)	0.29
Reoperation different compartment	8 (16.7%)	4 (16%)	
Symptomatic recurrence (PFDI)	14 (29.2%)	13 (52%)	0.08
Surgery for mesh erosion	2 (4%)	0	N/A

SUI stress urinary incontinence, *PGI-I* patient impression of improvement, *POP* pelvic organ prolapse, *PFDI* pelvic floor distress inventory

Table 3 Repeat surgery after index repair

	Perigee ($n = 48$)	Native tissue ($N = 25$)	P value
Midurethral sling	5	2	1
Posterior repair	4	4	1
Native anterior repair	0	1	1
Abdominal sacrocolpopexy	4	1	0.65
Division vaginal adhesions	2	0	0.54
Incision introitus	1	0	1
Abdominal paravaginal repair	1	0	1
Excision erosion	2	0	0.54
Vaginal mesh repair	0	2	0.11

undergoing further surgery for either de novo incontinence or recurrent prolapse during follow-up. The rate of mesh erosion was 11.6% although the need for surgical intervention was low (4%). This study is unusual in that it only includes women treated for recurrent prolapse and has a long follow-up period.

The long-term data on vaginal mesh repairs remains difficult to evaluate. There are few long-term series published, and they are heterogeneous involving primary and secondary cases, varying compartments and concomitant procedures [10–12], with varying follow-up. Long-term studies assessing a single procedure in a discrete population remain scarce. Heinonen published a long-term series with a similar follow-up period and protocol to the current study. Their study group was a mix of primary and recurrent (46%) prolapses in either the anterior, posterior or both compartments [12]. After a median of 7 years, they described a mesh erosion rate of 23% with 80% of women being satisfied with the procedure. Lo et al. described a subjective cure rate of 88.6% 3 years after surgery but combined their mesh repairs with a sacrospinous fixation [13]. Karmakar (2015) published a series of women with a 2-year median follow-up. They described cure rates (no anatomical recurrence or symptoms) of 91% in those with mesh repair for recurrent cystocele for an extrusion rate of 21% [11].

Mesh erosion rates were 11.6% with only two women in the study requiring surgical management for mesh erosion (4% of all women). This erosion rate was modest and it was expected that it might be higher in view of the length of follow-up and the fact that all the repairs were repeat procedures for a failed primary native tissue repair. The rate of mesh erosion described in this study is similar to that reported in the Cochrane review (12%) [6] and an equivalent rate to those from the Austrian database of 726 vaginal meshes who found mesh exposure of 12% at 1 year [14]. However, the current study has a much longer follow-up and would be expected to have a higher erosion rate.

There are additional risks unique to mesh repairs including mesh exposure and a longer operating time [6, 13]. The Cochrane 2016 found that by combining operation rates for mesh exposure, repeat prolapse surgery and surgery for stress incontinence, there was a higher reoperation rate in mesh repairs compared with native tissue repairs [6]. This was not found in the current study with no statistically significant difference in overall reoperation rate by this calculation. The MHRA concluded in 2014 that for the majority of women, the use of vaginal mesh implants is safe and effective [15].

Interestingly, despite some high-profile reports in the press, the women in this study were mostly unaware of any reports of complications relating to mesh. Only 19% of the women questioned reported being aware of concerns regarding vaginal mesh repair prior to being contacted for this study. Most of the women had been made aware by a family of a friend who had themselves suffered a complication of vaginal mesh repair. Overall, awareness of mesh controversy was low in this population but may be higher in a different patient group.

A high proportion of the women stopped sexual activity after the repair performed in this study. Discontinuation of sexual activity was similar in both the anterior mesh group and the native tissue repair with 46% of the anterior mesh group becoming sexually inactive and 40% of the native tissue repair becoming sexually inactive. Although sexual activity was noted in the study, much more information would have been obtained if a validated sexual function questionnaire had been used. Unfortunately, this was not a focus of research when the initial surgery was performed up to 8.8 years before this study was performed.

There are certain criticisms that could be made of this study. The study size might not appear large when compared to other studies, but many other studies contain primary cases and short follow-up. The post hoc power calculation suggested that the study might be slightly underpowered to show a difference in the PGI-I although this was not born out in the study results. No pre-operative questionnaires were available for direct comparison of symptoms and so there may be some reporting bias especially due to the long follow-up period. The follow-up time was significantly longer in the mesh arm despite attempts to match the cohorts. This might result in lower satisfaction in the mesh arm due to the need for further surgery for recurrence or new complications found later in the follow-up period. The results suggest the reverse with a lower symptomatic recurrence in the mesh arm. It may therefore be possible that the benefits of mesh might be underestimated due to the longer follow-up in this group. This was a single-center single-surgeon retrospective study and this may limit generalisability. However, in the absence of high-quality data from randomised controlled trials, this remains the best evidence currently available. The follow-up rate in the mesh cohort was excellent with 48/50 women seen (96%). The follow-up in the colporrhaphy group was similar to commonly seen in long-term studies with 66% contacted but this might introduce bias. The results presented concentrate on subjective data with the PGI-I but more qualitative data would have been useful.

Conclusions

The authors of this study stopped using anterior vaginal wall mesh procedures after 2011 as the operation was perceived to be risky and of no definite benefit. On the basis of the findings of this study, this decision should be reviewed. In the hands of the authors, the anterior mesh repair operation has a durable success rate with low morbidity and is probably superior to a native tissue repair. Unfortunately, this specific mesh is no longer marketed. The erosion rate is similar to studies with shorter follow-up. There may, given these findings, be a role for an anterior vaginal mesh repair performed by a trained surgeon in the carefully counselled woman.

Abbreviations
PGI-I: Patient global impression of improvement; POP: Pelvic organ prolapse

Author's contributions
N Curtiss examined and interviewed all women and wrote the manuscript. J Duckett developed the concept and edited the manuscript. Both authors read and approved the final manuscript.

Competing interests
The work was supported by a grant from American Medical Systems. They had no input in analysing the results or producing the manuscript.

References
1. Digesu G, Chaliha C, Salvatore S, Hutchings A, Khullar V (2005) The relationship of vaginal prolapse severity to symptoms and quality of life. BJOG 112:971–976
2. Jelovesk J, Barber M (2006) Women seeking treatment for advanced pelvic organ prolapse have decreased body image and quality of life. Am J Obstet Gynecol 194:1455–1461
3. Olsen A, Smith V, Bergstrom J, Colling J, Clark A (1997) Epidemiology of surgically managed pelvic organ prolapse and urinary incontinence. Obstet Gynecol 89:501–506
4. Beck R, McCormick S, Nordstrom L (1991) A 25-year experience with 519 anterior colporrhaphy procedures. Obstet Gynecol 78:1011–1018
5. NICE (2008) Surgical repair of vaginal wall prolapse using mesh. Retrieved from http://www.nice.org.uk/IPG267
6. Maher C, Feiner B, Baessler K, Christmann-Schmid C, Haya N, Marjoribanks J Transvaginal mesh or grafts compared with native tissue repair for vaginal prolapse. Cochrane Database Syst Rev 2016, Issue 2. Art. No.: CD012079. https://doi.org/10.1002/14651858.CD012079
7. Food, Drug Administration (FDA) Urogynecologic surgical mesh: update on the safety and effectiveness of transvaginal mesh placement for pelvic organ prolapse. https://www.fda.gov/downloads/medicaldevices/safety/.../ucm262760.pdf
8. The Scottish Independent Review of the Use, Safety and Efficacy of Transvaginal Mesh Implants in the Treatment of Stress Urinary Incontinence and Pelvic Organ Prolapse in Women: Interim Report. www.gov.scot/About/Review/Transvaginal-Mesh-Implants
9. Haylen BT, de Ridder D, Freeman RM, Swift SE, Bergmans B, Lee J et al (2010) An International Urogynecological Association (IUGA)/International Continence Society (ICS) joint report on the terminology for female pelvic floor dysfunction. Int Urogynecol J 21:5–26
10. Cooper J, Bondili A, Deguara C, Siraj N (2013) Vaginal repair with polypropylene mesh compared to traditional colporrhaphy for pelvic organ prolapse: medium-term follow-up. J Gynecol Surg 29:1–6
11. Karmakar D, Hayward L, Smalldridge J, Lin S (2015) Vaginal mesh for prolapse: a long-term prospective study of 218 mesh kit from a single centre. Int Urogynaecol J 26:1161–1170
12. Heinonen P, Aaltonen R, Joronen K, Ala-Nissila S (2016) Long-term outcome after transvaginal mesh repair of pelvic organ prolapse. Int Urogynecol J 27:1069–1074
13. Lo TS, Pue LB, Tan YL, PY W (2014) Long-term outcomes of synthetic transobturator nonabsorbable anterior mesh versus anterior colporrhaphy in symptomatic, advanced pelvic organ prolapse surgery. Int Urogynecol J 25:257–264
14. Bjelic-radisic V, Aigmueller T, Preyer O, Ralph G, Geiss I, Muller G et al (2014) Vaginal prolapse surgery with transvaginal mesh: results of the Austrian registry. Int Urogynecol J 25:1047–1052
15. Medicines and Healthcare Products Regulatory Agency (MHRA) (2014) A summary of the evidence on the benefits and risks of vaginal mesh implants. https://www.gov.uk/government/publications/vaginal-mesh-implants-summary-of-benefits-and-risks. Accessed Dec 2017

30

Incidence and predictors of failed second-generation endometrial ablation

Jordan Klebanoff[1]*(iD), Gretchen E. Makai[2], Nima R. Patel[2] and Matthew K. Hoffman[1]

Abstract

Background: The need for any treatment following an endometrial ablation is frequently cited as "failed therapy," with the two most common secondary interventions being repeat ablation and hysterectomy. Since second-generation devices have become standard of care, no large cohort study has assessed treatment outcomes with regard to only these newer devices. We sought to determine the incidence and predictors of failed second-generation endometrial ablation, defined as the need for surgical re-intervention.

We performed a retrospective cohort study at a single academic-affiliated community hospital. Subjects included women undergoing second-generation endometrial ablation for benign indications between October 2003 and March 2016. Second-generation devices utilized during the study period included the radiofrequency ablation device (RFA), hydrothermal ablation device (HTA), and the uterine balloon ablation system (UBA).

Results: Five thousand nine hundred thirty-six women underwent endometrial ablation at a single institution (3757 RFA (63.3%), 1848 HTA (31.1%), and 331 UBA (5.6%)). The primary outcome assessed was surgical re-intervention, defined as hysterectomy or repeat endometrial ablation. Of the total 927 (15.6%) women who required re-intervention, 822 (13.9%) underwent hysterectomy and 105 (1.8%) underwent repeat endometrial ablation. Women who underwent re-intervention were younger (41.6 versus 42.9 years, $p < .001$), were more often African-American (21.8% versus 16.2%, $p < .001$), and were more likely to have had a primary radiofrequency ablation procedure (hazard ratio 1.37; 95%CI 1.01 to 1.86). Older age was associated with decreased risk for treatment failure with women older than 45 years of age having the lowest risk for failure ($p < .001$). Age between 35 and 40 years conferred the highest risk of treatment failure (HR 1.59, 95% CI 1.32–1.92). Indications for re-intervention following ablation included menorrhagia (81.8%), abnormal uterine bleeding (27.8%), polyps/fibroids (18.7%), and pain (9.5%).

Conclusion: Surgical re-intervention was required in 15.6% of women who underwent second-generation endometrial ablation. Age, ethnicity, and radiofrequency ablation were significant risk factors for failed endometrial ablation, and menorrhagia was the leading indication for re-intervention.

Keywords: Endometrial ablation, Treatment failure, Hysterectomy, Risk factors

Background

Endometrial ablation, a surgical procedure to decrease or control heavy menstrual bleeding, is generally intended for premenopausal women who have failed, or are not candidates for, medical therapy. Ablation is contraindicated in women with undiagnosed abnormal bleeding and those who desire future fertility [1]. While hysteroscopic resection and ablation became the gold standard for endometrial ablation in the 1980s and 1990s, "second-generation"

endometrial ablation devices were developed in the late 1990s and early 2000s in order to improve ease, safety, and uniformity of ablation procedures [2]. The uterine balloon ThermaChoice® (UBA) (Gynecare, Somerville, New Jersey) received its first FDA approval in 1997, while the Hydro-ThermAblator® hydrothermal ablation (HTA) (Boston Scientific, Marlborough, Massachusetts) and NovaSure® radiofrequency ablation (RFA) (Hologic Inc., Marlborough, Massachusetts) devices gained their approvals in 2001 [3].

The need for any treatment following an endometrial ablation is frequently cited as "failed therapy," with the two most common secondary interventions being repeat ablation and hysterectomy [4–10]. In a longitudinal

* Correspondence: jklebanoff@christianacare.org
[1]Department of Obstetrics & Gynecology, Christiana Care Health System, 4755 Ogletown-Stanton Road, Suite 1905, Newark, DE 19718, USA
Full list of author information is available at the end of the article

5-year follow-up study of 139 women randomized to either RFA or HTA, rates of subsequent surgery were high (24% of the entire group) while relative risk was 0.43 for women in the RFA group compared to HTA [11]. The majority of the women who underwent subsequent surgery had a hysterectomy, as opposed to repeat ablation.

Surgical re-intervention rates above 20% suggest there is opportunity to improve outcomes of the primary intervention; one approach would be to improve patient selection for ablation. Risk factors previously identified for failed endometrial ablation include younger age at initial procedure, history of cesarean delivery, tubal ligation, and abnormal uterine findings on radiologic assessment including leiomyoma, thickened endometrial stripe, and polyps [5, 6, 8]. Since second-generation devices have become standard of care, no large cohort study has assessed treatment outcomes with regard to only these newer devices. The purpose of this study is to establish the rate of failed second-generation endometrial ablation, defined as subsequent hysterectomy or repeat ablation, in a large US-based cohort.

Methods

After obtaining approval by the Institutional Review Board, we performed a retrospective cohort study of women who had undergone an endometrial ablation from October 2003 through March 2016. Patients were identified using a contemporaneous electronic database. Data was extracted by using relevant International Classification of Diseases—Ninth revision (ICD-9) codes as well as Current Procedural Terminology (CPT) codes. Women were included if they had undergone RFA, HTA, or UBA for benign indications at a single academic-affiliated community hospital (choice of device utilized was based on physician preference).

Women were excluded if they had a diagnosis related to any gynecologic malignancy; if the ablation was performed by any modality other than RFA, HTA, or UBA; or if the indication for the ablation was postmenopausal bleeding.

The initial cohort of women identified was then re-analyzed, using relevant ICD-9 and CPT codes, to isolate any patient who underwent either a hysterectomy or repeat endometrial ablation at a date after their initial endometrial ablation. Subjects' electronic health records were further analyzed by reviewing operative reports to verify successful performance of the initial endometrial ablation procedure as well as any re-intervention. Women whose index ablation or subsequent re-intervention could not be confirmed in detailed operative reports were excluded.

The primary outcome evaluated was the incidence of surgical re-intervention, defined as either hysterectomy or repeat ablation. Exposures examined include influence of age, body mass index, race/ethnicity, ablation device type, concomitant or history of tubal ligation, indication for endometrial ablation, and concomitant uterine or adnexal surgery. All pertinent patient data were either extracted from the electronic health record or identified by review of operative reports. The data was initially analyzed using univariate modeling, using Stata 14.0 (College Station, TX). Recognizing that different ablation technologies were popularized at different time periods, Cox proportional hazard testing was used to adjust for the time to failure.

Results

Between October 2003 and March 2016, we identified 6299 women who underwent an endometrial ablation at a single academic-affiliated community hospital. After excluding 363 women due to missing information from the electronic health record or failure to undergo their scheduled ablation, 5936 women were eligible for analysis. Procedure distribution was as follows: 3757 RFA (63.3%), 1848 HTA (31.1%), and 331 UBA (5.6%) (Fig. 1). The mean age (± standard deviation) was 42.7 ± 5.7 years. The mean BMI was 29.9 ± 7.8 kg/m^2. The majority of women included were Caucasian (79.3%), with the remainder predominantly African-American (17%) (Table 1).

Surgical re-intervention was required in 927 women in the cohort (15.6%). Hysterectomy was performed in 822 women (13.8%) and endometrial ablation in 105 women (1.8%). Women who were younger and women who were African-American were more likely to require re-intervention (Table 1). Subjects were further stratified into five groups based on age at initial ablation: group 1, age < 35 years; group 2, age 35–39 years; group 3, age 40–44 years; group 4, age 45–49 years; and group 5, age ≥ 50 years (Fig. 2). Women in groups 1, 2, and 3 were more likely to require re-intervention compared to women in groups 4 and 5 ($p < .001$). The incidence of re-intervention for women in groups 1, 2, and 3 were 18.8, 19.7, and 16.4% respectively. Women in group 2 (age 35–39) had the highest likelihood of re-intervention (HR 1.59, 95% CI 1.32–1.92). Neither BMI, nor BMI category, affected the rates of re-intervention. Main indications for surgical re-intervention following ablation were menorrhagia (81.8%), abnormal uterine bleeding (27.8%), polyps or fibroids (18.7%), and pain (9.5%) (note: patients could have more than one diagnosis listed).

Recognizing that introduction of ablation procedure types occurred at differing times, Cox proportional hazard modeling was used to assess the efficacy of each

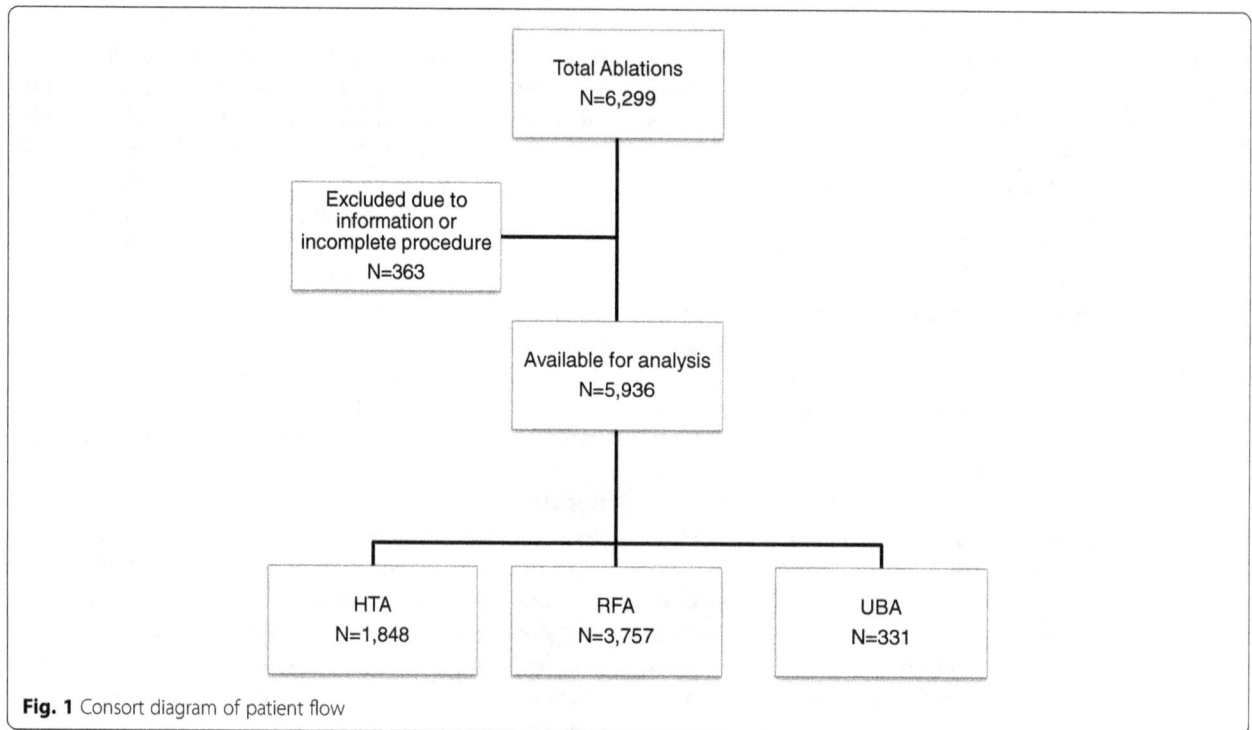

Fig. 1 Consort diagram of patient flow

of the three methods utilized in our study. When examined from the perspective of logistic regression, being African-American increased the risk of re-operation (OR 1.40; 95%CI 1.17 to 1.67), while being in the age group of 45–49 years (OR 0.72; 95%CI 0.61 to 0.85) or ≥50 years (OR 0.49; 95%CI 0.37 to 0.65) significantly lowered the risk. Having a primary RFA conferred a higher likelihood of treatment failure compared to both the HTA and UBA (hazard ratio 1.37; 95%CI 1.01 to 1.86). When pathological specimens were evaluated following hysterectomy, African-American women were significantly more likely to have a diagnosis of fibroid or polyp than women identifying as Caucasian or other ($p < .001$). Survival analysis was performed using data from patients with re-intervention ($n = 927$) to evaluate for differences between endometrial ablation procedures regarding time to failure. No statistically significant differences were found (Fig. 3). Overall incidence of re-intervention was 5, 10.5, and 13.3% at year 1, 3, and 5 respectively (Fig. 4).

Conclusions

Of the 5936 women included in the study, 927 (15.6%) underwent re-intervention with 822 (13.8%) undergoing hysterectomy and 105 (1.8%) undergoing repeat endometrial ablation. These re-intervention rates are similar to what has previously been published, with earlier large cohort studies reporting rates greater than 20%, while summaries of randomized controlled trials report rates increasing from

4.2% to over 20% based upon time from the primary procedure [3, 6].

Our study found that younger age at the time of ablation was a significant risk factor for surgical re-intervention. This risk was highest for women aged 35–39 years at the time of ablation; however, risk was increased in all women younger than 45 years. This is consistent with a majority of previous studies [4, 6, 8].

Our study did not find that indication for endometrial ablation was associated with risk of failed treatment. Menorrhagia was the most common indication for ablation in our cohort, while structural uterine anomalies (fibroid/polyp) represented the primary indication in 18% of cases. Structural uterine anomalies have been identified as risk factors for failed endometrial ablation. In the study by Wishall et al., any known structural uterine anomaly at the time of endometrial ablation was associated with hysterectomy following ablation [10]. This is believed to be due to distorted anatomy rendering the endometrial ablation less effective. Bansi-Matharu et al. published data from a retrospective review that found women with polyps present at the time of initial endometrial ablation were more likely to undergo repeat endometrial ablation [4].

Interestingly, our study identified African-American race as an independent risk factor for re-intervention following endometrial ablation. The African-American race is a known risk factor for the presence of uterine fibroids [12]. Thus, it is possible that this higher rate of treatment failure is associated with a higher incidence of

Table 1 Univariable analysis of risk factors for re-intervention

Variable	Re-intervention (%)	No Re-intervention (%)	p value
Total patients	927 (15.6)	5009 (84.4)	
Age (years)			
Mean	41.59	42.94	< .001
Age band < 35	90 (9.7)	388 (7.8)	
35–40	223 (24.1)	908 (18.1)	
40–45	324 (35.0)	1647 (32.9)	
45–50	233 (25.1)	1516 (30.3)	
> 50	57 (6.2)	550 (11.0)	
Race			
Asian	3 (0.3)	35 (0.7)	< .001
Black	202 (21.8)	809 (16.2)	
White	685 (73.9)	4020 (80.3)	
Other	37 (4.0)	145 (2.9)	
Weight (kg)	80.84	80.71	.60
Height (cm)	163.70	164.33	.07
BMI (kg/m^2)			
Mean	30.17	29.89	.75
< 18	1 (9.1)	10 (90.9)	
18–25	95 (10.3)	830 (89.7)	
25–30	113 (11.8)	845 (88.2)	
30–35	90 (13.9)	556 (86.1)	
35–40	46 (10.9)	375 (89.1)	
> 40	35 (11.2)	279 (88.9)	
Ablation technique			
Uterine balloon	47 (14.2)	284 (85.8)	
Hydrothermablation	349 (18.9)	1499 (81.1)	
Radiofrequency	531 (14.1)	3226 (85.9)	< .001

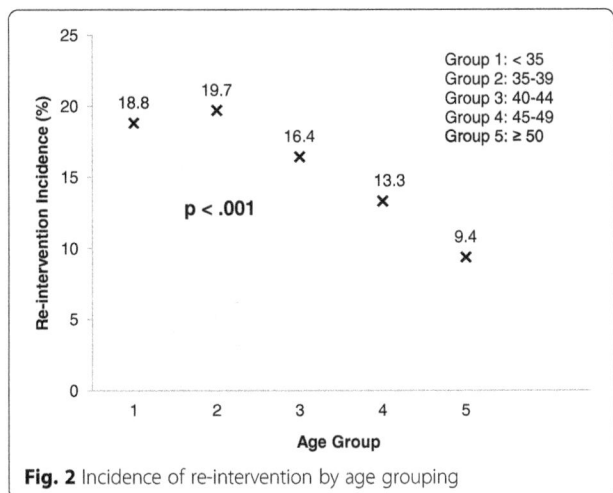

Fig. 2 Incidence of re-intervention by age grouping

uterine fibroids inherent among African-American women. This is further supported by our study, in that African-American women were significantly more likely to have fibroids or polyps on final pathology at the time of subsequent hysterectomy. Due to limitations in study design, we could not account for size, number, or location of fibroids or polyps present in women at the time of their index ablation.

The radiofrequency system conferred a higher likelihood of surgical re-intervention regardless of age, race, or procedural indication when compared to two other second-generation devices. This data differs from that of El-Nashar et al., who found in a population-based cohort study that there was no statistically significant difference in failure rates between UBA and RFA ($p = .26$) [13]. However, median follow-up in that study was 2.2 years and only included 200 patients undergoing UBA. It is possible our data are different given the larger total number of endometrial ablations, larger number of UBA, and the longer patient follow-up. It is also possible that physicians who prefer the radiofrequency device may have a lower threshold to diagnose treatment failure and surgically intervene. Based on the survival analysis, there was no statistically significant difference between the endometrial ablation devices utilized in this study with regard to time to re-intervention. Approximately half of the patients in this study failed at the 24-month period regardless of the ablation device utilized.

We found that BMI was not a risk factor for treatment failure. This is consistent with published data from Wishall et al., who performed a retrospective chart review of all endometrial ablations at Hahnemann University Hospital and the Hospital of the University of Pennsylvania from January 2006 to May 2013 [10]. Wishall found that BMI was not statistically significantly associated with treatment failure following endometrial ablation. Smithling et al. analyzed data from 968 women and had previously reported that a BMI > 30 was a statistically significant risk factor for treatment failure and re-intervention ($p = .003$) [9]. As Smithling's data included both first- and second-generation ablation devices, it may be that the efficacy of second-generation devices can overcome risks or limitations conferred by BMI.

The overall incidence of re-intervention at years 1, 3, and 5 found in this study is lower than what has previously been published. In a large cohort study by Longinotti et al., the overall incidences of hysterectomy at years 1 and 5 were 9.3 and 22.2%, respectively [6]. That study included women undergoing both first- and second-generation endometrial ablations which could explain the lower incidences found in this study of newer second-generation ablation devices.

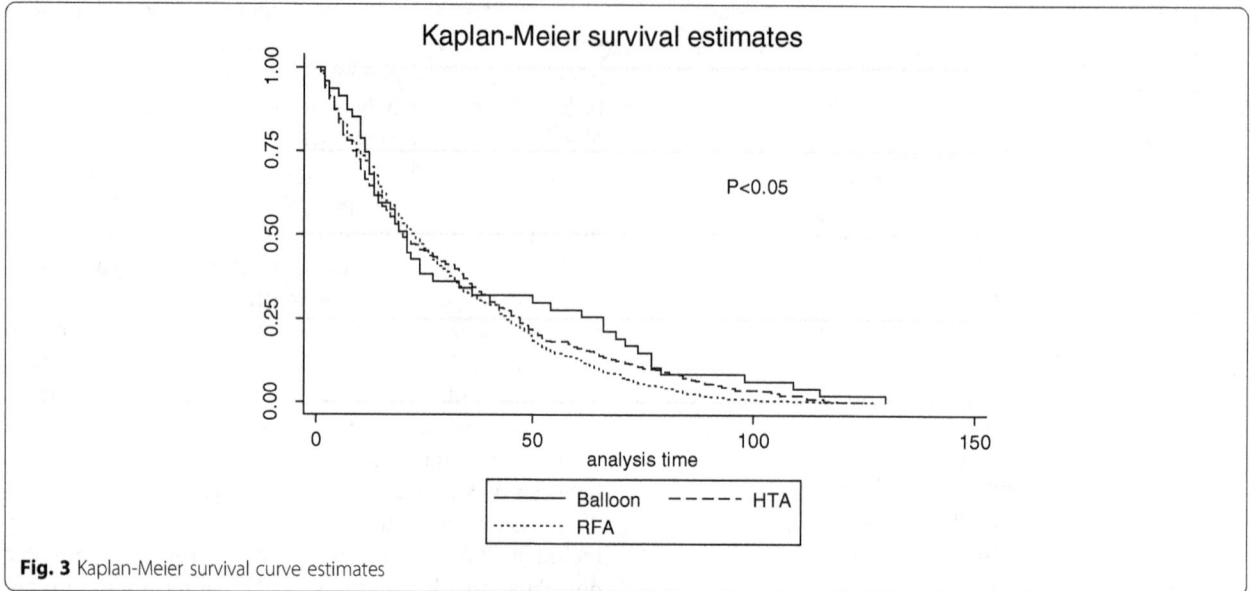

Fig. 3 Kaplan-Meier survival curve estimates

Due to data limitations, we are unable to comment whether tubal ligation affected long-term treatment outcome. Results regarding the effect of tubal ligation on outcome after endometrial ablation vary, with numerous reports documenting no effect [8, 14]. However, conflicting data suggest that women with a history of tubal ligation are more likely to experience treatment failure after endometrial ablation compared to women without a history of tubal ligation [5, 9]. Our study is limited in that women with a tubal ligation performed at an outside institution would not have been captured in this analysis.

Limitations of our study include those inherent in its retrospective nature. Data abstraction was dependent on procedural coding, which can be subject to bias and inaccuracies. We identified 363 (5.8%) women who had

inaccurate coding regarding their initial or subsequent procedure. The potential for loss to follow-up was unavoidable as there was no way to identify women who may have had an initial endometrial ablation at the study center and had a re-intervention at an outside institution. Strengths of this study include its large sample size as well as the utilization of individual chart review to ensure accurate data abstraction. This is also the only study to date to include only second-generation ablation devices. This can impact patient counseling, as much of the existing data included first-generation ablation techniques, which have largely fallen out of favor.

We conclude that the use of second-generation endometrial ablation in the community is successful for over 80% of women. Providers should consider a patient's age, race, and their own device preference at

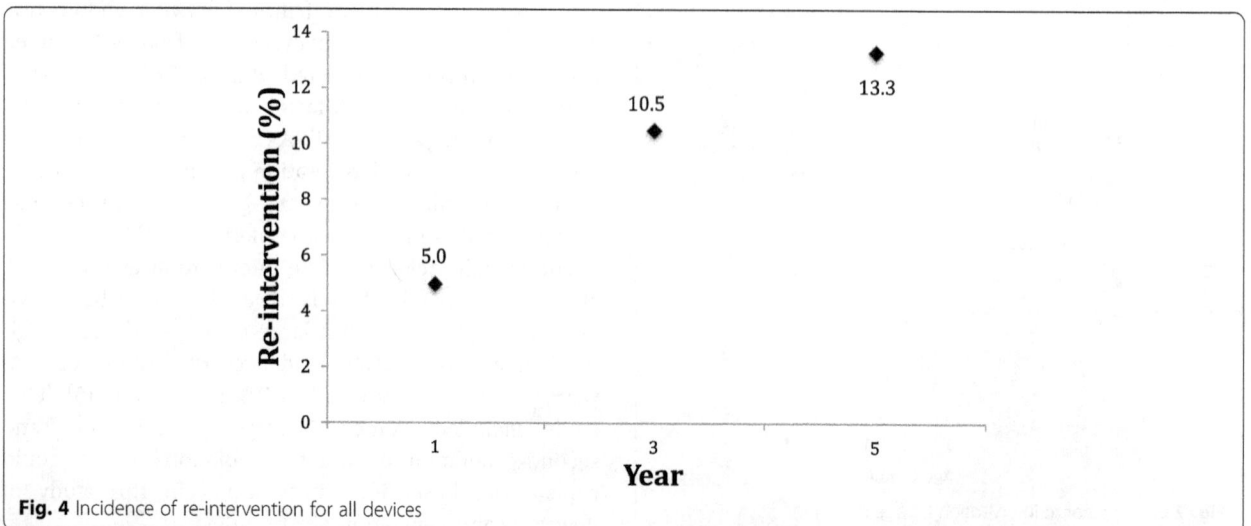

Fig. 4 Incidence of re-intervention for all devices

the time of endometrial ablation when counseling patients regarding likelihood of re-intervention. Over the last decade, it does not appear that the incidence of surgical re-intervention after endometrial ablation has significantly decreased despite evidence identifying patient risk factors. Improved patient selection could serve to lower this incidence.

Abbreviations
CPT: Current Procedural Terminology; HTA: Hydrothermal ablation device; ICD-9: International Classification of Diseases—Ninth revision; RFA: Radiofrequency ablation; UBA: Uterine balloon ablation system; BMI: Body mass index

Acknowledgements
Not applicable

Prior presentation
Klebanoff J, Makai GE, Patel NR, Hoffman MK. "Incidence and Predictors of Failed Second Generation Endometrial Ablation." 45th AAGL Global Congress of Minimally Invasive Gynecology. Orlando, FL, 2016 Nov.

Funding
Not applicable

Authors' contributions
Author JK carried out all the aspects of this study including design, chart review, statistical analysis, manuscript writing, editing, and submission. Authors GM, NP, and MK were intimately involved in the study design, statistical analysis, manuscript writing, and editing. All authors read and approved the final manuscript.

Competing interests
The authors declare that they have no competing interests.

Author details
[1]Department of Obstetrics & Gynecology, Christiana Care Health System, 4755 Ogletown-Stanton Road, Suite 1905, Newark, DE 19718, USA. [2]Division of Minimally Invasive Gynecology, Christiana Care Health System, Newark, DE, USA.

References
1. American College of Obstetrics & Gynecology (2007) ACOG practice bulletin no. 81: endometrial ablation. Obstet Gynecol 109:1233–1248
2. Cooper JM, Erickson ML (2000) Global endometrial ablation technologies. Obstet Gynecol Clin N Am 27(2):385–396
3. Lethaby A, Penninx J, Hickey M, Garry R, Majoribanks J (2013) Endometrial resection and ablation techniques for heavy menstrual bleeding, Cochrane database of systematic reviews issue 8. Art. No.: CD001501. doi:10.1002/14651858.CD001501.pub4
4. Bansi-Matharu L, Gurol-Urganci I, Mahmood TA, Templeton A, van der Meulen JH, Cromwell DA (2013) Rates of subsequent surgery following endometrial ablation among English women with menorrhagia: population-based cohort study. BJOG 120:1500–1507
5. El-Nashar SA, Hopkins MR, Creedon DJ, St Sauver JL, Weaver AL, McGree ME, Cliby WA, Famuyide AO (2009) Prediction of treatment outcomes after global endometrial ablation. Obstet Gynecol 113:97–106
6. Longinotti MK, Jacobson GF, Hung YY, Learman LA (2008) Probability of hysterectomy after endometrial ablation. Obstet Gynecol 112:1214–1220
7. Riley KA, Davies MF, Harkins GJ (2013) Characteristics of patients undergoing hysterectomy for failed endometrial ablation. JSLS 17:503–507
8. Shavell VI, Diamond MP, Senter JP, Kruger ML, Johns DA (2012) Hysterectomy subsequent to endometrial ablation. J Minim Invasive Gynecol 19(4):459–464
9. Smithling KR, Savella G, Raker CA, Matteson KA (2014, 211) Preoperative uterine bleeding pattern and risk of endometrial ablation failure. Am J Obstet Gynecol:556.e1–556.e6
10. Wishall KM, Price J, Pereira N, Butts SM, Della Badia CR (2014) Postablation risk factors for pain and subsequent hysterectomy. Obstet Gynecol 124:904–910
11. Penninx JP, Herman MC, Mol BW, Bongers MY (2011) Five-year follow-up after comparing bipolar endometrial ablation with hydrothermablation for menorrhagia. Obstet Gynecol 118:1287–1292
12. Marshall LM, Spiegelman D, Barbieri RL, Goldman MB, Manson JE, Colditz GA, Willett WC, Hunter DJ (1997) Variation in the incidence of uterine leiomyoma among premenopausal women by age and race. Obstet Gynecol 90:967–973
13. El-Nashar SA, Hopkins MR, Creedon DJ, Cliby WA, Famuyide AO (2009) Efficacy of bipolar radiofrequency endometrial ablation vs thermal balloon ablation for management of menorrhagia: a population-based cohort. J Minim Invasive Gynecol 16:692–699
14. Kreider SE, Starcher R, Hoppe J, Nelson K, Salas N (2013) Endometrial ablation: is tubal ligation a risk factor for hysterectomy. J Minim Invasive Gynecol 20(5):616–619

31

Implementation of laparoscopic hysterectomy for endometrial cancer over the past decade

Tim Wollinga[1,2], Nicole P. M. Ezendam[3,4], Florine A. Eggink[5], Marieke Smink[2], Dennis van Hamont[6], Brenda Pijlman[7], Erik Boss[8], Elisabeth J. Robbe[9], Huy Ngo[10], Dorry Boll[11], Constantijne H. Mom[12], Maaike A. van der Aa[13], Roy F. L. P. Kruitwagen[14,15], Hans W. Nijman[5] and Johanna M. A. Pijnenborg[2,16*] ⓘ

Abstract

Background: Laparoscopic hysterectomy (LH) for the treatment of early-stage endometrial carcinoma/cancer (EC) has demonstrated to be safe in several randomized controlled trials. Yet, data on implementation of LH in clinical practice are limited. In the present study, implementation of LH for EC was evaluated in a large oncology network in the Netherlands.

Results: Retrospectively, a total of 556 EC patients with FIGO stage I-II were registered in the selected years. The proportion of LH gradually increased from 11% in 2006 to 85% in 2015. LH was more often performed in patients with low-grade EC and was not related to the studied patient characteristics. The introduction of TLH was frequently preceded by LAVH. Patients treated in teaching hospitals were more likely to undergo a LH compared to patients in non-teaching hospitals. The conversion rate was 7.7%, and the overall complication rates between LH and AH were comparable, but less postoperative complications in LH.

Conclusions: Implementation of laparoscopic hysterectomy for early-stage EC increased from 11 to 85% in 10 years. Implementation of TLH was often preceded by LAVH and was faster in teaching hospitals.

Keywords: Endometrial cancer, Laparoscopic hysterectomy, Implementation

Background

Endometrial carcinoma/cancer (EC) is the most common malignancy of the female genital tract, with an increasing incidence in western countries [1]. In the Netherlands, about 1900 women are diagnosed with EC yearly. Due to the fact that most patients are diagnosed at an early stage, outcome is relatively favorable. However, 400 women die of this disease annually in the Netherlands [2]. Primary treatment consists of a total hysterectomy and bilateral salpingo-oophorectomy. Routine lymphadenectomy is not beneficial in early-stage, low-risk EC [3]. Historically, hysterectomy for EC was performed by laparotomy. In

1989, Harry Reich performed the first laparoscopic hysterectomy (LH) for a benign gynecological disease [4]. Subsequently, LH became an alternative approach for abdominal surgery with the advantage of an increased recovery time and reduced blood loss [5]. In 2006, the results from the Laparoscopic Approach to Carcinoma of the Endometrium (LACE) trial, a randomized controlled trial (RCT) including 509 patients with stage I EC, were published. This study demonstrated a similar survival in patients treated by total laparoscopic hysterectomy (TLH) compared to those who underwent abdominal hysterectomy (AH). The benefits of a laparoscopic approach included shorter hospital stay, less analgesics, and reduced perioperative morbidity [6]. These data were confirmed by a Dutch RCT including 283 patients with stage I EC, who were also randomized between TLH and AH [7]. The benefits of a laparoscopic approach seem to be even more relevant in

---
* Correspondence: Hanny.MA.Pijnenborg@radboudumc.nl
[2]Department of Obstetrics and Gynecology, Elisabeth-Tweesteden Hospital, Tilburg, The Netherlands
[16]Department of Obstetrics and Gynecology, Radboud University Medical Centre, 791, P.O. Box 9101, 6500 HB Nijmegen, The Netherlands
Full list of author information is available at the end of the article

obese patients with an increased risk of surgical morbidity [8]. This is particularly relevant in EC, as obesity is an important risk factor for the development of EC [9]. Yet, especially in morbidly obese patients, laparoscopic surgery for EC requires a well-trained team, with a completed learning curve of the surgeon, and anesthesiologists that are used to steep Trendelenburg position during surgery [10]. Over the last decades, the percentage of LH as a primary surgical treatment in EC has increased [11]. Factors that might influence the adoption of LH in clinical practice have been reported to be related to age and sex of the gynecologist and the presence of gynecology residents [12–14].

Previous studies have focused on the implementation of laparoscopy in general gynecology in the Netherlands and have shown a slowly increase of LH from 3% in 2007 to 10% in 2012 [15]. However, these data are based on questionnaires sent to gynecologists about their performed surgeries. So far, only a few studies have focused on the implementation of LH in the surgical treatment of EC. In a recent study, out of 5239 hysterectomies for EC in the USA, 51% was performed by laparoscopy in 2012 [16]. Bogani et al. demonstrated in a single-center study the implementation of laparoscopic surgery in the management of all types of gynecological cancers and showed an increase from 10 to 82% in a 10-year time period [17]. The aim of the present study was to evaluate the implementation of LH in the treatment of early-stage EC over the past 10 years in a large clinical oncology network and to determine which patient-, hospital-, and surgeon-related factors contributed to the implementation of LH. In addition, we evaluated the conversion and complication rates as well as the duration of laparoscopic surgery in relation to the annual number of EC surgeries per hospital.

Methods
Setting
A retrospective cohort study was performed in the Gynecological Oncology Centre South (GOCS), a clinical oncology network in the south of the Netherlands. The GOCS comprises eight collaborating hospitals: two oncological referral centers, four teaching hospitals, and two non-teaching hospitals. According to Dutch guidelines, surgical staging and lymph node dissection in clinical stage I, endometrioid-type EC are recommended only in case of clinical suspicion of lymph node metastasis or in case of high-grade histology, i.e., grade 3 endometrioid-type and all non-endometrioid-type EC cases. Adjuvant therapy consists of radiotherapy by either external beam radiation or vaginal vault brachytherapy, depending on the patient's age, myometrial invasion, LVSI, and tumor grade on final pathology [18, 19].

Patients
All patients that underwent primary surgical treatment for EC in 2006, 2009, 2012, or 2015 within the GOCS were included. Patients planned for a hysterectomy for another reason ($n = 13$), e.g., uterine myomas, but were diagnosed postoperatively with EC, were documented, but were excluded for analysis since the planned surgery was not based on the preoperative diagnosis of EC. Patients that received neoadjuvant chemotherapy, radiotherapy, or hormonal therapy were excluded ($n = 5$), as well as patients that were diagnosed with other uterine tumors ($n = 10$). Patients were classified according to the 2009 International Federation of Gynecology and Obstetrics (FIGO) staging system [20, 21]. Routine preoperative work-up in the Netherlands consists of a chest X-ray for low-risk (grade 1–2) endometrioid-type EC, and computed tomography scan for high-risk tumors, and only in low-grade EC when there is clinical suspicion of extended disease. Determination of myometrial invasion is not routinely performed (www.oncoline.nl).

Data extraction
Patient and tumor characteristics were extracted from patient files, pathology reports, and anesthesiological screenings. The following patient characteristics were collected: body mass index (BMI), comorbidity, previous surgery, and smoking habit. Both the planned and the performed surgical approaches were registered. LH was categorized into TLH and laparoscopic-assisted vaginal hysterectomy (LAVH). TLH was defined as a complete laparoscopic surgical approach including closure of the vaginal vault. When part of the procedure was done vaginally, including closure of the vaginal vault, it was recorded as LAVH. For patients that were planned for a laparoscopic approach but underwent AH, the reason for conversion was documented according to the following factors: adhesions, limited exposure, anesthesiological difficulties due to Trendelenburg position, and uncontrolled bleeding. In addition, complications during surgery and postoperatively were documented.

Outcome
Primary outcome was defined as the percentage of laparoscopic hysterectomies in all patients with FIGO stage I–II EC in 2006, 2009, 2012, and 2015, compared to the percentage of abdominal hysterectomies. Secondary outcomes were the determination of predictive factors for a laparoscopic approach and the relation between annual surgical volume and duration of surgery. Predictive factors for the laparoscopic approach were classified as patient, hospital, and surgeon related (age and gender). The type of hospital was classified as teaching and non-teaching hospital. Surgeon-related factors were age and gender of the surgeon. The duration of the surgical

procedures (LH and AH) was related to the annual number of patients undergoing surgery for EC within the hospitals.

Statistical analysis

Descriptive analyses were used to describe patients treated with LH and AH. Differences in characteristics between patients treated with LH and AH were assessed using Student's t tests for continuous variables and the chi-square test for categorical data. A multivariable logistic regression was performed to determine the association of the following patient-, hospital-, and surgeon-related factors with the likelihood of a laparoscopic hysterectomy: age of the patient, previous abdominal surgery, BMI, and diabetes mellitus. Patients who could potentially receive either LH or AH were included, i.e., those treated in 2012 and 2015, since LH was implemented in most hospitals in these years and those patients with a grade I and stage I and II endometrial cancer [11]. Statistical analyses were conducted using IBM SPSS Statistics, version 20 (SPSS Inc., Chicago, IL, USA). p values < 0.05 were considered statistically significant, and all statistical tests were two-sided.

Results

Patient cohort

A total of 662 patients were diagnosed with EC within the selected years: 2006, 2009, 2012, and 2015. Twenty-

eight patients were excluded due to other tumor types ($n = 10$), neoadjuvant chemotherapy ($n = 5$), and unexpected EC ($n = 13$). Subsequently, for analysis, only patients with FIGO stage I–II EC were included, resulting in 556 eligible patients, as demonstrated in Fig. 1. Patient and tumor characteristics are demonstrated in Table 1. There were no differences between patients that underwent a LH or AH with respect to age, BMI, parity, smoking, or duration of surgery. There were 19 conversions to laparotomy (7.7%): 14 due to adhesions, two due to uncontrolled bleeding, two due to anesthesiological difficulties, and one due to limited exposure. The conversions were different over time: 2006 (25.0%), 2009 (3.3%), 2012 (10.0%), and 2015 (6.9%). Previous abdominal surgery was not a risk factor for conversion to laparotomy ($p = 0.722$). Although there was no difference in the overall complication rate between LH and AH, perioperative complications were observed more frequently in the LH group, whereas postoperative complications were observed more frequently in the AH group. Complications during surgery in the AH group consisted of the following: intestinal wall injury ($n = 3$), bleeding ($n = 3$), and damage to the obturator nerve ($n = 1$). Complications in the LH group consisted of the following: intestinal wall injury ($n = 10$), bleeding ($n = 4$), injury to the bladder ($n = 2$), rupture of the cervix ($n = 2$), and uterine rupture ($n = 1$). Postoperative complications in the

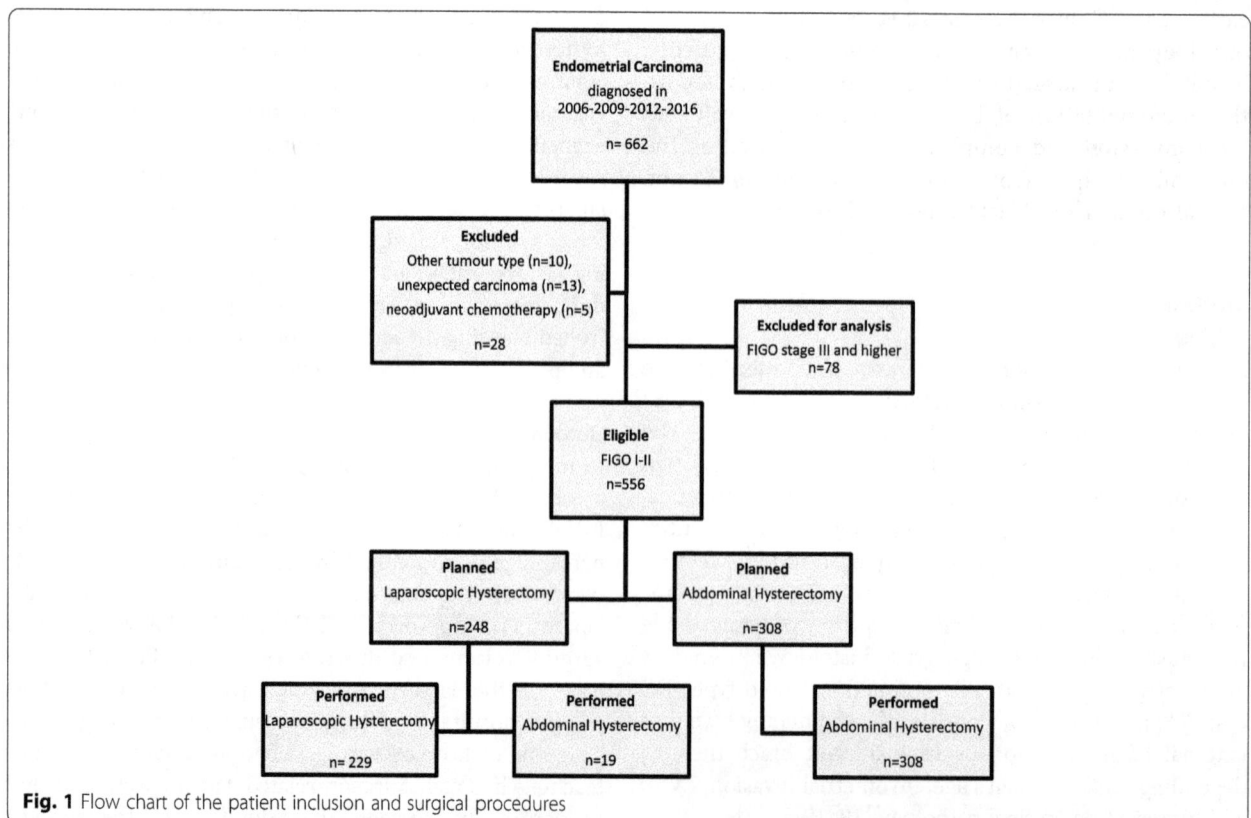

Fig. 1 Flow chart of the patient inclusion and surgical procedures

Table 1 Patient and tumor characteristics in relation to the type of performed surgical procedure

Treatment characteristics of all included patients	Total, n = 556	LH, n = 248	AH, n = 308	p value
Age in years (mean, SD)	65.8 (9.6)	65.3 (9.8)	66.4 (9.4)	0.166
BMI (mean, SD)	29.6 (6.7)	29.8 (7.0)	29.3 (6.3)	0.429
Parity (mean, SD)	2.0 (1.4)	2.03 (1.4)	2.02 (1.3)	0.909
Previous abdominal surgery	184	80	104	0.585
Comorbidity				
Hypertension	178	77	101	0.582
Type II diabetes	83	30	53	0.093
FIGO stage				0.364
IA	336	158	178	
IB	195	80	115	
II	25	10	15	
Histology				0.002
Endometrioid	502	231	271	
Non-endometrioid				
Serous	28	15	13	
Clear cell	8	2	6	
Carcinosarcoma	15	0	15	
Stromal cell sarcoma	3	0	3	
Tumor grade				0.000
1	279	151	128	
2	175	63	112	
3	102	34	68	
Treatment				
Hysterectomy and BSO	556	305	241	0.196
Additional staging/ lymphadenectomy	80	10	70	0.000
Conversion to laparotomy	19	19	–	
Duration of surgery, min (mean, SD)	101 (41.9)	116 (39.3)	90 (40.4)	0.204
Complications				
During surgery	26	19	7	0.004
After surgery	30	6	24	0.005

LH laparoscopic hysterectomy, *AH* abdominal hysterectomy

AH group consisted of wound dehiscence (*n* = 18), urinary tract infection (*n* = 3), wound infection (*n* = 2), and postoperative bleeding (*n* = 1). Complications after surgery in the LH group consisted of wound infection (*n* = 4), urinary tract infection (*n* = 1), and wound dehiscence (*n* = 1).

Surgical procedure during the years

During the study period, a steady rise of both LAVH and TLH was demonstrated, as illustrated in Fig. 2. In 2006, only eight (11%) patients underwent surgery by the laparoscopic approach, compared to 30 (19.7%) in 2009, 93 (60%) in 2012, and 117 (85%) in 2015. One teaching hospital introduced the laparoscopic approach for the treatment of EC in 2006. The remaining teaching hospitals started performing laparoscopic surgery between 2006 and 2015. The two non-teaching hospitals initiated LH for EC between 2012 and 2015. In five hospitals, the introduction of LAVH preceded the implementation of TLH.

Predictors of laparoscopic hysterectomy

There was no relation between patient-related factors, such as BMI (OR 1.00, 95% CI 0.98–1.0), previous abdominal surgery (OR 1.06, 95% CI 0.89–1.26), age (OR 0.98, 95% CI 0.97–1.00), type II DM (OR 0.59, 95% CI 0.34–1.02), and hypertension (OR 1.00, 95% CI 0.66–1.50) with the type of surgical approach. In addition, there was no relation between surgeon-related factors and type of surgery. Patients that underwent surgery in teaching hospitals were more likely to be operated by a laparoscopic approach compared to non-teaching hospitals (OR 4.65, 95% CI 2.59–8.36).

Duration of surgery

For all hospitals, the mean duration of surgery was calculated for LH and AH and related to the number of EC patients operated annually. As illustrated in Fig. 3, the mean duration of AH was independent of the number of performed procedures. Yet, for the duration of LH, there was a trend towards a longer operating time when less EC patients were treated per year.

Discussion

This study showed an imposing increase in laparoscopic treatment of early-stage EC from 11% of the procedures in 2006 to 85% in 2015, reflecting that LH was well implemented in the past decade in the studied clinical oncology network in the Netherlands. The introduction of TLH was frequently preceded by LAVH. The only predictive factor for a laparoscopic approach was treatment in a teaching hospital.

To the best of our knowledge, this is the first study that reports upon the implementation of LH in the treatment of EC over a 10-year period since the publication of the LACE trial in 2006. In a recently published study, results over a 4-year time span demonstrated an increase in minimally invasive hysterectomy of 22% in 2007 to 51% in 2011 in the USA [22]. Data are in line with results from Bogani et al. who compared the type of surgical approach for gynecological malignancies during the years 2000–2003 with 2008–2011 and showed a comparable increase from 10 to 82%. Yet, these data were from a single center and included large numbers that might

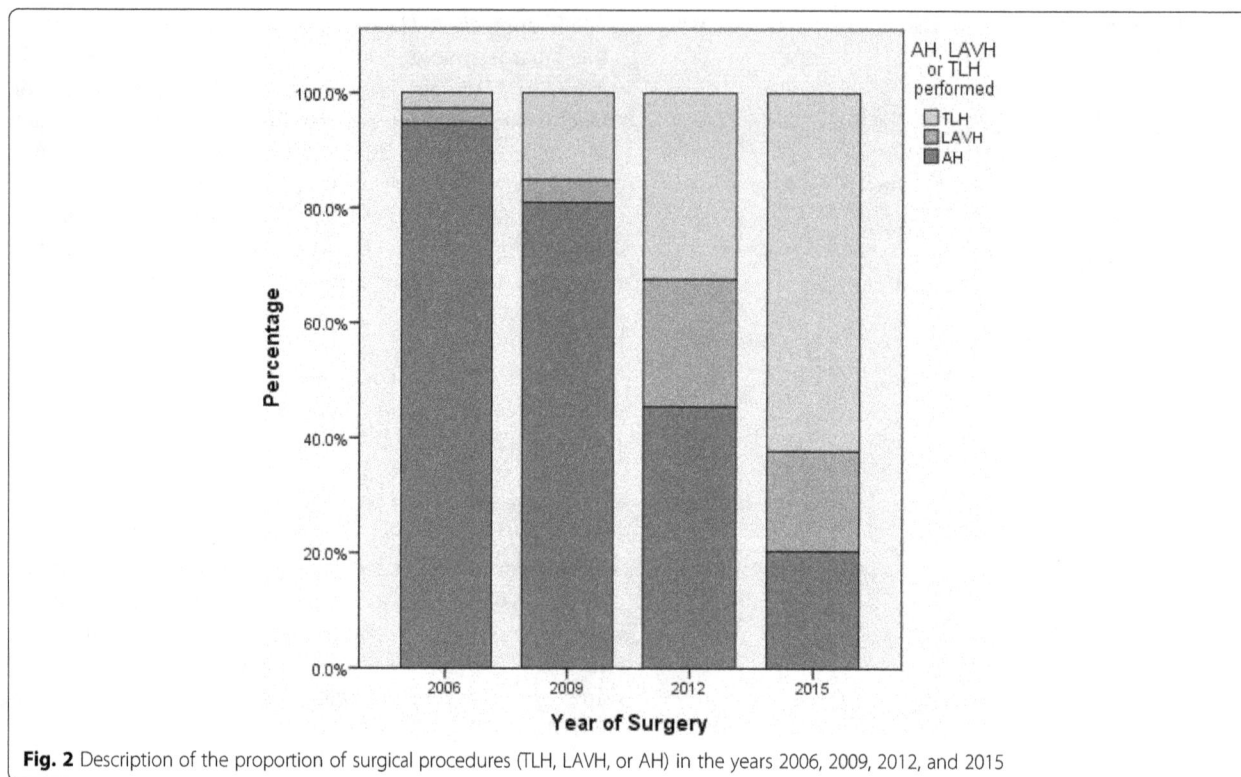

Fig. 2 Description of the proportion of surgical procedures (TLH, LAVH, or AH) in the years 2006, 2009, 2012, and 2015

explain a faster increase in implementation [17]. In comparison, the implementation of LH in the Netherlands was relatively late when compared to that in other countries, possibly due to the lack of centralization of EC treatment resulting in many hospitals treating small numbers [23]. Implementation in the Netherlands might have been facilitated by the Dutch RCT, published in 2010 [7].

The observed conversion rate changed over time and was 6.9% in the last year of our study, quite in line with the previous Dutch RCT that reported conversion rates of 10.8%, but higher than the reported 2.4% in the LACE trial [6, 7]. Even in 2015, this number is still relatively

high. Possible explanations are as follows: (1) variations in the time of the start of LH between hospitals that may not have reached the optimal surgical performance at the time of analysis, (2) relatively small numbers per hospital, and (3) a substantial proportion of obese patients (40.6%), since these are associated with increased conversion rate [23, 24]. The overall comparable complication rates support our assumption that laparoscopic surgeons in the GOCS region were sufficiently trained to perform a LH. The absence of a decrease in the rate of complications with the implementation of LH during the 10-year period can be explained by the fact that more surgeons started to perform LH for endometrial cancer,

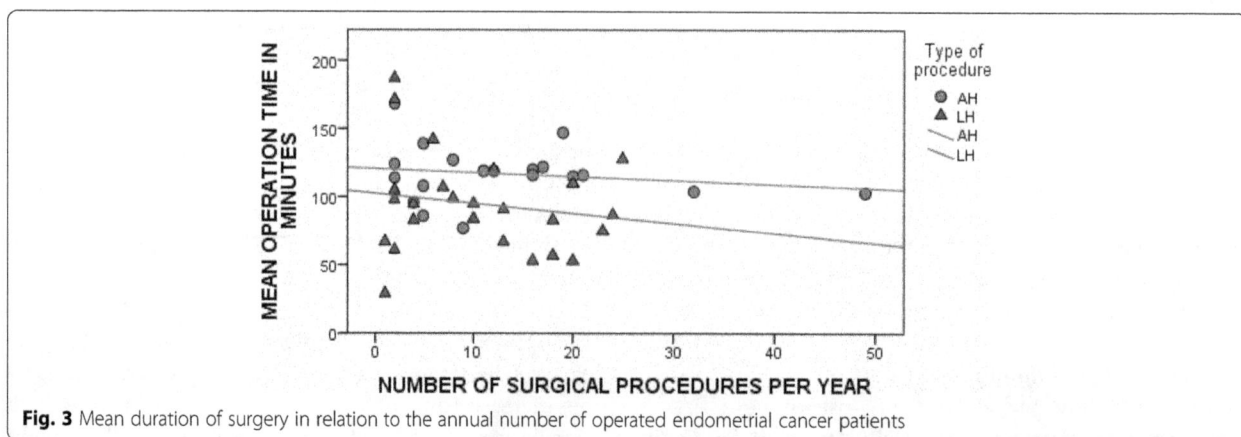

Fig. 3 Mean duration of surgery in relation to the annual number of operated endometrial cancer patients

each going through their individual learning curve. Analyses of an *overall* learning curve are thus a mixture of several *individual* learning curves. The observed trend towards an increased duration of surgery with less LH cases per year suggests that surgical volume might be relevant. However, since surgeons that perform LH of endometrial cancer also perform LH for benign indications, these numbers should be included for a proper analysis. The observation that the introduction of a TLH was frequently preceded by a LAVH approach may illustrate a step-wise adaptation of laparoscopic surgery. Although we hypothesized, according to previous findings, that patient-related factors such as BMI and previous abdominal surgery were predictive for the type of surgical approach, we could not confirm this in our study [24, 25]. In our study cohort, 72.6% of the patients were overweight, with 40.6% being obese. The Dutch RCT was conducted between 2007 and 2009, and training of the surgical team including the anesthesiologist may have improved in recent years, resulting in reduced conversion rate. Interestingly, the type of hospital was related to the implementation of a laparoscopic approach. In 2015, all hospitals had implemented the LH, but implementation was faster in teaching hospitals compared to that in non-teaching hospitals. This is in line with the study of Pijnenborg and ter Haar who demonstrated the important contribution of residents in teaching hospitals in the implementation of LH in clinical practice [12]. We did not observe a relation between the age or gender of surgeon and the type of primary surgical approach in line with previous data [13, 14]. The safety of laparoscopy in the treatment of EC is established in eight RCTs that included mainly early-stage, low-grade EC [11]. There is strong evidence for the role of laparoscopy in the management of low-grade EC, yet for high-grade EC, data are still limited. In a recently published study, it was shown that LH and laparoscopic lymph node dissection were equally safe when compared to open procedures in high-grade EC [26]. Although numbers are relatively small, these data illustrate the shift of the indication towards the laparoscopic approach in high-grade EC treatment. This is supported by a follow-up date of the Gynecologic Oncology Group (GOG) LAP2 trial, which demonstrated that the outcome of patients with high-risk histology, including grade 3 endometrioid-type, serous, and clear cell carcinosarcoma, was not related to the type of surgical approach [27]. In our study cohort, only 10 EC patients underwent a LH with lymphadenectomy, since surgical staging was implemented from 2015 onward. Yet, since numbers of high-grade EC with laparoscopic surgery are limited, there is still a need to continue monitoring whether a laparoscopic approach can be extended to high-grade EC patients. This switch from open to laparoscopic surgery has

great impact on the costs for healthcare. Even robotic-assisted laparoscopic hysterectomy was shown to be 17% cheaper when compared to AH, mainly due to a shorter hospital stay [28]. This benefit may be even more when conventional laparoscopic hysterectomy is performed and dependent on the use of expensive disposable supplies [29]. Whether advanced-stage EC can be treated by a minimal invasive procedure equally safe has not been studied so far.

This study has some limitations that need to be addressed. The surgical treatment of EC in the Netherlands is not centralized, and consequently, the current data reflect the clinical practice in one clinical oncology network in the Netherlands [23]. Since 2015, the surgical approach for EC is documented in the Netherlands Cancer Registry, demonstrating that 79% (66–83%) of the patients in 2015 with early-stage, low-grade EC were operated by a LH (data not shown). Based on our findings, we recommend to add the conversion rate and BMI to this Netherlands Cancer Registry database to monitor these in relation to annual cases in order to further improve the quality of care. Both the years of experience of individual surgeons with laparoscopic hysterectomy for benign indication and the experience of the surgical team have not been taken into account, while this may have influenced our data.

Conclusions

In conclusion, LH has been well implemented in the surgical treatment of early-stage EC in a clinical oncology network in the Netherlands. Currently, 85% of the early-stage EC patients are operated by LH, mainly patients with low-grade tumor. Additional monitoring of conversion and complication rates might contribute to improved quality of care in the shift towards a laparoscopic approach for the treatment of EC.

Abbreviations
AH: Abdominal hysterectomy; BMI: Body mass index; EC: Endometrial carcinoma/cancer; FIGO: International Federation of Gynecology and Obstetrics; LAVH: Laparoscopic-assisted vaginal hysterectomy; LH: Laparoscopic hysterectomy; TLH: Total laparoscopic hysterectomy; RCT: Randomized controlled trial

Acknowledgements
We would like to thank the Dutch Cancer Society for the financial support for this study.

Funding
This work was supported by the Dutch Cancer Society grant RUG 2014-7117 to HW Nijman.

Authors' contributions
We acknowledge all authors have contributed to the submitted manuscript. The author attestation report, containing the authors' individual contribution,

is added as supplementary document. All authors read and approved the final manuscript.

Authors' information

- HN is a professor of gynecological oncology and a principal investigator of the Dutch Cancer Society grant for "Quality of oncological care in endometrial cancer." The current study was part of this grant and performed on behalf of the interest of the Dutch Cancer Society to learn about the clinical implementation of endometrial cancer treatment in the Netherlands.
- MvdA is the head of the Research Department of the Dutch Comprehensive Cancer Centre (IKNL), and as an epidemiologist, she has extensive experience on population-based studies in gynecological cancer.
- JP is a member of the ESGE and chair elective of the European Network of Individual Treatment in Endometrial Cancer. She is working on many international collaborative studies both clinical and translational. She is the head of a large endometrial research group of the Radboud University Medical Centre Nijmegen, The Netherlands.

Competing interests

The authors declare that they have no competing interests.

Author details

[1]Medical Faculty, Erasmus University, Rotterdam, The Netherlands. [2]Department of Obstetrics and Gynecology, Elisabeth-Tweesteden Hospital, Tilburg, The Netherlands. [3]Department of Medical and Clinical Psychology, Tilburg University, Tilburg, The Netherlands. [4]Netherlands Comprehensive Cancer Organisation, Utrecht, The Netherlands. [5]Department of Obstetrics and Gynecology, University Medical Centre Groningen, University of Groningen, Groningen, The Netherlands. [6]Department of Obstetrics and Gynecology, Amphia Hospital, Breda, The Netherlands. [7]Department of Obstetrics and Gynecology, Jeroen Bosch Hospital, 's-Hertogenbosch, The Netherlands. [8]Department of Obstetrics and Gynecology, Máxima Medical Centre, Veldhoven, The Netherlands. [9]Department of Obstetrics and Gynecology, St. Anna Hospital, Geldrop, The Netherlands. [10]Department of Obstetrics and Gynecology, Elkerliek Hospital, Helmond, The Netherlands. [11]Department of Obstetrics and Gynecology, Catharina Hospital, Eindhoven, The Netherlands. [12]Department of Gynecologic Oncology, Gynecological Oncology Centre Amsterdam, Amsterdam, The Netherlands. [13]Department of Research, Netherlands Comprehensive Cancer Organisation, Utrecht, The Netherlands. [14]Department of Obstetrics and Gynecology, Maastricht University Medical Centre, Maastricht, The Netherlands. [15]GROW-School for Oncology and Developmental Biology, Maastricht University, Maastricht, The Netherlands. [16]Department of Obstetrics and Gynecology, Radboud University Medical Centre, 791, P.O. Box 9101, 6500 HB Nijmegen, The Netherlands.

References

1. Ferlay J, Soerjomataram I, Dikshit R, Eser S, Mathers C, Rebelo M et al (2015) Cancer incidence and mortality worldwide: sources, methods and major patterns in GLOBOCAN 2012. Int J Cancer 136:E359–E386. https://doi.org/10.1002/ijc.29210
2. Boll D, Karim-Kos HE, Verhoeven RH, Burger CW, Coebergh JW, Van De Poll-Franse LV et al (2013) Increased incidence and improved survival in endometrioid endometrial cancer diagnosed since 1989 in the Netherlands: a population based study. Eur J Obstet Gynecol Reprod Biol 166:209–214. https://doi.org/10.1016/j.ejogrb.2012.10.028
3. Frost JA, Webster KE, Bryant A, Morrison J (2015) Lymphadenectomy for the management of endometrial cancer. Cochrane Database Syst Rev 9: CD007585. https://doi.org/10.1002/14651858.CD007585 pub3
4. Reich H, DeCaprio J, McGlynn F (1989) Laparoscopic hysterectomy. J Gynecol Surg 5:213–216. https://doi.org/10.1089/gyn.1989.5.213
5. Nieboer TE, Johnson N, Lethaby A, Tavender E, Curr E, Garry R et al (2009) Surgical approach to hysterectomy for benign gynaecological disease. Cochrane Database Syst Rev. https://doi.org/10.1002/14651858.CD003677 pub4
6. Janda M, Gebski V, Forder P, Jackson D, Williams G, Obermair A (2006) Total laparoscopic versus open surgery for stage 1 endometrial cancer: the LACE randomized controlled trial. Contemp Clin Trials 27:353–363. https://doi.org/10.1016/j.cct.2006.03.004
7. Mourits MJE, Bijen CB, Arts HJ, ter Brugge HG, van der Sijde R, Paulsen L et al (2010) Safety of laparoscopy versus laparotomy in early-stage endometrial cancer: a randomised trial. Lancet Oncol 11:763–771. https://doi.org/10.1016/S1470-2045(10)70143-1
8. Bouwman F, Smits A, Lopes A, Das N, Pollard A, Massuger L et al (2015) The impact of BMI on surgical complications and outcomes in endometrial cancer surgery—an institutional study and systematic review of the literature. Gynecol Oncol 139:369–376. https://doi.org/10.1016/j.ygyno.2015.09.020
9. Reeves KW, Carter GC, Rodabough RJ, Lane D, McNeeley SG, Stefanick ML et al (2011) Obesity in relation to endometrial cancer risk and disease characteristics in the Women's Health Initiative. Gynecol Oncol 121:376–382
10. Janssen PF, Brölmann HAM, Huirne JAF (2013) Causes and prevention of laparoscopic ureter injuries: an analysis of 31 cases during laparoscopic hysterectomy in the Netherlands. Surg Endosc Other Interv Tech 27:946–956. https://doi.org/10.1007/s00464-012-2539-2
11. Galaal K, Bryant A, Fisher AD, Kew F, Al-Khaduri M, et al. Laparoscopy versus laparotomy for the management of early stage endometrial cancer (review). 2014:2012–4. doi:https://doi.org/10.1002/14651858.CD006655.pub2.Copyright
12. Pijnenborg JM, ter Haar JF (2011) Innovations in surgery: the role of residents in the implementation of laparoscopic hysterectomy. J Laparoendosc Adv Surg Tech A 21:615–619. https://doi.org/10.1089/lap.2010.0443
13. Huang CC, Wu MP, Huang YT (2012) Gynecologists' characteristics associated with the likelihood of performing laparoscopic-assisted hysterectomy: a nationwide population-based study. Eur J Obstet Gynecol Reprod Biol 161:209–214. https://doi.org/10.1016/j.ejogrb.2011.12.024
14. Einarsson JI, Matteson KA, Schulkin J, Chavan NR, Sangi-Haghpeykar H (2010) Minimally invasive hysterectomies—a survey on attitudes and barriers among practicing gynecologists. J Minim Invasive Gynecol 17:167–175. https://doi.org/10.1016/j.jmig.2009.12.017
15. Kolkman W, Trimbos-Kemper TCM, Jansen FW (2007) Operative laparoscopy in the Netherlands: diffusion and acceptance. Eur J Obstet Gynecol Reprod Biol 130:245–248. https://doi.org/10.1016/j.ejogrb.2006.01.019
16. Mannschreck DB, Matsuno R, Dowdy SC, Sinno AK, Tanner EJ, Stone RL et al (2016) Poor nationwide utilization of minimally invasive surgery in early-stage uterine cancer: an HCUP-National Inpatient Sample database study. Gynecol Oncol 141:13–14. https://doi.org/10.1016/j.ygyno.2016.04.062
17. Bogani G, Cromi A, Serati M, Di Naro E, Casarin J, Pinelli C et al (2015) Improving standard of care through introduction of laparoscopy for the surgical management of gynecological malignancies. Int J Gynecol Cancer 25:741–750. https://doi.org/10.1097/IGC.0000000000000406
18. Creutzberg CL, van Putten WL, Koper PC, Lybeert ML, Jobsen JJ, Wárlám-Rodenhuis CC et al (2000) Surgery and postoperative radiotherapy versus surgery alone for patients with stage-1 endometrial carcinoma: multicentre randomised trial. PORTEC Study Group. Post Operative Radiation Therapy in Endometrial Carcinoma. Lancet 355:1404–1411. S0140673600021395
19. Nout RA, Smit VT, Putter H, Jürgenliemk-Schulz IM, Jobsen JJ, Lutgens LC et al (2010) Vaginal brachytherapy versus pelvic external beam radiotherapy for patients with endometrial cancer of high-intermediate risk (PORTEC-2): an open-label, non-inferiority, randomised trial. Lancet 375:816–823. https://doi.org/10.1016/S0140-6736(09)62163-2
20. Haltia UM, Bützow R, Leminen A, Loukovaara M (2014) FIGO 1988 versus 2009 staging for endometrial carcinoma: a comparative study on prediction of survival and stage distribution according to histologic subtype. J Gynecol Oncol 25:30–35. https://doi.org/10.3802/jgo.2014.25.1.30
21. Pecorelli S, Zigliani L, Odicino F (2009) Revised FIGO staging for carcinoma of the cervix. Int J Gynecol Obstet 105:107–108. https://doi.org/10.1016/j.ijgo.2009.02.009
22. Fader AN, Weise RM, Sinno AK, Tanner EJ, Borah BJ, Moriarty JP et al (2016) Utilization of minimally invasive surgery in endometrial cancer care: a quality and cost disparity. Obstet Gynecol 127:91–100. https://doi.org/10.1097/AOG.0000000000001180
23. Becker JH, Ezendam NPM, Boll D, Van Der Aa M, Pijnenborg JMA (2015) Effects of surgical volumes on the survival of endometrial carcinoma. Gynecol Oncol 139:306–311. https://doi.org/10.1016/j.ygyno.2015.09.003

24. Fanning J, Hossler C (2010) Laparoscopic conversion rate for uterine cancer surgical staging. Obstet Gynecol 116:1354–1357. https://doi.org/10.1097/AOG.0b013e3181fae272

25. Bijen CBM, De Bock GH, Vermeulen KM, Arts HJG, Ter Brugge HG, Van Der Sijde R et al (2011) Laparoscopic hysterectomy is preferred over laparotomy in early endometrial cancer patients, however not cost effective in the very obese. Eur J Cancer 47:2158–2165. https://doi.org/10.1016/j.ejca.2011.04.035

26. Koskas M, Jozwiak M, Fournier M, Vergote I, Trum H, Lok C et al (2016) Long-term oncological safety of minimally invasive surgery in high-risk endometrial cancer. Eur J Cancer 65:185–191. https://doi.org/10.1016/j.ejca.2016.07.001

27. Fader AN, Java J, Tenney M, Ricci S, Gunderson CC, Temkin SM et al (2016) Impact of histology and surgical approach on survival among women with early-stage, high-grade uterine cancer: an NRG Oncology/Gynecologic Oncology Group ancillary analysis. Gynecol Oncol 143:460–465. https://doi.org/10.1016/j.ygyno.2016.10.016

28. Herling SF, Palle C, Møller AM, Thomsen T, Sørensen J (2016) Cost-analysis of robotic-assisted laparoscopic hysterectomy versus total abdominal hysterectomy for women with endometrial cancer and atypical complex hyperplasia. 95:299–308. https://doi.org/10.1111/aogs.12820

29. Desille-gbaguidi H, Hebert T, Paternotte-villemagne J, Gaborit C (2013) Overall care cost comparison between robotic and laparoscopic surgery for endometrial and cervical cancer. Eur J Obstet Gynecol Reprod Biol 171:348–352. https://doi.org/10.1016/j.ejogrb.2013.09.025

32

A randomized control trial to evaluate the importance of pre-training basic laparoscopic psychomotor skills upon the learning curve of laparoscopic intra-corporeal knot tying

Carlos Roger Molinas[1][*], Maria Mercedes Binda[1], Cesar Manuel Sisa[2] and Rudi Campo[3]

Abstract

Background: Training of basic laparoscopic psychomotor skills improves the acquisition of more advanced laparoscopic tasks, such as laparoscopic intra-corporeal knot tying (LICK). This randomized controlled trial was designed to evaluate whether pre-training of basic skills, as laparoscopic camera navigation (LCN), hand-eye coordination (HEC), and bimanual coordination (BMC), and the combination of the three of them, has any beneficial effect upon the learning curve of LICK. The study was carried out in a private center in Asunción, Paraguay, by 80 medical students without any experience in surgery. Four laparoscopic tasks were performed in the ENCILAP model (LCN, HEC, BMC, and LICK). Participants were allocated to 5 groups (G1–G5). The study was structured in 5 phases. In phase 1, they underwent a base-line test (T_1) for all tasks (1 repetition of each task in consecutive order). In phase 2, participants underwent different training programs (30 consecutive repetitions) for basic tasks according to the group they belong to (G1: none; G2: LCN; G3: HEC; G4: BMC; and G5: LCN, HEC, and BMC). In phase 3, they were tested again (T_2) in the same manner than at T_1. In phase 4, they underwent a standardized training program for LICK (30 consecutive repetitions). In phase 5, they were tested again (T_3) in the same manner than at T_1 and T_2. At each repetition, scoring was based on the time taken for task completion system.

Results: The scores were plotted and non-linear regression models were used to fit the learning curves to one- and two-phase exponential decay models for each participant (individual curves) and for each group (group curves). The LICK group learning curves fitted better to the two-phase exponential decay model. From these curves, the starting points ($Y0$), the point after HEC training/before LICK training ($Y1$), the Plateau, and the rate constants (K) were calculated. All groups, except for G4, started from a similar point ($Y0$). At $Y1$, G5 scored already better than the others (G1 $p = .004$; G2 $p = .04$; G3 $p < .0001$; G4 NS). Although all groups reached a similar Plateau, G5 has a quicker learning than the others, demonstrated by a higher K (G1 $p < 0.0001$; G2 $p < 0.0001$; G3 $p < 0.0001$; and G4 $p < 0.0001$).

Conclusions: Our data confirms that training improves laparoscopic skills and demonstrates that pre-training of all basic skills (i.e., LCN, HEC, and BMC) shortens the LICK learning curve.

Keywords: Laparoscopy, Training, Intra-corporeal knot tying, Psychomotor skills, Education, Training box, ENCILAP model, LASTT model

* Correspondence: roger.molinas@neolife.com.py
[1]NEOLIFE—Medicina y Cirugía Reproductiva, Avenida Brasilia 760, 1434
Asunción, Paraguay
Full list of author information is available at the end of the article

Background

The ideal method for training in laparoscopic surgery is continuously debated, and several systems have been proposed and developed based upon different models, target population, local institutional characteristics, medical specialty, and others [1, 2].

In spite of the controversies and differences, most specialists in surgical education agree that the traditional apprentice-tutor model is no longer useful for training all skills necessary for laparoscopic surgery. Indeed, to achieve proficiency through this model seems unacceptable for both practical and ethical reasons, such as the limited number of tutors, the fewer surgical cases in daily practice, the increased operating time, the higher complication rate, and the long learning curves [3, 4].

Furthermore, laparoscopic surgery demands both surgical and psychomotor skills that not necessarily should be trained together [3, 4], with increasing evidence suggesting that psychomotor skills must be trained earlier and outside the operating room [5–10].

Following this philosophy, the European Academy of Gynecological Surgery has developed the LASTT (Laparoscopic Skills Training and Testing) model for training basic laparoscopic psychomotor skills, such as laparoscopic camera navigation (LCN), hand-eye coordination (HEC), and bimanual coordination (BMC). The feasibility, face validity, and construct validity of this model have been demonstrated [11–13], and together with other tools (i.e., SUTT model, HYSTT model, E-Knot model, The Winner Project [14]), the LASTT model is also currently used for certification purposes [3, 4, 15, 16].

In the LASTT model, it has also been confirmed that training improves the laparoscopic skills, and it has been demonstrated that HEC training with both hands (dominant hand and non-dominant hand) improves the acquisition and retention of more complex laparoscopic tasks, such as intra-corporeal knot tying (LICK) [12, 17], shortening the LICK learning curve [18]. Therefore, this study was designed to evaluate whether pre-training of basic skills, as LCN, HEC or BMC, and the combination of the three of them, has any beneficial effect upon the learning curve of LICK.

Methods

Participants and venue

The study was approved by the Institutional Review Board and performed at *Universidad del Pacífico Privada* in Asunción, Paraguay, in 2012 by 80 last-year medical students without any experience in surgery. The sample size was calculated based on the LICK scores. Taking into account base-line scores of 500 ± 250 (mean $\pm$ SD) reported in novices [12] and to be able to detect a 50%difference with a power of 80% and a two-tailed level of significance of .05, some 12 participants per group would be required.

Instruments and materials and laparoscopic tasks

A novel model (*ENtrenamiento en CIrugía LAParoscópica*: ENCILAP) adapted from the LASTT [13] and the SUTT models was developed (Fig. 1). The model consists in a platform (30×30 cm) with several hollows for storing tools and fitting working modules (rectangular blocks of $10 \times 2.5 \times 1$ cm). Some modules are covered with a soft pad, whereas others have three circular wells (1×0.5 cm) with a picture or a color bottom. The modules can be fitted at $45°/90°$ at different locations of the platform. The ENCILAP was placed into the Szabo trainer box (Fig. 2). All tasks were performed with a 10-mm 30° optic connected to a laparoscopic tower and with standard laparoscopic instruments as described for each task (Karl Storz, Tuttlingen, Germany).

For LCN, the ENCILAP model was fitted with 6 modules at 45° (3 at the right and 3 at the left). Participants navigated the camera with the preferred hand in order to identify 12 figures, which comprise a large and a small symbol. The supervisor indicated the first symbol to be shown, which was identifiable from a panoramic viewpoint. Participants looked throughout the model for this symbol, found it, and focused on the small symbol situated next to it, which was shown on the center of the screen from a close-up viewpoint. This small symbol indicated the next large symbol to be identified. Following this order, participants continued till the identification of the last small symbol (Additional file 1: Video 1).

For HEC, the ENCILAP model was fitted with six modules at 45° (three at each side). One well of each module was filled in with a color pushpin with the tail upwards. Six color rings (4 mm with an opening of 2 mm) were placed in the center of the platform. Participants held and navigated the camera with one hand and held a 5-mm Kelly forceps with the other hand. One by one, the rings were grasped and introduced in the tails of the pushpin of the same color (Additional file 2: Video 2). The task was performed and scored alternatively with the dominant hand (DH) and the non-dominant hand (NDH), which was defined by the hand holding the forceps.

For BMC, the ENCILAP model was fitted with six modules at 45° (three at each side). One well of each module at the left was filled in with a color pushpin with the tail upwards. An assistant navigated the camera according to the participant's instructions. One by one, the pushpins were grasped and lifted with a 5-mm Kelly forceps held with the DH, re-grasped with a similar forceps held with the NDH, and introduced into empty wells of the same color at the right of the model. Then, the pushpins were transferred in the inverse order (from right to left) (Additional file 3: Video 3 and Additional file 4: Video 4).

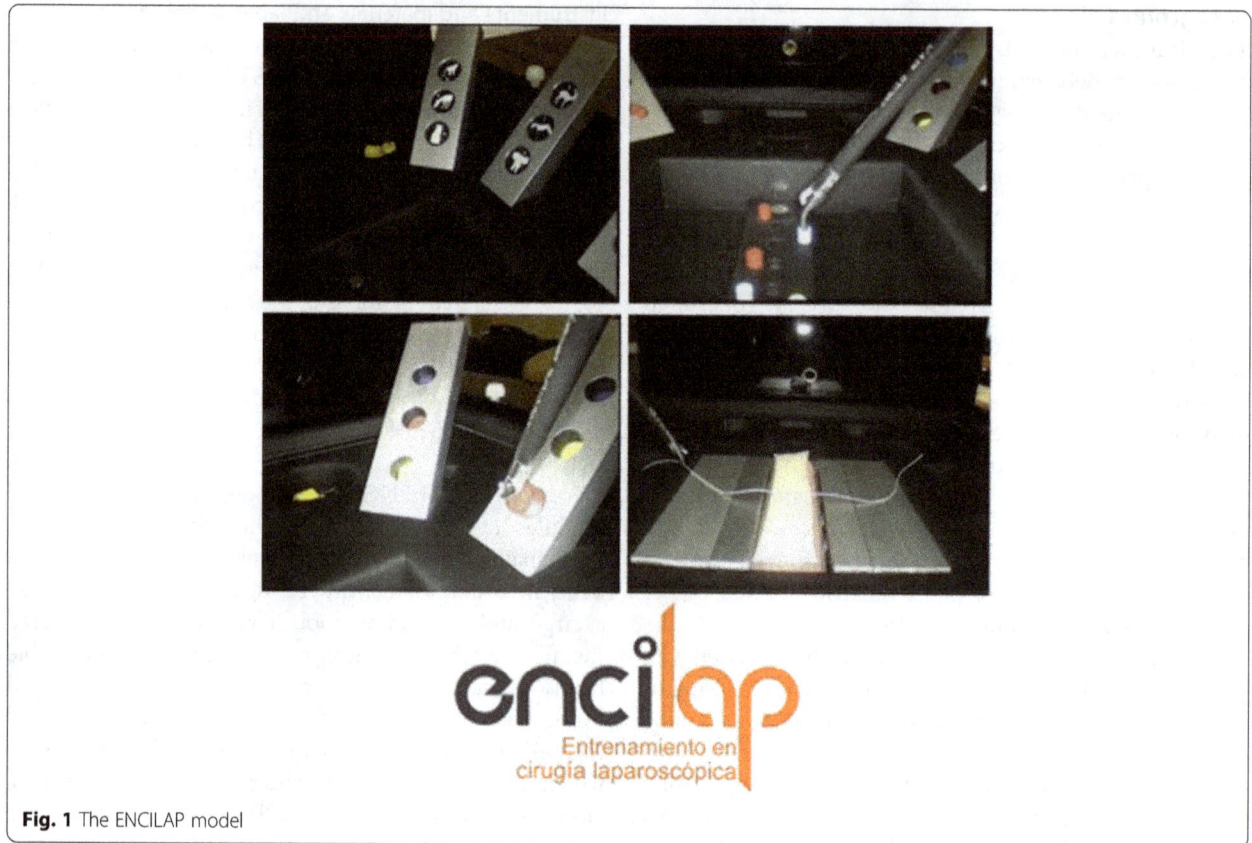

Fig. 1 The ENCILAP model

For LICK, the ENCILAP model was fitted with the soft module at 0° in the center of the platform, which was mounted with a suture (vicryl 2-0, 20 cm length) with 1 cm between entry and exit sites and with tails equally distributed to both sides. An assistant navigated the camera according to the participant's instructions, who held a 5-mm Koh needle holder with the DH and a similar one with the NDH. The tip of the thread was grasped with the left needle holder and the thread was pulled through the pad, leaving a 2-cm tail on the opposite side. Then, a double counter-clockwise knot was made, followed by a single clockwise knot, and, finally, by a single counter-

clockwise knot (Additional file 5: Video 5). The time for each repetition was limited to 300 s. The repetition ended either when the knot was accomplished or when the time limit expired. The supervisor controlled the knot quality and only flat and square knots were considered correctly performed.

Scoring system

The scoring was based in the time taken for task completion system. Each repetition of each task was scored by a supervisor, as explained below. For LCN, HEC, and BMC, the time for each repetition was limited to 180 s. The repetition ended either when all objectives (12 figures identified for LCN, 6 rings transported for HEC, 6 pushpins transported for BMC) were accomplished or when the time limit expired. The quality of the objectives was obvious, and thus, the supervisor just counted the number of objectives accomplished. If within the time limit at least one objective was achieved, the score was calculated dividing the time actually used (1–180) by the number of objectives accomplished (LCN 1–12, HEC 1–6, BMC 1–6). If in the maximum time any objective was achieved, a penalty score of 360 was given.

For LICK, the time for each repetition was limited to 300 s. The repetition ended either when the knot

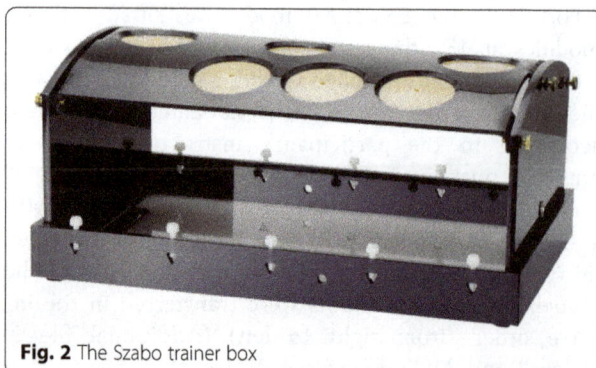

Fig. 2 The Szabo trainer box

was accomplished or when the time limit expired. Since the quality of the knot can be debatable, the supervisor controlled the quality and only flat and square knots were considered correct. If within the time limit the knot was successfully executed, the score was the time actually used (1–300). If in the maximum time the knot was not successfully executed, a penalty score of 600 was given.

Experimental design

Participants were randomly allocated to five groups (G1, G2, G3, G4, or G5; $n = 16$ per group). Within each group, they worked in fixed pairs throughout the study. Working sessions of 1–3 h were performed 2–3 times a week. A supervisor was present at the working station in all sessions to ascertain the setup

was correctly ensembled and to score the tasks. The study was structured in five phases (Fig. 3).

Phase 1

In the first session, participants filled in a questionnaire reporting age, gender, dominant hand side, hands' size according to the gloves' size (small 6.0–6.5, medium 7.0–7.5, large 8.0–8.5), interest in surgery, and experience in video games according to a visual analogue scale from 0 (no) to 10 (a lot). Then, video demonstration and full explanation of the different tasks were provided only one time. Finally, participants performed a baseline test (T_1), consisting in one repetition of LCN, HEC, BMC, and LICK in consecutive order and which were scored by the supervisor, as explained above.

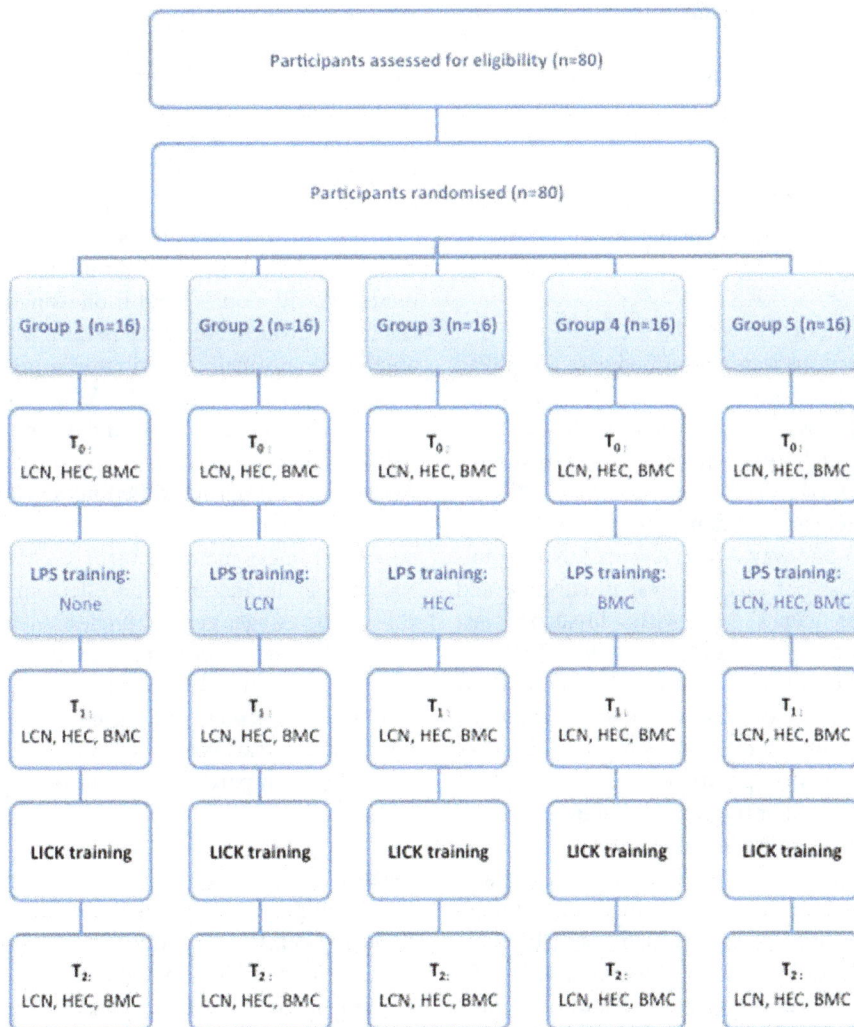

Fig. 3 Flow chart. LPS laparoscopic psychomotor skills, LCN laparoscopic camera navigation, HEC hand-eye coordination, BMC bimanual coordination, LICK laparoscopic intra-corporeal knot tying

Phase 2

Participants underwent differentiated training for basic skills according to the group they belong to, which consisted in 30 consecutive repetitions of the relevant task (G1: none; G2: LCN; G3: HEC; G4: BMC; and G5: LCN, HEC, and BMC in consecutive order). These were done in as many sessions as necessary according to participants' group and skills, spread in 1–2 weeks for G2, G3, and G4 and in 3–6 weeks for G5. All these repetitions were scored by the supervisor, as explained above.

Phase 3

After completion of basic skills training and before LICK training, participants were tested again (T_2) in the same manner than at T_1 in one single session.

Phase 4

All participants underwent a standardized training program for LICK, which consisted in 30 consecutive repetitions of the task. This was done in as many sessions as necessary according to participants' skills, spread in 1–2 weeks. All these repetitions were scored by the supervisor, as explained above.

Phase 5

After completion of LICK training, participants were tested again (T_3) in the same manner than at T_1 and T_2 in one single session.

Statistics and curve fitting

All statistical comparisons were performed with GraphPad Prism 6.00 (GraphPad Software, San Diego, California, USA) and SAS (SAS Institute Inc., Cary, North Carolina, USA). A two-tailed p value of $< .05$ was considered statistically significant.

Intergroup differences in demographic parameters were evaluated with one-way ANOVA with Tukey's multiple comparison post-test (age, interest in surgery, and experience in video games) and with chi-square test (gender, dominant hand side, and hand size).

The effect of the different pre-training conditions upon the LICK performance was evaluated in two ways: firstly, inter- and intragroup differences in the real scores registered at the evaluation points only (T_1, T_2, and T_3) and secondly, inter- and intragroup differences in the calculated scores at the entire learning curves.

The real scores registered by each group at T_1, T_2, and T_3 (continuous variable) were not normally distributed, and therefore, they are presented as medians (interquartile range). To evaluate intergroup differences at T_1, T_2, and T_3, the Kruskal-Wallis test (with Dunn's multiple comparison post-test) was used. To evaluate intragroup differences (T_1 vs. T_2, T_2 vs. T_3), the Wilcoxon matched-pairs signed rank test was used.

The real scores registered at all points were plotted to produce the learning curves for each student (individual learning curves) and for each group (group learning curves). Non-linear regression models were used to fit the curves to the one- and two-phase exponential decay models. The one-phase exponential decay model is expressed as $Y = (Y0 - \text{Plateau}) \times \exp. (- K \times X) + \text{Plateau}$. The two-phase exponential decay model is expressed as $Y = \text{Plateau} + \text{SpanFast} \times \exp. (- K\text{Fast} \times X) + \text{SpanSlow} \times \exp. (- K\text{Slow} \times X)$, where $\text{SpanFast} = (Y0 - \text{Plateau}) \times \text{PercentFast} \times .01$ and $\text{SpanSlow} = (Y0 - \text{Plateau}) \times (100 - \text{PercentFast}) \times .01$. Y is a dependent variable (score) and X is an independent variable (number of the repetition of the task). $Y0$ is the Y value when X is zero (the starting point before any training or T_1). Plateau is the Y value at infinite times, expressed in the same units as Y (the theoretical best score that can be achieved with infinite practice). K, $K\text{Fast}$ and $K\text{Slow}$ are rate constants, expressed in reciprocal of the X units and which measures the steepness of the curve (higher values of K indicates faster learning). Span is the difference between $Y0$ and Plateau, expressed in the same units as Y values. PercentFast is the fraction of the Span accounted for by the faster of the two components. For LICK, the $Y1$, which represents the Y extrapolated value from $X1$ (the first point of the curve immediately after HEC training/before LICK training or $T2$), was also calculated.

The extra sum-of-squares F test was used to evaluate which model fits better (one-phase vs. two-phase exponential decay models) and if one single curve adequately fits for all groups. All curve parameters (continuous variable) were normally distributed and therefore they are presented as means $\pm$ SEM. To evaluate intergroup differences at each curve parameter, the one-way ANOVA (with Tukey's multiple comparison post-test) was used. To evaluate intragroup differences ($Y0$ vs. $Y1$), the paired t test was used.

General linear methods (proc GLM) was performed to evaluate simultaneously the effect of independent variables such as age, gender (male/female), dominant hand side (right/left), level of interest in surgery (0–10), level of experience in video games (0–10), hand size (small/medium/large), and study group (G1 to G5) upon the speed of the learning (rate constant K), which was obtained for each participant from his/her individual learning curve.

Results

The demographics of the five groups are presented in Table 1. No intergroup differences were detected for any of the demographic parameters.

The results of the basic tasks (LCN, HEC, and BMC) were disregarded for the aims of this publication to avoid the presentation of so many data that could make the understanding of LICK data more confusing and

Table 1 Demographics

	Group				
	G1	G2	G3	G4	G5
Age	24.2 ± 0.7	22.3 ± 0.4	22.0 ± 0.3	22.5 ± 0.4	23.9 ± 1.1
Gender					
Male	7 (44%)	7 (44%)	6 (38%)	5 (31%)	9 (56%)
Female	9 (56%)	9 (56%)	10 (62%)	11 (69%)	7 (44%)
Dominant hand					
Right	13 (81%)	12 (75%)	14 (88%)	16 (100%)	15 (94%)
Left	3 (19%)	4 (25%)	2 (12%)	0 (0%)	1 (6%)
Hands size					
Small	7 (44%)	5 (31%)	7 (44%)	7 (44%)	2 (12%)
Medium	8 (50%)	8 (50%)	6 (38%)	7 (44%)	12 (75%)
Large	1 (6%)	3 (19%)	3 (18%)	2 (12%)	2 (12%)
Interest in surgery	7.4 ± 0.5	7.7 ± 0.6	5.8 ± 0.6	6.6 ± 0.6	7.4 ± 0.7
Experience in video games	3.7 ± 0.9	6.5 ± 0.8	5.1 ± 0.7	4.6 ± 0.7	5.2 ± 1.0

Age, interest in surgery, and experience in video games are presented as mean ± SEM. Gender, dominant hand, and hand size are presented as number (%)

unclear. Therefore, only the LICK results are presented here.

The baseline scores before any training (T_1) were similar in all groups (NS). Immediately before LICK training (T_2), the scores decreased in all groups compared to T_1 (G1 $p = .01$; G2 $p = .01$; G3 $p = .0005$; G4 $p = .0005$; G5 $p < .0001$). At this point, G5 scored better than G1 ($p < .05$), G2 ($p < .05$), G3 (NS), and G4 (NS). After LICK training (T_3), the scores further decreased in all groups compared to T_2 (G1 $p < .0001$; G2 $p < .0001$; G3 $p = .0002$; G4 $p < .0001$; G5 $p < .0001$). At this point, G5 scored better than G1 (NS), G2 (NS), G3 ($p < .05$), and G4 (NS) (Table 2).

The individual learning curves were fitted to one- and two-phase exponential decay models. Most individual curves fitted better the one-phase model, whereas few of them fitted better to two-phase model or were ambiguous (did not fit to any model) (Fig. 4).

The group learning curves were also fitted to the one- and two-phase exponential decay models. G1 and G2 fitted to both models but fitted better to the two-phase model (G1 $p = .0005$; G2 $p = .01$). G3, G4, and G5 fitted only to the one-phase model. Therefore, the one-phase exponential decay model was used for comparisons. One single type of curve did not adequately fit for all groups ($p < .0001$).

All groups had comparable starting points ($Y0$) (NS), except for G4 that started from a lower $Y0$ than G1 ($p < 0.01$), G3 ($p < 0.05$), and G5 ($p < 0.01$). At the next curve value ($Y1$), which represents the value immediately before LICK training, the scores decreased in G1 ($p = .004$), G2 ($p = .04$), G3 ($p < .0001$), G4 (NS), and G5 ($p < .0001$) compared to $Y0$. At this point, G5 scored better than G1 ($p < .0001$), G2 ($p < .0001$), G3 ($p < .001$), and G4 ($p < .0001$), whereas G4 scored better than G1 ($p < .001$) and G2 ($p < .05$), and G3 scored better than G1 ($p < .0001$) and G2 ($p < .0001$). All

Table 2 Laparoscopic intra-corporeal knot tying scores at the evaluation points (T_1, T_2, and T_3) and learning curve parameters

Score	Groups				
	G1	G2	G3	G4	G5
T_1	600 (600–600)	600 (348–600)	600 (277–600)	600 (238–600)	600 (420 – 600)
T_2	425 (165–600)[a#]	289 (188–600)[a#]	213 (90–525)[a]	163 (82–294)[a]	156 (101 – 186)[a]
T_3	49 (40–57)[a]	55 (48–62)[a]	65 (53–80)[a#]	49 (38–59)[a]	47 (35 – 57)[a]
$Y0$	503.2 ± 23.3[+]	459.9 ± 22.7	467.9 ± 27.1[+]	381.7 ± 21.0	503.0 ± 10.9[+]
$Y1$	416.0 ± 15.1[a#+o]	402.4 ± 16.1[a#+o]	289.5 ± 16.8[a#]	342.3 ± 15.6[#]	196.6 ± 9.2[a]
Plateau	70.3 ± 7.6	70.3 ± 10.3	92.9 ± 5.5	63.7 ± 12.1	63.0 ± 2.0
K	0.22 ± 0.02[#o]	0.16 ± 0.02[#o]	0.65 ± 0.09[#]	0.13 ± 0.02[#o]	1.19 ± 0.07

Scores T_1, T_2, and T_3 are presented as medians (interquartile range). Curve parameters ($Y0$, $Y1$, Plateau, and K) are presented as means ± SEM
*Intragroup differences ($p < .05$): T_1 vs. T_0, T_2 vs. T_1, and Y_1 vs. Y_0
oIntergroup differences ($p < .05$): vs. G3
+Intergroup differences ($p < .05$): vs. G4
#Intergroup differences ($p < .05$): vs. G5

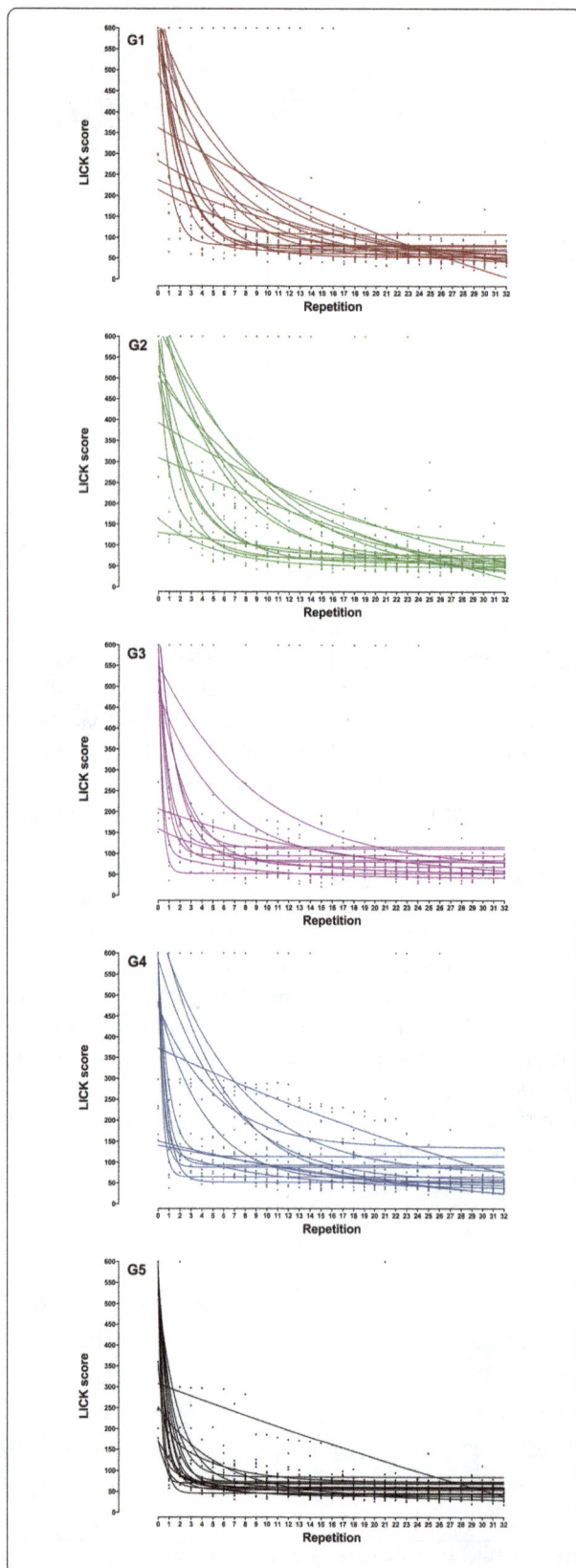

Fig. 4 Laparoscopic intra-corporeal knot tying (LICK). Individual learning curves. Each participant performed 33 consecutive repetitions (R0–R32) of LICK. The scores were plotted, and individual learning curves were observed. Most of them fitted to the one-phase exponential decay model, whereas some of them to the two-phase exponential decay model and some did not fit at all to any model

groups reached a similar plateau (NS) but at different speeds, as demonstrated by the different K values ($p < .0001$). Indeed, G5 has a significantly higher K than G1 ($p < 0.0001$), G2 ($p < 0.0001$), G3 ($p < 0.0001$), and G4 ($p < 0.0001$), whereas G3 has a significantly higher K than G1 ($p < 0.0001$), G2 ($p < 0.0001$), and G4 ($p < 0.0001$) (Table 2 and Fig. 5).

When the effect of the different variables (age, gender, dominant hand side, hand size, interest in surgery, experience in video game, and training group) upon the learning process (evaluated with the learning constant K) was computed, only the training group was shown to be significant ($p = .0005$).

Discussion

This study was performed under the frame of a general project aiming to evaluate factors that potentially can influence laparoscopic skills acquisition, which was initially done in the LASTT model [11–13]. The specific aim of the study was to characterize the LICK learning curve under different pre-training conditions (i.e., one control group with no pre-training, three study groups with pre-training of only one basic skill each (LCN, HEC, or BMC) and one study group with pre-training of the three basic skills (LCN, HEC, and BMC)). This was done in order to define whether pre-training of one basic skill shortens the LICK learning curve and moreover if pre-training of all basic skills has some additive beneficial effect.

For each participant, the scores registered at all points were plotted and individual and group learning curves were observed. For most individuals, as well as for most groups, the one-phase exponential decay was the best-fitted model. From the group curves, the starting point before any training ($Y0$), the point before LICK training ($Y1$), the Plateau, and the learning constant (K) were calculated. The $Y1$ was included to evaluate specifically the impact of previous training. Although the real values at baseline of all groups were comparable, the calculated values at $Y0$ were surprisingly different, being better/lower for G4. All other groups had comparable starting points ($Y0$) and improved their scores at the next evaluated point of the curve (i.e., $Y1$). Since this effect was observed even for G1, the influence of repetition cannot be neglected. This effect was more pronounce in G2 and even more in G3 and G4, indicating the importance of training LCN, HEC, and BMC, respectively.

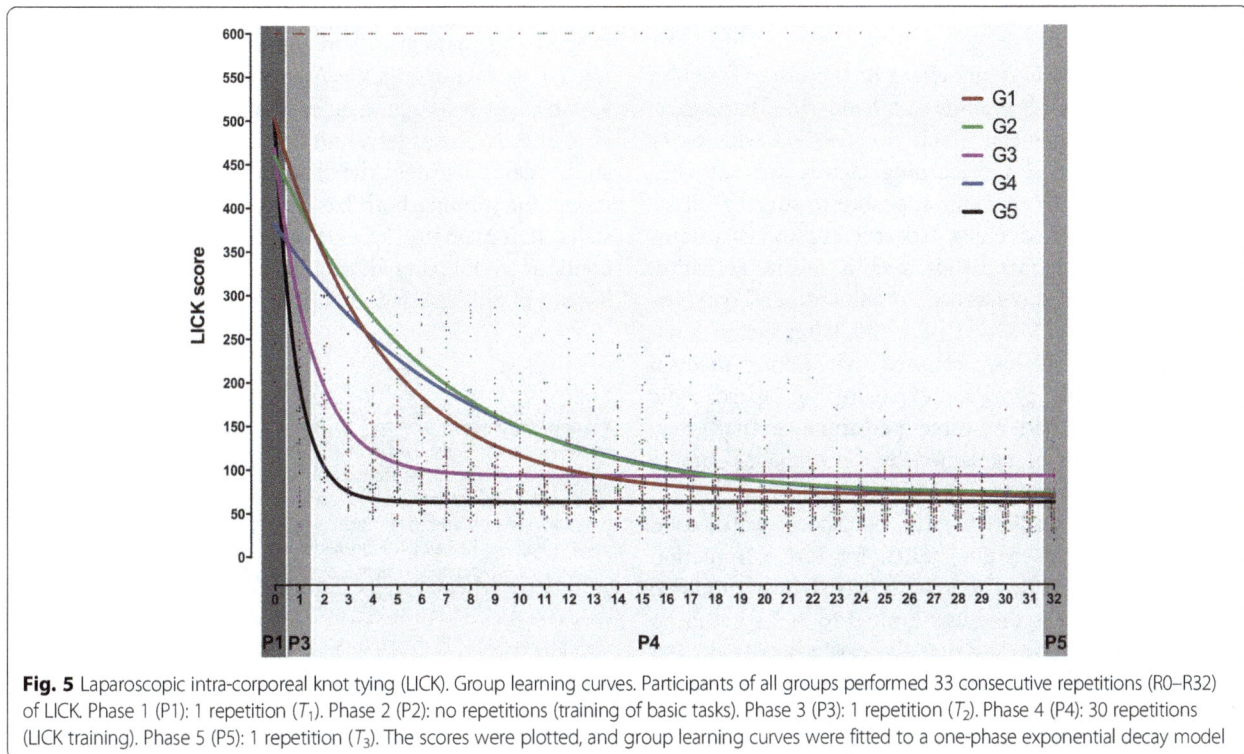

Fig. 5 Laparoscopic intra-corporeal knot tying (LICK). Group learning curves. Participants of all groups performed 33 consecutive repetitions (R0–R32) of LICK. Phase 1 (P1): 1 repetition (T_1). Phase 2 (P2): no repetitions (training of basic tasks). Phase 3 (P3): 1 repetition (T_2). Phase 4 (P4): 30 repetitions (LICK training). Phase 5 (P5): 1 repetition (T_3). The scores were plotted, and group learning curves were fitted to a one-phase exponential decay model

However, the greater effect was observed in G5, which also scored significantly better than all other groups. In spite of these differences at the beginning of the curve, all groups reached a similar Plateau but at different speed. Indeed, G5 has a quicker learning as demonstrated by the higher learning constant (K). All these together indicate the relevance of training all laparoscopic psychomotor skills first in order not only to start the LICK training from a better point but also to achieve proficiency sooner.

It has been sufficiently proved that training improves laparoscopic skills [19], which also applies specifically to training in box models as recently reported in a meta-analysis, at least in trainees with no previous laparoscopic experience [20]. The majority of the studies base this conclusion upon measurements performed at two or few points (before and after training). The effect of training however can be better appreciated if several points are taken into consideration, allowing tracking the improvement in performance over time, which is defined as a learning curve [21]. Although learning curves have been observed for many health technologies [22], only recently they have become regularly used and reported for laparoscopic procedures [13, 23–27].

Our data about LICK learning curves are consistent with previous studies. Vossen et al. have reported in 29 trainees learning curves with mono- or bi-exponential decay, the latter fitting their experimental points only marginally better [25]. Zhou et al. [28] and Thiyagarajan

et al. [29] have also reported in 20 trainees learning curves with an exponential decay shape.

There are few studies evaluating the effect of previous training upon LICK. Consistent with our study, Stefanidis et al. demonstrated in 20 novices that training basic laparoscopic skills (bean drop, running string, block move, checkerboard, and endostitch) shortened the learning curve of a more complex laparoscopic task like suturing. They have also claimed the additional benefit of substantial cost savings because the trained group required significantly less active instruction and less overall costs of the suture material [30]. In spite that learning curves were not reported, Fried et al. have also demonstrated in 215 surgeons that training a basic task (i.e., pegboard transfer) improves significantly the performance of LICK [31].

We believe that one of the strength of our study derives from the study population. Indeed, our sample size was larger than required to achieve our objectives and comprises medical students without experience in practicing surgery (neither laparotomy nor laparoscopy), which ascertains that the skills acquired derive exclusively from the training offered by this study, guaranteeing the purity of the data without external influences. Furthermore, the fact of being last-year students provides them with sufficient knowledge to define their interest in surgical practice. This issue was specifically evaluated, and in spite of the overall great interest reported in the general population, we failed to demonstrate an effect in the results, in contrast with previous studies reporting better results in trainees with higher interest in surgery [27].

We also did not find any effect of the other variables evaluated (age, gender, dominant hand side, hand size, interest in video games), which is consistent with other studies showing that the learning curves are not substantially affected by previous exposure to surgery, either by assisting or by watching laparoscopic interventions, nor by personal characteristics, such as leisure activities, eye dysfunction, eye correction, dominant hand, personality, and gender [25, 27, 31]. For this latter factor, however, Thorson et al. have claimed that among medical students with no previous exposure to laparoscopic trainers, women had a worse performance than men [32], which might be explained by their smaller sample size than in our study ($n = 32$ vs. 80 participants).

As in previous studies [11, 13], our scores were based upon the widely used time taken for task completion system [9, 20, 26, 33]. The system was slightly modified in the sense that the time was limited to 300 s based on previous results indicating that the vast majority of participants would have finished the task within these limits [12]. This was done because it would be practically impossible to carry out a large-scale measurement without time restrictions. It can be argued that this scoring system could be a limitation for our conclusions. We have to admit that time alone is not necessarily an accurate assessment of surgical skills and that accuracy and precision should be incorporated into the scoring system. In our system, however, these factors were implicitly incorporated because only knots correctly performed were scored without penalty.

For the aims of this and future studies, we developed a novel box trainer model, the ENCILAP model, based on the LASTT model [13] in order to make it more versatile and portable and with a more rigorous and precise design. Since the tasks performed were the same as those reported and validated in the LASTT model [11–13] and since this new model is basically the same, except for the design, a specific validation was not necessary. The experience gathered during this and other studies still being conducted, and the data reported, indicates that the simple concept of rectangular block modules placed at different places of a platform, and fitted accordingly, is feasible for training not only the basic skills (i.e., LCN, HEC, BMC) but also LICK, and that can be used as an alternative to the LASTT model or to any other box trainer developed with this aim.

Conclusions

In conclusion, our study confirms that training improves laparoscopic skills and demonstrates that pre-training of at least one basic task shortens the LICK learning curve and moreover that this beneficial effect is additive and more pronounce when the three basic tasks are pre-trained. Our data also demonstrate that the LICK learning curve is not significantly affected by confounding variables such as age, gender, dominant hand side, hand size, interest in surgery, and interest in video games. The study demonstrates the feasibility of the ENCILAP model for training both basic and advanced laparoscopic skills. It remains to be elucidated the potential effect of continuous tutoring during training and moreover the impact of all these factors upon real surgery in humans.

Acknowledgements

We would like to thank the Universidad del Pacífico Privada (Asunción, Paraguay) for offering their facilities, Architect Jorge Jury for designing and building the ENCILAP model, and Karl Storz (Tuttlingen, Germany) for providing the instruments and materials. We thank Anna Ivanova from the Leuven Statistics Research Centre, Katholieke Universiteit Leuven (Leuven, Belgium) for her support in statistical analysis, Mrs. Rossana Paredes and Alicia Amarilla for their support in collecting the data, Drs. Christian Leith and Victor Oviedo for their support as supervisors, and all medical students who actively participated in the study.

Funding

This study did not receive any funding and was funded by the authors' own resources.

Authors' contributions

CRM contributed in protocol/project development, data collection and management, data analysis, and manuscript writing/editing. MMB contributed in data analysis and manuscript writing/editing. CMS contributed in data collection and management. RC contributed in protocol/project development. All authors read and approved the final manuscript.

Competing interests

The authors declare that they have no competing interests.

Author details

[1]NEOLIFE—Medicina y Cirugía Reproductiva, Avenida Brasilia 760, 1434 Asunción, Paraguay. [2]Faculty of Medicine, Universidad del Pacífico Privada, Avenida San Martín 961, 1813 Asunción, Paraguay. [3]The European Academy of Gynaecological Surgery, Diestsevest 43, bus 0001, B3000 Leuven, Belgium.

References

1. Willaert W, Van De Putte D, Van RK, Van NY, Ceelen W, Pattyn P (2013) Training models in laparoscopy: a systematic review comparing their effectiveness in learning surgical skills. Acta Chir Belg 113:77–95
2. Thinggaard E, Kleif J, Bjerrum F et al (2016) Off-site training of laparoscopic skills, a scoping review using a thematic analysis. Surg Endosc 30:4733–4741
3. Campo R, Wattiez A, Tanos V et al (2016) Gynaecological endoscopic surgical education and assessment. A diploma programme in

gynaecological endoscopic surgery. Eur J Obstet Gynecol Reprod Biol 199:183–186

4. Campo R, Wattiez A, Tanos V et al (2016) Gynaecological endoscopic surgical education and assessment. A diploma programme in gynaecological endoscopic surgery. Gynecol Surg 13:133–137

5. Diesen DL, Erhunmwunsee L, Bennett KM et al (2011) Effectiveness of laparoscopic computer simulator versus usage of box trainer for endoscopic surgery training of novices. J Surg Educ 68:282–289

6. Escamirosa FP, Flores RM, Garcia IO, Vidal CR, Martinez AM (2015) Face, content, and construct validity of the EndoViS training system for objective assessment of psychomotor skills of laparoscopic surgeons. Surg Endosc 29:3392–3403

7. Hofstad EF, Vapenstad C, Chmarra MK, Lango T, Kuhry E, Marvik R (2013) A study of psychomotor skills in minimally invasive surgery: what differentiates expert and nonexpert performance. Surg Endosc 27:854–863

8. Munro MG (2012) Surgical simulation: where have we come from? Where are we now? Where are we going? J Minim Invasive Gynecol 19:272–283

9. Mulla M, Sharma D, Moghul M et al (2012) Learning basic laparoscopic skills: a randomized controlled study comparing box trainer, virtual reality simulator, and mental training. J Surg Educ 69:190–195

10. Sroka G, Feldman LS, Vassiliou MC, Kaneva PA, Fayez R, Fried GM (2010) Fundamentals of laparoscopic surgery simulator training to proficiency improves laparoscopic performance in the operating room—a randomized controlled trial. Am J Surg 199:115–120

11. Campo R, Reising C, Van Belle Y, Nassif J, O'Donovan P, Molinas CR (2010) A valid model for testing and training laparoscopic psychomotor skills. Gynecol Surg 7:133–141

12. Molinas CR, Campo R (2010) Defining a structured training program for acquiring basic and advanced laparoscopic psychomotor skills in a simulator. Gynecol Surg 7:427–435

13. Molinas CR, De Win G, Ritter O, Keckstein J, Miserez M, Campo R (2008) Feasibility and construct validity of a novel laparoscopic skills testing and training model. Gynecol Surg 5:281–290

14. The Winners Project, A new educational program developed by the IRCAD's gynaecology team led by professor Wattiez in collaboration with the European academy of Gynaecological surgery (2017). https://www.websurg.com/winners/get/

15. Campo R, Molinas CR, De Wilde RL et al (2012) Are you good enough for your patients? The European certification model in laparoscopic surgery. Facts Views Vis Obgyn 4:95–101

16. Campo R, Wattiez A, De Wilde RL, Molinas CR (2012) Training in laparoscopic surgery: from the lab to the OR. Zdrav Var 51:285–298

17. Molinas CR, Campo R (2016) Retention of laparoscopic psychomotor skills after a structured training program depends on the quality of the training and on the complexity of the task. Gynecol Surg 13:395–402

18. Molinas CR, Binda MM, Campo R (2017) Dominant hand, non-dominant hand, or both? The effect of pre-training in hand-eye oordination upon the learning curve of laparoscopic intra-corporeal knot tying. Gynecol Surg 14(1):12 1015-3

19. Torricelli FC, Barbosa JA, Marchini GS (2016) Impact of laparoscopic surgery training laboratory on surgeon's performance. World J Gastrointest Surg 8:735–743

20. Nagendran M, Toon CD, Davidson BR, Gurusamy KS (2014) Laparoscopic surgical box model training for surgical trainees with no prior laparoscopic experience. Cochrane Database Syst Rev 2014:CD010479

21. Cook JA, Ramsay CR, Fayers P (2007) Using the literature to quantify the learning curve: a case study. Int J Technol Assess Health Care 23:255–260

22. Ramsay CR, Grant AM, Wallace SA, Garthwaite PH, Monk AF, Russell IT (2001) Statistical assessment of the learning curves of health technologies. Health Technol Assess 5:1–79

23. Brunner WC, Korndorffer JR Jr, Sierra R et al (2004) Laparoscopic virtual reality training: are 30 repetitions enough? J Surg Res 122:150–156

24. Molinas CR, Binda MM, Mailova K, Koninckx PR (2004) The rabbit nephrectomy model for training in laparoscopic surgery. Hum Reprod 19:185–190

25. Vossen C, Van BP, Shaw RW, Koninckx PR (1997) Effect of training on endoscopic intracorporeal knot tying. Hum Reprod 12:2658–2663

26. Rodriguez-Sanjuan JC, Manuel-Palazuelos C, Fernandez-Diez MJ et al (2010) Assessment of resident training in laparoscopic surgery based on a digestive system anastomosis model in the laboratory. Cir Esp 87:20–25

27. Kolozsvari NO, Andalib A, Kaneva P et al (2011) Sex is not everything: the role of gender in early performance of a fundamental laparoscopic skill. Surg Endosc 25:1037–1042

28. Zhou M, Tse S, Derevianko A, Jones DB, Schwaitzberg SD, Cao CG (2012) Effect of haptic feedback in laparoscopic surgery skill acquisition. Surg Endosc 26:1128–1134

29. Thiyagarajan M, Ravindrakumar C (2016) A comparative study in learning curves of two different intracorporeal knot tying techniques. Minim Invasive Surg 2016:3059434

30. Stefanidis D, Hope WW, Korndorffer JR Jr, Markley S, Scott DJ (2010) Initial laparoscopic basic skills training shortens the learning curve of laparoscopic suturing and is cost-effective. J Am Coll Surg 210:436–440

31. Fried GM, Feldman LS, Vassiliou MC et al (2004) Proving the value of simulation in laparoscopic surgery. Ann Surg 240:518–525

32. Thorson CM, Kelly JP, Forse RA, Turaga KK (2011) Can we continue to ignore gender differences in performance on simulation trainers? J Laparoendosc Adv Surg Tech A 21:329–333

33. Fransen SA, Mertens LS, Botden SM, Stassen LP, Bouvy ND (2012) Performance curve of basic skills in single-incision laparoscopy versus conventional laparoscopy: is it really more difficult for the novice? Surg Endosc 26:1231–1237

33

Feasibility of sentinel lymph node fluorescence detection during robotic laparoendoscopic single-site surgery in early endometrial cancer: a prospective case series

Liliana Mereu[*], Alice Pellegrini, Roberta Carlin, Erica Terreno, Claudia Prasciolu and Saverio Tateo

Abstract

Background: In the last few decades, the introduction of technologies such as single-site surgery, robotics, and sentinel lymph node detection has reduced invasiveness in the treatment and staging of endometrial cancer patients. The goal of the present prospective cohort study is to evaluate the feasibility of lymph node fluorescence detection with robotic single-site approach in low-risk endometrial cancer.

Results: Fifteen non consecutive low-risk endometrial atypical hyperplasia (EAH) patients underwent sentinel lymph node (SLN) biopsy and total hysterectomy utilizing the Da Vinci Si Single-Site Surgical. System and Firefly 3D imaging. Indications for surgery included eight (53.3%) IA FIGO stage G1 EC, three (20%) IA FIGO stage G2 EC, and four (26.6%) EAH. Mean operative time was 155 min (range 112–175). One vaginal laceration was the only perioperative complication encountered, and all patients were discharged within 48 h of surgery.
SLN was detected in 86.6% of cases; 1/29 (3.4%) SLN results were positive for isolated tumor cells (ITCs) at immunohistochemical analysis.

Conclusions: The present study demonstrates the feasibility and applicability of robotic single-site approach with SLN fluorescence detection for the staging of low-risk endometrial cancer.

Keywords: Single-site surgery, Robotic, Fluorescence, Sentinel lymph node, Low-risk endometrial cancer, Minimal invasive surgery

Background

Surgery is considered the gold standard for staging and treating women with endometrial carcinoma (EC). The surgical treatment of endometrial cancer has quickly evolved since the late 1980s with the introduction of laparoscopy. In 2005, the US Food and Drug Administration approved the da Vinci robotic platform (Intuitive Surgical Inc., Sunnyvale, CA, USA) for gynecology, adding another tool for the management of EC.

Even if robotic surgery shows some disadvantages, such as size, number of port sites, and costs, it has obtained an important role in gynecologic surgery, due to its short learning curve, comfortable ergonomics, and improved intra- and postoperative outcomes.

The laparoendoscopic single-site surgery (LESS) is an alternative to conventional laparoscopic or robotic surgery, as it provides the improved cosmetic benefits of minimally invasive surgery while avoiding the potential morbidity related to multiple incisions. Although LESS is innovative, it nevertheless presents some challenges, requiring specific laparoscopic skills. The combination of robotics and single-site surgery appears to be the perfect fusion between the two techniques, enhancing the advantages and reducing the limitations.

* Correspondence: liliana_mereu@yahoo.com
Department of Obstetrics and Gynecology, Santa Chiara Hospital, Largo Medaglie d'Oro 9, 38122 Trento, Italy

Recent studies demonstrate that the robotic single-site (RSS) technique applied to total extra-fascial hysterectomy and even pelvic lymphadenectomy is a feasible and reproducible technique for the staging of endometrial cancer without the need of additional ports or conversion to laparoscopy [1–8]. Since 2015, the development of a fluorescence robotic camera for the RSS console makes it possible to apply the sentinel lymph node (SLN) protocol with RSS approach as described by Sinno et al. [9–11] and Silva E Silva [12].

SLN mapping may be an acceptable surgical strategy placed in between lymphadenectomy and no nodal evaluation in patients with endometrial cancer [13, 14]. As underlined by Abu-Rustum, the main point of SLN mapping is to reduce the number of nodes removed for staging, by targeting those most likely to contain metastasis and still maintaining the ability to find microscopic nodal disease [13]. Despite the low incidence of nodal disease in low-risk EC, omitting extra-peritoneal evaluation would result in an inadequate staging precluding adjuvant therapy when necessary; SLN can be an efficient alternative to the selection of patients to be surgically staged based on the intrauterine risk factor identification by means of frozen sections [15, 16].

The aim of this study is to evaluate the feasibility of robotic single-site hysterectomy (RSSH) plus sentinel node biopsy for the staging of endometrial endometrioid cancer.

Methods

This is a prospective, cohort study on nonconsecutive low-risk endometrial cancer patients treated with RSS hysterectomy plus bilateral salpingo-oophorectomy and SLN detection with the da Vinci Si Surgical System. All 15 patients were operated at the Gynecological Unit in S. Chiara Hospital by two senior surgeons (ST and LM) using the same surgical team. The main inclusion criteria were a clinical diagnosis of low-risk endometrial cancer (IA FIGO stage, G1–G2) or atypical endometrial hyperplasia revealed by the preoperative exams (endometrial biopsy, pelvic ultrasound, and/or MRI). We excluded patients with anesthesiological contraindications for the minimally invasive approach, body mass index > 30, and large uterus.

The pre-treatment evaluation included medical history collection, physical examination, vaginal pelvic examination, chest X-ray, pelvic ultrasound scan, or pelvic magnetic resonance imaging scan. Informed consent to RSSH and SLN fluorescence detection was obtained from all patients in accordance with the local and international legislation (Declaration of Helsinki) [17]. Approval to conduct the study was obtained independently from the Azienda Provinciale Servizi Sanitari (APSS) Ethics Committee (reference number RGCS-I-2016).

Clinical patient characteristics including age, body mass index (BMI), pre-surgical clinical staging, comorbidity, prior abdominal surgery, and intraoperative parameters including operative time, blood loss, conversion rate, and complications were recorded.

The operating time was measured from the beginning of the skin incision to the completion of skin closure. The estimated blood loss was calculated using the difference between washed and suctioned solution. Postoperative parameters included short-term (within 30 days of the procedure) and long-term (more than 30 days after the procedure) complications and length of hospital stay. Complications were measured by the Clavien-Dindo scale [18].

All patients were administered antibiotic prophylaxis (cefoxitin 2 g intravenously) and postoperative low molecular weight enoxaparin (40 mg/day subcutaneously). During the procedure, the patient was placed in the lithotomy position and underwent general anesthesia. The vaginal cavity was cleaned with a povidone-iodine solution and a Foley catheter was placed in the bladder. A speculum was placed for cervical visualization, and 4 ml of indocyanine green (ICG) was diluted to 1.25 mg/mL and was injected 1 ml superficially and 1 ml deeply into the cervical stroma at 3 and 9 o'clock position. A 2.5-cm incision was made using all the umbilical scar length, opening the peritoneal cavity. The single-site port was inserted into the abdominal cavity using an atraumatic forceps. The pneumoperitoneum was induced at a pressure of 12 mmHg. Four specific cannulae were introduced in the port: two 250-mm-long curved 5-mm cannulae for robotic instruments, one 8.5-mm cannula for the high-definition three-dimensional endoscope, and one 5-mm assistant surgeon cannula. The patient was moved to the Trendelenburg position, and the bowel was placed above the pelvic brim with a laparoscopic grasper. After adhesiolysis, if necessary, cytologic fluid aspiration and coagulation of both tubes with standard laparoscopic instruments were performed, and a Hohl uterine manipulator (Karl Storz GmbH & Co. KG, Tuttlingen, Germany) was placed using a video guidance. The da Vinci® Si System (Intuitive Surgical, Sunnyvale, CA) was docked between the patient's legs. A 3D 8.5-mm Firefly endoscope was used in the camera arm, and a unipolar hook and bipolar Maryland forceps were used on the right and left hands respectively. Fluorescence imaging was used to visualize the ICG tracer in the lymphatic system (Fig. 1). A successful mapping was defined as finding a channel leading from the cervix directly to one lymph node in at least one hemi-pelvis. The identified sentinel lymph nodes were then retrieved, labeled for a location with a clip, and inserted in an EndoBag. Extra-fascial total hysterectomy and bilateral salpingo-oophorectomy were then performed following the technique previously described [8]. The uterus and SLNs were extracted from the abdominal cavity through the

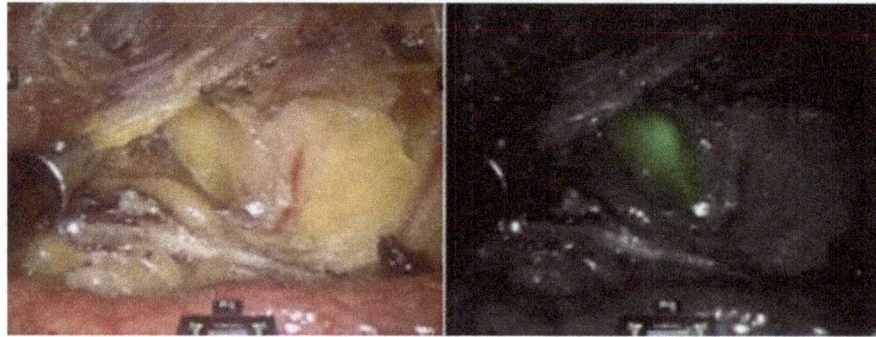

Fig. 1 Right external iliac SLN fluorescence detection

vagina. The vaginal cuff closure was performed internally with snaked single-port robotic needle holder and 0/0 barbed suture V-loc (Covidien Dublin, Ireland). The robot was undocked, and the single-site port was taken out. The umbilical incision was sutured in planes with number 1 Vicryl (Johnson & Johnson International, Belgium) on the aponeurosis, and Monocryl 3–0 (Johnson & Johnson International, Belgium) under the skin.

For the pathologic evaluation of SLNs in EC, the procedure used was the ultra-staging described by Abu-Rustum et al. [13].

Normally distributed data are presented as mean SD and confidence interval while skewed data are presented as median and range. Categorical variables are reported as absolute values and percentages.

Results

Between September 2015 and September 2017, 15 women underwent RSSH plus SLN fluorescence detection at the Gynecological Department of Santa Chiara Hospital, Trento, Italy.

Indications for surgery included eight (53.3%) IA FIGO stage, grade 1 endometrial cancer; three (20%) IA FIGO stage, grade 2 endometrial cancer; and four (26.6%) endometrial atypical hyperplasia, diagnosed by preoperative curettage and instrumental exams. Median patients' age was 60 (range 55–69), and body mass index was 23 kg/m^2 (range 21–33). Six (40%) patients had had prior abdominal surgery. Mean uterine weight was 113 g (range 50–230). The mean operative time was 155 min (range 112–175). An intraoperative vaginal laceration occurred in one patient, and all patients were discharged within 48 h of surgery.

SLN was detected in 86.6% of cases (two cases of no detection, nine cases of bilateral detection, and four cases of mono-lateral detection). Uterine frozen section was done only in case of no SLN detection to confirm myometrial invasion and grading. No systematic pelvic lymphadenectomy was required. In one case of no SLN detection, a vaginal laceration with vaginal valve occurred

soon after ICG intracervical injection (requiring vaginal suturing), and in one case, bilateral parametrial ICG diffusion has been observed. Twenty-nine SLNs were identified: 11 (37.9%) in the internal iliac region, 10 (34.5%) in the external iliac region, 5 (17.2%) in the obturator region, and 3 (10.4%) in the common iliac region (Table 1). 28/29 SLN proved negative at the final histological exam, in 1 (3.4%) SLN ITCs was detected by IHC. As shown in Table 2, upper staging occurred in 5/15 (33.3%) cases (3 endometrial atypical hyperplasia and 2 G1 endometrial cancer).

Discussion

The combination of robotic surgery, single umbilical access, and near-infrared fluorescence imaging makes it possible to minimize surgery and to apply SLN mapping at the same time, improving the intra- and postoperative outcome for the patients.

The technique used to perform a total hysterectomy and pelvic lymphadenectomy by RSS approach has already been described in our previous video article [8]. In the present case series, the closure of the vaginal cuff was performed internally with the utilization of robotic snaked needle holder. The 3D 8.5 mm Firefly™ fluorescence

Table 1 SLNs detection

Variable	N, frequency (%)
Mapping by pelvic	
Bilateral	9 (60.1)
Monolateral	4 (26.6)
None	2 (13.3)
SLN identified	29
Localization	
Internal iliac	11 (37.9)
External iliac	10 (34.5)
Obturator	5 (17.2)
Common iliac	3 (10.4)

Table 2 Pre- vs postsurgical staging

Variable	Preoperative, N (%)	Postoperative, N (%)
Endometrial atypical hyperplasia	4 (26.6)	1 (6.6)
Grading		
G1	8 (53.3)	8 (53.3)
G2	3 (20)	4 (26.6)
G3	0	2 (13.3)
Myometrial invasion		
M1	15 (100)	15 (100)
M2	0	0

endoscope (Intuitive Surgical) was utilized for the detection of SLN as already described by Sinno et al. [9–11].

The SLN detection rate was 86.6%, in line with the rate considered acceptable and reported to be from 80 to 90% or greater [19]. In two patients, SLN detection was not obtained in both hemi-pelvis: in one case, the vaginal laceration at the level of the right fornix could have promoted an IGC intraperitoneal diffusion, preventing the physiologic lymphatic spread of the dye; in the second case, bilateral parametrial diffusion probably obscured the visualization of the SLN.

During the research of the fluorescent lymph node, the two surgeons noted a less brilliant green than in standard robotic surgery, which required a reduction of the distance between the camera and the target organ. This event could have been due to the reduced diameter of the endoscope, as compared with the 3D 10-mm camera utilized in multiport robotic laparoscopy. In a study performed on pigs to determinate the optimal dosage of ICG of the robotic single-site instrumentation, Levison et al. evidenced that the optimal concentration of ICG is 250–500 µg per 0.5 ml [20]. Probably, the utilization of a concentration of 2.5 mg/mL instead of 1.25 mg/mL could improve the intensity and the identification of SLNs from the surrounding tissue.

The removal of the identified sentinel lymph node was possible in all cases using a bipolar forceps and a unipolar hook. In the study by Creasman et al., pelvic nodal metastases were found in 5% of patients with superficial myometrial invasion [21]. On the basis of the International Federation of Gynecology and Obstetrics (FIGO) 2009 staging system, Chi et al. found that 5.5% of patients with endometrioid histology, all grades, and myometrial invasion < 50%, had nodal metastasis [22]. More recent studies on low-risk EC and SLN detection revealed an incidence of lymph nodal metastases between 6 and 10% [15, 23–25]. Similarly, the occurrence of metastatic lymph nodal EC in patients with a preoperative diagnosis of EAH has been widely described before [15, 26, 27]. In the present study in 1/29 (3.4%) SLN, isolated tumor cells were found at IHC. One patient, with

endometrial cancer FIGO stage IA, grade 3, underwent adjuvant external beam radiotherapy.

Considering that classifying patients as EAH or low-risk EC based on pre- or intraoperative uterine factors alone may lead to an under-staging of 25–33% [23, 28, 29], in accordance with the previous studies we routinely performed SLN detection in EAH and low-risk EC. In this series of 15 patients, three cases of atypical hyperplasia became G1 and two cases of G1 endometrial cancer became G2 and G3 with the myometrial invasion of less than 50%.

Ten (66.6%) SLNs were detected in the internal iliac region, eight (53.3%) in the external iliac region, five (33.3%) in the obturator region, and three (20%) in the common iliac region; the present SLN mapping matches the SLN fluorescence detection with the Firefly system in stage I endometrial cancer reported by Abu-Rustum et al. [30]. The shortest single-port curve cannulae of 5×250 mm, 5-mm robotic single-site instruments (bipolar Maryland and monopolar hook), and standard docking made it possible to visualize and remove the SLNs also at the level of the common iliac vessels. The mean operative time of 155 min is longer than those reported by other studies, in which only a total hysterectomy without lymphadenectomy was performed [2, 3]. There is only one multicenter study on the feasibility of endometrial cancer by RSSL, where the mean time was 122 but pelvic lymphadenectomy was performed in only 17% of cases [7]. Following Sinno's algorithm [31], in two of 15 cases in which no SLNs were found, a frozen section analysis of the uterus was performed to confirm myometrial invasion and grading, without the need to perform systematic pelvic lymphadenectomy. In our institution, frozen section analysis of the SLN in EC patients is not routinely performed, because it may lead to high false-negative rates and may interfere with a proper ultra-staging at the permanent section.

As the technique did not require conversion, and as only one vaginal intraoperative laceration and no postoperative complications occurred, it may be considered safe for the patients and a valid and feasible alternative.

Conclusions

This preliminary study demonstrates the feasibility and applicability of robotic single-site approach with SLN fluorescence detection for the staging of low-risk endometrial cancer. A prospective multicenter case-control study is ongoing with the aim of comparing standard robotic vs single-site robotic approach for the treatment with SLN mapping of low-risk EC.

Further studies are needed to demonstrate the applicability of the SLN algorithm and to compare different minimally invasive approaches in higher risks endometrial cancer.

Abbreviations
APSS: Azienda Provinciale Servizi Sanitari; BMI: Body mass index; EAH: Endometrial atypical hyperplasia; EC: Endometrial cancer; ICG: Indocyanine green; IHC: Immunohistochemistry; ITC: Isolated tumor cell; LESS: Laparoendoscopic single-site surgery; RSS: Robotic single site; RSSH: Robotic single-site hysterectomy; SLN: Sentinel lymph node

Authors' contributions
ML is a surgeon, and she designed and wrote the paper and interpreted the data. AP contributed to the data acquisition, analysis, and interpretation. RC and ET contributed to the acquisition of data and wrote the paper. CP contributed to the acquisition of data and drafting of the paper. ST is a surgeon, and he contributed to the interpretation and supervision. All authors read and approved the final manuscript.

Competing interests
All authors declare that they have no competing interests.

References
1. Mereu L, Carri G, Khalifa H (2012) Robotic single port total laparoscopic hysterectomy for endometrial cancer patients. Gynecol Oncol 127:644
2. Cela V, Freschi L, Simi G, Ruggiero M, Tana R, Pluchino N (2013) Robotic single-site hysterectomy: feasibility, learning curve and surgical outcome. Surg Endosc 27:2638–2643
3. Vizza E, Corrado G, Mancini E et al (2013) Robotic single-site hysterectomy in low risk endometrial cancer: a pilot study. Ann Surg Oncol 20:2759–2764
4. Fagotti A, Corrado G, Fanfani F (2013) Robotic single-site hysterectomy (RSS-H) vs. laparoendoscopic single-site hysterectomy (LESS-H) in early endometrial cancer: a double-institution case-control study. Gynecol Oncol 30:219–223
5. Bogliolo S, Mereu L, Cassani I (2015) Robotic single-site hysterectomy: two institutions' preliminary experience. Int J Med Rob Comput Assisted Surg 11:159–165
6. Moukarzel LA, Fader AN, Tanner EJ (2017) Feasibility of robotic-assisted laparoendoscopic single-site surgery in the gynecologic oncology setting. J Minim Invasive Gynecol 24:258–263
7. Corrado G, Mereu L, Bogliolo S (2016) Robotic single site staging in endometrial cancer: a multi-institution study. Eur J Surg Oncol 42:1506–1511
8. Tateo S, Nozza A, Del Pezzo C (2014) Robotic single-site pelvic lymphadenectomy. Gynecol Oncol 134(3):631
9. Sinno AK, Fader AN, Tanner EJ 3rd (2015) Single site robotic sentinel lymph node biopsy and hysterectomy in endometrial cancer. Gynecol Oncol 137:190
10. Sinno AK, Tanner EJ (2015) Robotic laparoendoscopic single site radical hysterectomy with sentinel lymph node mapping and pelvic lymphadenectomy for cervical cancer. J Minim Invasive Gynecol 22:S115
11. Moukarzel LA, Sinno AK, Fader AN, Tanner EJ (2017) Comparing single-site and multiport robotic hysterectomy with sentinel lymph node mapping for endometrial cancer: surgical outcomes and costs. J Minim Invasive Gynecol 24:977–983
12. Silva E, Silva A, Fernandes RP (2017) Single-site robotic radical hysterectomy and sentinel lymphnode biopsy in cervical cancer: a case report. Rev Bras Ginecol Obstet 39:35–40
13. Abu-Rustum NR (2014) Sentinel lymph node mapping for endometrial cancer: a modern approach to surgical staging. J Natl Compr Canc Netw 12:288–229
14. Colombo N, Creutzberg C, Amant F (2015) ESMO-ESGO-ESTRO Endometrial Consensus Conference Working Group. ESMO-ESGO-ESTRO consensus conference on endometrial cancer: diagnosis, treatment and follow-up. Radiother Oncol 117:559–581
15. Papadia A, Gasparri ML, Siegenthaler F, Imboden S, Mohr S, Mueller MD (2017) FIGO stage IIIC endometrial cancer identification among patients with complex atypical hyperplasia, grade 1 and 2 endometrioid endometrial cancer: laparoscopic indocyanine green sentinel lymph node mapping versus frozen section of the uterus, why get around the problem? J Cancer Res Clin Oncol 143:491–497
16. Kim CH, Khoury-Collado F, Barber EL, Soslow RA, Makker V, Leitao MM Jr, Sonoda Y, Alektiar KM, Barakat RR, Abu-Rustum NR (2013) Sentinel lymph node mapping with pathologic ultrastaging: a valuable tool for assessing nodal metastasis in low-grade endometrial cancer with superficial myoinvasion. Gynecol Oncol 131:714–719
17. World Medical Association Declaration of Helsinki (1997) Recommendations guiding physicians in biomedical research involving human subjects. JAMA 277:925–926
18. Clavien PA, Barkun J, de Oliveira ML (2009) The Clavien-Dindo classification of surgical complications: five-year experience. Ann Surg 250:187–196
19. Khoury-Collado F, Glaser GE, Zivanovic O (2009) Improving sentinel lymph node detection rates in endometrial cancer: how many cases are needed? Gynecol Oncol 115:453–455
20. Levinson KL, Mahadi J, Escobar PF (2013) Feasibility and oprtimal indocianine green fluorescence for sentinel lympho node detection using robotic single-site instrumentation: preclinical study. J Min Invas Gynecol 20:691–696
21. Creasman WT, Morrow CP, Bundy BN, Homesley HD, Graham JE, Heller PB (1987) Surgical pathologic spread patterns of endometrial cancer: a gynecologic oncology group study. Cancer 60:2035–2041
22. Chi DS, Barakat RR, Palayekar MJ (2008) The incidence of pelvic lymph node metastasis by FIGO staging for patients with adequately surgically staged endometrial adenocarcinoma of endometrioid histology. Int J Gynecol Cancer 18:269–273
23. Darai E, Dubernard G, Bats AS (2015) Sentinel node biopsy for the management of early stage endometrial cancer: long-term results of the SENTI-ENDO study. Gynecol Oncol 136:64–59
24. Rossi EC, Kowalski LD, Scalici J (2017) A comparison of sentinel lymph node biopsy to lymphadenectomy for endometrial cancer staging (FIRES trial): a multicentre, prospective, cohort study. Lancet Oncol 18:384–392
25. Morotti M, Menada MV, Moioli M (2012) Frozen section pathology at time of hysterectomy accurately predicts endometrial cancer in patients with preoperative diagnosis of atypical endometrial hyperplasia. Gynecol Oncol 125:536–540
26. Trimble CL, Kauderer J, Zaino R (2006) Concurrent endometrial carcinoma in women with a biopsy diagnosis of atypical endometrial hyperplasia: a Gynecologic Oncology Group study. Cancer 106:812–819
27. Nugent EK, Bishop EH, Mathews CA (2012) Do uterine risk factors or lymph node metastasis more significantly affect recurrence in patients with endometrioid adenocarcinoma? Gynecol Oncol 125:94–98
28. Frumovitz M, Singh DK, Meyer L (2004) Predictors of final histology in patients with endometrial cancer. Gynecol Oncol 95:463–468
29. Daniel AG, Peters WA 3rd (1988) Accuracy of office and operating room curettage in the grading of endometrial carcinoma. Obstet Gynecol 71:612–614
30. Abu-Rustum NR, Khoury-Collado F, Pandit-Taskar N (2009) Sentinel lymph node mapping for grade 1 endometrial cancer: is it the answer to the surgical staging dilemma? Gynecol Oncol 113:163–169
31. Sinno AK, Peijnenburg E, Fader AN (2016) Reducing overtreatment: a comparison of lymph node assessment strategies for endometrial cancer. Gynecol Onco 143:281–286

34

A PET-positive rapidly growing mass of the abdominal wall after cesarean section with an unexpected diagnosis of vernix caseosa granuloma

Antonio Macciò[1*], Paraskevas Kotsonis[1], Fabrizio Lavra[1], Giacomo Chiappe[1], Ester Mura[2], Luca Melis[3] and Clelia Madeddu[4]

Abstract

Background: Abdominal wall tumors are rare and include heterogeneous diseases. Among them, desmoid tumors are the most frequent and are often diagnosed in young women during or early after pregnancy; inflammatory response after trauma or microtrauma, such as after cesarean section, may favor their growth.

Results: A 37-year-old woman presented with a progressive mass in the abdominal wall after a cesarean section. Positron emission tomography imaging confirmed a positive mass with a high maximum standardized uptake value; a biopsy suggested a myofibroblastic tumor. With continued tumor growth and worsening symptoms, the mass resembled a desmoid tumor; therefore, we proceed with its resection. The final diagnosis was foreign body granuloma as a reaction to the spillage of meconium and keratinous material in the amniotic fluid during cesarean section.

Conclusions: The present case provides information on an abdominal wall foreign body granuloma arisen from meconium and vernix caseosa after cesarean section, which presented an atypical clinical picture, mimicking a desmoid, thus requiring a careful diagnostic and treatment approach.

Keywords: Desmoid tumor, Foreign body granuloma, Cesarean section, Sarcoma, Meconium, Vernix caseosa

Background

In women, tumors of the anterior abdominal wall are rare and encompass very different pathologies, most commonly soft tissue sarcomas (mainly fibrosarcomas, dermatofibrosarcoma protuberans, and liposarcoma) and aggressive fibromatosis or desmoid tumors [1]. The differential diagnosis of abdominal wall tumors in women includes also sarcomatoid dissemination (particularly after conservative surgery in presence of occult leyomiosarcoma), metastases, or endometriosis implants [2]. Among these rare pathologies, desmoid tumors are the most frequent. They are very difficult to discriminate from sarcomas since they may present overlapping clinical behavior and radiological characteristics [2]. In fact,

rapid growth and pain represent the more typical symptoms of both these conditions. Notably, desmoids may develop in women of fertile age, especially during pregnancy and puerperium [3]. In addition, some abdominal wall sarcoma that developed in pregnancy has been described, particularly cases of dermatofibrosarcoma protuberans [4]. Even abdominal wall endometriosis may be related to pregnancy since it typically localizes at the surgical incision, such as cesarean section scars [5], and is associated with progressive pain.

Here, we describe a very rare case of a voluminous foreign body granuloma consequent to the spillage of meconium and keratinous material in the amniotic fluid developed in the abdominal wall after a cesarean section in a woman with previous myomectomy with morcellation for an atypical leyomioma.

* Correspondence: a.maccio@tin.it
[1]Department of Gynecologic Oncology, Azienda Ospedaliera Brotzu, via Edward Jenner, 09121 Cagliari, Italy
Full list of author information is available at the end of the article

Methods

The data of this case report was obtained through retrospective chart review. Written informed consent was obtained from the patient for the publication of the case report and the accompanying images.

Results

A 37-year-old woman (gravida 2, para 1) presented with a painful mass in the abdominal wall 1 month after a cesarean section delivery. Physical examination revealed a 3–4-cm palpable mass, which grew progressively with even more persistent pain; 15 days after the first check, the mass occupied all the lower quadrants of the abdominal wall. With the patient having a history of abdominal myomectomy for a large uterine leiomyoma (350 g, mitotic index 5/10 HPF; focal moderate atypia; Ki67, 15%) 2 years before, we hypothesized various possibilities based on our previous experience [6]: (a) recurrence of the previous myoma, (b) sarcomatoid degeneration of residuals of previously excised myoma, or (c) a desmoid tumor. Then, we performed computed tomography (CT), positron emission tomography (PET), and ultrasound-guided biopsy. CT showed an irregular formation in the lower part of the rectus muscles, consisting of a hyperdense ring that enclosed a hypodense area. This mass bordered in the adipose tissue on the anterior abdominal wall. To better assess its characteristics, etiology, and malignancy, the patient underwent PET/CT, which showed a large, irregular, and inhomogeneous high ^{18}F-fludeoxyglucose uptake (maximum standardized uptake value [SUV], 12.9) in the anterior abdominal wall. This area seemed to extend beyond the muscle tissue, possibly involving the omentum (Fig. 1). Histological examination of the Tru-cut needle biopsy showed loose connective tissue consisting of irregularly intersecting bundles of blended cells with modest nuclear atypia, intensely infiltrated by lymphoplasma cells (smooth muscle actin+/–; vimentin+; beta-catenin–; desmin–; Ki67 5%), suggesting a myofibroblastic tumor.

The mass continued to grow, and the associated symptomatology became increasingly worse and debilitating. The patient agreed to undergo surgical removal of the neoformation. Based on PET report, we started performing a diagnostic laparoscopy. After observing no connection between the mass and the abdominal cavity, we proceeded with a pubo-umbilical laparotomy and pointed out a voluminous yellow neoformation that started from the anterior sheath of the rectus muscles and extended to the subcutaneous adipose tissue (Fig. 2). We incised the sheath by involving approximately 2 cm of peripheral normal tissue using the LigaSure™ Small Jaw Open Sealer/Divider (Covidien, CO, USA). A good cleavage plan was found between the sheath and the rectus muscles, which were thus spared by excising the neoformation with the electric scalpel. The intraoperative histologic examination excluded a malignancy. The mass weighed approximately 300 g and measured 11 × 10 × 4 cm (Fig. 3). A biological mesh was applied. Final pathologic examination revealed the presence of striated muscular cells, a myofibroblastic

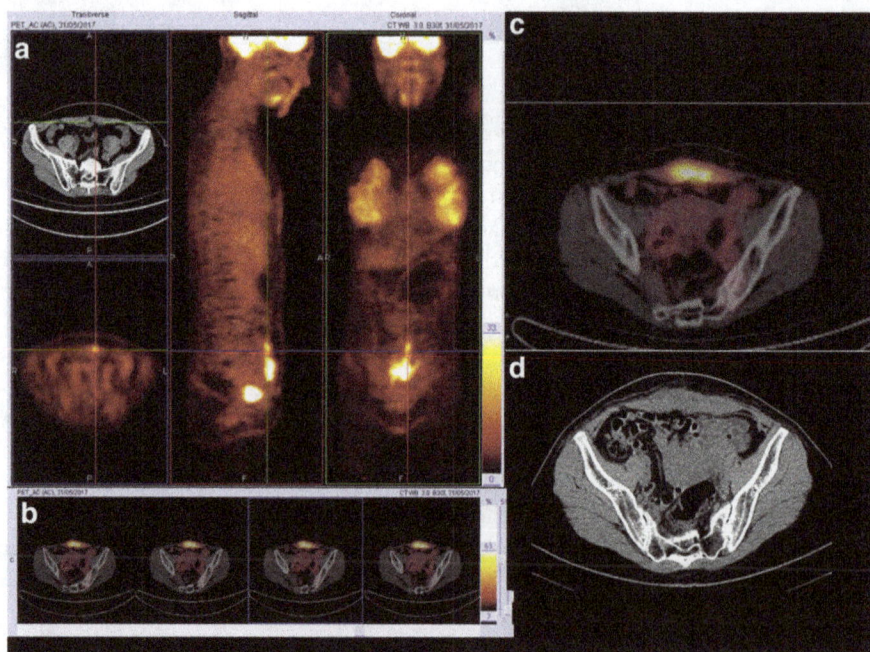

Fig. 1 Preoperative PET (**a–c**) and CT (**d**) scan showing the neoformation located in the in the context of the lower part of the rectus muscles of the abdomen. The PET showed an area of irregular and inhomogeneous hypercaptation in the context of the formation of the anterior abdominal wall with a very high maximum standardized uptake value (SUV max up to 12.9)

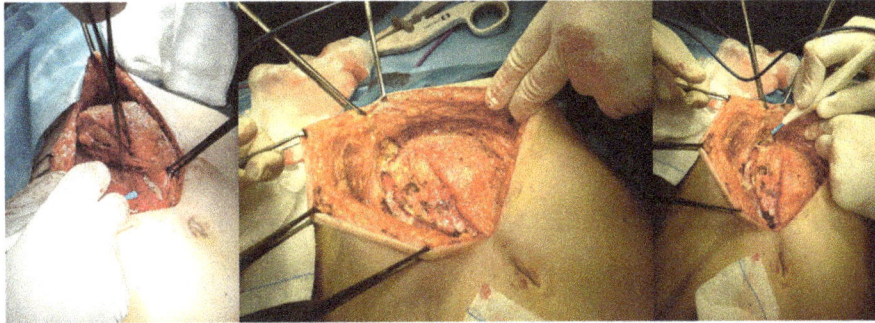

Fig. 2 Intraoperative pictures of surgery for abdominal wall neoformation. The mass started from the anterior sheath of the rectus muscle of the abdomen and extended to the adipose tissue of the subcutaneous layer

proliferation with giant cells resulting from foreign body reaction, granulocytes that infiltrated the adipose tissue (more typically present near sutures or centered on fetal squamous cells aggregates and keratin debris as observed in amniotic fluid (vernix caseosa), amorphous material compatible with meconium, and necrotic areas (Fig. 4). Immunohistochemistry showed positivity for smooth muscle actin and negativity for beta-catenin. Molecular analysis revealed a wild-type beta-catenin gene. Surgical margins were tumor-free. The final histological diagnosis was a foreign body granuloma.

To better characterize the inflammatory component of the neoformation, immediately after surgery, the cells obtained from mechanical and enzymatic degradation of the fresh tumor sample were separated by a discontinuous double density gradient (75–100% Ficoll-Hypaque), and their phenotype assessed by flow cytometry (Accuri C6, BD Biosciences, Erembodegem, Belgium) [7]. The cells isolated in the 75% gradient were threefold higher than those isolated in the 100% gradient. In the 100% gradient, cells were mainly activated T lymphocytes (CD3+/CD4+/Glut+, 47.6%; CD3+/CD8+/Glut+, 31.3%). Macrophages (CD14+) were the predominant cells (70%) in the 75% gradient; they were mostly M1 (CD14+/CD80+/Glut+, 48.9%) with less M2-polarized cells (CD14+/CD163+/Glut–, 20.4%) (M1/M2 ratio, 2.4). Additionally, in the 75% gradient, we found mesenchymal stem cells/fibrocytes (CD13+/CD14 –/Glut–, 13%; CD10+/CD33+/CD14–/Glut–, 10%).

Seven days following drainage removal, the patient presented with a subcutaneous effusion positive for *Klebsiella pneumoniae*. This required a percutaneous drainage within the fluid collection and infusion of 200 mg vancomycin in 10 mL saline solution through the drain twice a day for 7 days [8–10]. Since the problem did not resolve, we removed the mesh and used a medication with a single-use negative-pressure wound therapy system (PICO, Smith and Nephew, Hull, UK). Seven days after the removal of the wound therapy system, the patient was in optimal condition. Six months after surgery, she was disease-free.

Discussion

Tumors of the anterior abdominal wall constitute a rare class of neoplasia. A very important aspect of this clinical case is the unpredictability of its onset, making it unique and rare, being the case of a rare condition mimicking another rare conditions hence the need to describe it. In fact, the incidence of abdominal soft tissue sarcoma is about 2.8 cases per million per year (less than 5% of all soft tissue sarcomas) [1] similar to that of desmoid tumors, i.e., 2–4 cases per million per year [11], and the present case seems to be the first described in the literature. Desmoids preferentially develop in women of fertile age, especially during pregnancy and in puerperium. Hormonal factors such as pregnancy-related hyperestrogenism may favor their formation [3]. Since

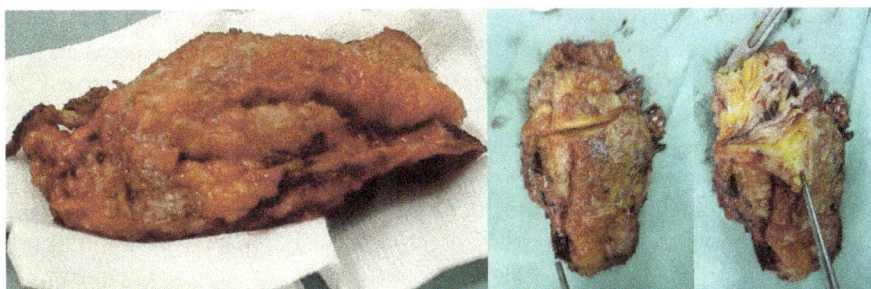

Fig. 3 Macroscopic view of the excised abdominal wall mass weighing approximately 300 g and sized 11 × 10 × 4 cm

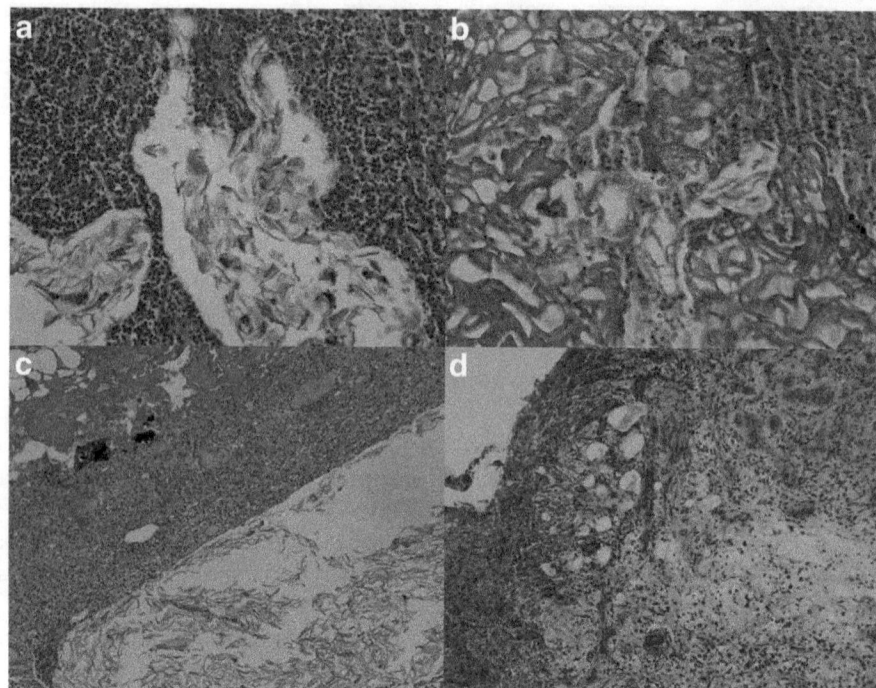

Fig. 4 Histological exam of the excised neoformation. **a** Keratin debris mixed with giant cells as for foreign body reaction (hematoxylin-eosin). **b** Keratin debris and meconium accompanied by inflammation that dissociates intensely edematous muscle tissue (hematoxylin-eosin). **c** Keratin debris surrounded by acute purulent inflammation, in the upper left amorphous brownish material referable to meconium (hematoxylin-eosin). **d** Granulation tissue and edema with evident neovascularization and presence of multinucleated giant cells (hematoxylin-eosin)

they may arise more frequently in the puerperium, traumas or microtraumas to the abdominal wall with consequent tissue correction may cause their onset [3]. Furthermore, surgery and inflammation may induce tumor growth. Typically, wound healing is a strictly controlled, self-limited process of tissue regeneration and remodeling. In response to tissue injury, mesenchymal cells are recruited to promote wound healing [12]; these pluripotent cells differentiate into fibroblasts, myofibroblasts, and endothelial cells. Therefore, the phenomena of repair, cicatrization, correction, and healing may lead to a series of events causing desmoid tumors, especially in people with a genetic predisposition to beta-catenin deregulation [11].

The present case showed a completely different clinical phenomenon. Although the symptomatic and growth characteristics of the neoformation resembled those of a desmoid tumor, the PET findings were positive, with a very high SUV. This influenced our presurgical diagnosis. In fact, desmoids are unlikely to be PET positive due to their low mitotic index, and if they are (but rarely), the SUV is very low [13]. One could also hypothesize a sarcoma caused by the sarcomatoid degeneration of residuals of the previous myomectomy. When a myomectomy is performed in confined spaces with the need for morcellation, the spillage of tissue components may occur, which over time, following adequate stimuli, may evolve into disseminated myomatosis and, in more serious cases, sarcomatoid degeneration

[6]. However, in our case, the preoperative biopsy did not confirm the suspicion of sarcoma but rather reinforced the hypothesis that it could be an atypical desmoid due to its high SUV index. According to the international guidelines [1], we performed a total surgical excision of the neoplasm. The definitive histology showed an extremely complex and rare problem; the desmoid nature was not confirmed (the lymphomonocytic component was prevalent, beta-catenin was negative, and the beta-catenin gene was wild type), but a foreign body granuloma was diagnosed. The foreign body consisted of amniotic fluid and meconium, suggesting either an inadequate cleaning of the cesarean incision site during suturing or, more probably, that these residuals triggered the generation of such peculiar inflammatory response in a likely predisposed woman. In fact, many women are exposed to meconium and amniotic fluid at the time of cesarean section, and the majority of them do not develop such an atypical inflammatory reaction. A foreign body reaction is usually characterized by inflammatory cell infiltration of mainly macrophages with foreign body giant cells, fibroblast activation, and peripheral fibrosis [14]. Macrophages have specific roles, including M1 or M2 polarization and the consequent difference in the storage of collagen and fibrosis [15]. At this regard, it should be emphasized our decision to proceed with the immunofluorescence analysis of the pseudotumor tissue by flow cytometry. We performed this peculiar, but greatly belonging to

A PET-positive rapidly growing mass of the abdominal wall after cesarean section...

227

our research expertise [7], assay specifically to understand the origin of the PET glucidic hypermetabolism and to better define the inflammatory component, considering that the intraoperative histology excluded the diagnosis of sarcoma. In our case, the analysis of the cell phenotype by flow cytometry demonstrated that M1-polarized Glut+ macrophages were the most dominant cell subsets. Therefore, the positive PET finding was certainly correlated to the high number of inflammatory cells, particularly CD14/Glut+ cells with high glucose uptake; meanwhile, the CD13+ and CD10+ cells were Glut–. These results confirm that the neoformation was an early granuloma that rapidly arose as a reaction to the spillage of meconium and keratinous material (vernix caseosa) present in the amniotic fluid in the subcutaneous tissue during cesarean section. The literature reports very rare cases of similar clinical conditions [16, 17], referred to as "organizing peritonitis, which included prominent collections of anucleate squamous cells in association with a foreign body-type granulomatous response" [16]. To our knowledge, this is the first case described in the literature.

Conclusions

The present paper provides information on an abdominal wall foreign body granuloma arisen from meconium and vernix caseosa after cesarean section, which is a unique and unpredictable condition that requires careful diagnosis and treatment. Different from sarcomas and desmoids, this atypical neoformation does not need a post-surgical follow-up and therefore it is essential to know how to diagnose it and not confuse it with other similar conditions. Thus, also atypical problems should be considered during the diagnostic and therapeutic phase emphasizing strongly a multidisciplinary approach to better planning its appropriate management.

Abbreviations
CT: Computed tomography; PET: Positron emission tomography; SUV: Standardized uptake value

Acknowledgements
The authors would like to thank Ivan Collu, Andreea Voicu, and Antonio Loffreda for their technical assistance. The work is supported by the "Associazione Sarda per la ricerca in Oncologia Ginecologica-ONLUS."

Authors' contributions
AM and CM contributed to the protocol development, data collection and management, data analysis, and manuscript writing/editing. PK, FL, GC, EM, and LM contributed to the data collection and management, data analysis, and manuscript editing. All authors read and approved the manuscript.

Competing interests
The authors declare that they have no competing interests.

Author details
[1]Department of Gynecologic Oncology, Azienda Ospedaliera Brotzu, via Edward Jenner, 09121 Cagliari, Italy. [2]Department of Pathology, Azienda Ospedaliera Brotzu, Cagliari, Italy. [3]Department of Nuclear Medicine, Azienda Ospedaliera Brotzu, Cagliari, Italy. [4]Department of Public Health and Medical Sciences, University of Cagliari, Cagliari, Italy.

References
1. Stojadinovic A, Hoos A, Karpoff HM, Leung DH, Antonescu CR, Brennan MF, Lewis JJ (2001) Soft tissue tumors of the abdominal wall: analysis of disease patterns and treatment. Arch Surg 136:70–79
2. Levy AD, Manning MA, Miettinen MM (2017) Soft-tissue sarcomas of the abdomen and pelvis: radiologic-pathologic features, part 2-uncommon sarcomas. Radiographics 37:797–812
3. Gurluler E, Gures N, Citil I, Kemik O, Berber I, Sumer A, Gurkan A (2014) Desmoid tumor in puerperium period: a case report. Clin Med Insights Case Rep 7:29–32
4. Har-Shai Y, Govrin-Yehudain J, Ullmann Y et al (1993) Dermatofibrosarcoma protuberans appearing during pregnancy. Ann Plast Surg 31:91–93
5. Ozel L, Sagiroglu J, Unal A, Unal E, Gunes P, Baskent E, Aka N, Titiz MI, Tufekci EC (2012) Abdominal wall endometriosis in the cesarean section surgical scar: a potential diagnostic pitfall. J Obstet Gynaecol Res 38(3):526–530
6. Macciò A, Chiappe G, Kotsonis P, Lavra F, Serra M, Demontis R, Madeddu C (2017) Abdominal leiomyosarcomatosis after surgery with external morcellation for occult smooth muscle tumors of uncertain malignant potential: a case report. Int J Surg Case Rep 38:107–110
7. Madeddu C, Gramignano G, Kotsonis P, Coghe F, Atzeni V, Scartozzi M, Macciò A (2018) Microenvironmental M1 tumor-associated macrophage polarization influences cancer-related anemia in advanced ovarian cancer: key role of Interleukin-6 [published online April 19, 2018]. Haematologica. https://doi.org/10.3324/haematol.2018.191551
8. Dietz UA, Spor L, Germer CT (2018) Management of mesh-related infections. Chirurg 82:208–217
9. Meagher H, Clarke Moloney M, Grace PA (2015) Conservative management of mesh-site infection in hernia repair surgery: a case series. Hernia 19:231–237
10. Narkhede R, Shah NM, Dalal PR, Mangukia C, Dholaria S (2015) Postoperative mesh infection-still a concern in laparoscopic era. Indian J Surg 77(4):322–326
11. Skubitz KM (2017) Biology and treatment of aggressive fibromatosis or desmoid tumor. Mayo Clin Proc 92:947–964
12. Wu Y, Chen L, Scott PG, Tredget EE (2007) Mesenchymal stem cells enhance wound healing through differentiation and angiogenesis. Stem Cells 25: 2648–2659
13. Basu S, Nair N, Banavali S (2007) Uptake characteristics of fluorodeoxyglucose (FDG) in deep fibromatosis and abdominal desmoids: potential clinical role of FDG-PET in the management. Br J Radiol 80:750–756
14. Williams GT, Williams WJ (1983) Granulomatous inflammation--a review. J Clin Pathol 36:723–733
15. Shapouri-Moghaddam A, Mohammadian S, Vazini H, Taghadosi M, Esmaeili SA, Mardani F, Seifi B, Mohammadi A, Afshari JT, Sahebkar A (2018) Macrophage plasticity, polarization, and function in health and disease. J Cell Physiol 233(9):6425–6440
16. George E, Leyser S, Zimmer HL, Simonowitz DA, Agress RL, Nordin DD (1995) Vernix caseosa peritonitis. An infrequent complication of cesarean section with distinctive histopathologic features. Am J Clin Pathol 103:681–684
17. Stuart OA, Morris AR, Baber RJ (2009) Vernix caseosa peritonitis - no longer rare or innocent: a case series. J Med Case Rep 3:60

35

Laparoscopic-guided transversus abdominis plane block versus trocar site local anesthetic infiltration in gynecologic laparoscopy

Ibrahim A. El sharkwy[*], Elsayed H. Noureldin, Ekramy A. Mohamed and Ali A. Mohamed

Abstract

Background: Relieving postoperative pain and prompt resumption of physical activity are of the utmost importance for the patients and surgeons. Infiltration of local anesthetic is frequently used methods of pain control postoperatively. Laparoscopically delivered transversus abdominis plane block is a new modification of ultrasound-guided transversus abdominis plane block.

This study was conducted to compare the efficacy of laparoscopic-guided transversus abdominis plane block with trocar site local anesthetic infiltration for pain control after gynecologic laparoscopy.

Results: No statistically significant difference between the two groups in mean visual analogue scale at 1, 18, and 24 h ($P = 0.34$, $P = 0.41$, and $P = 0.61$, respectively), while the mean visual analogue scale was significantly lower in the laparoscopic-guided transversus abdominis plane block group than in the trocar site local anesthetic infiltration group at 3, 6, and 12 h ($P = 0.049$, $P = 0.011$, and $P = 0.042$, respectively). No statistically significant difference was observed in the cumulative narcotics consumed at 3 h ($P = 0.52$); however, women with transversus abdominis plane block have consumed significantly less amount of narcotics than women with trocar site infiltration at 6, 12, and 24 h ($P = 0.04$, $P = 0.038$, and $P = 0.031$ respectively). Patient satisfaction was significantly higher in the laparoscopic-guided transversus abdominis plane block group ($P = 0.035$).

Conclusion: Laparoscopic-guided transversus abdominis plane block is more effective in reduction of both pain scores in the early postoperative period and the cumulative narcotics consumption than trocar site local anesthetic infiltration in gynecologic laparoscopy.

Keywords: Laparoscopic guided, Transversus abdominis plane block, Trocar site, Local anesthetic infiltration gynecologic laparoscopy

Background

Laparoscopic intervention, with very low mortality, minimal morbidity, fast recovery, the best cosmetic outcome, and the least postoperative pain, has gained a major participation in gynecologic surgery throughout the past two decades [1]. During laparoscopic surgery, inflation of the abdomen provides the surgeon a perfect view of the structures and a room to work [2]. Relieving postoperative pain and prompt resumption of physical activity are of the

utmost importance for the patients and surgeons [3]. Block of abdominal wall and infiltration of local anesthetic are frequently used methods of pain control postoperatively [4]. Transversus abdominis plane (TAP) block is a recent regional anesthetic modality that anesthetizes the afferent neural pathway of the anterior abdominal wall. This is mediated through injecting a local anesthetic between the transversus abdominis muscle and the internal oblique muscle [5]. TAP block was shown to be effective means for pain control after open and laparoscopic gynecological surgeries [6]. Laparoscopically delivered

* Correspondence: Ibrahimsharkwy@yahoo.com
Faculty of Medicine, Zagazig University, Zagazig, Egypt

TAP block is a new modification of ultrasound-guided TAP block, it allows injection of the local anesthetic in the appropriate place directed by the laparoscopic camera [7]. Local anesthetic infiltration at the site of the surgical wound was validated as a postoperative analgesia [8]. The aim of this study was to compare the efficacy of laparoscopic-guided transversus abdominis plane block with trocar site local anesthetic infiltration for pain control after gynecologic laparoscopy.

Methods

Our prospective single-blinded randomized controlled clinical trial was carried out in the Department of Obstetrics and Gynecology, Faculty of Medicine, Zagazig University, after approval by the University Ethics Committee. A written informed consent was provided by all participants.

Inclusion criteria included women who are scheduled for gynecological laparoscopic intervention and 18 years old and older. Women with chronic pain syndrome, allergy to local anesthetic, and postoperative intraperitoneal drain and women needed alteration to laparotomy were excluded from the study. Consenting eligible women were allocated randomly to either laparoscopic-guided transversus abdominis plane block or trocar site local anesthetic infiltration. Randomization was created by the computer. Allocation was concealed in opaque, sealed, and serially numbered envelopes. Patients and postoperative assistants were blinded to the procedure while, surgeons and anesthetists were not.

For laparoscopic-guided transversus abdominis plane block group, at the end of the procedure and before release of pneumoperitoneum, laparoscopic camera allowed direct internal visualization of the selected area, between the iliac crest and the costal margin in the mid-axillary line, where the TAP block will be inserted. The surgeon introduced a needle through the skin and felt the 2-pops representing the 2 fascial planes. Visualization helped the surgeon to reach the proper space between the internal oblique and transversus abdominis muscles. If the needle tip exceeded the transversus abdominis muscle and was directly beyond or penetrated the peritoneum, the surgeon should withdraw it back 3–5 mm to be in the correct place. Twenty to 25 ml of 0.25% bupivacaine with epinephrine was injected on each side after an initial negative aspiration. After completing injection, a bulge was demonstrated owing to pooling of the local anesthetic behind transversus abdominis muscles and the peritoneum.

For trocar site local anesthetic infiltration group, 10 ml of 0.25% bupivacaine with epinephrine was injected around the umbilical port opening. Five milliliters was injected around each one of the essential two and any extra 5-mm laparoscopic port openings at the end of the procedure.

Demographic and preoperative data like age, body mass index (BMI), type of operation, and the total operative time were collected. During surgery, all patients received the same intravenous analgesia according to body weight (fentanyl 1.5 mcg /kg) by the anesthesiologist. They did not receive analgesics, immediately after surgery, in the post anesthesia care unit till complete recovery. In the postoperative ward, they received the standard postoperative analgesics. Our department protocol is 1 g intravenous paracetamol every 8 h and intravenous meperidine 20 mg every time the patients need analgesia. Postoperative pain was assessed at 1, 3, 6, 12, 18, and 24 h with a 10-point visual analogue scale (VAS), with a range of 0 (indicating no pain) to 10 (indicating the worst pain). The cumulative meperidine consumed on request was calculated at 3, 6, 12, and 24 h. Patient satisfaction was reported on a scale from 0 (indicating very poor satisfaction) and 10 (indicating excellent satisfaction) at 24 h.

The primary outcome was the difference in pain scores at 1, 3, 6, 12, 18, and 24 h between the two groups. The secondary outcomes were the difference in the cumulative meperidine consumed at 3, 6, 12, and 24 h, in addition to the difference in patient satisfaction at 24 h between the two groups.

Sample size calculation was based on a previous suggestion that two-point difference in VAS between the two groups would be clinically expressive [9]. With a suggested standard deviation of difference to be 4, each group should contain 34 women to provide this difference with 80% power and statistical significance of 0.05. Five women were added to compensate for an assumed 15% dropout, so at least 39 women should be included in each group.

Results

Between May 2016 and June 2017, a total of 105 women were assessed for eligibility. Of them, 90 gave consent for the study. They were allocated randomly to laparoscopic-guided TAP block group ($n = 45$) or trocar site local anesthetic infiltration group ($n = 45$). Four women were excluded from analysis due to lack of visual analogue pain scores: one woman in the laparoscopic-guided TAP block group and three women in the trocar site local anesthetic infiltration group. Two women in each group were excluded from analysis due to insertion of intraperitoneal drain (Fig. 1).

Age, weight, time of operation, and type of operation in both groups were comparable. Patient satisfaction was significantly higher in the laparoscopic guided TAP block group than the trocar site local anesthetic infiltration group (Table 1).

There was no statistically significant difference between the two groups in mean visual analogue scale at 1, 18, and 24 h ($P = 0.34$, $P = 0.41$, and $P = 0.61$, respectively), while mean visual analogue scale was significantly lower in the laparoscopic-guided TAP block group than the trocar site local anesthetic infiltration group at 3, 6, and 12 h ($P = 0.049$, $P = 0.011$ and $P = 0.042$, respectively) (Table 2).

No statistically significant difference was observed in the cumulative meperidine consumed at 3 h between the laparoscopic-guided TAP block group 55 ± 18 mg and the trocar site local anesthetic infiltration group 76 ± 23 mg ($P = 0.52$). However, cumulative meperidine consumed in TAP block group was significantly less than trocar site infiltration group at 6, 12, and 24 h ($P = 0.04$, $P = 0.038$, and $P = 0.031$ respectively) (Table 3).

Discussion

Opioids, NSAIDs, and paracetamol are effective postoperative analgesics, but their use is not without complications [10]. Inclusion of TAP block in the postoperative multi-modal analgesia protocols has reduced the use of the other analgesics and the related side effects [11].

In the first described TAP block, a blunt needle was introduced blindly through the external and the internal oblique muscles, guided by the double- pop technique. The local anesthetic was injected between the transverse abdominis and the internal oblique muscles. This method has resulted in some penetrative injuries, and sometimes, it fails to gain the proper anesthetic effect [5]. Recently, ultrasound-guided TAP block has increased the efficacy and safety of the procedure through visualization of the needle tip and the local anesthetic injection site [12]. But, the technique needs great skills also; minimal complications have been described [13].

Previous randomized trials have reported the efficacy of the ultrasound-guided TAP block as a postoperative analgesia after open appendectomy, laparoscopic cholecystectomy, and abdominal hysterectomy [14–16]. Similarly, it has gained a specific analgesic advantage in gynecologic laparoscopic intervention where tissue trauma and pain were minimal to moderate [17–20]. Nevertheless, such postoperative analgesic efficacy of ultrasound-guided TAP block was not confirmed, when compared with trocar site local anesthetic infiltration

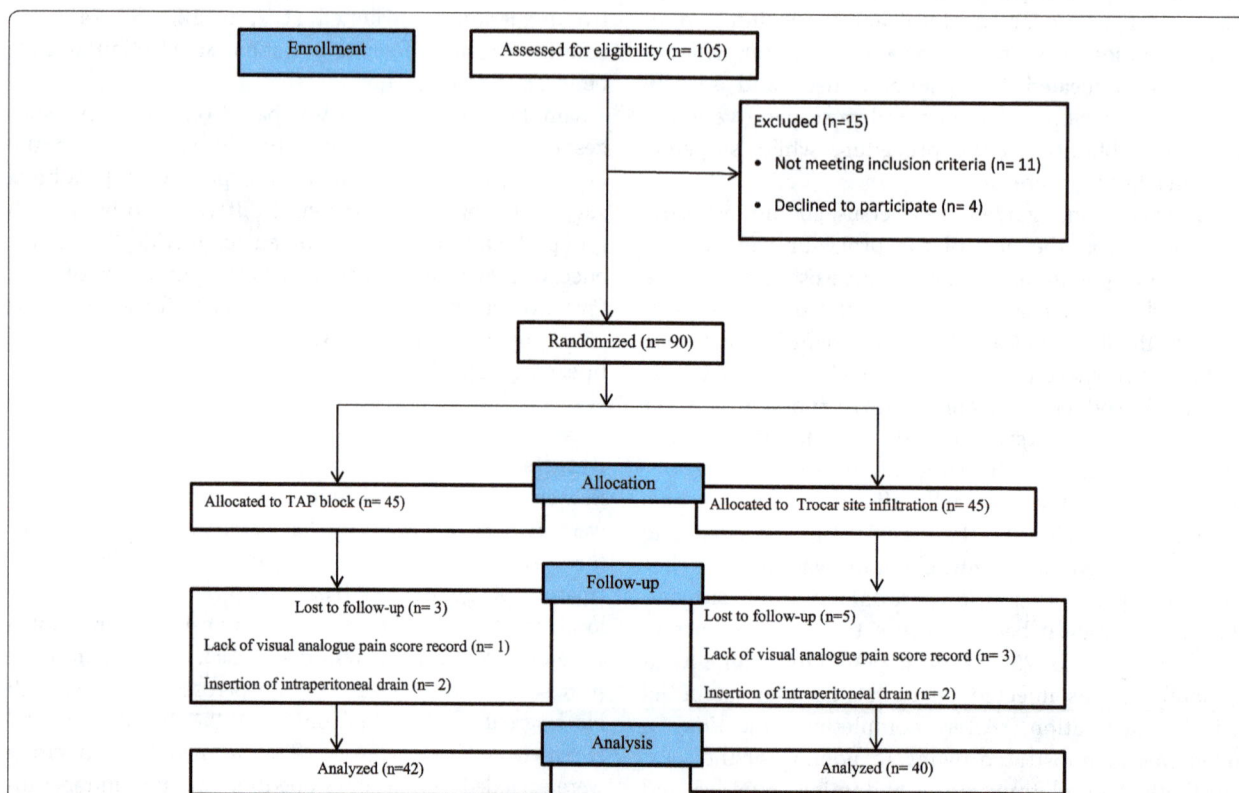

Fig. 1 Patient flowchart. A total of 105 women were assessed for eligibility. Of them, 90 gave consent for the study. They were allocated randomly to laparoscopic-guided TAP block group ($n = 45$) or trocar site local anesthetic infiltration group ($n = 45$). Four women were excluded from analysis due to lack of visual analogue pain scores: one woman in the laparoscopic-guided TAP block group and three women in the trocar site local anesthetic infiltration group. Two women in each group were excluded from analysis due to insertion of intraperitoneal drain

Laparoscopic-guided transversus abdominis plane block versus trocar site local anesthetic...

231

Table 1 Demographic and clinical characteristics of patients

	TAP block group (n = 42)	Trocar site group (n = 40)	P value
Age (years)	38.5 ± 9.1	38.8 ± 10.2	0.91
Weight (BMI)	26.9 ± 6.8	27.2 ± 6.6	0.87
Time of operation (min)	77.5 ± 35.1	84.6 ± 38.3	0.32
Type of operation			0.56
Ovarian cystectomy	8 (19%)	9 (22%)	
Salpingectomy	8 (19%)	5 (12%)	
LSH	5 (12%)	6 (15%)	
TLH	10 (24%)	12 (30%)	
Laparoscopic myomectomy	5 (12%)	3 (8%)	
Presacral neurectomy	3 (7%)	1 (3%)	
Sacrocolpopexy	3 (7%)	4 (10%)	
Patient satisfaction	7.6 ± 2.4	5.1 ± 2.3	0.035

BMI body mass index, LSH laparoscopic supracervical hysterectomy, TLH total laparoscopic hysterectomy

following laparoscopic cholecystectomy [21] and spinal morphine after cesarean delivery [22].

Local anesthetic injection in the neurovascular plane between the internal oblique and transversus abdominis muscles under laparoscopic vision was first described by Magee et al. [7]. Afterward, Chetwood et al. [23] used a similar method following laparoscopic nephrectomy which was safe and time saving. In addition, laparoscopic-guided TAP block has reduced postoperative pain scores after laparoscopic cholecystectomy [24, 25] and laparoscopic ventral hernia repair [26].

Favuzza and Delaney [27] stated that laparoscopic-guided TAP block has resulted in effective pain relief, reduction in narcotic requirement and short postoperative hospital stay in patients who underwent laparoscopic colorectal surgery. The addition of laparoscopic-guided TAP block to enhanced recovery pathway (ERP) was safe, effective, and allowed early discharge of patients following laparoscopic colorectal surgery [28–30].

Postoperative local anesthetic injection into trocar insertion sites after laparoscopic gynecologic surgery has reduced pain scores significantly in early postoperative period compared with placebo [31]. On the other hand, pain scores reduction was not significant [32].

Table 2 Mean visual analogue scale at different time points

Hour	TAP block group (n = 42)	Trocar site group (n = 40)	P value
1	1.3 ± 0.7	1.6 ± 0.9	0.34
3	1.7 ± 1.1	2.14 ± 0.7	0.049
6	2.15 ± 0.2	3.1 ± 0.8	0.011
12	1.9 ± 0.2	2.7 ± 0.4	0.042
18	1.2 ± 0.6	1.6 ± 0.5	0.41
24	0.7 ± 0.8	0.9 ± 1.0	0.61

Table 3 Cumulative narcotics (meperidine in mg) consumed at different time points

Hour	TAP block group (n = 42)	Trocar site group (n = 40)	P value
3	55 ± 18	76 ± 23	0.52
6	71 ± 22	96 ± 21	0.04
12	99 ± 31	117 ± 28	0.038
24	111 ± 15	132 ± 23	0.031

Various studies have compared ultrasound-guided TAP block with trocar site local anesthetic infiltration. The results varied from significant reduction [33] to non-significant reduction [34] in cumulative morphine use at 24 h with TAP blocks compared with local anesthetic infiltration. A recent trial [35] has reported that ultrasound-guided TAP block has no significant clinical benefit over trocar site local anesthetic infiltration in laparoscopic nephrectomy. Huang et al. [36] found that the combination of TAP block and trocar sites local anesthetic infiltration provided better analgesic effect than TAP block alone.

To the best of our knowledge, few trials studied the efficacy of laparoscopic-guided TAP block. In consistence with our results, laparoscopic-guided TAP block decreased both postoperative pain and opioid use after laparoscopic ventral hernia repair [26]. Furthermore, it was safe and efficient analgesic in elderly patients who underwent elective laparoscopic cholecystectomy [25]. On the contrary, El Hachem et al. [37] found that neither laparoscopic-guided TAP block nor ultrasound-guided TAP block offered postoperative analgesic superiority over trocar site local anesthetic infiltration after four ports gynecologic laparoscopy. Although the local anesthetic was injected at the end of operation similar to our study, but this difference in the results could be attributed to the dissimilarity in local anesthetic doses or the special methodology of the other study. Patients were divided into two groups: one group consisted of unilateral anesthesiologist-administeredultrasound-guided TAP block and the other group consisted of unilateral surgeon- administered laparoscopic-guided TAP block. In both groups, the contralateral port sites were infiltrated with local anesthetic. VAS pain score was recorded on the TAP block and contralateral sides, using the patients as their own controls.

Conclusions

In conclusion, laparoscopic-guided TAP block is more effective in reduction of both pain scores in the early postoperative period and cumulative meperidine consumption than trocar site local anesthetic infiltration in gynecologic laparoscopy.

The present study had some limitations, pain scores on movement were not assessed, blinding of surgeons and anesthetists was difficult, and it did not focus on side effects. So, further properly blinded studies containing large number of patients and using different doses of local anesthetic are required to verify these results.

Abbreviations
BMI: Body mass index; ERP: Enhanced recovery pathway; LSH: Laparoscopic supracervical hysterectomy; NSAIDs: Non-steroidal anti-inflammatory drugs; TAP: Transversus abdominis plane; TLH: Total laparoscopic hysterectomy; VAS: Visual analogue scale

Acknowledgements
We would like to thank our unit's residents and nurses for help.

Authors' contributions
IAE and EHN participated in the project development and data collection. EAM and AAM participated in the data collection and manuscript writing. All authors read and approved the final manuscript.

Authors' information
I A Elsharkwy: His fields of interest are laparoscopy and feto-maternal medicine. Has many papers published in the field of obstetrics and gynecology.

Ethics approval and consent to participate

- Ethical Approval: The study was approved by the ethics Committee of Zagazig University
- Informed consent: Informed consent was obtained from all individual participants included in the study.
- Statement of human rights: All procedures performed in studies involving human participants were in accordance with the ethical standards of the institutional and/or national research committee and with the 1964 Helsinki declaration and its later amendments or comparable ethical standards.

Competing interests
The authors declare that they have no competing interests.

References
1. Nieboer TE, Hendriks JC, Bongers MY, Vierhout ME, Kluivers KB (2012) Quality of life after laparoscopic and abdominal hysterectomy: a randomized controlled trial. Obstet Gynecol 119:85–91
2. Garry R, Fountain J, Mason S et al (2004) The eVALuate study; two parallel randomised trials, one comparing laparoscopic with abdominal hysterectomy, the other comparing laparoscopic with vaginal hysterectomy. Br Med J 328:129
3. Kulen FT, Tihan D, Duman U, Bayam E, Zaim G (2016) Laparoscopic partial cholecystectomy: a safe and effective alternative surgical technique in difficult cholecystectomies. Turk J Surg 32:185–190
4. Bamigboye AA, Hofmeyr GJ (2010) Caesarean section wound infiltration with local anesthesia for postoperative pain relief - any benefit? S Afr Med J 100:313–319
5. Rafi AN (2001) Abdominal field block: a new approach via the lumbar triangle. Anesthesia 56:1024–1027
6. Sivapurapu V, Vasudevan A, Gupta S, Badhe AS (2013) Comparison of analgesic efficacy of transversus abdominis plane block with direct infiltration of local anesthetic into surgical incision in lower abdominal gynecological surgeries. J Anaesthesiol Clin Pharmacol 29:71–75
7. Magee C, Clarke C, Lewis A (2011) Laparoscopic TAP block for laparoscopic cholecystectomy: description of a novel technique. Surgeon 9:352–353

8. Gupta A (2005) Local anesthesia for pain relief after laparoscopic cholecystectomy–a systematic review. Best Pract Res Clin Anesthesiol 19:275–292
9. Farrar JT, Portenoy RK, Berlin JA, Kinman JL, Strom BL (2000) Defining the clinically important difference in pain outcome measures. Pain 88:287–294
10. Eslamian L, Jalili Z, Jamal A et al (2012) Transversus abdominis plane block reduces postoperative pain intensity and analgesic consumption in elective cesarean delivery under general anesthesia. J Anesth 26:334–338
11. Fusco P, Scimia P, Paladini G et al (2015) Transversus abdominis plane block for analgesia after cesarean delivery. A systematic review. Minerva Anestesiol 81:195–204
12. Lancaster P, Chadwick M (2010) Liver trauma secondary to ultrasound-guided transversus plane block. Br J An esth 104:509
13. Sandeman DJ, Bennett M, Dilley AV et al (2011) Ultrasound-guided transversus abdominis plane blocks for laparoscopic appendicectomy in children: a prospective randomized trial. Br J Anesth 106:882–886
14. Niraj G, Searle A, Mathews M, Misra V, Baban M, Kiani S et al (2009) Analgesic efficacy of ultrasound-guided transversus abdominis plane block in patients undergoing open appendicectomy. Br J Anesth 103:601–605
15. El-Dawlatly AA, Turkistani A, Kettner SC, Machata AM, Delvi MB, Thallaj A et al (2009) Ultrasound-guided transversus abdominis plane block: description of a new technique and comparison with conventional systemic analgesia during laparoscopic cholecystectomy. Br J Anesth 102:763–767
16. Carney J, McDonnell JG, Ochana A, Bhinder R, Laffey JG (2008) The transversus abdominis plane block provides effective postoperative analgesia in patients undergoing total abdominal hysterectomy. Anesth Analg 107:2056–2060
17. De Oliveira GS Jr, Fitzgerald PC, Marcus RJ, Ahmad S, McCarthy RJ (2011) A dose-ranging study of the effect of transversus abdominis block on postoperative quality of recovery and analgesia after outpatient laparoscopy. Anesth Analg 113:1218–1225
18. Pather S, Loadsman JA, Gopalan PD, Rao A, Philp S, Carter J (2011) The role of transversus abdominis plane blocks in women undergoing total laparoscopic hysterectomy: a retrospective review. Aust N Z J Obstet Gynaecol 51:544–547
19. Champaneria R, Shah L, Geoghegan J, Gupta JK, Daniels JP (2013) Analgesic effectiveness of transversus abdominis plane blocks after hysterectomy: a meta-analysis. Eur J Obstet Gynecol Reprod Biol 166:1–9
20. Kawahara R, Tamai Y, Yamasaki K, Okuno S, Hanada R, Funato T (2015) The analgesic efficacy of ultrasound-guided transversus abdominis plane block with mid-axillary approach after gynecologic laparoscopic surgery: a randomized controlled trial. J Anaesthesiol Clin Pharmacol 31:67–71
21. Ortiz J, Suliburk JW, Wu K, Bailard NS, Mason C, Minard CG et al (2012) Bilateral transversus abdominis plane block does not decrease postoperative pain after laparoscopic cholecystectomy when compared with local anesthetic infiltration of trocar insertion sites. Reg Anesth Pain Med 37:188–192
22. McMorrow RC, Ni Mhuircheartaigh RJ, Ahmed KA, Aslani A, Ng SC, Conrick-Martin I et al (2011) Comparison of transversus abdominis plane block vs spinal morphine for pain relief after Caesarean section. Br J Anesth 106:706–712
23. Chetwood A, Agrawal S, Hrouda D, Doyle P (2011) Laparoscopic assisted transversus abdominis plane block: a novel insertion technique during laparoscopic nephrectomy. Anesthesia 66:317–318
24. Elamin G, Waters PS, Hamid H, O'keeffe HM, Waldron RM, Duggan MS (2015) Efficacy of a laparoscopically delivered transversus abdominis plane block technique during elective laparoscopic cholecystectomy: a prospective, double-blind randomized trial. J Am Coll Surg 221:335–344
25. Tihan D, Totoz T, Tokocin M, Ercan G, Calikoglu TK, Vartanoglu T (2016) Efficacy of laparoscopic transversus abdominis plane block for elective laparoscopic cholecystectomy in elderly patients. Bosn J Basic Med Sci 16:139–144
26. Fields AC, Gonzalez DO, Chin EH, Nguyen SQ, Zhang LP, Divino CM (2015) Laparoscopic-assisted transversus abdominis plane block for postoperative pain control in laparoscopic ventral hernia repair: a randomized controlled trial. J Am Coll Surg 221:462–469
27. Favuzza J, Delaney CP (2013) Laparoscopic-guided transversus abdominis plane block for colorectal surgery. Dis Colon Rectum 56:389–391
28. Favuzza J, Delaney CP (2013) Outcomes of discharge after elective laparoscopic colorectal surgery with transversus abdominis plane blocks and enhanced recovery pathway. J Am Coll Surg 217:503–506
29. Alvarez MP, Foley KE, Zebley DM, Fassler SA (2014) Comprehensive enhanced recovery pathway significantly reduces postoperative length of stay and opioid usage in elective laparoscopic colectomy. Surg Endosc 29:1–6

30. Keller DS, Ermlich BO, Delaney CP (2014) Demonstrating the benefits of transversus abdominis plane blocks on patient outcomes in laparoscopic colorectal surgery: review of 200 consecutive cases. J Am Coll Surg 219: 1143–1148

31. Selcuk S, Api M, Polat M, Arinkan A, Aksoy B, Akca T et al (2016) Effectiveness of local anesthetic on postoperative pain in different levels of laparoscopic gynecological surgery. Arch Gynecol Obstet 293:1279–1285

32. Tam T, Harkins G, Wegrzyniak L, Ehrgood S, Kunselman A, Davies M (2014) Infiltration of bupivacaine local anesthetic to trocar insertion sites after laparoscopy: a randomized, double blind, stratified, and controlled trial. J Minim Invasive Gynecol 21:1015–1021

33. Park JS, Choi GS, Kwak KH, Jung H, Jeon Y, Park S (2015) Effect of local wound infiltration and transversus abdominis plane block on morphine use after laparoscopic colectomy: a nonrandomized, single-blind prospective study. J Surg Res 195:61–66

34. Bava EP, Ramachandran R, Rewari V, Chandralekha, Bansal VK, Trikha A (2016) Analgesic efficacy of ultrasound guided transversus abdominis plane block versus local anesthetic infiltration in adult patients undergoing single incision laparoscopic cholecystectomy: a randomized controlled trial. Anesth Essays Res 10:561–567

35. Araújo AM, Guimarães J, Nunes CS, Couto PS, Amadeu E (2017) Post-operative pain after ultrasound transversus abdominis plane block versus trocar site infiltration in laparoscopic nephrectomy: a prospective study. Rev Bras Anestesiol. https://doi.org/10.1016/j.bjan.2016.08.008

36. Huang S, Mi S, He Y, Li Y, Wang S (2016) Analgesic efficacy of trocar sites local anesthetic infiltration with and without transversus abdominis plane block after laparoscopic hysterectomy: a randomized trial. Int J Clin Exp Med 9:6518–6524

37. El Hachem L, Small E, Chung P, Moshier EL, Friedman K, Fenske SS et al (2015) Randomized controlled double-blind trial of transversus abdominis plane block versus trocar site infiltration in gynecologic laparoscopy. Am J Obstet Gynecol 212:182.e1–182.e9

36

Comparing self-assessment of laparoscopic technical skills with expert opinion for gynecological surgeons in an operative setting

Rami Kilani

Abstract

Background: Competence in laparoscopic skills is important for all gynaecological surgeons. Most residency programmes teach technical skills in the operating room and through lectures, where the evaluation of surgical skills is usually done through subjective evaluation. After graduating residency, most surgeons depend on themselves to decide if they are competent in performing a certain procedure. The objective of this study is to evaluate the accuracy of surgeon self-assessment compared with expert assessment of competence in laparoscopic surgical skills. A double-blind prospective cohort study was undertaken at Prince Hamza Hospital between January 2016 and April 2016 in Amman, Jordan. Eight practicing gynecologists and obstetricians performed and recorded 88 laparoscopic procedures including ovarian cystectomy, salpingectomy for ectopic pregnancy, salpingoophorectomy, resection of endometriosis, adhesiolysis and ovarian drilling. Participating gynecologists recorded the procedures and were asked to complete a Global Rating Index of Technical Skills (GRITS) evaluation after the surgery testing across multiple areas with a lowest score of 8 and a highest score of 40. Two well-versed laparoscopic experts in objective structured assessment of technical skills (OSATS) also independently scored all procedures using the same parameters. The correlation coefficient and internal consistency were calculated.

Results: The GRITS score was calculated for each participant with a mean assessment score of 3.47 for each parameter. Participants self-assessment scores were significantly higher than expert assessment scores (p<0.05). The correlation coefficient was calculated and it can be seen that there was high inter-expert correlation in assessment across all participants evaluations (ICC > 0.90).

Conclusion: Self-assessment of surgical laparoscopic skills is higher than expert evaluation of these technical skills. Quality assurance measures need to be revisited and restructured through more frequent assessments using peer and expert assessment alongside self-assessment. Gynecologists also need to undergo proper assessment prior to starting independently performing procedures that require new skills.

Keywords: Global Rating Index of Technical Skills (GRITS), Objective structured assessment of technical skills (OSATS), Intra-class correlation coefficient (ICC), Continuing Professional Development (CPD), Self-assessment, Surgical skills, Expert assessment

Correspondence: rkilani2000@yahoo.com
Hashemite University, Zarqa, Jordan

Background

Accurate self-assessment of knowledge and technical skills is essential for the safe and effective practice of medicine. Davis Boud defines self-assessment in his book "Enhancing Learning Through Self-Assessment" as the act of judging ourselves and making decisions about the next step. Boud's opinion is that assessment can only be conducted against specific benchmarks or criteria [1]. Gordon published a systematic review on trainees from different health professions, college students, and graduate trainees [2]. The researchers explored self-assessment relative to an objective standard or an expert's evaluation and concluded that self-assessment is fundamental to continuing medical competency and that self-assessment coupled with a specific set of criteria may lead to an improved outcome and more skilled professionals. Sullivan and Hall suggest that self-assessment promotes reflection on self-performance and motivates learners to react accordingly [3]. The application of the aforementioned concepts in medicine and specifically in laparoscopic surgery could lead to accurate self-assessment of performance by surgeons. This could eventually lead to the proper identification of strengths and weaknesses and allow the individual to create a plan for improvement.

Barnsley et al. looked at junior doctor self-assessment regarding confidence and competence of clinical skills versus objective assessment [4]. The researchers found no correlation between self-assessment and objective assessment. MacDonald et al. compared self-assessment of technical skills with simulator data in second and third year medical students with no previous exposure to laparoscopic training [5]. This selected task required the operator to pick up the target with one grasper and place it in the target box without releasing the target. Medical students were asked to evaluate their performance, and their evaluation was compared to the simulator data. The study found that self-assessment improves with repetition. Other researchers looked at resident self-assessment versus faculty assessment in performing laparoscopic procedures and found that residents were more critical of their performance than faculty members [6].

Arora et al. recently looked at self-assessment in technical and non-technical skills among surgical residents in a simulated environment [7]. Surgeons were asked to perform a laparoscopic cholecystectomy in a simulated laboratory. Two experts assessed the technical skills of surgeons, whereby the first expert watched the procedure live from a control room while the second expert evaluated technical skills after watching a video recording of the procedure. Both participants and experts used a validated objective tool. This study concluded that residents are accurate in self-assessment of their technical skills. However, that particular study and most literature examining this area of research face limitations to their experiments including small sample sizes and the use of simulated procedures rather than actual procedures. According to the data that was collected, no evidence was found of a published study investigating self-assessment of laparoscopic technical skills of practicing gynecological surgeons performing specific procedures and comparing the evaluation to an external evaluator assessment. Thus, the aim of this study is to examine the use of self-assessment comparatively between gynecologists and experts with a large pool of participants performing laparoscopic procedures in the operative setting.

Methods

Examination process

Jordanian surgeons have adopted minimally invasive surgical techniques similarly to their counterparts in different areas of the world. Most Jordanian surgeons acquire the new skills through attending courses, workshops, and shadowing colleagues who have more experience in minimally invasive procedures. Privileges to perform surgeries are granted by the hospital based on qualifications. There is no official Jordanian recertification program after passing the specialty board exams, and the continuous medical education program is still at the early stages of development which makes a surgeon's self-assessment of technical skills significantly more important.

The project is a prospective study. Participants are Jordanian board-certified obstetricians and gynecologists with privileges to practice at Prince Hamzah Hospital.

Candidates were approached by the primary investigator in the time period between January 2016 and April 2016 to participate in the study. They were supplied with an information leaflet explaining the research project, objectives, methods, and tasks involved. Surgeons who agreed to participate signed a consent form and were given a tutorial by the primary investigator on the Global Rating Index of Technical Skills (GRIT). This involved a 20-min session to familiarize them with the evaluation criteria and instructions on how to complete the evaluation form. An instruction sheet with all tutorial information was supplied to all participating surgeons. An example of a videotaped performance with predetermined scores was also shown to all participants.

Operative laparoscopic procedures including laparoscopic oophorectomy, laparoscopic ovarian cystectomy, laparoscopic salpingectomy, and adhesiolysis were evaluated. These procedures were chosen because they are the most common laparoscopic procedures performed at Prince Hamzah Hospital. Both gynecologists and external assessors were familiar with those procedures. The aforementioned procedures were also considered "short" procedures, thereby making the video assessment stage less time consuming.

The surgical lists at Prince Hamzah Hospital were reviewed the day prior to the surgery, and all participating gynecologists with operative laparoscopy cases were reminded to record the case and complete the GRIT. Emergency cases were also included, and the on-call gynecologist was asked to record the case and complete the form as well. The GRIT evaluation forms (Additional file 1) were available in all the gynecological operative suites. Extra copies were also available in a nearby office. The patients were not asked for permission to record the cases in accordance with the United Kingdom General Medical Council guidelines which states that a separate permission for recording a surgical procedure is not needed as long as the patient is anonymized.

Every participating gynecologist was assigned a number. Participating gynecologists recorded every procedure and were asked to complete the evaluation form after the surgery and included their assigned number and the procedure performed on every form. The form and DVD of the procedure were placed in personalized envelopes with the participant's number and collected daily.

The video recordings were sent to two of the external assessors who used the same GRIT to evaluate for technical skills. External assessors were blinded to which surgeon performed which procedure. The external assessors were experienced laparoscopic surgeons with experience in teaching and evaluating residents. They were familiar with the objective structured assessment of technical skill (OSAT) global rate scale. They scored separately and did not communicate during the scoring process.

Statistical analysis
Data used for the descriptive statistics were obtained from intraoperative video records. Shapiro-Wilk test was used as test of normality. Mann-Whitney U test and Student t test were also used to test for distribution. Cronbach's alpha was used to calculate internal consistency. Internal consistency is a measure of reliability and measures whether several items that propose to measure the same general construct produce similar scores. Intra-class correlation coefficient (ICC) and Pearson correlation were used to measure inter-expert assessment reliability. Guidelines for evaluating the level of agreement among scores were > 0.80 for excellent correlation, 0.60–0.80 for good correlation, 0.40–0.60 for fair correlation, and < 0.40 for poor correlation.

Results
A total of eight gynecologists met the inclusion criteria and agreed to participate in the study. Two surgeons were excluded due to the fact that they did not perform operative laparoscopy. The total number of procedures recorded during the study period was 88 cases. Ten cases were excluded; four recordings were incomplete and six were corrupted. This brought the total number

of procedures to 78 cases, collected from eight gynecologists. Qualifications and years of experience of the participating gynecologists can be seen in Table 1 which also highlights the number of surgical cases performed by the participating gynecologists. The videos varied widely in length from 8 min for an ovarian cyst aspiration procedure to 83 min for ablation of endometriosis procedure. The total length of all videos was 2655 min, and the mean was 37.4 min per video. The videos included mainly ovarian cystectomies, salpingectomies for ectopic pregnancy, salpingoophorectomies, resection of endometriosis, adhesiolysis, and ovarian drilling.

Internal consistency reliability was calculated for the GRIT without the communication skills, which were excluded due to the difficulty in observing this specific skill through video. Internal consistency reliability showed excellent reliability (Cronbach's alpha 0.883–0.904).

An initial descriptive analysis and normality test was carried out which indicated normal distribution of participants' scores with a Shapiro-Wilk normality test value of $p > 0.05$. In case of normal distribution, comparing means using t test is considered appropriate. The independent sample test was used since the populations were considered independent.

In Table 2, it can be seen that individual scores were evaluated significantly higher than expert evaluation ($p < 0.05$). Figure 1 demonstrates the mean scores for each measured component for all participants, expert 1 and expert 2.

ANOVA test was carried out to determine whether there are any significant differences between the means of the total scores of all participants, expert 1 and expert 2 groups in Table 3. It was found that there was a statistically significant difference between the total scores of the participant and the experts; self-assessment was significantly higher than expert assessment.

Inter-expert assessment reliability was evaluated using ICC. All analyses of the inter-expert assessment reliability indicated excellent correlation as can be seen in Table 4. The total inter-expert assessment reliability for the two expert scores was calculated looking at the ICC and excellent reliability was noted (ICC = 0.9630).

Discussion
Introspection and self-assessment are valuable traits for surgeons leading to comprehensive development of technical and personal skills. Overconfidence and lack of awareness of one's own abilities may lead to the inability to recognize limits and may endanger patients [8]. Self-assessment is thereby a significant measure of quality assurance that can potentially help improve patient safety and reduce error in the operating room.

Simulation learning has overtaken traditional methods in the training of new surgeons making self-assessment more important than ever. This type of teaching shifts learning

Table 1 Participants' qualifications and years of experience

	Years of experience	Cases performed	Cases excluded	Cases used
Participant 1	6	14	2	12
Participant 2	8	10	–	10
Participant 3	7	12	1	11
Participant 4	9	8	2	6
Participant 5	18	7	1	6
Participant 6	20	13	2	11
Participant 7	12	13	2	11
Participant 8	10	11	–	11

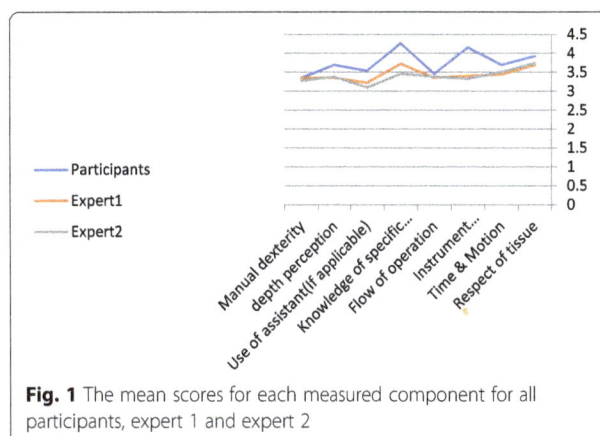

Fig. 1 The mean scores for each measured component for all participants, expert 1 and expert 2

towards self-direction. Thus, surgeons must be able to accurately assess their abilities to personalize their training according to their individual performance [9]. Furthermore, self-assessment is an important parameter of personal development through continuous learning and has been shown to be an important part of a consultant's yearly appraisal [10].

New procedures requiring different technical skills are being introduced regularly in the field of minimally invasive surgery. Surgeons are thereby depending regularly on self-evaluation to determine if they can perform these procedures. Insufficient learning and inadequate evaluation of a surgeon's capabilities may lead to harming the patients. The advent of laparoscopic cholecystectomy led to surgeons offering the procedure to their patients after only attending one course leading to a major spike in common bile duct injuries. Researchers thereby explored the amount of experience needed to adequately perform a laparoscopic cholecystectomy and found it to be approximately 50 cases, owing to the fact that most complications occur in the first 30 cases [11].

Improved teaching and application of the new technology leads to decreased complications in laparoscopic procedures; however, surgeons are still solely responsible for

determining their competence in performing new procedures [12]. Our study demonstrates a lack of agreement between self-assessment and expert assessment of surgical technical skills thereby indicating that current self-assessment measures are inadequate. We used the Global Rating Index of Technical Skills (GRIT) (Additional file 1) for the self-assessment as well as the external evaluator assessment since this tool is documented and proven to be feasible, reliable, and valid [13].

Similar research to our study was done by Evans et al. and found that surgeons are not capable of effectively evaluating their technical surgical skills [8]. The authors compared self-assessment with peer assessment and expert assessment and concluded that surgeons tend to overestimate their technical skills. Comparatively, the participants in our study were more likely to overestimate their technical skills. In contrast, two recent studies from the Imperial College London [7, 10] found moderate to high correlation between self-assessment and an expert assessment for technical skills. However, the imperial study looked at students rather than independent practicing physicians.

The results of this study also suggest similar findings to Pandey et al. that demonstrated that surgeons may inaccurately self-assess their own skills and have difficulty accepting that their performance may be suboptimal [14]. The results of this study should encourage surgeons to enroll in formal assessment prior to starting to perform surgeries that require new skills. The results should also encourage surgeons to use self-assessment to improve their skills and to identify their strengths and work on

Table 2 t test to compare the mean of participants and expert scores

The tested samples	t test for equality of means
All participants mean scores with expert 1 mean scores	p value 0.030
All participants mean scores with expert 2 mean scores	p value 0.017
All participants mean scores with the mean scores of both experts	p value 0.003

Table 3 ANOVA test for the total scores of the participants and experts

ANOVA score					
	Sum of squares	df	Mean square	F	Sig.
Between groups	188.838	2	94.419	4.405	.014
Within groups	2443.282	114	21.432		
Total	2632.120	116			

Table 4 Inter expert assessment reliability

Inter-expert assessment correlation	Intra-class correlation coefficient (ICC)
Participant 1 cases	0.962
Participant 2 cases	0.938
Participant 3 cases	0.975
Participant 4 cases	0.995
Participant 5 cases	0.975
Participant 6 cases	0.962
Participant 7 cases	0.938
Participant 8 cases	0.990

improving their weaknesses. Simulation labs would be an ideal environment to improve skills independently. This has been implemented in many different centers with promising results as shown in Arora et al. [7].

There is currently no true medical license recertification program in Jordan and several other countries in the Middle East and the rest of the world. Health officials and governing bodies need to consider developing a program or model for periodic evaluation of surgical skills encompassing cognitive and technical skills. To our knowledge, no systematic empirical research exist that measures self-assessment in an operative setting with qualified and experienced gynecologists with at least 7 years of experience. Our study is unique in the fact that it allows for measuring real-life technical skills of surgeons rather than assessment of simulation lab skills.

It is assumed that expert assessment is the gold standard as the best measure of evaluation. Many authors looked at verifying the claim that expert assessment is the best form of assessment when studying global rating scales [15]. They found contradicting results with most studies showing only moderate correlation between expert evaluation and raw scores [16]. It is difficult to find an alternative to expert assessment in medical education, which is why most studies, including this one, use experts as the measure for assessment.

The reliability of the expert assessment was also studied, and authors agree that experts are likely to agree among themselves given the chance to evaluate a short, structured, and simple task [17, 18]. Martin et al. also found high inter-reliability between experts watching a video recording of residents performing a standardized patient interview [9]. In this study, two experts scored the participants separately to improve the reliability of the expert assessment.

The limitations of our study include the use of means for comparison and sample size. Sample size in our study was limited since ethical approval was only obtained from Prince Hamzah Hospital in Amman; other hospitals and specialists thereby could not be included in the study. The comparison of group means as generated by the

participants and the experts may conceal individual differences [15]. This can also be seen in the research by Arnold et al. that examined subgroups of self-assessors. The authors found that high achievers tend to underestimate their performance while underachievers tend to overestimate their performance [19]. These findings may serve to reinforce the claim that there is a weak correlation between self-assessment scores and expert scores.

This study also focuses on the assessment of technical skills only. Non-technical skills are not evaluated since video recording of procedures is not considered a good tool for this type of evaluation. However, non-technical skills such as teamwork, leadership, situation awareness, decision making, task management, and communication are equally important, if not more important, than technical skills [20, 21]. Comparatively, studies that looked at self-assessment of non-technical skills showed that surgeons inadequately assess non-technical skills. It was also found that self-assessment of non-technical skills is significantly more overestimated when compared to expert evaluation with a sample of more experienced surgeons [7].

Conclusions

This study shows that there remains a significant difference between self-assessment and expert assessment in the evaluation of laparoscopic technical skills for gynecological surgeons. Accurate self-assessment of technical skills in laparoscopy is important for practicing gynecologist as well as trainees to identify their strengths and weaknesses and improve their performance. Adequate self-assessment measures should encourage gynecologist to improve their skills independently in a simulated environment. This study showed that experienced gynecologist overestimated their surgical skills when compared to expert assessment. Quality assurance measures need to be revisited and restructured through more frequent assessments using peer and expert assessment alongside self-assessment. Gynecologists also need to undergo proper assessment prior to starting to independently perform procedures that require new skills.

Abbreviations
ABOG: American Board of Obstetrics and Gynecology; CPD: Continuing professional development; GOALS: Global Operative Assessment of Laparoscopic Skills; IUD: Intra uterine device; JMC: Jordan Medical Council; MOC: Maintenance of Certificate; MOH: Ministry of Health; OSATS: Objective structured assessment of technical skills; OSCE: Objective Structured clinical Exam; RCOG: Royal College of Obstetricians and Gynaecologists; RMS: Royal Medical Services

Acknowledgements
We owe our deepest gratitude to Dr. Mazen Fraij and Dr. Osama Badran, Consultant Gynecologists, who offered to score the videos and managed to fit this difficult task in their very busy schedules with no financial gain. We also want to thank Prince Hamzah Hospital staff for their outstanding contribution.

Funding

No external source of funding. First author sponsored all printed and visual materials.

Author's contributions

RK designed the study, recruited the patients, analyzed the data, and wrote the paper. The author read and approved the final manuscript.

Author's information

Dr Rami Kilani is an Assistant Professor of Obstetrics and Gynecology at the Hashemite University-Zarqa, Jordan.

Competing interests

The author declares no competing interests.

References

1. Boud D, Falchikov N (1995) What does research tell us about self assessment. In: Enhancing learning through self assessment. Kogan Page, London
2. Gordon MJ (1991) A review of the validity and accuracy of self-assessments in health professions training. Acad Med 66(12):762–769
3. Sullivan K, Hall C (1997) Introducing students to self-assessment. Assess Eval High Educ 22(3):289–305
4. Barnsley L, Lyon PM, Ralston SJ, Hibbert EJ, Cunningham I, Gordon FC, Field MJ (2004) Clinical skills in junior medical officers: a comparison of self-reported confidence and observed competence. Med Educ 38(4):358–367
5. MacDonald J, Williams RG, Rogers DA (2003) Self-assessment in simulation-based surgical skills training. Am J Surg 185(4):319–322
6. Peyre SE, MacDonald H, Al-Marayati L, Templeman C, Muderspach LI (2010) Resident self-assessment versus faculty assessment of laparoscopic technical skills using a global rating scale. Int J Med Educ 1:37
7. Arora S, Miskovic D, Hull L, Moorthy K, Aggarwal R, Johannsson H, Gautama S, Kneebone R, Sevdalis N (2011) Self vs expert assessment of technical and non-technical skills in high fidelity simulation. Am J Surg 202(4):500–506
8. Evans AW, Leeson R, Petrie A (2007) Reliability of peer and self-assessment scores compared with trainers' scores following third molar surgery. Med Educ 41(9):866–872
9. Martin JA, Regehr G, Reznick R, MacRae H, Murnaghan J, Hutchison C, Brown M (1997) Objective structured assessment of technical skill (OSATS) for surgical residents. Br J Surg 84(2):273–278
10. Moorthy K, Munz Y, Orchard TR, Gould S, Rockall T, Darzi A (2004) An innovative method for the assessment of skills in lower gastrointestinal endoscopy. Surg Endosc Interv Tech 18(11):1608–1619
11. Ellison EC, Carey LC (2008) Lessons learned from the evolution of the laparoscopic revolution. Surg Clin N Am 88(5):927–941
12. Luchtefeld M, Kerwel TG (2012) Continuing medical education, maintenance of certification, and physician reentry. Clin Colon Rectal Surg 25(3):171
13. Doyle JD, Webber EM, Sidhu RS (2007) A universal global rating scale for the evaluation of technical skills in the operating room. Am J Surg 193(5):551–555
14. Pandey VA, Wolfe JHN, Black SA, Cairols M, Liapis CD, Bergqvist D (2008) Self-assessment of technical skill in surgery: the need for expert feedback. Ann R Coll Surg Engl 90(4):286–290
15. Ward M, Gruppen L, Regehr G (2002) Measuring self-assessment: current state of the art. Adv Health Sci Educ 7(1):63–80
16. Risucci DA, Tortolani AJ, Ward RJ (1989) Ratings of surgical residents by self, supervisors and peers. Surg Gynecol Obstet 169(6):519–526
17. Regehr G, MacRae H, Reznick RK, Szalay D (1998) Comparing the psychometric properties of checklists and global rating scales for assessing performance on an OSCE-format examination. Acad Med 73(9):993–997
18. Miller JD, McCain J, Lynam DR, Few LR, Gentile B, MacKillop J, Campbell WK (2014) A comparison of the criterion validity of popular measures of narcissism and narcissistic personality disorder via the use of expert ratings. Psychol Assess 26(3):958
19. Arnold L, Willoughby TL, Calkins EV (1985) Self-evaluation in undergraduate medical education: a longitudinal perspective. Acad Med 60(1):21–28
20. Salas E, Bowers CA, Edens E (eds) (2001) Improving teamwork in organizations: applications of resource management training. CRC press/Taylor and Fracis group. ISBN 9780805828450 - CAT# ER5855
21. Siu J, Maran N, Paterson-Brown S (2016) Observation of behavioural markers of non-technical skills in the operating room and their relationship to intra-operative incidents. Surgeon 14(3):119–128

37

Elective uterine artery embolization prior to laparoscopic resection of interstitial pregnancy: two cases

Iris Verbeeck[1] , Francesca Donders[1] , Pieter-Jan Buyck[2] , Dirk Timmerman[1] , Andries Van Holsbeeck[2] ,
Sandra A Cornelissen[2] , Anne-Sophie Van Rompuy[3] , Lien Van den Haute[5] , Sylvie Gordts[4] ,
Carla Tomassetti[1] and Jan Deprest[1,6*]

Abstract

Background: Interstitial pregnancies (IP) can be treated medically or surgically. The most common complication remains hemorrhage. The risk of that may be reduced by elective uterine artery embolization (UAE) prior to surgery, which we applied in two consecutive cases with high vascularization on ultrasound. We also reviewed larger series ($n \geq 10$) on medical as well as surgical management of IP on success and complication rates and reviewed the entire literature on UAE.

Results: A gravida 5 (two ectopic pregnancies treated by salpingectomy) para 1 (cesarean section complicated by a niche, earlier repaired) presented with an asymptomatic IP. Primary treatment consisted of systemic methotrexate (MTX). Because of raising β-hCG and persisting heart activity 1 week later, she was referred for surgery (β-hCG = 59,000 IU/L; CRL = 10.5 mm). Another gravida 5 para 3 presented with an asymptomatic evolutive IP on dating ultrasound. Because of the size (CRL = 24.5 mm), thin overlaying myometrium, and high β-hCG (121,758 IU/L), we opted for primary surgery. Both IPs were highly vascularized with high flow rates. To prevent bleeding, a bilateral UAE was performed. The surgery was nearly bloodless.

In the literature, a wide range of treatment regimens for IP is reported. Larger series report a success rate of 76% for primary systemic MTX, 88% for primary local medical treatment, and 94% for primary surgery. It was not possible to determine reliable hemorrhage or rupture rates following MTX administration. As to laparoscopic surgery, the blood transfusion rate for bleeding was 9% while the conversion rate for hemorrhage was 2%. The use of UAE to reduce the risk for hemorrhage before ($n = 2$) or after ($n = 19$) MTX administration was reported in 21 cases. This failed in two cases (90% success rate), and one patient required transfusion (5%). Two cases treated with UAE and primary surgery were reported, yet the exact indication for embolization was not elaborated. Alternative hemostatic techniques during surgical management have been proposed to reduce blood loss and operating time, yet individual outcomes were not identifiable.

Conclusion: We report on the use of elective UAE prior to laparoscopic resection of IP, because of signs of strong vascularization on ultrasound. This strategy coincided with a nearly bloodless operation. Literature review suggests that this is one of the effective methods to reduce blood loss intra-operatively.

Keywords: Ectopic pregnancy, Interstitial pregnancy, Embolization, Laparoscopy, Cornual resection, Cornuostomy

* Correspondence: jan.deprest@uzleuven.be
[1]Department Gynecology-Obstetrics, University Hospital Leuven, Herestraat 49, 3000 Leuven, Belgium
[6]Institute for Women's Health and Wellcome/EPSRC Centre for Interventional & Surgical Sciences (WEISS), University College London, Charles Bell House, 43-45 Foley Street, London W1W 7TS, UK
Full list of author information is available at the end of the article

Background

Ectopic pregnancy (EP) is any type of pregnancy in which the fertilized ovum implants outside the uterine cavity. The vast majority of EPs are situated in the fallopian tube, typically in the ampullary region (70%), less likely in the isthmic (12%), fimbrial (11%), or interstitial part (2–4%). Other uncommon locations include ovarian (1–3%), abdominal (< 1%), cervical (< 1%), rudimentary horn (< 0.5%), and cesarean scar pregnancies (1–3%) [1–4].

In 1989, EPs occurred at an estimated prevalence of 1–2% worldwide. This is two to three times higher than in 1970 [5]. The increase is presumably related to an increased prevalence of risk factors directly or indirectly leading to decreased tubal passage. The prevalence has since not significantly changed [6, 7].

Pregnancies that are situated in the interstitial portion of the fallopian tube are referred to as *interstitial* [8, 9]. The intramural or interstitial part of the tube is approximately 0.7 mm wide and 1–2 cm long, often with a tortuous course [8]. Interstitial pregnancies (IPs) are also referred to as "cornual," though some reserve this entity to pregnancies located within a rudimentary horn of an abnormal uterine cavity [8, 9]. While the generic risk factors displayed in Table 1 may also apply, specific risk factors to this type of EP are previous ipsilateral or bilateral salpingectomy, previous EP, in vitro fertilization, and tubal damage from previous EP [8]. Historically, the mortality rate of this condition was around 2.5%, which is approximately seven times higher than that of EPs in general. It is assumed that this can be explained by the greater expansion capacity at this location, the richer vascularization of the area, eventually leading to life-threatening hemorrhage when rupture occurs [8].

There is to our knowledge no consensus on the best treatment modality of IP. Herein, we provide a literature review which we did on the occasion of treating two patients with uterine artery embolization (UAE) immediately prior surgical treatment, because of an anticipated high risk for bleeding.

Two cases

A 28-year-old gravida 5 para 1 was referred for a second opinion on an evolutive IP. She had a history of a primary cesarean section for vasa previa, a spontaneous first trimester miscarriage, two EPs treated by salpingectomy, and a hysteroscopic cesarean scar niche repair. The latter niche repair was done because of ultrasound signs of fluid in the niche before starting in vitro fertilization (IVF) treatment. On hysteroscopy, blood and debris were confirmed and a repair was performed 4 months prior to the index event (IP). Control hysteroscopy 1 month after the procedure showed normal findings. The index pregnancy was by IVF. On early scan at 6 + 6 weeks, an IP was suspected. We confirmed this at 7 + 1 weeks to be a left IP with a gestational sac of 19 × 20 mm, CRL of 6.8 mm, β-hCG of 38,000 IU/L, and heart activity. There was no abdominal fluid. The referring center opted for a single-dose methotrexate (MTX) protocol (75 mg; 50 mg/m^2). She presented on day one post-injection with stinging and cramping abdominal pain, yet without hemodynamic impact or peritoneal signs. On day six post-injection, she was referred because of raising β-hCG and persisting heart activity, spotting, along with intermittent abdominal pain. Figure 1 displays the ultrasound, β-hCG, and hemoglobin findings over the reporting period. We decided to proceed with surgical intervention yet opted for prior bilateral UAE during the same general

Table 1 Risk factors of ectopic pregnancy [19–23]

Highly increased risk (OR = 4–40)	Moderately increased risk (OR = 2–20)
Previous tubal surgery	Infertility
Documented tubal pathology	Previous genital infections
History of EP	Multiple sexual partners
In-utero exposure to DES	
Use of IUD [22, 23]	
Minimally increased risk (OR = 1-4)	Other risk factors
Previous pelvic/abdominal surgery	Age (> 35–40 years)
Cigarette smoking	Assisted reproductive technologies
Vaginal douching	Anatomical uterine abnormality
Early age at first intercourse	Non-Caucasian
	Prior spontaneous or medically induced abortion

OR odds ratio, *EP* ectopic pregnancy, *DES* diethylstilbestrol, *IUD* intra-uterine device

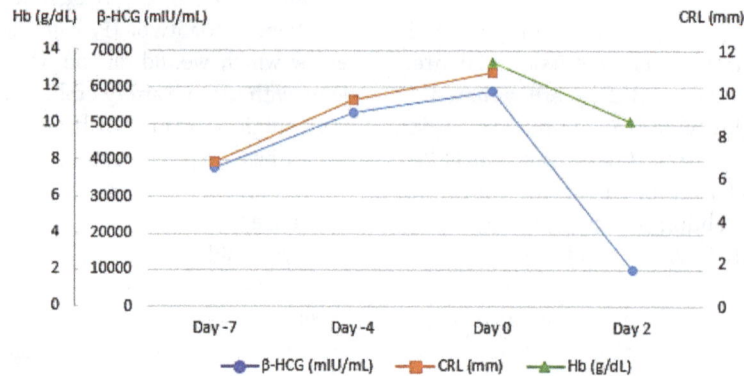

Fig. 1 Case 1: clinical, biochemical and ultrasound findings (day 0 = day of surgery)

anesthesia to reduce the risk for hemorrhage based on the apparent high vascularization around the pregnancy. Access was gained through the right femoral artery with catheterization of the left internal iliac artery followed by selective catheterization of the left uterine artery. Polyvinyl particles (Contour 250-350, Boston Scientific, Diegem, Belgium) were injected under 3D angiography control. The same procedure was followed on the contralateral side. Then, a laparoscopic cornual resection was performed and the uterine defect was closed in two layers using Vicryl 2-0 (Fig. 2). Blood loss was negligible, yet operating time was 140 min. Histopathology confirmed an IP. She was discharged on day two, and β-hCG became unmeasurable 4 weeks later. She had a withdrawal bleeding 3 weeks after the operation and had another period 5 weeks later. A waiting period of at least 6 months [10, 11] was advised to allow maximal healing of the uterus. She conceived 8 months after the IP in the first IVF cycle. She presented again with right fossa pain at 5 + 3 weeks, yet ultrasound confirmed an intracavitary position without any signs of IP.

A 32-year-old gravida 5 para 3 spontaneously conceived. She was referred because on elective dating ultrasound at 9 + 2 weeks a right evolutive IP was found. She had a history of a spontaneous first trimester miscarriage and three uncomplicated term vaginal deliveries. On ultrasound, the surrounding myometrium was 2.2 mm which was strongly vascularized (Fig. 3). Because of the size (CRL = 24.5 mm), the thin myometrial layer, and a β-hCG of 121,758 IU/L, we advocated immediate surgery, yet because of the vascularization we first offered bilateral UAE. Polyvinyl particles (Contour 355-500, Boston Scientific; Embosphere 500-700 and 700-900, Merit Medical, Brussels, Belgium) and spongostan plugs (Ethicon, Diegem, Belgium) were used (Fig. 4). On laparoscopy, a 6-cm pregnancy in the right uterine horn was observed. The pregnancy was removed by cornuostomy, and the myometrial defect was sutured in three layers (first V-loc 2-0, second and third Vicryl 2-0). Blood loss was negligible, and operating time was 180 min. Two months later she still had some brown vaginal discharge. Ultrasound showed normal findings with a strong proliferative endometrium along with a corpus luteum on the left ovary and a normal looking scar at the resection site. β-hCG was 3.2 IU/L.

Both patients explicitly consented to have their history being reported in the literature.

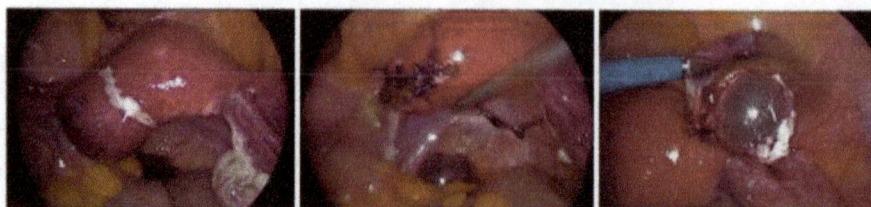

Fig. 2 Case 1: Left: left interstitial pregnancy, preventive coagulation around insertion line. Middle: status post cornual resection and closure of uterine defect with gestational sac in the pouch of Douglas. Right: gestational sac bulging out of resection piece

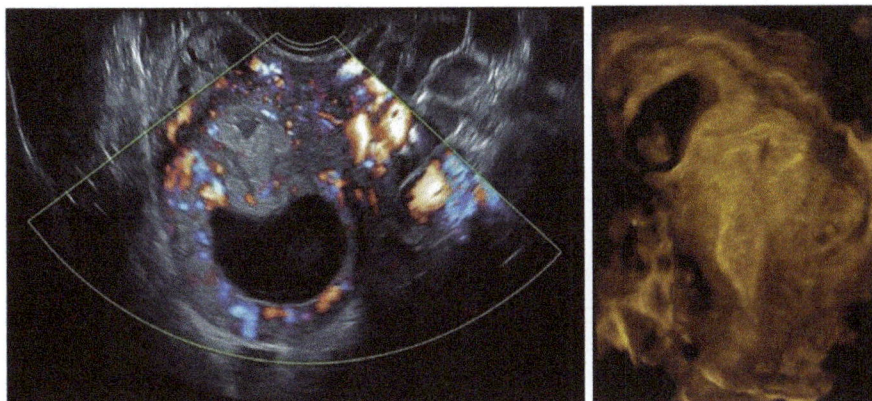

Fig. 3 Case 2: interstitial pregnancy on ultrasound: Left: 2D image showing high flow in the thin surrounding myometrium. Right: 3D rendered image showing the interstitial localization

Methods

For the literature review, we searched the PubMed on this matter, published until February 2018, using the following key terms "Pregnancy, Interstitial"[Mesh], "Therapeutics"[Mesh], "Interstitial Pregnancy," and "Pregnancy Treatment" (953 papers). Sources of relevant articles in the references were screened as well (> 100 papers). All English-, French-, Dutch- and German-language articles were retrieved and screened on title and abstract for relevance (Appendix 1, 2, 3, 4, 5, and 6). Articles in which the location of the EP was unclear or in which the outcome was not clearly specified or objectively measured were excluded. We empirically decided to further discuss outcomes of series with 10 patients or more as to have reasonable denominators for calculating overall outcomes. The only exception to that was Table 4, which displays the entire published experience with UAE. There was not a single series with ≥ 10 patients treated with UAE.

Results

There is considerable experience with primary systemic medical therapy in asymptomatic hemodynamically stable patients with IP. Table 2 summarizes studies describing ten or more patients with IP treated by primary *systemic* MTX. Dosing and regimen of MTX are inconsistent, and success rates are typically over 70%, except in one series [12]. In case of failure (persisting β-hCG leading to additional treatment), surgery was offered, except in one series by Hiersch et al., where second-line local MTX was combined with UAE. Out of five patients, two still required surgery as a third step. Tanaka et al. described 33 cases treated with a very consistent scheme of slowly intravenously injected, yet a fixed dose MTX. The success rate was 94%; two patients required surgery. The opposite was true in the experience of Kim et al. ($n = 30$) administering intramuscular MTX, yet with an inconsistent dosing regimen. Sixteen (53%) required additional surgery.

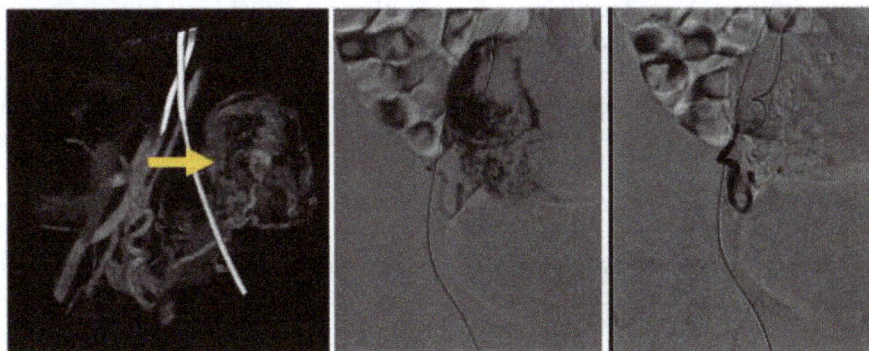

Fig. 4 Case 2: Left: 3D CT angiography after contrast injection in the right iliac artery visualizing the right interstitial pregnancy (arrow). Middle: before embolization of the right uterine artery. Right: after embolization of the right uterine artery

Table 2 Primary systemic MTX treatment of interstitial pregnancy

Author	N	Initial β-hCG	Systemic MTX treatment	Hospital stay	Negative β-hCG	Success
Jermy et al. [24]	17	32–31,381	50 mg/m² IM	0–40	3–13	16/17
Hiersch et al. [25]	14	15,764	1 mg/kg/d IM on day 1, 3, 5, 7	N/A	N/A	9/14
	3	< 2500	50 mg/m² IM	1	N/A	3/3
Tanaka et al. [26]	33	230–106,634	100 mg IV + 200 mg IV	1–4	3–19	31/33
Kim et al. [12]	5	375–102,970	1 mg/kg/d IM on day 1, 3, 5, 7	N/A	N/A	14/30
	24		50 mg/m² IM	N/A	N/A	
	1		100 mg IV in bolus followed by 200 mg IV	N/A	N/A	

N number of cases, *β-hCG* mIU/ml, *MTX* methotrexate, *IM* intramuscular, *IV* intravenous, *hospital stay* days, *negative β-hCG* weeks

Local injection of MTX, potassium chloride (KCL), etoposide, and actinomycin D under laparoscopic, ultrasound, or hysteroscopic guidance have all been reported as effective (Table 3 and Appendix 2). These injections are usually given into the gestational sac, occasionally in the surrounding myometrium or locally intra-arterial. These are invasive procedures, compared to systemic MTX. Benifla et al. used MTX for IP locations and KCl for heterotopic presentations, out of concerns for teratogenicity. Of the three eutopic pregnancies associated to a heterotopic location, two were eventually lost. Further details on outcomes are missing. The calculated success rate was 88%. Treatment failures were not offered a second MTX injection, yet successfully managed by surgery.

Table 4 displays reports on patients managed with *selective UAE* combined with any administration regimen of MTX. The actual indication for *secondary* UAE was refusal of surgery (Ophir et al., Yang et al.; each *n* = 1) or not mentioned (Deruelle et al., Tamarit et al., Berretta et al., Hiersch et al.). *Primary* UAE combined with MTX was either part of a standard protocol (*n* = 9; Krissi et al.) or because of the suspicion of increased risk for hemorrhage (*n* = 1; Valsky et al.). The paper does however not mention how that increased risk was estimated. Table 4 also includes two cases managed by UAE followed immediately by planned surgery (either laparoscopic or hysteroscopic). The argument for UAE was made based on increased vascularization on 3D CT angiography. In one of those two cases, a subsequent spontaneous conception and cesarean delivery of a healthy baby at 37 weeks was reported. Overall success rate in all the series in this table is 91%.

Table 5 displays the experience with *primary* surgery, typically by minimally invasive access. Success rate was 94%; transfusion need was 9%. Primary laparotomy was performed for tubal rupture, in case of severe adhesions (Tulandi et al.) or because of surgeon's preference (Hwang et al.). Conversions were because of significant hematoperitoneum or because of uncontrolled bleeding perioperatively (*n* = 7; 2%).

Discussion

Today the diagnosis of EP is usually made by ultrasound. In high-risk patients or countries where access to early ultrasound is easy, the diagnosis can be made *prior* to the development of symptoms. This allows careful planning of management. We surgically managed two cases of IP, which both were initially asymptomatic. One had typical risk factors and the other one did not. One had prior MTX therapy, and the second one had a very high β-hCG level. Both the ultrasound examination raised the suspicion of a highly vascularized lesion. Therefore, we decided to perform primarily bilateral UAE and surgery in the same anesthesia. This is different than the cases managed in Table 4. Though it is impossible to prove that UAE reduces the risk for hemorrhage, it seems that our surgery in both cases was nearly bloodless. Treatment was apparently also effective given that β-hCG levels fell as expected.

When systematically searching the literature, a gap of knowledge is identified on the use of UAE or in a broader perspective, the management of IP. This is probably because of the rarity of the condition. The data around do neither allow a proper meta-analysis, so that we limited ourselves to summarize the findings in somewhat larger series for each management option. There is quite some experience with primary medical therapy in asymptomatic hemodynamically stable patients. In analogy to other ectopic locations [13], the variability of MTX administration protocols is wide, including systemic single shot (either promptly or slowly infused), repetitive doses, and local administration [13]. Medical therapy has also been combined with UAE, mostly successful, yet Hiersch et al. reports on two cases where second line local MTX treatment combined with UAE failed. In those, we would guess the patient would have had more benefit of surgery.

Table 3 Primary local medical treatment of interstitial pregnancy

Author	N	Initial β-hCG	Local medical treatment	Hospital stay	Negative β-hCG	Complications	Success
Benifla et al. [27]	2	16,000–43,000	MTX 1 mg/kg + SMTX	3	6 (1/2)	Bleeding 1/2	1/2
	6	360–10,000	MTX 1 mg/kg	3	1–3	–	6/6
	3[a]	15,000–25,205	KCL 2 mEq in 2 ml volume	3	[a]	Miscarriage 2/3	3/3
Cassik et al. [28]	23	102–69,820	MTX 25 mg	N/A	3–14	–	21/23
Framarino et al. [29]	14	2800–3200	MTX 25 mg	N/A	Max. 8	–	14/14

N number of cases, β-hCG mIU/ml, (S)MTX (systemic) methotrexate, KCL potassium chloride, hospital stay days, negative β-hCG weeks
[a] Heterotopic pregnancy

Our literature review learns that the most frequent complication of surgery is hemorrhage, either with or without transfusion. The overall transfusion rate in IP is not judgeable since no reference to that outcome was made in any of the medically treated cases. However, 9% of laparoscopically managed IPs required blood transfusion. Therefore, it seems logical to take measures to reduce that risk. Surgically, one can use prophylactic coagulation by electrosurgery or ligation of the feeding artery, yet this may compromise viability of the tissue. Alternatively, vasoconstrictors have been described to reduce blood loss and operating time, yet they may have their own side effects and have only been reported to be effective for IPs with an average β-hCG of 10,000–25,000 IU/L [8, 14, 15]. Conversely, these are very cheap agents.

Modern invasive radiologic techniques are becoming increasingly popular, and those services become more widely accessible even in a semi-acute setting. Embolization techniques have found their place in modern obstetrics and gynecology. The experience with uterine myomas is meanwhile very large, and subsequent conception seems to be possible and relatively safe [16]. Torre et al. described an insignificant change in fertility rate and ovarian reserve after UAE for uterine fibroids in women with no other infertility factors [16]. Krissi et al. reported on the subsequent fertility after MTX administration with UAE in the treatment IP. Out of five women who tried to conceive, four did so, and three delivered successfully. Disadvantages of UAE are the higher cost in comparison to vasopressin, the longer duration of anesthesia, the more complicated logistics, and the additional local morbidity (e.g. ischemic pain, Asherman syndrome) [17, 18].

Conclusions

We report on the use of elective UAE prior to laparoscopic resection of IP, which coincided with a nearly bloodless operation. A literature search shows a wide variety of treatment options, yet most cases seem to be following the typical approach to EP. The overall success rate of surgical treatment of IP is higher than that of medical treatment. When performing laparoscopy, good hemostatic techniques are recommended since the operation takes place in a strongly vascularized region [8, 14, 15]. Our experience with two cases of UAE is yet another approach. It seems safe and reliable and does not preclude future conception.

Table 4 Primary and secondary treatment of interstitial pregnancy with elective UAE

Author	N	Initial β-hCG	Initial treatment	β-hCG pre- UAE	Treatment	Hospital stay	Negative β-hCG	Complications	Success
Valsky et al. [30]	1	11,695	–	–	MTX + UAE	N/A	5	–	1/1
Takeda et al. [31]	1	95,365	–	–	UAE + CR	8	6	–	1/1
Krissi et al. [32]	9	1667–46,923	–	–	UAE + S/LMTX	13	8	–	9/9
Takeda et al. [33]	1	44,917	–	–	UAE + TE + SMTX	N/A	13	–	1/1
Ophir et al. [34]	1	33,689	SMTX	51,098	UAE	7	8	–	1/1
Deruelle et al. [35]	1	17,785	SMTX	20,458	UAE	6	10	–	1/1
Yang et al. [17]	1	29,454	SMTX	35,654	UAE	6	4	–	1/1
Tamarit et al. [36]	2	4394–8970	SMTX	8689–10,164	UAE + LMTX	1	10	–	2/2
Berretta et al. [37]	1	49,997	SMTX	59,494	UAE	11	10	–	1/1
Hiersch et al. [25]	5	15,383	SMTX	N/A	UAE + LMTX	N/A	N/A	Transfusion 1/5 Rupture 2/5	3/5

N number of cases, β-hCG mIU/ml, S/LMTX systemic/local methotrexate, UAE uterine artery embolization, CR cornual resection (laparoscopic), TE transcervical evacuation (under laparoscopic guidance), hospital stay days, negative β-hCG weeks

246 Gynecological Surgery: New Frontiers

Table 5 Primary surgical treatment of interstitial pregnancy

Author	N	Initial β-hCG	Surgical treatment	Duration	Rupture	Hospital stay	Negative β-hCG	Complications	Success
Moon et al. [38]	3	1320–24,700	Laparoscopic CS°	52	No	N/A	N/A	–	3/3
	18	28.5–305,100	Laparoscopic CS°°	U:28; R:82	3/18	N/A	N/A	–	17/18
	3	4469–13,000	Laparoscopic CS°°°	35	No	N/A	N/A	–	3/3
Tulandi et al. [39]	13	11,471	Laparotomic CR	N/A	9/13	N/A	N/A	Transfusion 7/13	13/13
	8	2087	Laparoscopic CR	N/A	5/11	N/A	N/A	Transfusion 2/11	7/8
	3	2087	Laparoscopic CS	N/A	5/11	N/A	N/A	Transfusion 2/11	3/3
MacRae et al. [40]	3	3150–38,000	Laparoscopic CS	N/A	1/3	2	N/A	–	3/3
	8	0–21,352	Laparoscopic CR	N/A	3/8	2	N/A	Conversion: 1/8	7/8
Ng et al. [41]	53	N/A	Laparoscopic CS if IP 1–2 cm° / Laparoscopic CR if IP ≥ 3 cm°	67 (mean)	8/53	2	3	Conversion: 1/53 / Transfusion: 8/53	44/53
Moon et al. [14]	20	177–39,508	Laparoscopic CS°	N/A	2/20	N/A	N/A	–	19/20
Hwang et al. [42]	54	12,741	Laparotomic CR	71	19/54	6	N/A	Transfusion 25/54	54/54
	34	12,905	Laparoscopic CR	81	8/34	5	N/A	Transfusion 13/34	34/34
Cai et al. [43]	15	N/A	Laparoscopic CS°	30–80	N/A	2–5	2–5	–	15/15
	7	3000–32,000	TE, LG and HG	45–90	No	N/A	2–5	Perforation: 2/7	5/7
Zuo et al. [44]	16	14,696	Laparoscopic CR	25–120	No	3–4	N/A	Rupture: 1/16	16/16
Ahn et al. [45]	6	17,797–69,303	TE, UG	N/A	N/A	2–8	N/A	–	5/6
	9	20,319–50,271	Laparoscopic CR	N/A	N/A	4–7	N/A	Transfusion: 1/9	9/9
Douysset et al. [46]	13	369–45,780	Laparoscopic CR	N/A	9/18	5	N/A	Transfusion: 4/18	11/13
	5	369–45,780	Laparoscopic CS	N/A	9/18	5	N/A	Transfusion: 4/18	4/5
Watanabe et al. [47]	12	998–55,820	Laparoscopic CS°	61–160	2/12	N/A	N/A	–	12/12
	1	69	Laparoscopic CS°	N/A	Yes	N/A	N/A	–	1/1
Kim et al. [11]	13*	N/A	Laparoscopic CR	40–145	2/13	2–7	N/A	Rupture 1/11 / Transfusion: 2/13 / Miscarriage: 1/13	13/13
Nikodijevic et al. [48]	13	16,687	Laparoscopic CR	N/A	N/A	N/A	4–8	Conversion: 5/13 / Transfusion: 4/13	13/13
Nirgianakis et al. [49]	10	27,634	Laparoscopic CR~	115	N/A	3	N/A	Transfusion: 3/10	10/10
Wang et al. [50]	38	25,150	Laparoscopic CS°	71	11/38	3	N/A	–	35/38
Lee et al. [51]	53	575–64,831	Laparoscopic CR	77	N/A	N/A	N/A	–	49/53
	22	1454–62,422	Laparoscopic CS· °	59	N/A	N/A	N/A	–	21/22

N number of cases, β-hCG mIU/ml, CR cornual resection, CS cornuostomy, IP interstitial pregnancy, TE transcervical evacuation, HG under hysteroscopic guidance, LG under laparoscopic guidance, R ruptured, UR unruptured, duration minutes, hospital stay days, negative β-hCG weeks
Hemostatic technique: °vasopressin, °°endoloop, °°°encircling suture, *heterotopic pregnancy

Appendix 1

Table 6 Primary systemic MTX treatment of interstitial pregnancy

Author	N	Initial β-hCG	Systemic MTX treatment	Hospital stay	Negative β-hCG	Complications	Success
Tanaka et al. [52]	1	64,000	30 mg IM day 0 + 15 mg/d IM 5 days, 3 cycles	N/A	3	Liver function ↓	1/1
Benifla et al. [27]	2	364–5340	15 mg/d IM for 5 days	3	3 (1/2)	–	1/2
	2	430–450	1 mg/kg/d IM for 4 days	3	3–6	–	2/2
Hajenius et al. [53]	8	410–81,000	1 mg/kg/d IM on day 1, 3, 5, 7	N/A	7–21	–	8/8
Galimberti and Jones [54]	1	7072	50 mg/m² IM	N/A	N/A	–	0/1
Bernardini et al. [55]	1	12,470	100 mg IM	N/A	14	–	1/1
Fisch et al. [56]	1	102,000	50 mg/m² IM on day 1, 3, 5, 7	11	7	–	0/1
Sagiv et al. [57]	1	28,166	2 × 75 mg IM	4	N/A	–	0/1
Lalchandani et al. [58]	1	12,338	400 mg/w IV for 8 weeks	N/A	8	–	1/1
Verity et al. [59]	1	1060	2 × 75 mg IM	N/A	7	–	1/1
	1	5560	2 × 50 mg/m² IM, 48 h apart	N/A	8–9	–	1/1
	1	3510	1 mg/kg IM, 2 doses	N/A	4	–	1/1
	1	9070	1 mg/kg IM, 1 dose	–	6–7	–	1/1
Advincula and Senapati [60]	1	62,889	N/A	N/A	N/A	N/A	0/1
Jermy et al. [24]	17	32–31,381	50 mg/m² IM°	0–40	3–13	–	16/17
Ophir et al. [34]	1	33,689	50 mg/m² IM°	7	8	–	0/1
Reid and Buddha [61]	1	4680	50 mg/m² IM	N/A	7	–	1/1
Rodriguez et al. [62]	7	1592–75,868	50 mg/m² IM°	N/A	2–15	–	7/7
Tulandi et al. [39]	4	2627–6739	50 mg/m² IM	N/A	7 (2/4)	–	2/4
Cassik et al. [28]	5	793–41,150	2 × 50 mg/m² IM, 48 h apart	N/A	3–7	Obstipation 2/5 Neuropathy 1/5 Mild ↓ liver 1/5	4/5
Deruelle et al. [35]	1	17,785	2 × 1 mg/kg IM	6	10	–	0/1
Klemm et al. [63]	3	11,743–22,134	1 mg/kg/d IV on day 1, 3, 5, 7; 2 cycles	N/A	N/A	–	3/3
Araujo et al. [64]	1	4815	50 mg IM	N/A	N/A	–	0/1
Yang et al. [17]	1	29,454	1 mg/kg IM	6	4	–	0/1
Fujioka et al. [65]	1	11,430	50 mg/m² IM	N/A	N/A	–	0/1
Api and Api [66]	1	11,706	1 mg/kg IM	1	1	–	0/1
Günenç et al. [67]	1	8314	2 × 1 mg/kg IM	N/A	N/A	–	0/1
Tamarit et al. [36]	2	4394–8970	2 × 50 mg IM	1	10	–	0/2
Kato et al. [68]	1	90,000	50 mg/m² IM	N/A	N/A	–	0/1
Lee et al. [69]	1	3029	4 × 1 mg/kg IM	3	N/A	–	0/1
Gomez et al. [70]	2	3724–4116	70–75 mg + oral Mifepristone	2	5–7	–	2/2
Monia et al. [71]	3	3000–111,633	1–4× IM	N/A	2–6 (2/3)	–	2/3
Szylit et al. [72]	1	21,281	2 × 50 mg/m² IM, 48 h apart	N/A	N/A	–	0/1
Ahn et al. [45]	1	4478	Multiple doses	4	N/A	–	1/1
Berretta et al. [37]	1	49,997	2 × 80 mg IM	11	N/A	–	0/1
Sagiv et al. [73]	4	4304–28,166	50 mg/m² IM°	N/A	N/A	–	1/4
Surbone et al. [74]	3	2974–15,022	1 mg/kg IM	N/A	N/A	–	2/3
Fritz et al. [75]	1	8200	50 mg/m² IM	N/A	N/A	–	0/1
Hiersch et al. [25]	14	15,764	1 mg/kg/d IM on day 1, 3, 5, 7	N/A	N/A	–	9/14
	3	< 2500	50 mg/m² IM	1	N/A	–	3/3
Horne et al. [76]	5	2458–9730	50 mg/m² IM°	N/A	10	–	5/5
Meddeb et al. [77]	1	6320	Single dose	N/A	N/A	PTD	0/1
Corioni et al. [78]	1	8681	1 mg/kg IM	11	9	–	1/1
Kim et al. [79]	1	35,890	Every 2 days for 4 weeks	N/A	17	Pseudocyst	1/1

Table 6 Primary systemic MTX treatment of interstitial pregnancy *(Continued)*

Author	N	Initial β-hCG	Systemic MTX treatment	Hospital stay	Negative β-hCG	Complications	Success
Singh et al. [80]	1	89,000	1 mg/kg IM, 3 doses	21	12	–	1/1
Tanaka et al. [26]	33	230–106,634	100 mg IV in bolus followed by 200 mg IV	1–4	3–19	–	31/33
Nikodijevic et al. [48]	2	19,563	N/A	N/A	4	–	3/3
Kahramanoglu et al. [81]	1	1263	50 mg/m² IM	7	6	–	1/1
Kim et al. [12]	5	375–102,970	1 mg/kg/d IM on day 1, 3, 5, 7	N/A	N/A	N/A	14/30
	24		50 mg/m² IM	N/A	N/A	N/A	
	1		100 mg IV in bolus followed by 200 mg IV	N/A	N/A	N/A	

N number of cases, *β-hCG* mIU/ml, *MTX* methotrexate, *IM* intramuscular, *IV* intravenous, *hospital stay* days, *negative β-hCG* weeks, *PTD* persistent trophoblastic disease
°With a second injection, if β-hCG decrease is less than 15% from days 4 to 7

Appendix 2

Table 7 Primary local medical treatment of interstitial pregnancy

Author	N	Initial β-hCG	Local medical treatment	Hospital stay	Negative β-hCG	Complications	Success
Timor-Tritsch et al. [82]	1*	14,100	KCL 0.5 ml of 2 mEq/ml cornual	N/A	6 (*)	Miscarriage	1/1
	1	1400	MTX 25 mg cornual	4	5	–	1/1
Benifla et al. [27]	2	16,000–43,000	MTX 1 mg/kg intrasaccular, UG[1]	3 (1/2)	6 (1/2)	Bleeding 1/2	1/2
	6	360–10,000	MTX 1 mg/kg intrasaccular, UG/LG	3	1–3	–	6/6
	3*	15,000–25,205	KCL 2 mEq in 2 ml volume intrasaccular	3	*	Miscarriage 2/3	3/3
Baker et al. [83]	1*	18,423	MTX 12.5 mg with 1 ml of 20% KCL	0	*	–	1/1
Wilkinson et al. [84]	1	10,500	MTX 40 mg	N/A	N/A	–	1/1
Lin et al. [85]	1	3256	MTX 50 mg with diluted vasopressin	2	2	–	1/1
Oyawoye et al. [86]	1*	78,685	MTX	N/A	*	–	1/1
Verity et al. [59]	1	5780	MTX 50 mg, LG[2]	N/A	9	–	1/1
	1	5578	MTX 50 mg, LG	N/A	4	–	1/1
Tulandi et al. [39]	2	2627–6739	MTX, LG	N/A	7 (1/2)	–	1/2
	2		MTX	N/A	7	–	2/2
Cassik et al. [28]	23	102–69,820	MTX 25 mg, UG[3]	N/A	3–14	–	21/23
Chou et al. [87]	1	6413	KCL 2.5 mEq, UG	N/A	12	–	1/1
Narang and Kalu [88]	2	3700–40,000	MTX 50 mg/m²	N/A	N/A	–	2/2
Andrés et al. [89]	3	6193–21,999	MTX 50 mg intrasaccular, UG[4]	1	4–10	Leukopenia 1/3	2/3
Monia et al. [71]	2	7909–64,000	MTX 20–40 mg[5]	N/A	2	–	2/2
	1	8400	MTX 60 mg	N/A	4	–	1/1
Surbone et al. [74]	6	2974–15,022	MTX 1 mg/kg	N/A	N/A	–	5/6
Swank et al. [90]	1	90,504	MTX 50 mg[5]	7	7	–	1/1
Douysset et al. [46]	2	369–45,780	N/A	N/A	N/A	–	2/2
Framarino et al. [29]	14	2800–3200	MTX 25 mg	N/A	Max. 8	–	14/14
Yu et al. [91]	4*	N/A	MTX 1 mg/kg	N/A	N/A	–	4/4
Maçães et al. [92]	1	2776	MTX 25 mg with 2 mEq KCL	N/A	8	–	1/1
Leggieri et al. [93]	1	5055	MTX 25 mg	4	3	–	1/1
Nikodijevic et al. [48]	3	19,563	MTX[5]	N/A	4	–	2/2
	1		MTX	N/A	N/A	N/A	0/1
Kim et al. [12]	2	2292–59,090	MTX 1 mg/kg	N/A	N/A	N/A	7/8
	6		MTX 1 mg/kg[5]	N/A	N/A	N/A	

N number of cases, *β-hCG* mIU/ml, *KCL* potassium chloride, *MTX* methotrexate, *UG* under ultrasound guidance, *LG* under laparoscopic guidance, *hospital stay* days, *negative β-hCG* weeks
*Heterotopic pregnancy: 1: MTX 1 mg/kg/d IM 3 days after, 2: MTX 50 mg IM on days 2 and 4, 3: in viable pregnancies + KCL intracardially (5/23), 4 MTX 50 mg/m²IM (2/3 patients), 5: systemic MTX

Appendix 3

Table 8 Secondary/tertiary systemic/local medical treatment of interstitial treatment

Author	N	Initial β-hCG	Initial treatment	Medical treatment	Hospital stay	Negative β-hCG	Complications	Success
Fisch et al. [56]	1	102,000	SMTX	MTX 50 mg intrasaccular	11	7	–	1/1
Moon et al. [38]	1	47,200	Laparoscopic CS	MTX	N/A	N/A	N/A	1/1
Tulandi et al. [39]	1	2086	Laparoscopic CR	MTX	N/A	N/A	N/A	1/1
Takeda et al. [94]	1	16,100	Laparoscopic CS	MTX	30	N/A	N/A	1/1
Araujo et al. [64]	1	4815	SMTX	LMTX (50 mg), UG	N/A	N/A	·	1/1
Fujioka et al. [65]	1	11,430	SMTX	Dactinomycin 12 μg/kg IV	N/A	N/A	–	1/1
MacRae et al. [40]	1	7237	Laparoscopic CR	SMTX	N/A	N/A	N/A	1/1
Ng et al. [41]	9	N/A	Laparoscopy	SMTX	N/A	N/A	N/A	9/9
Sahoo et al. [95]	1	12,000	Laparoscopy	SMTX	N/A	N/A	–	1/1
Moon et al. [14]	1	9836	Laparoscopic CS	SMTX	N/A	N/A	N/A	1/1
Kato et al. [68]	1	90,000	SMTX	LMTX (25 mg)	N/A	6	–	1/1
Surbone et al. [74]	1	N/A	LMTX	SMTX	N/A	N/A	N/A	0/1
Douysset et al. [46]	2	N/A	Laparoscopic CR	MTX	N/A	N/A	N/A	2/2
	1	N/A	Laparoscopic CS	MTX	N/A	N/A	N/A	1/1
Poon et al. [96]	2	3658–89,968	Expectant	LMTX	N/A	N/A	N/A	2/2
Wang et al. [50]	1	N/A	Laparoscopic CS	MTX 20 mg IM for 5 days	N/A	4	–	1/1
Lee et al. [51]	5	N/A	Laparoscopy	MTX multiple dose regimen	N/A	N/A	–	5/5

N number of cases, *β-hCG* mIU/ml, *(S/L)MTX* (systemic/local) methotrexate, *CR* cornual resection, *CS* cornuostomy, *IM* intramuscular, *IV* intravenous, *UG* under ultrasound guidance, *hospital stay* days, *negative β-hCG* weeks

Appendix 4

Table 9 Primary surgical treatment of interstitial pregnancy

Author	N	Initial β-hCG	Surgical treatment	Operating time	Rupture	Hospital stay	Negative β-hCG	Complications	Success
Steadman [97]	1	N/A	Resection of GT	N/A	Yes	7	N/A	Transfusion	1/1
Bickerstaff [98]	1	N/A	CR	N/A	N/A	N/A	N/A	–	1/1
Farabow et al. [99]	1	N/A	Laparotomic CR	N/A	Yes	N/A	N/A	Transfusion	1/1
Iuchtman and Grunstein [100]	2	N/A	Laparotomic resection of GT	N/A	Yes	8	N/A	N/A	2/2
Hill et al. [101]	1	N/A	Laparoscopic resection of GT°	N/A	No	2	4–5	–	1/1
Reich et al. [102]	1	16,300	Laparoscopic CR	N/A	Yes	2	3	Transfusion	1/1
de Boer et al. [103]	1	N/A	Laparotomic CS	N/A	No	2	N/A	–	1/1
Pelosi [104]	1	N/A	Laparoscopic CR	45	N/A	1	N/A	–	1/1
Laury [105]	1	2450	Laparoscopic CS	N/A	No	0	N/A	–	1/1
Sherer et al. [106]	1*	N/A	Laparoscopic CR	N/A	Yes	3	*	Transfusion	1/1
Tulandi et al. [107]	4	4700–14,500	Laparoscopic CR°	N/A	No	N/A	N/A	–	5/5
	1	8000	Laparoscopic SS°	N/A	No	N/A	N/A	–	1/1
Woodland et al. [108]	1	11,061	Laparoscopic CR°	N/A	No	1	N/A	–	1/1
Katz and Lurie [109]	1	6300	Laparoscopic CS°	N/A	No	N/A	N/A	–	1/1
Groboman and Milad [110]	1	32,827	Laparoscopic CS°	N/A	No	N/A	6	–	1/1
Kasum et al. [111]	1*	5450	Laparoscopic resection of GT	N/A	Yes	N/A	*	–	1/1
Crvenkoviæ et al. [112]	1	8800	Laparoscopic CR°	60	No	4	2	–	1/1
Rahimi [113]	1	3672	Laparoscopic CS°	N/A	No	1	2	–	1/1
Moon et al. [38]	3	28.5–305,100	Laparoscopic CS°	52	No	N/A	N/A	–	3/3
	18		Laparoscopic CS°°	U:28; R:82	3/18	N/A	N/A		17/18
	3		Laparoscopic CS°°°	35	No	N/A	N/A	–	3/3
Vicino et al. [114]	1	21,800	Laparoscopic CR	N/A	No	N/A	2	–	1/1
Ayoubi et al. [115]	1*	N/A	Laparotomic resection of GT	N/A	Yes	N/A	*	–	1/1
Dumesic et al. [116]	1*	N/A	Laparotomic CR	N/A	Yes	N/A	N/A	Transfusion Miscarriage	1/1
Kun and Tung [117]	1	N/A	Laparotomic resection of GT	N/A	Yes	6	N/A	–	1/1
Osuga et al. [118]	3	14,352–19,457	Laparoscopic CR	N/A	N/A	N/A	N/A	–	3/3
Sagiv et al. [57]	1	N/A	Laparoscopic CS	N/A	Yes	1	N/A	Transfusion	1/1
DeWitt and Abbott [119]	1	N/A	CR	N/A	Yes	3	N/A	Transfusion	1/1
Sills et al. [120]	1*	N/A	Laparoscopic CS	< 60	No	3	*	–	1/1
Chang et al. [121]	1*	63,300	Laparotomic resection of GT	N/A	N/A	N/A	*	–	1/1
Habek et al. [122]	2	N/A	Laparotomic hysterectomy	N/A	Yes	8	N/A	Transfusion 1/2	2/2
Izquierdo et al. [123]	1	2500	CR	N/A	N/A	3	N/A	–	1/1
Katz et al. [124]	2	3467–9800	TE, LG and HG	N/A	No	N/A	N/A	–	2/2

Table 9 Primary surgical treatment of interstitial pregnancy (Continued)

Author	N	Initial β-hCG	Surgical treatment	Operating time	Rupture	Hospital stay	Negative β-hCG	Complications	Success
Yoo et al. [125]	4	39,245	Laparoscopic CS°	54	No	2	4	–	4/4
Gezer and Mutlu [126]	1	N/A	Laparoscopic CS	N/A	No	1	N/A	–	1/1
Grimbizis et al. [127]	1	821	Laparoscopic CR	N/A	Yes	1	3	–	1/1
Lee et al. [128]	1	45,000	Laparotomic CS	N/A	No	7	N/A	–	1/1
Savvidou et al. [129]	1	27,724	Laparoscopic resection of GT	N/A	Yes	4	3	Transfusion Conversion	1/1
Thakur et al. [130]	2	3356–17,735	TE, LG and UG	N/A	No	2	N/A	–	2/2
	2	N/A	TE, LG and UG	N/A	No	N/A	N/A	–	2/2
Tulandi et al. [39]	13	11,471	Laparotomic CR	N/A	9/13	N/A	N/A	Transfusion 7/13	13/13
	8	2087	Laparoscopic CR	N/A	5/11	N/A	N/A	Transfusion 2/11	7/8
	3	N/A	Laparoscopic CS	N/A	5/11	N/A	N/A	Transfusion 2/11	3/3
Zhang et al. [131]	3	8593–16,820	TE, LG	< 18	No	3 (max)	4	–	3/3
Huang et al. [132]	4	39,933–74,551	Laparoscopic CS	N/A	No	N/A	4	–	4/4
Kumakiri et al. [133]	1	9460	Laparoscopic CR°	84	No	2	4	–	1/1
Ross et al. [134]	2	23,480–45,780	TE, UG¹	N/A	No	2	4–8	–	2/2
Takeda et al. [94]	2	4250–15,500	Laparoscopic CR	44–98	Yes	6–11	N/A	Transfusion 2/2	2/2
	1	16,100	Laparoscopic CS	75	Yes	30	N/A	Transfusion	0/1
Ko et al. [135]	1	1356	Laparoscopic resection of GT	N/A	No	1	1	–	1/1
Lee et al. [136]	1	N/A	Laparotomic CS	N/A	No	3	N/A	–	1/1
Oliver et al. [137]	5	14,874	TE, LG and UG	N/A	No	N/A	N/A	–	5/5
Lialios et al. [138]	1*	N/A	Laparoscopic CR	N/A	Yes	2	*	–	1/1
Qin et al. [139]	1*	N/A	Laparoscopic CR^∞	N/A	No	N/A	*	–	1/1
Sherer et al. [140]	1	N/A	Laparotomic resection of GT	N/A	Yes	3	N/A	–	1/1
Casadio et al. [141]	1	9383	Laparoscopic CS	40	No	2	5	–	1/1
Cheng et al. [142]	1	59,959	Laparoscopic CS	N/A	No	6	5	–	1/1
Choi et al. [143]	8	3400–74,060	Laparoscopic CS°	35–80	No	N/A	2–5	–	8/8
Duong et al. [144]	1	N/A	Laparotomic resection of GT	N/A	Yes	7	N/A	Transfusion	1/1
MacRae et al. [40]	3	3150–38,000	Laparoscopic CS	N/A	1/3	2	N/A	–	3/3
	8	0–21,352	Laparoscopic CR	N/A	3/8	2	N/A	Conversion 1/8	7/8
Ng et al. [41]	53	N/A	Laparoscopic CS if IP 1–2 cm°, Laparoscopic CR if IP 3 cm or more°	67 (mean)	8/53	2	3	Conversion 1/53 Transfusion 8/53	44/53
Pluchino et al. [145]	1	N/A	Laparoscopic CS	N/A	Yes	2	N/A	–	1/1
Moon et al. [14]	20	177–39,508	Laparoscopic CS°	N/A	2/20	N/A	N/A	–	19/20
Pan et al. [146]	1	79,194	Bilateral CR (bilateral IP)	N/A	No	10	N/A	–	1/1
Pistofidis et al. [147]	1	18,900	Laparoscopic resection of GT	N/A	Yes	2	N/A	–	1/1
Tinelli et al. [148]	3	7600–12,500	Laparoscopic CS	45 (mean)	1/3	1	2	–	3/3

Table 9 Primary surgical treatment of interstitial pregnancy (Continued)

Author	N	Initial β-hCG	Surgical treatment	Operating time	Rupture	Hospital stay	Negative β-hCG	Complications	Success
Vignali et al. [149]	3	431–3252	Laparoscopic CR	36–60	No	1	N/A	–	3/3
Walid et al. [150]	1	N/A	Laparoscopic resection of GT°	N/A	N/A	N/A	N/A	–	1/1
Yan [151]	1	3600	Laparoscopic resection of GT°	60	No	N/A	N/A	–	1/1
Aust et al. [152]	1*	N/A	Laparoscopic CR	N/A	No	0	*	Miscarriage	1/1
Cerviño et al. [153]	1	20,940	TE, UG²	N/A	No	N/A	5	–	1/1
Chachan et al. [154]	1*	N/A	Laparoscopic CS	N/A	No	1	*	–	1/1
Hwang et al. [42]	54	12,741	Laparotomic CR	71	19/54	6	N/A	Transfusion 25/54	54/54
	34	12,905	Laparoscopic CR	81	8/34	5	N/A	Transfusion 13/34, Bowel injury 1/34	34/34
Lazard et al. [155]	2	4900–14,720	Laparoscopic CR	25–35	No	2–3	2–3	–	2/2
Lodhi et al. [156]	1	6041	Laparoscopic CR	N/A	No	2	N/A	–	1/1
Yamamoto et al. [157]	1	N/A	Laparoscopic CR	N/A	Yes	2	N/A	Transfusion	1/1
Ahsan Akhtar et al. [158]	1	16,740	Laparoscopic CR°	N/A	No	1	N/A	–	1/1
Cai et al. [43]	15	N/A	Laparoscopic CS°	25	No	1	3	–	15/15
Cucinella et al. [159]	7	3000–32,000	TE, LG, and HG	30–80	No	2–5	2–5	Perforation 2/7	5/7
Garavaglia et al. [160]	5	1286–20,680	Laparoscopic CR^oooo	45–90	No	N/A	3–4	–	5/5
Muglu et al. [161]	1	2173	Laparoscopic CS	31–46	N/A	N/A	N/A	–	1/1
Rheinboldt et al. [162]	1	N/A	Laparoscopic resection of GT	N/A	N/A	N/A	N/A	–	1/1
Zuo et al. [44]	16	14,696	Laparoscopic CR	25–120	No	3–4	N/A	Rupture 1/16	16/16
Ahn et al. [45]	6	17,797–69,303	TE, UG	N/A	No	2–8	N/A	–	5/6
MacKenna et al. [163]	9	20,319–50,271	Laparoscopic CR°	4–7	N/A	4–7	2	Transfusion 1/9	9/9
Mooij and Van Dillen [164]	1	5820	Laparoscopic CR°	N/A	No	1	N/A	N/A	1/1
Sagiv et al. [73]	3	3282–13,260	Laparoscopic CR	N/A	N/A	N/A	N/A	–	3/3
Surbone et al. [74]	2	21,930–88,270	Laparoscopic CS	N/A	N/A	N/A	N/A	Conversion 1/2	2/2
Warda et al. [165]	2	2974–15,022	Laparoscopic CR	N/A	N/A	N/A	N/A	–	2/2
Wright et al. [166]	3	1455–27,052	TE, UG¹	N/A	No	6–12	6–12	–	3/3
Zhang and Yuan [167]	2	2808–14,030	Laparoscopic CR°	45–95	No	6–7	<1	–	2/2
Chandran [168]	1	N/A	Laparotomic CR	N/A	No	5	N/A	–	1/1
Douysset et al. [46]	13	369–45,780	Laparoscopic CR	N/A	9/18	5	N/A	Transfusion 4/18	11/13
	5	N/A	Laparoscopic CS	N/A	9/18	5	N/A	Transfusion 4/18	4/5
Garretto et al. [169]	1	26,476	Laparoscopic CR	N/A	No	1	N/A	–	1/1
Manea et al. [11]	2	2238–8915	Laparoscopic resection of GT	N/A	Yes	N/A	N/A	–	2/2

Table 9 Primary surgical treatment of interstitial pregnancy (Continued)

Author	N	Initial β-hCG	Surgical treatment	Operating time	Rupture	Hospital stay	Negative β-hCG	Complications	Success
Nezhat et al. [170]	1	6892	Laparoscopic CR⁻	N/A	Yes	N/A	N/A	–	1/1
	1	N/A	TE⁶ UG + LG	N/A	No	1	5	–	1/1
Wang et al. [171]	8	636–13,310	Laparoscopic CS°	40–100	No	2	N/A	–	8/8
	1	N/A	Laparoscopic CS°	N/A	No	2	N/A	–	1/1
Warda et al. [172]	4	N/A	Laparoscopic CS°	N/A	No	N/A	N/A	–	4/4
Watanabe et al. [47]	12	998–55,820	Laparoscopic CS°°	61–160	2/12	N/A	N/A	–	12/12
	1	69	Laparoscopic CS°	N/A	Yes	N/A	N/A	–	1/1
Yu et al. [91]	4*	N/A	Laparotomic resection of GT	N/A	N/A	N/A	*	Miscarriage 1/4	4/4
Ansari et al. [173]	1	65,000	Laparoscopic CS°	78	No	0	12	–	1/1
Afifi et al. [174]	2	3890–17,445	Laparoscopic CS°⁶ °°°°°	55–65	1/2	1	1–2	–	2/2
Faioli et al. [10]	3	10,119–18,765	Laparoscopic CR	28	No	N/A	3	–	3/3
Grindler et al. [175]	1	39,745	TE, UG	N/A	No	0	N/A		1/1
Jeon et al. [176]	9*	N/A	Laparotomy	N/A	N/A	N/A	N/A	N/A	9/9
Kim et al. [177]	13*	N/A	Laparoscopic CR	40–145	2/13	2–7	N/A	Rupture 1/11; Transfusion 2/13; Miscarriage 1/13	13/13
Mallick et al. [178]	2	2304–14,480	Laparoscopic CS	N/A	1/2	0	N/A	–	2/2
	2	N/A	Laparoscopic CS	N/A	No	1	N/A	–	2/2
Nikodijevic et al. [48]	13	16,687	Laparoscopic CR	N/A	N/A	N/A	4–8	Conversion 5/13; Transfusion 4/13	13/13
Nirgianakis et al. [49]	10	27,634	Laparoscopic CR⁻	115	N/A	3	N/A	Transfusion 3/10	10/10
Said [179]	4	N/A	Laparoscopic resection of GT⁻	40–60	N/A	2	N/A	–	4/4
	1*	N/A	Laparoscopic resection of GT	N/A	Yes	N/A	*	–	1/1
Wang et al. [50]	38	25,150	Laparoscopic CS°	71	11/38	3	N/A	–	35/38
Xu et al. [180]	1	N/A	Resection of GT	N/A	Yes	N/A	N/A	Transfusion	1/1
Kahramanoglu et al. [81]	1	> 10,000	Laparotomic resection of GT	N/A	Yes	3	N/A	Transfusion	1/1
	1	9277	TE, UG	N/A	No	0	4	–	1/1
	1	N/A	TE, LG	N/A	No	1	1	–	1/1
Lee et al. [51]	53	575–64,831	Laparoscopic CR³	77	N/A	N/A	N/A	–	49/53
	22	1454–62,422	Laparoscopic CS⁻ °	59	N/A	N/A	N/A	–	21/22

N number of cases, β-hCG mIU/ml, CR cornual resection, CS cornuostomy, TE transcervical evacuation, SS salpingostomy, GT gestational tissue, R ruptured, U unruptured, UG under ultrasound guidance, LG under laparoscopic guidance, HG under hysteroscopic guidance, IP interstitial pregnancy, operating time minutes, hospital stay days, negative β-hCG weeks
*Heterotopic pregnancy, hemostatic technique: °vasopressin, °°endoloop, °°°encircling suture, °°°°Purse-string" suture, °°°°°stitch at the uterine fundus and in the mesosalpinx, ⁶local injection of diluted adrenaline
(1/4)—1: MTX 50 mg/m^2 IM; 2: MTX 1 mg/kg IM; 3: +/− postoperative prophylactic MTX

Appendix 5

Table 10 Secondary/tertiary surgical treatment of interstitial pregnancy

Author	N	Initial β-hCG	Initial treatment	Surgical treatment	Operating time	Rupture	Hospital stay	Negative β-hCG	Complication	Success
Benifla et al. [27]	1	5340	SMTX	Laparotomic CR	N/A	N/A	N/A	N/A	N/A	1/1
	1	43,000	LMTX	Laparotomic CR	N/A	Yes	N/A	N/A	N/A	1/1
Galimberti and Jones [54]	1	7072	SMTX	Laparotomy	N/A	N/A	N/A	N/A	–	1/1
Hamada et al. [181]	1	8000	Expectant	Laparotomic HE	N/A	No	N/A	N/A	–	1/1
Sungurtekin and Uyar [182]	1	31,737	SMTX	Laparotomy	N/A	No	N/A	N/A	–	1/1
Bremner et al. [183]	1	92	Expectant	Laparoscopic CS	N/A	No	0	N/A	Ileus	1/1
Sagiv et al. [57]	1	28,166	SMTX	Laparoscopic CS	N/A	Yes	4	N/A	–	1/1
Advincula et al. [60]	1	62,889	SMTX	Laparotomic CR	N/A	N/A	N/A	N/A	–	1/1
Coric et al. [184]	1	1770	Expectant + aspiration	Laparoscopic CR	60	No	5	N/A	–	1/1
Jermy et al. [24]	1	> 10,000	SMTX	Laparotomy	N/A	No	N/A	N/A	–	1/1
Tulandi et al. [39]	2	2627–6739	SMTX	Laparoscopy	N/A	No	N/A	N/A	N/A	2/2
	1		LMTX	Laparotomy	N/A	No	N/A	N/A	N/A	1/1
Cassik et al. [28]	1	41,150	SMTX	Laparotomic CR	N/A	N/A	N/A	N/A	N/A	1/1
	2	102–69,820	LMTX	N/A	N/A	N/A	N/A	N/A	N/A	2/2
Api and Api [66]	1	18,654	SMTX	Laparoscopic CS	N/A	No	1	1	–	1/1
Günenç et al. [67]	1	8314	SMTX	Laparoscopic CS	N/A	No	N/A	5	–	1/1
Lee et al. [69]	1	14,273	SMTX	Laparoscopic CR	90	No	3	N/A	–	1/1
Lodhi et al. [156]	1	19,714	MTX	Laparoscopic CR	N/A	No	2	N/A	–	1/1
Andrés et al. [89]	1	6193	LMTX	Laparoscopy	N/A	Yes	N/A	N/A	–	1/1
Monia et al. [71]	1	94,000	SMTX	Laparoscopic CR	N/A	N/A	N/A	N/A	–	1/1
Szylit et al. [72]	1	21,281	SMTX	Laparoscopic CR	N/A	N/A	2	N/A	–	1/1
Sagiv et al. [73]	2	4304–4987	SMTX	Laparoscopic CR	N/A	N/A	N/A	N/A	–	2/2
	1	28,166	SMTX	Laparoscopic CS	N/A	N/A	N/A	N/A	–	1/1
Surbone et al. [74]	1	N/A	SMTX	Laparoscopic CS	N/A	N/A	N/A	N/A	N/A	1/1
	1	N/A	L/SMTX	Laparoscopic CS	N/A	N/A	N/A	N/A	N/A	1/1
Fritz et al. [75]	1	8200	SMTX	TE, LG	N/A	No	0	3	–	1/1
Hiersch et al. [25]	2	15,383	SLMTX + UAE	N/A	N/A	Yes	N/A	N/A	–	2/2
Meddeb et al. [77]	1	6320	SMTX	Laparoscopic CR	N/A	No	N/A	N/A	PTD	1/1
Tanaka et al. [26]	2	8500–63,000	SMTX	N/A	N/A	Yes	N/A	N/A	–	2/2
Nikodijevic et al. [48]	1	19,563	LMTX	N/A	N/A	No	N/A	N/A	–	1/1
Wang et al. [50]	2	176-N/A	Surgery	Repeat laparoscopy	N/A	Scar	Day 3	3–4	–	2/2

N number of cases, *β-hCG* mIU/ml, *(S/L)MTX* (systemic/local) methotrexate, *UAE* uterine artery embolization, *CR* cornual resection, *CS* cornuostomy, *HE* hysterectomy, *operating time* minutes, *hospital stay* days, *negative β-hCG* weeks, *PTD* persistent trophoblastic disease

Appendix 6

Table 11 Recurrent interstitial pregnancy and its treatment

Author	N	β-hCG	Treatment 1st IP	Success	β-hCG	Treatment 2nd IP	Success	β-hCG	Treatment 3rd IP	Success
Sungurtekin and Uyar [182]	1	32	SMTX	1/1	31,737	SMTX	0/1	–	–	–
Sagiv et al. [57]	1	15,400	LMTX	1/1	2577	Laparoscopic CS°	1/1	–	–	–
Vilos [185]	1	12,000	Laparoscopic CR	1/1	4700	Laparoscopic CR	1/1	–	–	–
Sahoo et al. [95]	1	N/A	Laparotomy	1/1	N/A	Laparoscopy	0/1	N/A	Laparoscopic CR	1/1
Siow and Ng [186]	2	N/A	Laparoscopic CS	2/2	N/A	Laparoscopic CR	2/2	–	–	–
	1	N/A	Laparoscopy	1/1	N/A	Laparoscopic CR	1/1	–	–	–
	1	N/A	Laparoscopic CR	1/1	N/A	Laparoscopic CR	1/1	N/A	Laparoscopic CR	1/1

N number of cases, *β-hCG* mIU/ml, *IP* interstitial pregnancy, *S/LMTX* systemic/local methotrexate, *CR* cornual resection, *CS* cornuostomy
Hemostatic technique: °vasopressin

Abbreviations

EP: Ectopic pregnancy; IP: Interstitial pregnancy; IVF: In vitro fertilization; KCL: Potassium chloride; MTX: Methotrexate; UAE: Uterine artery embolization

Authors' contributions

IV, FD, PJB, DT, AVH, SAC, ASVR, LVDH, SG, CT, and JDP did the clinical management of the patients involved. IV and FD did the data collection. IV and JDP did the data analysis. All authors contributed to the manuscript writing and read and approved the final manuscript.

Authors' information

JD was a fundamental clinical researcher for the Fonds Wetenschappelijk Onderzoek Vlaanderen (2001–2016). He is now funded by the Great Ormond Street Hospital Charity Fund, London, UK.

Competing interests

The authors declare that they no competing interests.

Author details

[1]Department Gynecology-Obstetrics, University Hospital Leuven, Herestraat 49, 3000 Leuven, Belgium. [2]Department Radiology, University Hospital Leuven, Herestraat 49, 3000 Leuven, Belgium. [3]Department Pathology, University Hospital Leuven, Herestraat 49, 3000 Leuven, Belgium. [4]Department Reproductive medicine LIFE, General Hospital Heilig Hart Ziekenhuis, Naamsestraat 105, 3000 Leuven, Belgium. [5]Department Gynecology-Obstetrics, General Hospital Onze-Lieve-Vrouwziekenhuis, Moorselbaan 164, 9300 Aalst, Belgium. [6]Institute for Women's Health and Wellcome/EPSRC Centre for Interventional & Surgical Sciences (WEISS), University College London, Charles Bell House, 43-45 Foley Street, London W1W 7TS, UK.

References

1. Bouyer J, Coste J, Fernandez H, Pouly JL, Job-Spira N (2002) Sites of ectopic pregnancy: a 10 year population-based study of 1800 cases. Hum Reprod 17(12):3224–3230.
2. Ramkrishna J, Kan GR, Reidy KL, Ang WC, Palma-Dias R (2017) Comparison of management regimens following ultrasound diagnosis of nontubal ectopic pregnancies: a retrospective cohort study. BJOG 125(5):567–575.
3. Chetty M, Elson J (2009) Treating non-tubal ectopic pregnancy. Best Pract Res Clin Obstet Gynaecol 23(4):529–538.
4. Alalade AO, Smith FJE, Kendall CE, Odejinmi F (2017) Evidence-based management of non-tubal ectopic pregnancies. J Obstet Gynaecol 37(8): 982–991.
5. Goldner TE, Lawson HW, Xia Z, Atrash HK (1993) Surveillance for ectopic pregnancy - United States 1970-1989. Morbidity and Mortality Weekly Report: Surveillance Summaries 42:73–85.
6. Jurkovic D, Wilkinson H (2011) Diagnosis and management of ectopic pregnancy. BMJ 342:d3397.
7. Alkatout I, Honemeyer U, Strauss A, Tinelli A, Malvasi A, Jonat W et al (2013) Clinical diagnosis and treatment of ectopic pregnancy. Obstet Gynecol Surv 68(8):571–581.
8. Moawad NS, Mahajan ST, Moniz MH, Taylor SE, Hurd WW (2010) Current diagnosis and treatment of interstitial pregnancy. Am J Obstet Gynecol 202(1):15–29.
9. Lau S, Tulandi T (1999) Conservative medical and surgical management of interstitial ectopic pregnancy. Fertil Steril 72(2):207–215.
10. Faioli R, Berretta R, Dall'Asta A, Di Serio M, Galli L, Monica M et al (2016) Endoloop technique for laparoscopic cornuectomy: a safe and effective approach for the treatment of interstitial pregnancy. J Obstet Gynaecol Res 42(8):1034–1037.
11. Manea C, Pavlidou E, Urias AA, Bouquet de la Joliniere J, Dubuisson JB, Feki A (2014) Laparoscopic management of interstitial pregnancy and fertility outcomes after ipsilateral salpingectomy - three case reports. Front Surg 1:34.
12. Kim MJ, Cha JH, Bae HS, Kim MK, Kim ML, Yun BS et al (2017) Therapeutic outcomes of methotrexate injection in unruptured interstitial pregnancy. Obstet Gynecol Sci 60(6):571–578.
13. Panelli DM, Phillips CH, Brady PC (2015) Incidence, diagnosis and management of tubal and nontubal ectopic pregnancies: a review. Fertil Res Pract 1:15.
14. Moon HS, Kim SG, Park GS, Choi JK, Koo JS, Joo BS. Efficacy of bleeding control using a large amount of highly diluted vasopressin in laparoscopic treatment for interstitial pregnancy. Am J Obstet Gynecol 2010;203(1):30 e1–6.
15. Cucinella G, Calagna G, Rotolo S, Granese R, Saitta S, Tonni G et al (2014) Interstitial pregnancy: a 'road map' of surgical treatment based on a systematic review of the literature. Gynecol Obstet Investig 78(3):141–149.
16. Torre A, Fauconnier A, Kahn V, Limot O, Bussierres L, Pelage JP (2017) Fertility after uterine artery embolization for symptomatic multiple fibroids with no other infertility factors. Eur Radiol 27(7):2850–2859.
17. Yang SB, Lee SJ, Joe HS, Goo DE, Chang YW, Kim DH (2007) Selective uterine artery embolization for management of interstitial ectopic pregnancy. Korean J Radiol 8(2):176–179.
18. Song D, Liu Y, Xiao Y, Li TC, Zhou F, Xia E (2014) A matched cohort study comparing the outcome of intrauterine adhesiolysis for Asherman's syndrome after uterine artery embolization or surgical trauma. J Minim Invasive Gynecol 21(6):1022–1028.
19. Li C, Zhao WH, Zhu Q, Cao SJ, Ping H, Xi X et al (2015) Risk factors for ectopic pregnancy: a multi-center case-control study. BMC Pregnancy Childbirth 15:187.
20. Bouyer J, Coste J, Shojaei T, Pouly J-L, Fernandez H, Gerbaud L et al (2003) Risk factors for ectopic pregnancy: a comprehensive analysis based on a large case-control, population-based study in France. Am J Epidemiol 157(3):185–194.
21. Ankum WM, Mol BWJ, Van der Veen F, Bossuyt PMM (1996) Risk factors for ectopic pregnancy: a meta-analysis**supported in part by grant OG 93/007 from the Ziekenfonds-Raad, Amstelveen, the Netherlands. Fertil Steril 65(6):1093–1099.
22. Backman T, Rauramo I, Huhtala S, Koskenvuo M (2004) Pregnancy during the use of levonorgestrel intrauterine system. Am J Obstet Gynecol 190(1):50–54.
23. Xiong X, Buekens P, Wollast E (1995) IUD use and the risk of ectopic pregnancy: a meta-analysis of case-control studies. Contraception 52(1):23–34.
24. Jermy K, Thomas J, Doo A, Bourne T (2004) The conservative management of interstitial pregnancy. BJOG 111(11):1283–1288.
25. Hiersch L, Krissi H, Ashwal E, From A, Wiznitzer A, Peled Y (2014) Effectiveness of medical treatment with methotrexate for interstitial pregnancy. Aust N Z J Obstet Gynaecol 54(6):576–580.
26. Tanaka K, Baartz D, Khoo SK (2015) Management of interstitial ectopic pregnancy with intravenous methotrexate: an extended study of a standardised regimen. Aust N Z J Obstet Gynaecol 55(2):176–180.
27. Benifla JL, Fernandez H, Sebban E, Darai E, Frydman R, Madelenat P (1996) Alternative to surgery of treatment of unruptured interstitial pregnancy: 15 cases of medical treatment. Eur J Obstet Gynecol Reprod Biol 70(2):151–156.
28. Cassik P, Ofili-Yebovi D, Yazbek J, Lee C, Elson J, Jurkovic D (2005) Factors influencing the success of conservative treatment of interstitial pregnancy. Ultrasound Obstet Gynecol 26(3):279–282.
29. Framarino-dei-Malatesta M, Piccioni MG, Derme M, Polidori NF, Tibaldi V, Iannini I et al (2014) Transabdominal ultrasound-guided injection of methotrexate in the treatment of ectopic interstitial pregnancies. J Clin Ultrasound 42(9):522–526.
30. Valsky DV, Hamani Y, Verstandig A, Yagel S (2007) The use of 3D rendering, VCI-C, 3D power Doppler and B-flow in the evaluation of interstitial pregnancy with arteriovenous malformation treated by selective uterine artery embolization. Ultrasound Obstet Gynecol 29(3):352–355.

31. Takeda A, Koyama K, Imoto S, Mori M, Sakai K, Nakamura H (2009) Successful management of interstitial pregnancy with fetal cardiac activity by laparoscopic-assisted cornual resection with preoperative transcatheter uterine artery embolization. Arch Gynecol Obstet 280(2):305–308.
32. Krissi H, Hiersch L, Stolovitch N, Nitke S, Wiznitzer A, Peled Y (2014) Outcome, complications and future fertility in women treated with uterine artery embolization and methotrexate for non-tubal ectopic pregnancy. Eur J Obstet Gynecol Reprod Biol 182:172–176.
33. Takeda A, Koike W, Hayashi S, Imoto S, Nakamura H (2015) Magnetic resonance imaging and 3-dimensional computed tomographic angiography for conservative management of proximal interstitial pregnancy by hysteroscopic resection after transcatheter arterial chemoembolization. J Minim Invasive Gynecol 22(4):658–662.
34. Ophir E, Singer-Jordan J, Oettinger M, Odeh M, Tendler R, Feldman Y et al (2004) Uterine artery embolization for management of interstitial twin ectopic pregnancy: case report. Hum Reprod 19(8):1774–1777.
35. Deruelle P, Lucot J-P, Lions C, Robert Y (2005) Management of interstitial pregnancy using selective uterine artery embolization. Obstet Gynecol 106(5):1165–1167.
36. Tamarit G, Lonjedo E, Gonzalez M, Tamarit S, Domingo S, Pellicer A. Combined use of uterine artery embolization and local methotrexate injection in interstitial ectopic pregnancies with poor prognosis. Fertil Steril 2010;93(4):1348 e1–4.
37. Berretta R, Merisio C, Dall'Asta A, Verrotti C, Rolla M, Bruni S et al (2014) Conservative treatment for interstitial monochorionic twin pregnancy: case report and review of the published work. J Obstet Gynaecol Res 40(3):829–832.
38. Moon HS, Choi YJ, Park YH, Kim SG (2000) New simple endoscopic operations for interstitial pregnancies. Am J Obstet Gynecol 182(1).
39. Tulandi T, Al-Jaroudi D (2004) Interstitial pregnancy: results generated from the Society of Reproductive Surgeons Registry. Obstet Gynecol 103(1):47–50.
40. MacRae R, Olowu O, Rizzuto MI, Odejinmi F (2009) Diagnosis and laparoscopic management of 11 consecutive cases of cornual ectopic pregnancy. Arch Gynecol Obstet 280(1):59–64.
41. Ng S, Hamontri S, Chua I, Chern B, Siow A (2009) Laparoscopic management of 53 cases of cornual ectopic pregnancy. Fertil Steril 92(2):448–452.
42. Hwang JH, Lee JK, Lee NW, Lee KW (2011) Open cornual resection versus laparoscopic cornual resection in patients with interstitial ectopic pregnancies. Eur J Obstet Gynecol Reprod Biol 156(1):78–82.
43. Cai Z, Wang F, Cao H, Xia Q, Chen X, Cai Y (2012) The value of laparoscopy alone or combined with hysteroscopy in the treatment of interstitial pregnancy: analysis of 22 cases. Arch Gynecol Obstet 285(3):727–732.
44. Zuo X, Shen A, Chen M (2012) Successful management of unruptured interstitial pregnancy in 17 consecutive cases by using laparoscopic surgery. Aust N Z J Obstet Gynaecol 52(4):387–390.
45. Ahn JW, Lee SJ, Lee SH, Kang SP, Won HS (2013) Ultrasound-guided transcervical forceps extraction of unruptured interstitial pregnancy. BJOG 120(10):1285–1288.
46. Douysset X, Verspyck E, Diguet A, Marpeau L, Chanavaz-Lacheray I, Rondeau S et al (2014) Interstitial pregnancy: experience at Rouen's hospital. Gynecol Obstet Fertil. 42(4):216–221.
47. Watanabe T, Watanabe Z, Watanabe T, Fujimoto K, Sasaki E (2014) Laparoscopic cornuotomy for interstitial pregnancy and postoperative course. J Obstet Gynaecol Res 40(8):1983–1988.
48. Nikodijevic K, Bricou A, Benbara A, Moreaux G, Nguyen C, Carbillon L et al (2016) Cornual pregnancy: management and subsequent fertility. Gynecol Obstet Fertil 44(1):11–16.
49. Nirgianakis K, Papadia A, Grandi G, McKinnon B, Bolla D, Mueller MD (2017) Laparoscopic management of ectopic pregnancies: a comparison between interstitial and "more distal" tubal pregnancies. Arch Gynecol Obstet 295(1):95–101.
50. Wang J, Huang D, Lin X, Saravelos SH, Chen J, Zhang X et al (2016) Incidence of interstitial pregnancy after in vitro fertilization/embryo transfer and the outcome of a consecutive series of 38 cases managed by laparoscopic cornuostomy or cornual repair. J Minim Invasive Gynecol 23(5):739–747.
51. Lee MH, Im SY, Kim MK, Shin SY, Park WI (2017) Comparison of laparoscopic cornual resection and cornuotomy for interstitial pregnancy. J Minim Invasive Gynecol 24(3):397–401.
52. Tanaka T, Hayashi H, Kutsuzawa T, Fujimoto S, Ichinoe K (1982) Treatment of interstitial ectopic pregnancy with methotrexate: report of a successful case. Fertil Steril 37(6):851–852.
53. Hajenius PJ, Voigt RR, Engelsbel S, Mol BWJ, Hemrika DJ, Van der Veen F (1996) Serum human chorionic gonadotropin clearance curves in patients with interstitial pregnancy treated with systemic methotrexate**supported in part by grant OG 93/007 from the Health Insurance Funds Council, Amstelveen, the Netherlands. Fertil Steril 66(5):723–728.
54. Galimberti A, Jones MR (1997) Failure of conservative treatment with methotrexate for interstitial pregnancy despite progressive decrease of serial serum betaHCG. J Obstet Gynaecol 17(4):407–408.
55. Bernardini L, Valenzano M, Foglia G (1998) Spontaneous interstitial pregnancy on a tubal stump after unilateral adenectomy followed by transvaginal colour Doppler ultrasound. Hum Reprod 13(6):1723–1726.
56. Fisch JD, Ortiz BH, Tazuke SI, Chitkara U, Giudice LC. Medical management of interstitial ectopic pregnancy: a case report and literature review. 1998; 13(7):1981–1986.
57. Sagiv R, Golan A, Arbel-Alon S, Glezerman M (2001) Three conservative approaches to treatment of interstitial pregnancy. J Am Assoc Gynecol Laparosc. 8(1):154–158.
58. Lalchandani S, Geary M, O'Herlihy C, Sheil O (2003) Conservative management of placenta accreta and unruptured interstitial cornual pregnancy using methotrexate. Eur J Obstet Gynecol Reprod Biol 107(1):96–97.
59. Verity L, Ludlow J, Dickinson JE (2003) Interstitial ectopic pregnancy: a contemporary case series. Aust NZ J Obstet Gynecol 43:232–235.
60. Advincula AP, Senapati S (2004) Interstitial pregnancy. Fertil Steril 82(6):1660–1661.
61. Reid P, Buddha L (2004) Hysteroscopic diagnosis of interstitial ectopic pregnancy. BJOG 111:89–90.
62. Rodriguez L, Takacs P, Kang J (2004) Single-dose methotrexate for the management of interstitial ectopic pregnancy. Int J Gynaecol Obstet 84(3):271–272.
63. Klemm P, Koehler C, Eichhorn KH, Hillemanns P, Schneider A (2006) Sonographic monitoring of systemic and local methotrexate (MTX) therapy in patients with intact interstitial pregnancies. J Perinat Med 34(2):149–157.
64. Araujo Junior E, Zanforlin Filho SM, Pires CR, Guimaraes Filho HA, Massaguer AA, Nardozza LM et al (2007) Three-dimensional transvaginal sonographic diagnosis of early and asymptomatic interstitial pregnancy. Arch Gynecol Obstet 275(3):207–210.
65. Fujioka S, Yamashita Y, Kawabe S, Kamegai H, Terai Y, Ohmichi M (2009) A case of a methotrexate-resistant ectopic pregnancy in which dactinomycin was effective as a second-line chemotherapy. Fertil Steril 91(3):929 e13–929 e15.
66. Api M, Api O (2010) Laparoscopic cornuotomy in the management of an advanced interstitial ectopic pregnancy: a case report. Gynecol Endocrinol 26(3):208–212.
67. Gunenc Z, Bingol B, Celik A, Bozkurt S, Ozekici U (2010) Laparoscopic surgery of interstitial (cornual) pregnancy, a case report. J Turk Ger Gynecol Assoc 11(2):102–104.
68. Kato S, Tanaka T, Terai Y, Yamashita Y, Ohmichi M (2011) Interstitial pregnancy treated by transcervical aspiration of the gestational sac combined with systemic and local administration of methotrexate. J Obstet Gynaecol Res 37(9):1250–1254.
69. Lee ES, Hahn HS, Park BJ, Ro DY, Kim JH, Kim YW (2011) Single-port laparoscopic cornual resection for a spontaneous cornual ectopic pregnancy following ipsilateral salpingectomy. Fertil Steril 96(2):e106–e110.
70. Gomez Garcia MT, Aguaron Benitez G, Barbera Belda B, Callejon Rodriguez C, Gonzalez Merlo G (2012) Medical therapy (methotrexate and mifepristone) alone or in combination with another type of therapy for the management of cervical or interstitial ectopic pregnancy. Eur J Obstet Gynecol Reprod Biol 165(1):77–81.
71. Monia M, Atef Y, Manel M, Fethi B, Khaled N, Hedi R (2012) Traitement médicale des grossesses interstitielles non rompues. Tunis Méd 90(5):421–423.
72. Szylit N, Podgaec S, Traina E, Oliveira R (2012) Video laparoscopic intervention for an interstitial pregnancy after failure of clinical treatment. Sao Paulo Med J 130(3):202–207.
73. Sagiv R, Debby A, Keidar R, Kerner R, Golan A (2013) Interstitial pregnancy management and subsequent pregnancy outcome. Acta Obstet Gynecol Scand 92(11):1327–1330.
74. Surbone A, Cottier O, Vial Y, Francini K, Hohlfeld P, Achtari C (2013) Interstitial pregnancies' diagnosis and management: an eleven cases series. Swiss Med Wkly 143:w13736.

75. Fritz RB, Rosenblum N, Gaither K, Sherman A, McCalla A (2014) Successful laparoscopically assisted transcervical suction evacuation of interstitial pregnancy following failed methotrexate injection in a community hospital setting. Case Rep Obstet Gynecol 2014:695293.

76. Horne AW, Skubisz MM, Tong S, Duncan WC, Neil P, Wallace EM et al (2014) Combination gefitinib and methotrexate treatment for non-tubal ectopic pregnancies: a case series. Hum Reprod 29(7):1375–1379.

77. Meddeb S, Rhim MS, Zarrouk W, Bibi M, Yacoubi MT, Khairi H (2014) Unusual gestational choriocarcinoma arising in an interstitial pregnancy. Int J Surg Case Rep 5(11):787–788.

78. Corioni S, Perelli F, Bianchi C, Cozzolino M, Maggio L, Masini G et al (2015) Interstitial pregnancy treated with a single-dose of systemic methotrexate: a successful management. J Res Med Sci 20(3):312–316.

79. Kim TH, Lee HH (2015) Pseudocyst development after treatment for interstitial ectopic pregnancy. Taiwan J Obstet Gynecol 54(1):107–108.

80. Singh N, Tripathi R, Mala Y, Batra A (2015) Diagnostic dilemma in cornual pregnancy- 3D ultrasonography may aid!! J Clin Diagn Res 9(1):QD12–QD13.

81. Kahramanoglu I, Mammadov Z, Turan H, Urer A, Tuten A (2017) Management options for interstitial ectopic pregnancies: a case series. Pak J Med Sci 33(2):476–482.

82. Timor-Tritsch IE, Monteagudo A, Matera C, Veit C (1992) Sonographic evolution of cornual pregnancies treated without surgery. Obstet Gynecol 79(6):1044–1049.

83. Baker VL, Givens CR, Martin Cadieux MC (1997) Transvaginal reduction of an interstitial heterotopic pregnancy with preservation of the intrauterine gestation. Am J Obstet Gynecol 176:1384–1385.

84. Wilkinson C, Petrucco O, Pachulicz M, Furness M (1998) Interstitial ectopic pregnancy - management with laparoscopically-guided local methotrexate infiltration. Aust NZ J Obstet Gynaecol 38(4):434–437.

85. Lin Y, Hwang J, Huang L, Chou C (2002) Conservative treatment for a ruptured interstitial pregnancy. Acta Obstet Gynecol Scand 81:179.

86. Oyawoye S, Chander B, Pavlovic B, Hunter J, Gadir AA (2003) Heterotopic pregnancy: successful management with aspiration of cornual/interstitial gestational sac and instillation of small dose of methotrexate. Fetal Diagn Ther 18(1):1–4.

87. Chou MM, Tseng JJ, Yi YC, Chen WC, Ho ES (2005) Diagnosis of an interstitial pregnancy with 4-dimensional volume contrast imaging. Am J Obstet Gynecol 193(4):1551–1553.

88. Narang L, Kalu G (2009) Laparoscopic salpingocentesis using methotrexate in combination with oral mifepristone for successful treatment of interstitial pregnancy: a case report. Fertil Steril 92(6):2038 e5–2038 e7.

89. Andres MP, Campillos JM, Lapresta M, Lahoz I, Crespo R, Tobajas J (2012) Management of ectopic pregnancies with poor prognosis through ultrasound guided intrasacular injection of methotrexate, series of 14 cases. Arch Gynecol Obstet 285(2):529–533.

90. Swank ML, Harken TR, Porto M (2013) Management of interstitial ectopic pregnancies with a combined intra-amniotic and systemic approach. Obstet Gynecol 122(2 Pt 2):461–464.

91. Yu Y, Xu W, Xie Z, Huang Q, Li S (2014) Management and outcome of 25 heterotopic pregnancies in Zhejiang, China. Eur J Obstet Gynecol Reprod Biol 180:157–161.

92. Macaes A, Fernandes S, Rodrigues C, Branco M (2015) Interstitial ectopic pregnancy managed with local methotrexate. BMJ Case Rep. 2015. https://doi.org/10.1136/bcr-2015-212563.

93. Leggieri C, Guasina F, Casadio P, Arena A, Pilu G, Seracchioli R (2016) Hysteroscopic methotrexate injection under ultrasonographic guidance for interstitial pregnancy. J Minim Invasive Gynecol 23(7):1195–1199.

94. Takeda A, Manabe S, Mitsui T, Nakamura H (2006) Management of patients with ectopic pregnancy with massive hemoperitoneum by laparoscopic surgery with intraoperative autologous blood transfusion. J Minim Invasive Gynecol 13(1):43–48.

95. Sahoo S, Jose J, Shah N, Opemuyi I (2008) Recurrent cornual ectopic pregnancies. Gynecol Surg 6(4):389–391.

96. Poon LC, Emmanuel E, Ross JA, Johns J (2014) How feasible is expectant management of interstitial ectopic pregnancy? Ultrasound Obstet Gynecol 43(3):317–321.

97. Steadman H (1956) Ruptured interstitial pregnancy following homolateral salpingectomy. Obstet Gynecol 7(5):572–575.

98. Bickerstaff H (1957) Homolateral interstitial pregnancy following salpingectomy. Obstet Gynecol 10(4):422–424.

99. Farabow W, Cater C, Brame R (1969) Interstitial pregnancy: presentation of two cases and review of salient clinical features. South Med J 62:859–862.

100. Iuchtman M, Grunstein S (1987) Acute abdomen in ruptured interstitial pregnancy following unilateral salpingectomy. Eur J Obstet Gynecol Reprod Biol 26:165–168.

101. Hill GA, Segars JH, Herbert CM (1989) Laparoscopic management of interstitial pregnancy. J Gynecol Surg 5:209–212.

102. Reich H, McGlynn F, Budin R, Tsoutsoplides G, DeCaprio J (1990) Laparoscopic treatment of ruptured interstitial pregnancy. J Gynecol Surg 6(2):135–138.

103. de Boer C, van Dongen P, Willemsen W, Klapwijk C (1992) Ultrasound diagnosis of interstitial pregnancy. Eur J Obstet Gynecol Reprod Biol 47:164–166.

104. Pelosi M (1994) Successful taparoscopic removal of an interstitial ectopic pregnancy. J Am Assoc Gynecol Laparosc. 1(4):S28.

105. Laury D (1995) Laparoscopic treatment of an interstitial pregnancy. J Am Assoc Gynecol Laparosc. 2:219–212.

106. Sherer DM, Scibetta JJ, Sanko SR (1995) Heterotopic quadruplet gestation with laparoscopic resection of ruptured interstitial pregnancy and subsequent successful outcome of triplets. Am J Obstet Gynecol 172:216–217.

107. Tulandi T, Vilos G, Gomel V (1995) Laparoscopic treatment of interstitial pregnancy. Obstet Gynecol 85(3):465–467.

108. Woodland M, DePasquale S, Molinari J, Sagullo C (1996) Laparoscopic approach to interstitial pregnancy. J Am Assoc Gynecol Laparosc. 3(3):439–441.

109. Katz Z, Lurie S (1997) Laparoscopic cornuostomy in the treatment of interstitial pregnancy with subsequent hysterosalpingography. BJOG 104:955–956.

110. Grobman WA, Milad MP (1998) Conservative laparoscopic management of a large cornual ectopic pregnancy. Hum Reprod 13(7):2002–2004.

111. Kasum M, Grizelj V, Simunic V (1998) Combined interstitial and intrauterine pregnancies after in-vitro fertilization and embryo transfer. Hum Reprod 13(6):1547–1549.

112. Crvenkoviæ G, Barišiæ D, Æorušiæ A, Nola M (1999) Laparoscopic management of the cornual pregnancy. Croatian Med J 40(1).

113. Rahimi M (1999) A new laparoscopic approach for the treatment of interstitial ectopic pregnancy. J Am Assoc Gynecol Laparosc 6(2):205–207.

114. Vicino M, Loverro G, Resta L, Bettocchi S, Vimercati A, Selvaggi L (2000) Laparoscopic cornual excision in a viable large interstitial pregnancy without blood flow detected by color Doppler ultrasonography. Fertil Steril 74(2):407–409.

115. Ayoubi J-M, Fanchin R, Fo O, Fernandez H, Pons J-C (2001) Tubal curettage: a new conservative treatment for haemorrhagic interstitial pregnancies: case report. Hum Reprod 16(4):780–781.

116. Dumesic DA, Damario MA, Session DR (2001) Interstitial heterotopic pregnancy in a woman conceiving by in vitro fertilization after bilateral salpingectomy. Mayo Clin Proc 76(1):90–92.

117. Kun W, Tung W (2001) On the look out for a rarity: interstitial/cornual pregnancy. Eur J Emerg Med 8:147–150.

118. Osuga Y, Tsutsumi O, Fujiwara T, Kugu K, Fujimoto A, Taketani Y (2001) Usefulness of long-jaw forceps in laparoscopic cornual resection of interstitial pregnancies. J Am Assoc Gynecol Laparosc. 8(3):429–432.

119. DeWitt C, Abbott J (2002) Interstitial pregnancy: a potential for misdiagnosis of ectopic pregnancy with emergency department ultrasonography. Ann Emerg Med 40(1):106–109.

120. Sills ES, Perloe M, Kaplan CR, Sweitzer CL, Morton PC, Tucker MJ (2002) Uncomplicated pregnancy and normal singleton delivery after surgical excision of heterotopic (cornual) pregnancy following in vitro fertilization/embryo transfer. Arch Gynecol Obstet 266:181–184.

121. Chang Y, Lee JN, Yang CH, Hsu SC, Tsai EM (2003) An unexpected quadruplet heterotopic pregnancy after bilateral salpingectomy and replacement of three embryos. Fertil Steril 80(1):218–220.

122. Habek D, Mrcela M, Rubin M, Hrgovic Z (2003) Ruptured interstitial pregnancy. Arch Gynecol Obstet 267:170–172.

123. Izquierdo LA, Nicholas MC (2003) Three-dimensional transvaginal sonography of interstitial pregnancy. J Clin Ultrasound 31(9):484–487.

124. Katz DL, Barrett JP, Sanfilippo JS, Badway DM (2003) Combined hysteroscopy and laparoscopy in the treatment of interstitial pregnancy. Am J Obstet Gynecol 188(4):1113–1114.

125. Yoo E-H, Chun S-H, Kim J-I (2003) Endoscopic treatment of interstitial pregnancy. Acta Obstet Gynecol Scand 82:189–191.

126. Gezer A, Mutlu H (2004) Laparoscopic management of cornual pregnancy without sutures. Arch Gynecol Obstet 270(3):194–196.

127. Grimbizis G (2004) Case report: laparoscopic treatment of a ruptured interstitial pregnancy. Reprod BioMed Online 9(4):447–451.

128. Lee GS, Hur SY, Kown I, Shin JC, Kim SP, Kim SJ (2005) Diagnosis of early intramural ectopic pregnancy. J Clin Ultrasound 33(4):190–192.

129. Savvidou MD, Setchell TE, Sieunarine K, Smith JR (2006) Conservative surgical management of ruptured interstitial pregnancy. Acta Obstet Gynecol Scand 85(5):629–631.

130. Thakur Y, Coker A, Morris J, Oliver R (2004) Laparoscopic and ultrasound-guided transcervical evacuation of cornual ectopic pregnancy: an alternative approach. J Obstet Gynaecol 24(7):809–810.

131. Zhang X, Liu X, Fan H (2004) Interstitial pregnancy and transcervical curettage. Obstet Gynecol 104(5 Pt 2):1193–1195.

132. Huang MC, Su TH, Lee MY (2005) Laparoscopic management of interstitial pregnancy. Int J Gynaecol Obstet 88(1):51–52.

133. Kumakiri J, Takeuchi H, Kitade M, Kikuchi I, Shimanuki H, Kubo M et al (2005) Interstitial pregnancy with huge adenomyosis uteri managed laparoscopically by using pre-operative and intra-operative imaging: case report. BJOG 112(11):1578–1580.

134. Ross R, Lindheim SR, Olive DL, Pritts EA (2006) Cornual gestation: a systematic literature review and two case reports of a novel treatment regimen. J Minim Invasive Gynecol 13(1):74–78.

135. Ko ML, Jeng CJ, Chou CS, She BC, Chen SC, Tzeng CR (2007) Laparoscopic electrodessication of an interstitial pregnancy. Fertil Steril 88(3):705 e19–705 e20.

136. Lee W, Chen C, Chang T, Chen R, Chow S. Interstitial pregnancy with a retained intrauterine device. Taiwan J Obstet Gynecol 2007;46(4):442–4.

137. Oliver R, Malik M, Coker A, Morris J (2007) Management of extra-tubal and rare ectopic pregnancies: case series and review of current literature. Arch Gynecol Obstet 276(2):125–131.

138. Lialios GA, Kallitsaris A, Kabisios T, Messinis IE (2008) Ruptured heterotopic interstitial pregnancy: rare case of acute abdomen in a Jehovah's Witness patient. Fertil Steril 90(4):1200 e15–1200 e17.

139. Qin L, Li S, Tan S (2008) Laparoscopic loop ligature for selective therapy in heterotopic interstitial and intrauterine pregnancy following in-vitro fertilization and embryo transfer. Int J Gynaecol Obstet 101(1):80–81.

140. Sherer DM, Dalloul M, Sokolovski M, Borawski D, Granderson F, Abulafia O (2009) Interstitial pregnancy undetected during earlier first-trimester screening for fetal aneuploidy at 13 weeks' gestation. J Clin Ultrasound 37(3):168–170.

141. Casadio P, Formelli G, Spagnolo E, De Angelis D, Marra E, Armillotta F et al (2009) Laparoscopic treatment of interstitial twin pregnancy. Fertil Steril 92(1):390 e13–390 e17.

142. Cheng Z, Xu L, Zhu Y, Dai H, Qu X, Gong J (2009) Laparoscopic uterine vessels occlusion for the treatment of interstitial pregnancy. J Laparoendosc Adv Surg Tech A 19(4):509–512.

143. Choi YS, Eun DS, Choi J, Shin KS, Choi JH, Park HD (2009) Laparoscopic cornuotomy using a temporary tourniquet suture and diluted vasopressin injection in interstitial pregnancy. Fertil Steril 91(5):1933–1937.

144. Duong D, Baker WE, Adedipe A (2009) Clinician-performed ultrasound diagnosis of ruptured interstitial pregnancy. Am J Emerg Med 27(9):1170 e1–1170 e2.

145. Pluchino N, Ninni F, Angioni S, Carmignani A, Genazzani AR, Cela V (2009) Spontaneous cornual pregnancy after homolateral salpingectomy for an earlier tubal pregnancy: a case report and literature review. J Minim Invasive Gynecol 16(2):208–211.

146. Pan J, Qian Y, Wang J (2010) Bilateral interstitial pregnancy after in vitro fertilization and embryo transfer with bilateral fallopian tube resection detected by transvaginal sonography. J Ultrasound Med 29:1829–1832.

147. Pistofidis G, Bardis NS, Koukoura OG, Balinakos P (2010) Spontaneous intraoperative rupture of interstitial pregnancy. Laparoscopic management. J Minim Invasive Gynecol 17(6):191.

148. Tinelli A, Malvasi A, Pellegrino M, Pontrelli G, Martulli B, Tsin DA (2010) Laparoscopical management of cornual pregnancies: a report of three cases. Eur J Obstet Gynecol Reprod Biol 151(2):199–202.

149. Vignali M, Bertazzoli E, Natale A, Alabiso G, Barbisetti De Prun A, Ciocca E (2010) Three cases of interstitial tubal pregnancy after ipsilateral salpingectomy for a previous ectopic pregnancy. J Minim Invasive Gynecol 17(6):158.

150. Walid MS, Heaton RL (2010) Diagnosis and laparoscopic treatment of cornual ectopic pregnancy. Arch Gynecol Obstet 8. https://doi.org/10.3205/000105.

151. Yan CM (2010) Laparoscopic management of three rare types of ectopic pregnancy. Hong Kong Med J 16(2):132–136.

152. Aust T, O'Neill A, Cario G (2011) Purse-string suture technique to enable laparoscopic management of the interstitial gestation of a heterotopic pregnancy. Fertil Steril 95(1):261–263.

153. Cervino E, Ramon YCCL, Perez P, Couceiro E (2011) Ultrasound-guided transcervical evacuation of interstitial twin pregnancy. Fertil Steril 96(4):927–930.

154. Chachan S, Waters N, Kent A (2011) Laparoscopic management of cornual heterotopic pregnancy with the use of Harmonic ACE®—a case report. Gynecol Surg 8(2):243–246.

155. Lazard A, Poizac S, Courbiere B, Cravello L, Gamerre M, Agostini A. Cornual resection for interstitial pregnancy by laparoendoscopic single-site surgery. Fertil Steril 2011;95(7):2432 e5–8.

156. Lodhi W, Andersen K, Yoong W (2011) Laparoscopic cornuectomy revisited: a case series of 3 patients using the Multifire Endo GIA Stapler. Eur J Obstet Gynecol Reprod Biol 159(2):477–478.

157. Yamamoto MP, Zaritsky EF (2011) Total laparoscopic management of a 13 week cornual ectopic pregnancy. J Minim Invasive Gynecol 18(6).

158. Ahsan Akhtar M, Izzat F, Keay SD (2012) Laparoscopic management of interstitial pregnancy with automatic stapler. BMJ Case Rep 2012. https://doi.org/10.1136/bcr-2012-006851.

159. Cucinella G, Rotolo S, Calagna G, Granese R, Agrusa A, Perino A (2012) Laparoscopic management of interstitial pregnancy: the "purse-string" technique. Acta Obstet Gynecol Scand 91(8):996–999.

160. Garavaglia E, Quaranta L, Pasi F, Redaelli A, Colombo G, Candiani M (2012) Interstitial pregnancy after in vitro fertilization and embryo transfer following bilateral salpingectomy: report of two cases and literature review. Int J Fertil Steril 6(2):131–134.

161. Muglu J, Uchil D, Sau A, Zamblera D, Jolaoso A (2012) Recurrent uterine rupture after laparoscopic surgery for interstitial ectopic pregnancy. J Gynecol Surg 28(2):169–171.

162. Rheinboldt M, Ibrahim S (2013) Atypical presentation of a large interstitial pregnancy. Emerg Radiol 20(3):251–254.

163. Mackenna A, Fernandez E, Fernandez C (2013) Treatment of interstitial pregnancy by laparoscopic cornual resection. J Minim Invasive Gynecol 20(4):406–407.

164. Mooij R, van Dillen J (2013) Een jonge vrouw met acute buikpijn. Ned Tijdschr Geneesk 157:A5496.

165. Warda H, Mamik MM, Ashraf M, Abuzeid MI (2013) Laparoscopic cornuostomy for a large interstitial ectopic pregnancy. J Minim Invasive Gynecol 20(6):742–743.

166. Wright SD, Busbridge RC, Gard GB (2013) A conservative and fertility preserving treatment for interstitial ectopic pregnancy. Aust N Z J Obstet Gynaecol 53(2):211–213.

167. Zhang K, Yuan P (2013) Laparoscopy-assisted vaginal cornual resection for the treatment of large interstitial pregnancy. J Laparoendosc Adv Surg Tech A. 23(9):783–786.

168. Chandran JR (2014) Cornual pregnancy and its management: a case report. IJSS Case Reports & Reviews 1(6):1–3.

169. Garretto D, Lee LN, Budorick NE, Figueroa R (2015) Interstitial twin pregnancy: a unique case presentation. J Clin Ultrasound 43(7):447–450.

170. Nezhat CH, Dun EC (2014) Laparoscopically-assisted, hysteroscopic removal of an interstitial pregnancy with a fertility-preserving technique. J Minim Invasive Gynecol 21(6):1091–1094.

171. Wang YL, Weng SS, Huang WC, Su TH (2014) Laparoscopic management of ectopic pregnancies in unusual locations. Taiwan J Obstet Gynecol. 53(4): 466–470.

172. Warda H, Mamik MM, Ashraf M, Abuzeid MI (2014) Interstitial ectopic pregnancy: conservative surgical management. JSLS 18(2):197–203.

173. Ansari A, Ahmad S, James J, Jeppson C, Holloway R (2015) Robotic-assisted laparoscopic resection of cornual ectopic pregnancy a case report. J Reprod Med 60(1):58–64.

174. Afifi Y, Mahmud A, Fatma A (2016) Hemostatic techniques for laparoscopic management of cornual pregnancy: double-impact devascularization technique. J Minim Invasive Gynecol 23(2):274–280.

175. Grindler NM, Ng J, Tocce K, Alvero R (2016) Considerations for management of interstitial ectopic pregnancies: two case reports. J Med Case Rep 10(1):106.

176. Jeon JH, Hwang YI, Shin IH, Park CW, Yang KM, Kim HO (2016) The risk factors and pregnancy outcomes of 48 cases of heterotopic pregnancy from a single center. J Korean Med Sci 31(7):1094–1099.

177. Kim MJ, Jung YW, Cha JH, Seok HH, Han JE, Seong SJ et al (2016) Successful management of heterotopic cornual pregnancy with laparoscopic cornual resection. Eur J Obstet Gynecol Reprod Biol 203:199–202.

178. Mallick R, Ajala T (2016) A new technique in the laparoscopic resection of cornual ectopic pregnancies: a case series. Gynecol Surg 13(3):147–151.

179. Said TH (2016) Laparoscopic management of interstitial ectopic using simple and safe technique: case series and review of literature. J Obstet Gynaecol India 66(Suppl 1):482–487.

180. Xu Y, Lu Y, Chen H, Li D, Zhang J, Zheng L (2016) Heterotopic pregnancy after in vitro fertilization and embryo transfer after bilateral total salpingectomy/tubal ligation: case report and literature review. J Minim Invasive Gynecol 23(3):338–345.
181. Hamada S, Nakah O, Morideh N, Higuchih K, Takahashih H (1997) Ultrasonography and magnetic resonance imaging findings in a patient with an unruptured interstitial pregnancy. Eur J Obstet Gynecol Reprod Biol 73:107–201.
182. Sungurtekin U, Uyar Y (1998) Recurrent interstitial pregnancy. Aust NZ J Obstet Gynecol. 38(4):438–440.
183. Bremner T, Cela V, Luciano AA (2000) Surgical management of interstitial pregnancy. J Am Assoc Gynecol Laparosc. 7(3):387–389.
184. Coric M, Barisic D, Strelec M (2004) Laparoscopic approach to interstitial pregnancy. Arch Gynecol Obstet 270(4):287–289.
185. Vilos GA (2001) Laparoscopic ligation and resection of two ipsilateral interstitial pregnancies in the same patient. J Am Assoc Gynecol Laparosc. 8(2):299–302.
186. Siow A, Ng S (2011) Laparoscopic management of 4 cases of recurrent cornual ectopic pregnancy and review of literature. J Minim Invasive Gynecol 18(3):296–302.

Permissions

All chapters in this book were first published in GS, by Springer; hereby published with permission under the Creative Commons Attribution License or equivalent. Every chapter published in this book has been scrutinized by our experts. Their significance has been extensively debated. The topics covered herein carry significant findings which will fuel the growth of the discipline. They may even be implemented as practical applications or may be referred to as a beginning point for another development.

The contributors of this book come from diverse backgrounds, making this book a truly international effort. This book will bring forth new frontiers with its revolutionizing research information and detailed analysis of the nascent developments around the world.

We would like to thank all the contributing authors for lending their expertise to make the book truly unique. They have played a crucial role in the development of this book. Without their invaluable contributions this book wouldn't have been possible. They have made vital efforts to compile up to date information on the varied aspects of this subject to make this book a valuable addition to the collection of many professionals and students.

This book was conceptualized with the vision of imparting up-to-date information and advanced data in this field. To ensure the same, a matchless editorial board was set up. Every individual on the board went through rigorous rounds of assessment to prove their worth. After which they invested a large part of their time researching and compiling the most relevant data for our readers.

The editorial board has been involved in producing this book since its inception. They have spent rigorous hours researching and exploring the diverse topics which have resulted in the successful publishing of this book. They have passed on their knowledge of decades through this book. To expedite this challenging task, the publisher supported the team at every step. A small team of assistant editors was also appointed to further simplify the editing procedure and attain best results for the readers.

Apart from the editorial board, the designing team has also invested a significant amount of their time in understanding the subject and creating the most relevant covers. They scrutinized every image to scout for the most suitable representation of the subject and create an appropriate cover for the book.

The publishing team has been an ardent support to the editorial, designing and production team. Their endless efforts to recruit the best for this project, has resulted in the accomplishment of this book. They are a veteran in the field of academics and their pool of knowledge is as vast as their experience in printing. Their expertise and guidance has proved useful at every step. Their uncompromising quality standards have made this book an exceptional effort. Their encouragement from time to time has been an inspiration for everyone.

The publisher and the editorial board hope that this book will prove to be a valuable piece of knowledge for researchers, students, practitioners and scholars across the globe.

List of Contributors

Liliana Mereu, Roberta Carlin, Francesca Guasina and Saverio Tateo
Department of Gynecology and Obstetrics, St. Chiara Hospital of Trento, Trento, Italy

Alice Pellegrini and Valeria Berlanda
Department of Gynecology and Obstetrics, St. Chiara Hospital of Trento, Trento, Italy
Department of Gynecology and Obstetrics, University of Verona, Verona, Italy

Afsaneh Tehranian, Roghayeh Hassani Zangbar, Faezeh Aghajani, Saeedeh Rafiei and Tayebe Esfidani
Department of Obstetrics and Gynecology, Roointan-Arash Women's Hospital, Tehran University of Medical Sciences, Tehran, Iran

Mahdi Sepidarkish
Department of Epidemiology and Reproductive Health, Reproductive Epidemiology Research Center, Royan Institute for Reproductive Biomedicine, ACECR, Tehran, Iran

Pietro Gambadauro
Centre for Reproduction, Uppsala University Hospital, 751 85 Uppsala, Sweden
Karolinska Institute, LIME/NASP-C7, 17177 Stockholm, Sweden
Department of Women's and Children's Health, Uppsala University, 751 85 Uppsala, Sweden

Johannes Gudmundsson
Centre for Reproduction, Uppsala University Hospital, 751 85 Uppsala, Sweden
Department of Women's and Children's Health, Uppsala University, 751 85 Uppsala, Sweden

Carlos Roger Molinas and Maria Mercedes Binda
Neolife – Medicina y Cirugia Reproductiva, Avenida Brasilia 760, 1434 Asuncion, Paraguay

Rudi Campo
European Academy of Gynaecological Surgery, Leuven, Belgium

Helen Jefferis, Natalia Price and Simon Jackson
Department of Gynaecology, The Women's Centre 8 John Radcliffe Hospital, Oxford University Hospitals NHS Trust 9, Headley Way, Oxford OX3 9DU 10, UK

Tamer A. Hosny
Department of Obstetrics and Gynecology, Alexandria University Hospital, 16A Mohamed Said Pasha street, San Stefano, Alexandria 21411, Egypt

Amal Alsalamah and Nazar Amso
School of Medicine, College of Biomedical and Life Sciences, Cardiff University, Office 220, 45 Salisbury road, Cathays, Cardiff CF24 4AB, UK

Yves Van Belle and Rudi Campo
European Academy of Gynaecological Surgery, Leuven, Belgium

Vasilios Tanos
Aretaeion Medical Center, Nicosia, Cyprus

Gregoris Grimbizis
First Department Obstetrics/Gynecology, Aristotle University of Thessaloniki, Thessaloniki, Greece

Kerenza Hood
Centre for Trials Research, College of Biomedical and Life Sciences, Cardiff University, Cardiff, UK

Neil Pugh
Department of Medical Physics and Radiology, University Hospital of Wales, Cardiff and Vale University Health Board, Cardiff, UK

N. Mak, S. A. Slockers and J. W. M. Maas
Department of Obstetrics and Gynaecology, Máxima Medical Centre, Veldhoven, The Netherlands

M. Y. Bongers
Department of Obstetrics and Gynaecology, Máxima Medical Centre, Veldhoven, The Netherlands
Department of Obstetrics and Gynaecology, GROW—School for Oncology and Developmental Biology, Maastricht University Medical Centre, Maastricht, The Netherlands

I. M. A. Reinders
Department of Obstetrics and Gynaecology, VieCuri Medical Centre, Venlo, The Netherlands
Department of Obstetrics and Gynaecology, GROW—School for Oncology and Developmental Biology, Maastricht University Medical Centre, Maastricht, The Netherlands

E. H. M. N. Westen
Department of Obstetrics and Gynaecology, Rode Kruis Hospital, Beverwijk, The Netherlands

Vered H. Eisenberg, Nissim Arbib, Eyal Schiff, Reuven Achiron, Motti Goldenberg and David Soriano
Department of Obstetrics and Gynecology, Sheba Medical Center, Tel-Hashomer, Tel-Aviv University, 52621 Ramat Gan, Israel

Juan L. Alcazar
Department of Obstetrics and Gynecology, Clinica Universidad de Navarra, University of Navarra, Pamplona, Spain

Fabio Imperato
Villa Del Rosario, Rome, Italy. 2Gemelli Hospitals, Università Cattolica, Rome, Italy

Anastasia Ussia
Villa Del Rosario, Rome, Italy
Gemelli Hospitals, Università Cattolica, Rome, Italy

Larissa Schindler and Arnaud Wattiez
Latifa Hospital, Dubai, United Arab Emirates

Philippe R. Koninckx
Department of Obstetrics and Gynecology, Catholic University Leuven, University Hospital, Gasthuisberg, B-3000 Leuven, Belgium. Vuilenbos 2 3360, Bierbeek, Belgium

Samuel W. King
Department of Urogynaecology, Oxford University Hospitals, Oxford, UK
Oxford Medical School, John Radcliffe Hospital, University of Oxford, Oxford, UK
John Radcliffe Hospital, Oxford University Hospitals NHS Foundation Trust, Oxford, UK
Harrogate District Hospital, Lancaster Park Rd, Harrogate, UK

Helen Jefferis, Simon Jackson and Natalia Price
Department of Urogynaecology, Oxford University Hospitals, Oxford, UK
John Radcliffe Hospital, Oxford University Hospitals NHS Foundation Trust, Oxford, UK

Alexander G. Marfin
John Radcliffe Hospital, Oxford University Hospitals NHS Foundation Trust, Oxford, UK

Sara Câmara, Filipa de Castro Coelho, Cláudia Freitas and Lilia Remesso
Department of Obstetrics and Gynecology, Hospital Dr. Nélio Mendonça, Avenida Luís de Camões n° 57, Funchal 9004-514, Portugal

R. Fusun Sirkeci
St George's, University of London, London, UK

Anna Maria Belli
Department of Radiology, St George's Healthcare NHS Foundation Trust, St George's, University of London, London, UK

Isaac T. Manyonda
Department of Obstetrics and Gynecology, St George's Healthcare NHS Foundation Trust, St George's, University of London, Blackshaw Road, Tooting, SW17 0QT London, UK

Kathy Niblock and Geoff McCracken
Craigavon Area Hospital, 68 Lurgan Rd, Portadown, Craigavon, BT63 5QQ, Northern Ireland

Keith Johnston and Emily Bailie
Antrim Area Hospital, 45 Bush Rd, Antrim BT41 2RL, Northern Ireland

Lilian Ugwumadu, Rima Chakrabarti, Elaine Williams-Brown, John Rendle, Ian Swift, Babbin John, Heather Allen-Coward and Emmanuel Ofuasia
Croydon Endometriosis Centre, Croydon University Hospital, 530 London Road, Croydon CR7 7YE, UK

E. A. Roovers, A. A. Kraayenbrink, C. I. M. Aalders, F. Hartog and F. P. H. L. J. Dijkhuizen
Department of Obstetrics and Gynecology, Rijnstate hospital, Wagnerlaan 55, 6815 AD Arnhem, The Netherlands

W. J. van Weelden
Department of Obstetrics and Gynecology, Rijnstate hospital, Wagnerlaan 55, 6815 AD Arnhem, The Netherlands
Department of Obstetrics and Gynecology, Radboud University Nijmegen Medical Center, Geert Grooteplein-Zuid 22, 6525 GA Nijmegen, The Netherlands

B. B. M. Gordon
Department of Obstetrics and Gynecology, Radboud University Nijmegen Medical Center, Geert Grooteplein-Zuid 22, 6525 GA Nijmegen, The Netherlands

Maria Mercedes Binda
Department of Obstetrics and Gynaecology, KU Leuven – Catholic University of Leuven, 3000 Leuven, Belgium

Roberta Corona
Department of Obstetrics and Gynaecology, KU Leuven – Catholic University of Leuven, 3000 Leuven, BelgiumBarbados Fertility Centre, Seaston House, Hastings, Barbados

Philippe R. Koninckx
Department of Obstetrics and Gynaecology, KU Leuven – Catholic University of Leuven, 3000 Leuven, Belgium
KU Leuven, Vuilenbosstraat 2, 3360 Bierbeek, Belgium

Leila Adamyan
Department of Reproductive Medicineand Surgery, Moscow State University of Medicine and Dentistry, Moscow, Russia

Victor Gomel
Department of Obstetrics and Gynecology, University of British Columbia, Women's Hospital, Vancouver, British Columbia, Canada

Lennart Van der Veeken, Francesca Maria Russo and Luc De Catte
Academic Department of Development and Regeneration, Woman and Child, Biomedical Sciences, and Clinical Department of Obstetrics and Gynaecology, KU Leuven, Herestraat 49, 3000, Leuven, Belgium

Jan Deprest
Academic Department of Development and Regeneration, Woman and Child, Biomedical Sciences, and Clinical Department of Obstetrics and Gynaecology, KU Leuven, Herestraat 49, 3000, Leuven, Belgium
TOTAL (Tracheal Occlusion To Accelerate Lung Growth Trial) Consortium, Leuven, Belgium
European Reference Network on Rare and Inherited Congenital Anomalies "ERNICA", Rotterdam, The Netherlands

Eduard Gratacos
TOTAL (Tracheal Occlusion To Accelerate Lung Growth Trial) Consortium, Leuven, Belgium
BCNatal – Barcelona Center for MaternaleFetal and Neonatal Medicine (Hospital Clínic and Hospital Sant Joan de Déu), IDIBAPS, University of Barcelona, and Centre for Biomedical Research on Rare Diseases (CIBER-ER), Barcelona, Spain

Alexandra Benachi
TOTAL (Tracheal Occlusion To Accelerate Lung Growth Trial) Consortium, Leuven, Belgium
Department of Obstetrics, Gynaecology and Reproductive Medicine, Hôpital Antoine-Béclère, University Paris Sud, Clamart, France
European Reference Network on Rare and Inherited Congenital Anomalies "ERNICA", Rotterdam, The Netherlands

Yves Ville
TOTAL (Tracheal Occlusion To Accelerate Lung Growth Trial) Consortium, Leuven, Belgium

Fetal Medicine Unit, Obstetrics and Fetal Medicine Department, Necker-Enfants Malades Hospital, Université Paris Descartes, Sorbonne Paris Cité, Paris, France

Kypros Nicolaides
TOTAL (Tracheal Occlusion To Accelerate Lung Growth Trial) Consortium, Leuven, Belgium
Harris Birthright Centre, King's College Hospital, London, UK

Christoph Berg
TOTAL (Tracheal Occlusion To Accelerate Lung Growth Trial) Consortium, Leuven, Belgium
Division of Fetal Surgery, Department of Obstetrics and Prenatal Medicine, University of Bonn, Bonn, Germany
Department of Obstetrics and Gynecology, University of Cologne, Cologne, Germany

Glenn Gardener
TOTAL (Tracheal Occlusion To Accelerate Lung Growth Trial) Consortium, Leuven, Belgium
Mater Health Services, Mater Research UQ, Brisbane, Australia

Nicola Persico
TOTAL (Tracheal Occlusion To Accelerate Lung Growth Trial) Consortium, Leuven, Belgium
Department of Obstetrics and Gynecology, "L. Mangiagalli, " Fondazione IRCCS "Ca' Granda" - Ospedale Maggiore Policlinico, Milan, Italy

Pietro Bagolan
TOTAL (Tracheal Occlusion To Accelerate Lung Growth Trial) Consortium, Leuven, Belgium
Neonatal Surgery Unit, Department of Medical and Surgical Neonatology, Bambino Gesù Children's Hospital, IRCCS, Piazza S. Onofrio, 4, 00165 Rome, Italy
European Reference Network on Rare and Inherited Congenital Anomalies "ERNICA", Rotterdam, The Netherlands

Greg Ryan
TOTAL (Tracheal Occlusion To Accelerate Lung Growth Trial) Consortium, Leuven, Belgium
Fetal Medicine Unit, Mt Sinai Hospital, University of Toronto, Toronto, Canada

Michael A. Belfort
TOTAL (Tracheal Occlusion To Accelerate Lung Growth Trial) Consortium, Leuven, Belgium
Department of Obstetrics and Gynecology, Baylor College of Medicine and Texas Children's Fetal Center, Houston, Texas, USA

Xin Sun, Min Xue, Xinliang Deng, Yun Lin, Ying Tan and Xueli Wei
Department of Obstetrics and Gynecology, The 3rd Xiangya Hospital of Central South University, 138 Tongzipo Rd, Changsha, Hunan 410013, China

S. H. Walker and L. Gokhale
Department of Obstetrics and Gynaecology, Royal Gwent Hospital, Aneurin Bevan University Health Board, Newport, UK

Evelien M. Sandberg, Sara R. C. Driessen and Evelien A. T. Bak
Department of Gynecology, Leiden University Medical Centre, Leiden, the Netherlands

Judith P. Berger
Department of Gynecology, Leiden University Medical Centre, Leiden, the Netherlands
Department of Gynecology, Haaglanden Medical Centre, the Hague, the Netherlands

Frank Willem Jansen
Department of Gynecology, Leiden University Medical Centre, Leiden, the Netherlands
Department BioMechanical Engineering, Delft University of Technology, Delft, the Netherlands
Department of Gynecology, Minimally Invasive Surgery, Leiden University Medical Centre, RC, Leiden, the Netherlands

Nan van Geloven
Department of Medical Statistics, Leiden University Medical Centre, Leiden, the Netherlands

Mathilde J. G. H. Smeets and Johann P. T. Rhemrev
Department of Gynecology, Haaglanden Medical Centre, the Hague, the Netherlands

Vasilios Tanos
St. Georges Medical School, Nicosia University, Nicosia, Cyprus
Department of Obstetrics and Gynaecology, Aretaeio Hospital, Nicosia, Cyprus

Hans Brölmann
Departmentof Obstetrics and Gynaecology, VU University Medical Centre, De Boelelaan 1117, 1181HV Amsterdam, The Netherlands

Rudi Leon DeWilde
Clinic of Gynaecology, Obstetrics and Gynaecological Oncology, University Hospital for Gynaecology, Pius-Hospital Oldenburg, Medical Campus University of Oldenburg, Oldenburg, Germany

Peter O'Donovan
Obstetrics and Gynaecological Oncology Yorkshire Clinic, Bradford Road, Bingley, West Yorkshire BD16 1TW, UK

Elina Symeonidou
Nicosia, Cyprus

Rudi Campo
European Society Gynaecological Endoscopy, European Academy for Gynaecological Surgery, LIFE, Tiensevest, 168, 3000 Leuven Leuven, Belgium

Karlien Vossaert, Susanne Housmans, Stefaan Pacquée, Geertje Callewaert and Laura Cattani
Pelvic Floor Unit Department of Gynaecology, University Hospitals Leuven, Leuven Herestraat 49, 3000 Leuven, Belgium

Jan Deprest
Pelvic Floor Unit Department of Gynaecology, University Hospitals Leuven, Leuven Herestraat 49, 3000 Leuven, Belgium
Institute for Women's Health, University College London, London, UK

Frank Van der Aa
Department of Urology, University Hospitals Leuven, Leuven, Belgium

Albert Wolthuis and André D'hoore
Department of Abdominal Surgery, University Hospitals Leuven, Leuven, Belgium

Philip Roelandt
Departments of Gastroenterology, University Hospitals Leuven, Leuven, Belgium
Academic Department of Development and Regeneration, Group Biomedical Sciences, Katholieke Universiteit Leuven, Leuven, Belgium

Antonio Macciò, Paraskevas Kotsonis, Giacomo Chiappe, Fabrizio Lavra and Ivan Collu
Department of Gynecologic Oncology, Azienda Ospedaliera Brotzu, via Jenner, 09100 Cagliari, Italy

Clelia Madeddu
Department of Medical Sciences and Public Health, University of Cagliari, Cagliari, Italy

Roberto Demontis
Department of Medical Sciences and Public Health, Section of Forensic Medicine, University of Cagliari, Cagliari, Italy

Tjalina W. O. Hamerlynck, Hannelore Van der Veken and Steven Weyers
Women's Clinic, Ghent University Hospital, C. Heymanslaan 10, 9000 Ghent, Belgium

Jan Bosteels
Women's Clinic, Ghent University Hospital, C. Heymanslaan 10, 9000 Ghent, Belgium
Department of Gynaecology, Imelda Hospital, Imeldalaan 9, 2820, Bonheiden, Belgium

Dora Meyers
Faculty of Medicine and Health Sciences, Ghent University, C. Heymanslaan 10, 9000 Ghent, Belgium

Chou Phay Lim
Obstetrics and Gynaecology, Royal Victoria Infirmary, Newcastle upon Tyne Hospitals NHS Foundation Trust, Newcastle Upon Tyne NE1 4LP, UK

Mark Roberts and Tony Chalhoub
Royal Victoria Infirmary, Newcastle Upon Tyne, UK

Jason Waugh
Obstetrics and Gynaecology, Northern Deanery, HEE (NE), Newcastle Upon Tyne, UK

Laura Delgaty
Newcastle University, Newcastle Upon Tyne, UK

Rebecca Mallick and Funlayo Odejinmi
Department of Gynaecology, Barts Health NHS Trust, Whipps Cross University Hospital, London E11 1NR, UK

Géraldine Brichant, Marie Denef, Linda Tebache, Gaëlle Poismans, Valérie Dechenne and Michelle Nisolle
University Department of Obstetrics and Gynecology, CHR La Citadelle, Boulevard du Douzième de Ligne, 1, 4000 Liège, Belgium

Serena Pinzauti
UO Ostetricia e Ginecologia, Ospedale Santa Maria alla Gruccia, Arezzo, Montevarchi, Italy

Natasha Curtiss and Jonathan Duckett
Department of Obstetrics and Gynaecology, Medway Maritime Hospital, Windmill Road, Gillingham, Kent ME7 5NY, UK

Jordan Klebanoff and Matthew K. Hoffman
Department of Obstetrics and Gynecology, Christiana Care Health System, 4755 Ogletown-Stanton Road, Suite 1905, Newark, DE 19718, USA

Gretchen E. Makai and Nima R. Patel
Division of Minimally Invasive Gynecology, Christiana Care Health System, Newark, DE, USA

Tim Wollinga
Medical Faculty, Erasmus University, Rotterdam, The Netherlands
Department of Obstetrics and Gynecology, Elisabeth-Tweesteden Hospital, Tilburg, The Netherlands

Marieke Smink
Department of Obstetrics and Gynecology, Elisabeth-Tweesteden Hospital, Tilburg, The Netherlands

Johanna M. A. Pijnenborg
Department of Obstetrics and Gynecology, Elisabeth-Tweesteden Hospital, Tilburg, The Netherlands
Department of Obstetrics and Gynecology, Radboud University Medical Centre, 791, 6500 HB Nijmegen, The Netherlands

Nicole P. M. Ezendam
Department of Medical and Clinical Psychology, Tilburg University, Tilburg, The Netherlands
Netherlands Comprehensive Cancer Organisation, Utrecht, The Netherlands

Florine A. Eggink and Hans W. Nijman
Department of Obstetrics and Gynecology, University Medical Centre Groningen, University of Groningen, Groningen, The Netherlands

Dennis van Hamont
Department of Obstetrics and Gynecology, Amphia Hospital, Breda, The Netherlands

Brenda Pijlman
Department of Obstetrics and Gynecology, Jeroen Bosch Hospital, 's-Hertogenbosch, The Netherlands

Erik Boss
Department of Obstetrics and Gynecology, Máxima Medical Centre, Veldhoven, The Netherlands

Elisabeth J. Robbe
Department of Obstetrics and Gynecology, St. Anna Hospital, Geldrop, The Netherlands

Huy Ngo
Department of Obstetrics and Gynecology, Elkerliek Hospital, Helmond, The Netherlands

Dorry Boll
Department of Obstetrics and Gynecology, Catharina Hospital, Eindhoven, The Netherlands

Constantijne H. Mom
Department of Gynecologic Oncology, Gynecological Oncology Centre Amsterdam, Amsterdam, The Netherlands

Maaike A. van der Aa
Department of Research, Netherlands Comprehensive Cancer Organisation, Utrecht, The Netherlands

Roy F. L. P. Kruitwagen
Department of Obstetrics and Gynecology, Maastricht University Medical Centre, Maastricht, The Netherlands GROW-School for Oncology and Developmental Biology, Maastricht University, Maastricht, The Netherlands

Carlos Roger Molinas and Maria Mercedes Binda
NEOLIFE—Medicina y Cirugía Reproductiva, Avenida Brasilia 760, 1434 Asunción, Paraguay

Cesar Manuel Sisa
Faculty of Medicine, Universidad del Pacífico Privada, Avenida San Martín 961, 1813 Asunción, Paraguay

Rudi Campo
The European Academy of Gynaecological Surgery, Diestsevest 43, bus 0001, B3000 Leuven, Belgium

Liliana Mereu, Alice Pellegrini, Roberta Carlin, Erica Terreno, Claudia Prasciolu and Saverio Tateo
Department of Obstetrics and Gynecology, Santa Chiara Hospital, Largo Medaglie d'Oro 9, 38122 Trento, Italy

Antonio Macciò, Paraskevas Kotsonis, Fabrizio Lavra and Giacomo Chiappe
Department of Gynecologic Oncology, Azienda Ospedaliera Brotzu, via Edward Jenner, 09121 Cagliari, Italy

Ester Mura
Department of Pathology, Azienda Ospedaliera Brotzu, Cagliari, Italy

Luca Melis
Department of Nuclear Medicine, Azienda Ospedaliera Brotzu, Cagliari, Italy

Clelia Madeddu
Department of Public Health and Medical Sciences, University of Cagliari, Cagliari, Italy

Ibrahim A. El sharkwy, Elsayed H. Noureldin, Ekramy A. Mohamed and Ali A. Mohamed
Faculty of Medicine, Zagazig University, Zagazig, Egypt

Rami Kilani
Hashemite University, Zarqa, Jordan

Iris Verbeeck, Francesca Donders, Dirk Timmerman and Carla Tomassetti
Department Gynecology-Obstetrics, University Hospital Leuven, Herestraat 49, 3000 Leuven, Belgium

Jan Deprest
Department Gynecology-Obstetrics, University Hospital Leuven, Herestraat 49, 3000 Leuven, Belgium Institute for Women's Health and Wellcome/EPSRC Centre for Interventional and Surgical Sciences (WEISS), University College London, Charles Bell House, 43-45 Foley Street, London W1W 7TS, UK

Pieter-Jan Buyck, Andries Van Holsbeeck and Sandra A Cornelissen
Department Radiology, University Hospital Leuven, Herestraat 49, 3000 Leuven, Belgium

Anne-Sophie Van Rompuy
Department Pathology, University Hospital Leuven, Herestraat 49, 3000 Leuven, Belgium

Sylvie Gordts
Department Reproductive medicine LIFE, General Hospital Heilig Hart Ziekenhuis, Naamsestraat 105, 3000 Leuven, Belgium

Lien Van den Haute
Department Gynecology-Obstetrics, General Hospital Onze-Lieve-Vrouwziekenhuis, Moorselbaan 164, 9300 Aalst, Belgium

Index

www.ingramcontent.com/pod-product-compliance
Lightning Source LLC
Chambersburg PA
CBHW080457200326
41458CB00012B/4000